# HALLUX VALGUS AND FOREFOOT SURGERY

# HALLUX VALGUS AND FOREFOOT SURGERY

Edited by

## Vincent J. Hetherington, D.P.M., M.S., Dip.A.B.P.S., F.A.C.F.A.S.

Dean for Academic Affairs
Professor and Former Chairman
Department of Surgery
Ohio College of Podiatric Medicine
Cleveland, Ohio

*Formerly Associate Dean for Clinical Affairs*
*College of Podiatric Medicine and Surgery*
*University of Osteopathic Medicine and Health Sciences*
*Des Moines, Iowa*

Churchill Livingstone
New York, Edinburgh, London, Madrid, Melbourne, Milan, Tokyo

**Library of Congress Cataloging-in-Publication Data**

Hallux valgus and forefoot surgery / edited by Vincent J.
  Hetherington.
        p.   cm.
    Includes bibliographical references and index.
    ISBN 0-443-08775-X
    1. Hallux valgus—Surgery.  2. Toes—Surgery.  3. Toes-
  -Abnormalities.    I. Hetherington, V.
    [DNLM:  1. Hallux Valgus—surgery.  2. Forefoot, Human—surgery.
  WE 883 H193 1994]
  RD787.H35  1994
  617.5′85—dc20
  DNLM/DLC
  for Library of Congress                                       94-19069
                                                                CIP

© **Churchill Livingstone Inc. 1994**

Distributed in the United Kingdom by Churchill Livingstone, Robert Stevenson House, 1–3 Baxter's Place, Leith Walk, Edinburgh EH1 3AF, and by associated companies, branches, and representatives throughout the world.

Accurate indications, adverse reactions, and dosage schedules for drugs are provided in this book, but it is possible that they may change. The reader is urged to review the package information data of the manufacturers of the medications mentioned.

The Publishers have made every effort to trace the copyright holders for borrowed material. If they have inadvertently overlooked any, they will be pleased to make the necessary arrangements at the first opportunity.

Acquisitions Editor: *Carol Bader*
Copy Editor: *David Terry*
Production Supervisor: *Sharon Tuder*
Cover Design: *Paul Moran*

Printed in the United States of America

First published in 1994      7   6   5   4   3   2   1

# Contributors

**Richard J. Bogdan, D.P.M., Dip.A.B.P.S.**
Private practice, La Jolla, California; formerly, Associate Professor and Chairman, Department of Biomechanics and Orthopedics, Ohio College of Podiatric Medicine, Cleveland, Ohio

**Allan M. Boike, D.P.M., Dip.A.B.P.S., F.A.C.F.A.S.**
Associate Professor, Department of Surgery, Ohio College of Podiatric Medicine; Podiatry Staff, Department of Podiatric Surgery, Mt. Sinai Medical Center, Cleveland, Ohio

**John H. Bonk, D.P.M., Dip.A.B.P.S., F.A.C.F.A.S.**
Adjunct Clinical Faculty, Department of Surgery, Ohio College of Podiatric Medicine, Cleveland, Ohio

**Domenick A. Calise, D.P.M.**
Assistant Professor, Department of Surgery, Ohio College of Podiatric Medicine; Director of Surgery, Cleveland Foot and Ankle Clinic, Ohio College of Podiatric Medicine, Cleveland, Ohio

**Edward L. Chairman, D.P.M., Dip.A.B.P.S., F.A.C.F.A.S.**
Podiatric Surgeon, Division of Podiatric Surgery, Department of Orthopaedics, Graduate Hospital, Philadelphia, Pennsylvania

**Bao-Xing Chen, M.D.**
Visiting Professor, Department of Orthopedic Surgery, Beijing Medical University; Professor, Department of Orthopedic Surgery, Beijing Institute of Foot Surgery, Beijing, China

**Gloria Christin, D.P.M., A.A.C.F.A.S.**
Private practice, Toledo, Ohio

**Paul S. Cwikla, D.P.M., Ph.D.**
Graduate, Ohio College of Podiatric Medicine, Cleveland, Ohio

**J. Colin Dagnall, L.H.D., F.Ch.S.**
Member, Advisory Committee, Center for the History of Foot Care and Footwear, Pennsylvania College of Podiatric Medicine, Philadelphia, Pennsylvania; Friend, The Wellcome Institute for the History of Medicine, London, England; Chiropodist, War Pensions Directorate, Blackpool, Lancashire, England

**Michael A. Feist, D.P.M., M.S.**

Former Resident, California College of Podiatric Medicine, San Francisco, California

**Michael Gerber, D.P.M.**

Assistant Professor, Department of Surgery, Ohio College of Podiatric Medicine, Cleveland, Ohio

**Charles Gudas, D.P.M.**

Clinical Professor, Department of Surgery, University of Chicago Division of the Biological Sciences Pritzker School of Medicine, Chicago, Illinois

**Vincent J. Hetherington, D.P.M., M.S., Dip.A.B.P.S., F.A.C.F.A.S.**

Dean for Academic Affairs, and Professor and Former Chairman, Department of Surgery, Ohio College of Podiatric Medicine, Cleveland, Ohio; formerly Associate Dean for Clinical Affairs, College of Podiatric Medicine and Surgery, University of Osteopathic Medicine and Health Sciences, Des Moines, Iowa

**Tadao Ishizuka, M.D., Ph.D.**

Chief Director, Jonan Hospital; Counselor, Japanese Society for the Medical Study of Footwear, Tokyo, Japan

**Ronald E. Johnson, D.P.M.**

Associate Dean, College of Podiatric Medicine and Surgery, University of Osteopathic Medicine and Health Sciences, Des Moines, Iowa

**Michael Korbol, D.P.M., P.T., F.A.C.F.A.S.**

Private practice, Raleigh, North Carolina; formerly Assistant Clinical Professor, Department of Surgery, Ohio College of Podiatric Medicine, Cleveland, Ohio

**D.N. Kreibich, M.B.**

Senior Registrar, Department of Orthopaedic Surgery, Royal Victoria Infirmary, Newcastle, England

**John E. Laco, D.P.M., Dip.A.B.P.O., Dip.A.B.P.P.C.**

Associate Professor, Department of Podiatric Medicine, College of Podiatric Medicine and Surgery, Des Moines, Iowa; Residency Director, Primary Podiatric Care Program, Minnesota Extension, College of Podiatric Medicine and Surgery, Eagan, Minnesota

**David M. LaPorta, D.P.M., Dip.A.B.P.S., F.A.C.F.A.S.**

Staff Physician, Department of Podiatric Surgery, Monmouth Medical Center, Long Branch, New Jersey

**Janis E. Lehtinen, D.P.M.**

Attending Physician, Department of Surgery, Lutheran General Hospital, Park Ridge, Illinois; Associate, Department of Surgery, Lake Forest Hospital, Lake Forest, Illinois

**Francis Lynch, D.P.M., Dip.A.B.P.S., F.A.C.F.A.S.**

Director, Achilles Foot Health Center, North Haven, Connecticut

**Maria Malone, D.P.M.**

Graduate, Ohio College of Podiatric Medicine, Cleveland, Ohio

**Praya Mam, D.P.M.**

Former Second-Year Surgical Resident, Ohio College of Podiatric Medicine, Cleveland, Ohio

**Denise M. Mandracchia, D.P.M., A.A.C.F.A.S.**

Adjunct Assistant Professor, Department of Podiatric Medicine, College of Podiatric Medicine and Surgery, University of Osteopathic Medicine and Health Sciences, Des Moines, Iowa

**Vincent J. Mandracchia, D.P.M., M.S., F.A.C.F.A.S.**

Associate Professor, Department of Podiatric Medicine, College of Podiatric Medicine and Surgery, University of Osteopathic Medicine and Health Sciences, Des Moines, Iowa; formerly Chairman, Department of Podiatric Surgery, Springfield Hospital, Springfield, Pennsylvania

**Thomas V. Melillo, D.P.M., Dip.A.B.P.S., F.A.C.F.A.S.**

Professor, Department of Podiatric Surgery, and President, Ohio College of Podiatric Medicine, Cleveland, Ohio

**Tracy A. Merrell, D.P.M.**

Graduate, College of Podiatric Medicine and Surgery, University of Osteopathic Medicine and Health Sciences, Des Moines, Iowa

**Stephen J. Miller, D.P.M., Dip.A.B.P.S., Dip.A.B.P.O., F.A.C.F.A.S.**

Teaching Faculty, The Podiatry Institute, Tucker, Georgia; Co-Founder, Northwest Podiatric Foundation, Seattle, Washington; Adjunct Faculty, Department of Surgery, Pennsylvania College of Podiatric Medicine, Philadelphia, Pennsylvania; Active Staff, Island Hospital, Anacortes, Washington

**Vincent J. Muscarella, D.P.M.**

Clinical Instructor, Department of Surgery, Pennsylvania College of Podiatric Medicine; Chairman, Department of Podiatric Surgery, Suburban General Hospital, Norristown, Pennsylvania

**Bonnie J. Nicklas, D.P.M., Dip.A.B.P.S., F.A.C.F.A.S.**

Associate Professor and Chair, Department of Surgery, Ohio College of Podiatric Medicine, Cleveland, Ohio

**Lawrence M. Oloff, D.P.M**

Professor, Department of Surgery; Vice-President and Dean for Academic Affairs; Co-Director, Special Problems Clinic, California College of Podiatric Medicine, San Francisco, California; Clinical Assistant Professor, Podiatric Section, Division of Orthopedic Surgery, Department of Functional Restoration, Stanford University School of Medicine, Stanford, California

**Lawrence Osher, D.P.M.**

Associate Professor, Department of Medicine, and Director, Department of Radiology, Ohio College of Podiatric Medicine, Cleveland, Ohio

**Gordon W. Patton, D.P.M., Dip.A.B.P.S., F.A.C.F.A.S.**

Teaching Faculty, Podiatry Institute, Northlake Regional Medical Center, Tucker, Georgia

**Daryl Phillips, D.P.M.**

Professor, Department of Podiatric Medicine, College of Podiatric Medicine, University of Osteopathic Medicine, Des Moines, Iowa

**Bernard Regnauld, M.D.**

Private practice, Nantes, France; formerly, Medical Intern, Department of Orthopaedics, University Hospital Centre, Nantes, France

**Patrick D. Roberto, D.P.M.**

Private practice, Delmont, Pennsylvania

**Brad G. Samojla, D.P.M.**

Assistant Professor, Department of Podiatric Medicine, Ohio College of Podiatric Medicine, Cleveland, Ohio

**T.W.D. Smith, M.B., F.R.C.S., F.R.C.S.E.**

Consultant Surgeon, Department of Orthopaedic Surgery, Northern General Hospital, Sheffield, England

**Alan J. Snyder, D.P.M.**

Private practice, North Wales, Pennsylvania; formerly, Surgical Fellow, Department of Surgery, Ohio College of Podiatric Medicine, Cleveland, Ohio

**David Stanley, M.B., F.R.C.S., F.R.C.S.E.**

Consultant Surgeon, Department of Orthopaedic Surgery, Northern General Hospital, Sheffield, England

**Gunther Steinböck, M.D.**

Orthopedic Hospital, Vienna, Austria

**Richard M. Stess, D.P.M., Dip.A.B.P.S., Dip.A.B.P.O., F.A.C.F.A.S.**
Asssistant Clinical Professor, Department of Medicine, University of California, San Francisco, School of Medicine; Associate Clinical Professor, Department of Podiatric Medicine, California College of Podiatric Medicine; Chief, Department of Podiatry, and Director of Podiatric Education, Department of Veterans Affairs Medical Center, San Francisco, California

**William F. Todd, D.P.M., Dip.A.B.P.S., F.A.C.F.A.S.**
Director, Diabetic Foot Center, and Member, Residency Training Committee, Monsignor Clement Kern Hospital for Special Surgery, Warren, Michigan

**Randall K. Tom, D.P.M.**
Second-Year Resident, Monsignor Clement Kern Hospital for Special Surgery, Warren, Michigan

**Rodney Tomczak, D.P.M., Ed.D., Dip.A.B.P.S., F.A.C.F.A.S.**
Professor, Department of Podiatry, University of Osteopathic Medicine, Des Moines, Iowa

**John V. Vanore, D.P.M.**
Attending Medical Staff, Doctors Hospital of Hyde Park; private practice, Chicago, Illinois

**George F. Wallace, D.P.M., Dip.A.B.P.S., Dip.A.B.P.O.**
Clinical Instructor, Department of Podiatry, and Chairman and Residency Director of Podiatric Surgery, University of Medicine and Dentistry of New Jersey, Hasbrough Heights, New Jersey

**Marilyn J. Waller, D.P.M.**
Private practice, Hayward, California

**John M. White, D.P.M.**
Private practice, New Boston, Texas

**Kendrick A. Whitney, D.P.M.**
Clinical Instructor, Department of Orthopaedics, Pennsylvania College of Podiatric Medicine; Co-Director, Diabetic Foot Clinic, and Instructor, Department of Orthopaedics, Foot and Ankle Institute of the Pennsylvania College of Podiatric Medicine, Philadelphia, Pennsylvania

**James E. Zelichowski, D.P.M.**
Staff Member, Department of Surgery, Henry General Hospital, Stockbridge, Georgia; Former Chairman, Department of Surgery, and Externship Director, Atlanta Hospital, Atlanta, Georgia

# Foreword

It is my extreme pleasure to have the opportunity to write the foreword for *Hallux Valgus and Forefoot Surgery*. This book is a marvelous amalgamation of basic and clinical sciences from the perspective of a diverse and expert international group of contributing authors. The diversity and caliber of these authors make this text valuable and interesting.

Since the 1980s there has been an enormous volume of material written about forefoot and hallux valgus surgery. This book provides a systematic approach to forefoot surgery with topics ranging from surgical anatomy, pathology, biomechanics, biomaterials, fixation and criteria based surgical techniques, and complications. It is an important and very readable text that discusses the scientific materials commonly seen in the busy foot and ankle surgical practice; it provides a fine perspective of surgical approaches—both the time honored classic procedures and state-of-the-art cutting edge innovations. The most commonly confronted pathology in the forefoot is brilliantly discussed and illustrated in this comprehensive book. International input adds to the scope and freshness of the overall presentation.

Dr. Hetherington, the consummate educator, has held many academic positions and is currently the Dean for Academic Affairs and Professor of Surgery at the Ohio College of Podiatric Medicine. Having known Dr. Hetherington since his residency days, I have had the joy of witnessing his emergence as a preeminent authority on research and education as it relates to foot and ankle pathology on an international level.

*Hallux Valgus and Forefoot Surgery* is an outstanding text that is a must for any practitioner of foot and ankle surgery.

*David C. Novicki, D.P.M., F.A.C.F.A.S.*
*President, American College of Foot and*
*Ankle Surgeons, Park Ridge, Illinois*
*Attending Clinical Physician*
*Veterans Administration Hospital*
*West Haven, Connecticut*

# Preface

*Hallux Valgus and Forefoot Surgery* brings together a group of physicians interested in the care of the foot who unselfishly share their experience, expertise, and knowledge with those of similar interest. Deformities of the forefoot are complex, causing varying degrees of pain and suffering. Such deformities also contribute to overall functional disability in many patients suffering from the variety of deformities affecting the foot. This is especially true of older patients for whom mobility equates with independence.

This book addresses the clinical aspects of deformity of the forefoot, focusing primarily on hallux valgus. Presented in separate chapters are the anatomy of the forefoot, biomechanics of the hallux valgus deformity, and clinical and radiographic evaluation of the forefoot. These initial chapters are then followed by a series of chapters on procedures for the management of hallux valgus; these chapters address criteria for procedure selection based on clinical, radiographic, and biomechanical foundations. They include soft tissue procedures, phalangeal, distal, and proximal metatarsal osteotomy, and procedures involving the cuneiform. Each addresses a specific type of procedure in detail including indications and complications. Some repetition of material may occur in several of the chapters; this was done to allow for completeness of presentation of the material in the individual chapters and to reinforce some of the radiographic, biomechanical, and other principles relative to the specific procedures described. The terms *hallux valgus* and *hallux abducto valgus* have been used interchangeably throughout the text and for practical purposes refer to the same deformity.

The text would not be complete without addressing other deformities associated with hallux valgus that accompany the painful forefoot. These include hallux limitus and rigidus, hallux varus, nail and digital deformity, metatarsalgia, as well as neuroma and nerve entrapment syndromes. Separate chapters deal with management of diabetic and rheumatoid patients. An international perspective is added to demonstrate the similarity and diversity of the approaches to the management of hallux valgus. It is my hope that this text will become a useful resource to students, residents, and practitioners.

I would like to thank all of the contributing authors for their generous commitment of time, knowledge, and patience; it is for this reason that I dedicate the book to them.

I would also like to acknowledge the contributions made by Joan Lannoch for her artwork, Donna Perzeski, who was invaluable with her library research assistance, Carol Bader and David Terry of Churchill Livingstone, and my secretary Laura Fisher for her assistance. I especially thank my wife, Jo, and daughter, Nancy, for their patience in enduring the time that the book has taken away from them and for their support during the preparation of this text.

*Vincent J. Hetherington, D.P.M., M.S.*
*Dip.A.B.P.S., F.A.C.F.A.S.*

# Contents

# 1

# Introduction

## J. COLIN DAGNALL

*This condition [hallux valgus] is peculiar to civilized man except in isolated cases where it is the result of direct violence to or disease of the metatarsophalangeal joint. Its most frequent cause is the habitual wearing of a pointed shoe.*
*—Otto F. Schuster[1]*

*The etiology of hallux valgus may include congenital, arthritis, hereditary (most common), biomechanical and trauma. The deformity usually progresses due to the biomechanics of walking. Shoes as an etiology is a myth.*
*—Lawrence B. Harkless and Steven M. Krych[2]*

When I first thought about my approach to the history of hallux valgus surgery, the task seemed relatively easy. The problem would involve taking the vast literature and condensing it into only a few pages. My approach to the history of hallux valgus surgery was to be a traditional one, a biographic, chronologic, and bibliographic study. The more I considered this approach, however, the more uncertain I became. Thus, I have started with two quotations that demonstrate the controversy involving the etiology of hallux valgus. Two opposing viewpoints exist—that the etiology of hallux valgus is the habitual wearing of pointed shoes, and that the etiology includes hereditary, congenital, biomechanical, and traumatic causes, but not the wearing of shoes—and over the years, studies have found evidence to support both claims (see Ch. 3).

As Kelikian[3] has noted, "a staggering number of articles" have been written on the etiology of hallux valgus, and in wading through what has been written, one finds a number of stock statements that need reappraisal. Kelikian writes[6]:

The literature is cluttered with numerous conjectures concerning the causation of malformed toes; greater emphasis is being placed on evolutionary antecedents and on heredity, and less on civilized habits. It has become fashionable to overlook the obvious—shoes as one of the major causes of malformed toes—and indulge in conjectures. Theories that are not universally accepted by professional anthropologists and embryologists have been flaunted by clinicians as established facts. It is understandable that the sophomore sibling who wanted to follow the footsteps of Darwin or Bardeen, but somehow got sidetracked into the unglamorous avocation of treating twisted toes, should—out of sheer nostalgia or in response to the secret whisperings of his suppressed desire—attempt to relate his thought with those of his student-day idols. There is nothing wrong in trying to connect clinical observations with the general body of scientific knowledge, provided that he who attempts such correlation is well versed in both fields, or at least has studied the pros and cons of the controversial question. When the clinician starts with a fixed idea and seeks confirmation in the work of a scientist, he is liable to be misled, and if influential, in his turn mislead others.

An influential orthopedic surgeon started the trend in the twenties; he surmised that hallux valgus—

1

rather, metatarsus primus varus—might be a 'reversion to the branch-grasping Simian type great toe, described by Morton.' He did not seem aware that Morton's theory had been subjected to severe criticism by more than one professional anthropologist. He also suspected 'a persistence of the embryo great toe, described by Lebloc' and did not appear to have taken sufficient pain to spell embryologist Leboucq's name correctly.

Many theories have been published regarding the etiology of hallux valgus. The influence of footgear is commonly cited as a factor in its development, and the classic explanation is "that the toes are pressed out of position by wearing tight or pointed shoes," but Wiles (1949)[4] noted that "in recent years there had been marked improvement in the design of children's footwear and an increasing awareness amongst parents of its importance, but no corresponding decrease in the incidence of hallux valgus."

No definitive study on the etiology of hallux valgus exists, and other factors including biomechanics, arthritis, and trauma have all been considered to be the cause. Root (1977)[5] stated that hallux abducto valgus "is an acquired deformity caused by abnormal mechanics at the first metatarso-phalangeal joint which occurs during the propulsive period of the stance phase of gait."

The cause of hallux valgus may be multifactorial with footwear a contributing factor in a foot that is predisposed to develop hallux valgus.[6]

. . . up to this point we have carefully avoided facing up to the influence of footwear upon the great toe, but inexorably it appears as though we must be driven back to the ideas which for a long time were considered to be unscientific and unfashionable. That is not to suggest that we throw overboard all the ideas which have been gathered over the years. Many of these are indeed complementary, and it is probable that we shall eventually agree that there is no one, all-embracing, cause of hallux valgus, even though we are at the same time forced to agree that footwear is the trigger that fires the gun. 'No footwear, no hallux valgus' is extraordinarily difficult to refute, and all evidence we have points to the fact that the greater the delay in starting footwear, the greater the chance of escaping hallux valgus, or at least the longer will its onset be delayed.

# TREATMENT OF HALLUX VALGUS

If one were to list all the procedures that have been described for the correction of this deformity of the great toe, one would not contribute anything to the total of human endeavor but would confuse the issue even further.[7]

Volkman (1856) "complained that the 'affection' that 'not only deforms the foot in a most clumsy way but also makes the gait uncertain and continuous walking painful' had not received from surgeons the attention it deserved. According to their social status, patients with what we now call hallux valgus were relegated to barbers to have their calluses trimmed, or to bootmakers to have their shoes adjusted. Hallux valgus was considered as belonging to a 'low class of surgery.' "[3]

Treatment of hallux valgus includes both conservative and surgical procedures. "The future of the treatment of many of the common disabilities of the foot lies, doubtless, in re-education of function rather than in reinforcement by mechanical contrivances or more drastic treatment by the refinements of surgical technique."[8]

Surgical techniques for the treatment of hallux valgus have existed since the 1800s and include arthroplasty, osteotomies, and joint destructive procedures. "Metcalf (1912) summarized 15 different operations; Timmer (1930) mentioned 25; Verbrugge (1933) outlined 51; Perrot (1946) counted 68; and McBridge (1952) named 58." McBride wrote that such a variety of methods "can mean but one thing, namely that hallux valgus is a recalcitrant disorder."[3] Kelikian[3] argues:

This is a discreet understatement, not the whole truth. Most surgical procedures on record have scant, extremely tenuous, often untenable principles to support them. A number of operations are possible only on paper, in drawings or blueprints. Behind some of them lurks the desire of the progenitor to perpetuate his name by linking it to a supposedly new method. Lack of historical perspective might have led some of these authors to claim originality for a procedure that had been tried in the past and justly or unjustly relegated to limbo. Frequently one favored technique is applied to all grades of deformities: the cases are not objectively studied and surgically individualized.

Although I am not a surgeon, I recognize that podiatric surgeons have done much to ensure that hallux valgus no longer belongs to a "low class of surgery." Each case must be objectively studied and surgically individualized. The foot remains a vulnerable part of the body on which to operate, and hallux valgus remains a "recalcitrant disorder." The lesson the surgeon can learn from the history of hallux valgus is, first, do no harm. Although the present trend is to discount the role of footwear in the etiology of hallux valgus, history shows us that a foot in the years following surgery is in need of the right shoe for the right occasion.

## PALLIATIVE METHODS OF TREATMENT OF HALLUX VALGUS

From ancient times, the bursal cyst (and often an overlying corn or a keratotic plug in the sinus) associated with hallux valgus received treatment. Theodorice (1267)[9] taught that "it should be excavated all around, and then extirpated down to its roots . . . afterwards the spot cauterized." Many writers subsequently described the many variations of ways to remove the corn or plug and reduce the bursitis.

Durlacher (1845)[10] gave a rational approach that still stands:

> The best mode of treatment in such a case would be to reduce the inflammation by rest, and by the application of cold lotions, after which the corns may be carefully extracted, and a plaster, made with soap cerate and adhesive plaster, applied over the joint. If the great toe is inclined obliquely towards the others, a piece of sponge, or a pledget made with tape or linen of sufficient thickness, should be placed between the first and the great toe, so as to bring the latter in a parallel line with the joint and the metatarsal bone. In this manner, the patient wearing a properly-made shoe, a cure may be soon effected, but the plaster must be retained over the joint for some time after the pain and inflammation have subsided.

In the treatment of the corn and its underlying sac, or to destroy the sinus, Durlacher considered the use of silver nitrate to be a specific.

In the nineteenth century, there was much interest in mechanical devices to influence the deformity. Peck (1871)[11] followed Meyer's (1863)[12] work and wrote, overconfidently, on "how distorted great toe can be straightened." Many were the springs, protective pads, splints, and toe posts in shoes. Much physical therapy was tried; Thomsen (1944)[13] discussed, exhaustively, exercises to mobilize the toes and correct established deformity. His book also had a lengthy section on corrective shoes and supplementary appliances. American and British chiropodists developed to a fine art the palliative treatment of the bursitis and the fabrication of replaceable protective devices; Runting (1925),[14] Woolf (1937),[15] and Budin (1941)[16] can be consulted with profit today. When surgery is not considered appropriate, or is not acceptable to the patient, the condition can be stabilized and the patient rendered symptom free.

## DEVELOPMENT OF HALLUX VALGUS SURGERY

Before the introduction of anaesthesia (general in 1846; local in 1884), and the work of Lister from 1867, using antisepsis and then asepsis to reduce the risk of infection, operating on the joint was both agonizing for the patient as well as hazardous in the extreme.

One of the earliest hints of a definitive surgical approach to hallux valgus was given by Boyer (1826)[17] when he recommended ablation of the "cyst." In 1836, Fricke (1837)[18] operated on two cases of "exostosis of the ball of the foot . . . excision of the bones which form the metatarsodigital joint of the great toe was performed with great success." Resection of the joint was subsequently reported by Pancoast (1844),[19] Hilton (1853),[20] and Butcher (1859).[21] Rose (1874)[22] also removed the sesamoids in addition to the resection of the head of the first metatarsal and the base of the proximal phalanx. Nélaton (1859)[23] recommended tenotomy of the long extensor of the great toe, and thus set the scene for subsequent tenotomies and tendon transplants of infinite variety.

Others must have done so before, but Reverdin (1881)[24] popularized the removal of just the so-called exostosis alone. He was not satisfied with the result, and then did in addition an osteotomy through the distal portion of the first metatarsal. The base of the wedge of bone removed was directed medially and its apex touched the lateral cortex; the toe was straightened and the capital piece was sutured to the shaft. Subsequently, many surgeons experimented with many similar techniques, but few mention Reverdin. Broca (1852)[25] performed an arthrodesis of the first metatarsophalangeal joint for hallux valgus. He stressed the importance of judging the angle at which the joint is fixed, to allow a measure of dorsiflexion.

There are several versions as to who first put into practice resection of the proximal part of the proximal phalanx of the hallux, but Keller (1904)[26] generally gets the credit. In a second paper 8 years later, Keller[27] reported the results of 26 operations (a surprisingly small series); he adopted an eyebrow incision and removed more of the exostosis. Ironically, considering that this operation became a standard procedure, Keller was not very interested in it and went on to work in general surgery.

Mayo (1908)[28] removed the head of the first metatarsal, and used a locally fashioned fascial flap to cover the denuded articular end of the remodeled bone. Holden (1954)[29] wrote:

> When there is severe deformity of the hallux and other toes, the Keller procedure gives poor results. In selected cases, arthrodesis of the first metatarsophalangeal joint, with correction of toe deformities and excision of the displaced metatarsal heads, gives gratifying results.

The work that followed Keller and Mayo indicates the versatility of the human imagination. The many contributions to the treatment of this recalcitrant problem made by podiatric surgeons are set out in this volume. Humility, clinical judgment, careful assessment of the individual patient, and delicate operating technique are required, rather than the invention of ever more "new" procedures.

# REFERENCES

1. Schuster OF: Foot Orthopaedics. First Institute of Podiatry, New York, 1927
2. Harkless LB, Krych SM: Handbook of Common Foot Problems. Churchill Livingstone, New York, 1990
3. Kelikian H: Hallux Valgus, Allied Deformities of the Forefoot and Metatarsalgia. WB Saunders, Philadelphia, 1965
4. Wiles P: Essentials of Orthopaedics. JA Churchill, London, 1949
5. Root ML, Orien WP, Weed JH: Normal and Abnormal Function of the Foot. Clinical Biomechanics Corp., Los Angeles, 1977
6. England MD: The problem of hallux valgus. Chiropodist 9:275, 1954
7. Giannestras NJ: Foot Disorders: Medical and Surgical Management. Lea & Febiger, Philadelphia, 1973
8. Jones FW: Structure and Function as seen in the foot. Baillière, Tindall London, 1944
9. Theodorice B (Bishop of Cervia): The Surgery of Theodorice (translated from Latin by Campbell E, Colton J), Vol. II, p. 110. Appelton-Century-Crofts, New York, 1955–1960 (original published in 1267)
10. Durlacher L: A Treatise on Corns, Bunions, the Diseases of Nails, and the General Management of the Feet. Simpkin Marshall, London, 1845
11. Peck JL: Dress and Care of the Feet. SR Wells, New York, 1871
12. Meyer GH: Why the Shoe Pinches. RT Trall, New York, 1863
13. Thomsen W: Kampf der Fusschwaeche. JF Lehmanns, Munich, 1944
14. Runting EGV: Practical Chiropody. Scientific Press, London, 1925
15. Woolf WH: Toe Casting and Liquid Rubber Technic. Harriman Printing, New York, 1937
16. Budin HA: Principles and Practice of Orthodigita. Strathmore Press, New York, 1941
17. Boyer A: Traité des Maladies Chirurgicales. Migneret, Paris, 1826
18. Fricke JLG: Exostosis of the ball of the foot. J Med Sci 11:497, 1837
19. Pancoast J: A Treatise on Operative Surgery. Carey and Hart, Philadelphia, 1844
20. Hilton J: Resection of the metatarso-phalangeal joint of the great toe. Med Tms Gaz 7:141, 1853
21. Butcher: Excision of the metatarso-phalangeal articulation of the great toe; recovery, with perfect use of the foot. Dublin Quart J Med Sci 27:48, 1859
22. Rose A: Resection considered as a remedy for abduction of the great toe—hallux valgus—and bunion. Med Rec 9:200, 1874
23. Nélaton A: Elémens de Pathologie Chirurgicale. G Bailliére, Paris, 1859
24. Reverdin J: De la déviation en dehors du gros orteil (hallux valgus, vulg 'oignon,' 'bunions,' 'Ballen') et de son traitment chirurgical. Trans Int Med Congr 2:408, 1881
25. Broca P: Des difformités de la partie antérieure du pied produite par l'action de la chaussure. Bull Soc Anat 27:60, 1852
26. Keller WL: The surgical treatment of bunions and hallux valgus. New York Med J 80:741, 1904

27. Keller WL: Further observations on the surgical treatment of hallux valgus and bunions. New York Med J 95:696, 1912

28. Mayo CH: The surgical treatment of bunions. Ann Surg 48:300, 1908

29. Holden NT: The operative treatment of hallux valgus—a review of the Keller procedure. Guy's Hosp Rep 103:274, 1954

# 2

# Normal Anatomy of the Forefoot

*BRAD G. SAMOJLA*

## LIMB DEVELOPMENT

There are many different types of deformities that may present in the foot. Many congenital deformities can be explained by problems occurring during development of the lower limb.[1] Some of the most common congenital deformities include syndactyly, missing digits, and duplication of digits.[2–4] There are other deformities, however, that may be more difficult to identify, such as missing or abnormal muscles, absent or undersized vessels, and anomalous nerves.[3,5]

The limbs start to appear in the early stages of the embryonic period of development (fourth to eighth intrauterine [IU] week) as condensations of mesenchyme. The upper limb appears a few days before the lower limb. By the end of the embryonic period, the embryo has become distinctly human. Furthermore, all the limbs are formed with all the fingers and toes fully developed (Fig. 2-1). The fetal period (9 weeks IU to birth) is characterized by further growth of the fetus. From the time of birth through the first 6 years of life, the skeleton not only grows in size, with the legs elongating faster than the arms, but undergoes rotational and torsional changes as well.[6] These rotational and torsional changes usually are complete by the sixth year. Skeletal maturity occurs when all growth plates have closed.[7,8]

During the first week of the embryonic period (fourth week IU), small elevations appear on the ventrolateral aspect of the embryo (Fig. 1). These elevations, called limb buds, consist of a mass of mesenchyme covered with ectoderm. During the sixth IU week, the mesenchyme within the center of the limb bud condenses. This mass rapidly undergoes chondrification to form hyaline cartilage, and by the end of the

embryonic period ossification has started in most of the long bones of the body. When first formed, the feet are paddle-shaped plates. By the end of the seventh IU week, however, the mesenchymal tissue starts to condense into digital rays and the mesenchyme between the digits eventually degenerates. By the end of this week, the embryo has free movable toes.

Limb rotation occurs between the seventh and eighth IU weeks. It is during this time the embryo takes on the familiar "fetal position." Previous to limb rotation the knees and the elbows are both directed laterad. When rotation occurs, the knee rotates craniad, such that it is now anterior. The elbow rotates in a caudal direction such that it is directed posterior (see Fig. 2-1).

Simultaneously, the mesenchyme immediately surrounding the potential bone develops into a ventral and dorsal mass. These masses eventually form the dorsal and ventral groups of muscles in the limb. The ventral rami of adjacent spinal cord segments grow into these future muscles and form myotomes, some of which persist in the adult.

The arterial supply to the developing lower limb starts as a capillary plexus off the dorsal side of the umbilical artery and the internal iliac artery.[7] The artery formed from this plexus is the *axial artery* and is located in the dorsal aspect of the leg. The axial artery terminates by passing through the sinus tarsi and forming a plantar capillary network. The *femoral artery* forms from the external iliac artery. It descends the limb along the ventral aspect of the thigh and terminates on the dorsum of the foot. During its development, the femoral artery communicates with the axial artery in many locations. Gradually, between the end of the embryonic period and birth, the axial artery

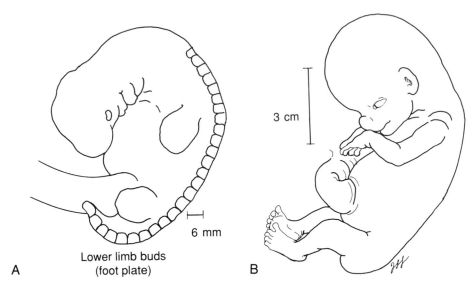

**Fig. 2-1.** Development of the limbs in the embryo. (**A**) Early embryonic period. The limb buds have formed and the embryo is approximately 6 mm long. (**B**) End of the embryonic period. All the digits have formed, and the limbs have rotated. The embryo is approximately 3 cm long.

degenerates and persists as the popliteal and peroneal arteries.

Skeletal growth is a long process that begins in the seventh IU week and ends as late as 30 years of life. Skeletal growth begins with the appearance of a *primary center of ossification*. All bones that are formed by cartilage have a primary center of ossification. In long bones, primary centers are located in the shaft and appear between the twelfth and fifteenth IU week.[6,7] Short bones, usually develop from a single center of ossification that may appear as late as 5 years after birth.[6,7] *Secondary centers of ossification* are additional centers of ossification. In long bones, secondary centers usually appear in the ends of the bones.

**Table 2-1.** Ossification Centers for the Bones of the Foot

| Bone | Primary Center | Secondary Centers (years) | Fusion (years) |
|---|---|---|---|
| Metatarsals | Shaft 2–4, 9th week IU | Head, 1–2 | 18–20 |
| | Shaft 1, 10th week IU | Base, 1–2 (head, 10) | 18–20 |
| | Shaft 5, 10th week IU | Head, 1–2 (base, 7–10) | 18–20 |
| Phalanges | Distal shaft, 9–12 weeks IU | Base, 2–8 | 18–20 |
| | Proximal shaft, 11–15 weeks IU | Base, 2–8 | 18–20 |
| | Middle shaft, 15 weeks IU | Base, 2–8 | 18–20 |
| Calcaneus | 3rd month IU | Calcaneal tuberosity, 6–8 | 14–16 |
| Talus | Body, 6–7 months IU | (lateral tubercle, 8–9 years) | |
| Cuboid | Birth | | |
| Lateral cuneiform | 6 months | | |
| Medial cuneiform | 1–2 years | | |
| Intermediate cuneiform | 1.5–2 years | | |
| Navicular | 2.5–5 years | (tuberosity, 10 years) | |
| Hallucal sesamoids | 7–8 years | (bipartite sesamoids, two centers) | |

(Data from Netter,[6] Clemente,[7] Sarrafian,[8] Draves,[9] and Edeiken.[10])

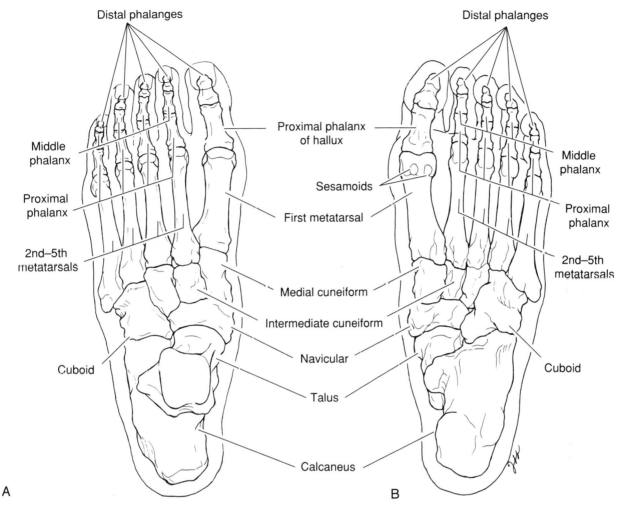

**Fig. 2-2.** Skeletal structure of the foot. (**A**) Dorsal view. (**B**) Plantar view.

The *growth plate* (epiphyseal plate) is a cartilaginous area between a primary center of ossification and the secondary center of ossification. In long bones, this occurs between the shaft and the ends.

The ossification centers for each bone appear at characteristic locations and times. More important than the exact time of appearance of an ossification center is the order in which these centers appear (Table 2-1). [6-10] As a general rule, the order of fusion of a secondary center to the primary center is opposite to their order of appearance; for example, the last secondary center to appear is the first to fuse to the primary center.

## OSTEOLOGY

The main function of the foot is to support the body during locomotion and quiet standing. In anatomic position, the foot is at a right angle to the leg with the feet straight ahead. The "at ease" or neutral stance position is with the foot at a right angle to the leg, but the feet are slightly abducted. In either case, the midline of the foot is through the second metatarsal.

The bones of the foot consist of the calcaneus, talus, navicular, 3 cuneiforms, cuboid, 5 metatarsals, and 14 phalanges. These 26 bones of the foot are divided into the tarsus, metatarsus, and phalanges (Fig. 2-2). The 7

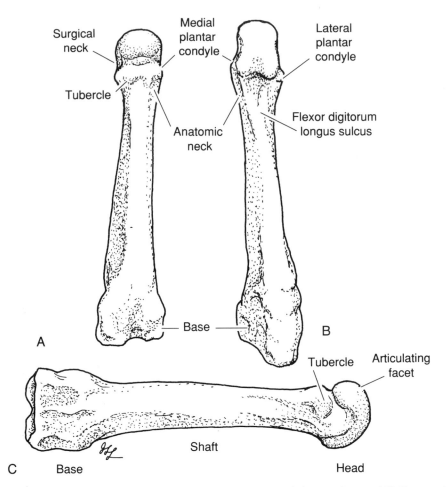

**Fig. 2-3.** General features of a metatarsal. (**A**) Side view. (**B**) Dorsal view. (**C**) Plantar view.

tarsal bones are short bones that connect the metatarsals to the leg. The 5 metatarsals are weight-bearing bones and provide a foundation for the digits. The phalanges provide the skeletal structure for the digits.

Functionally, the bones of the foot can also be grouped into the rearfoot (which consists of the calcaneus and talus), the midfoot (which consists of the navicular, cuboid, and the three cuneiforms), and the forefoot (which consists of the metatarsals and their respective phalanges). The foot bones can also be grouped into a medial or lateral column. The medial column consists of the talus, navicular, the three cuneiforms, the first to third metatarsals, and the respective phalanges. The lateral column consists of the calcaneus, cuboid, the fourth and fifth metatarsals, and the phalanges.

## The Metatarsal Bones

### General Characteristics

There are a total of five metatarsals, which are numbered from I to V in a medial to lateral fashion. Each metatarsal is a long bone presenting with a base, shaft, and head (Fig. 2-3). The metatarsals extend anteriorly from the foot and are nearly parallel to each other (0°–8°).[11] The first metatarsal is the shortest in absolute length while the second is the longest (see Fig. 2-2). Straus[11] showed that the first metatarsal is approximately 83 percent of the length of the second metatarsal. More commonly, one refers to the protrusion of a metatarsal in the articulated foot (relative length). For example, the second metatarsal protrudes the most distal and is considered to be the longest. Because the fifth metatarsal does not protrude as far as any of the other metatarsals, in the articulated skeleton, it is considered the shortest. The formula most commonly cited referring to the protrusion or relative length of the metatarsals is 2 (longest) > 3 > 1 > 4 > 5 (shortest) (see Fig. 2-2).[8,9]

## Base

The base is the most proximal end of the metatarsal and articulates with the tarsus and the other metatarsals (see Fig. 2-3). The base is usually wedge shaped, presenting with five surfaces. The superior and inferior surfaces are rough for the attachment of ligaments. The medial and lateral surfaces present with both flat articular and nonarticular areas. The articular facets are for either the tarsus or metatarsus. The posterior surface is slightly concave and is covered with an articular facet for articulation with the tarsus.

## Shaft

When viewed along their dorsal surfaces, the shaft of each metatarsal extends directly anteriorly from the base and tapers distad. The fifth metatarsal shaft differs slightly from the others in that the shaft has a small degree of lateral bowing. When viewed from the side the bone is curved, being convex dorsal and concave plantar (see Fig. 2-3). The shaft of each metatarsal varies in thickness; however, each is roughly pyramidal in section. Further, within each metatarsal there is a degree of torsion between the base and the head of the bone. The amount and direction of the torsion varies among the five metatarsals.[8,11]

## Head

The head of a metatarsal presents with a smooth convex facet covered with hyaline cartilage that extends farther on the plantar surface than the dorsal surface (see Fig. 2-3). The plantar surface is characterized by two condyles separated by a small shallow groove for the passage of the flexor tendons. The *lateral plantar condyle* is larger than the *medial plantar condyle*. Both condyles are continuous with the articular surface of the head.

Dorsally, a depression known as the *surgical neck* is present immediately posterior to the articular surface. Posterior to the surgical neck are a *medial* and *lateral tubercle* for the attachment of metatarsophalangeal

collateral ligaments. Finally, posterior to these tubercles is another depression known as the *anatomic neck* that represents the point where the primary and secondary centers of ossification have fused.

## Development

All the metatarsals develop from two centers of ossification (see Table 2-1).[6–10] The primary centers appear in the shafts of the second, third, and fourth metatarsals before the primary centers in the first and fifth metatarsals. Secondary centers or the epiphysis appear in all the heads of the metatarsals except the first, where the secondary center is located in the base. Occasional centers of ossification appear in the head of the first and in the tuberosity of the fifth metatarsals.

## The First Metatarsal

Located on the most medial aspect of the foot, the first metatarsal has two regular articulations, the proximal phalanx distad and the medial cuneiform proximad. On occasion, however, the first metatarsal articulates laterally with the second metatarsal. The first metatarsal is the shortest and broadest, and probably the most mobile metatarsal.

The posterior surface of the base presents with a kidney-shaped facet for articulation with the anterior surface of the medial cuneiform (Fig. 2-4). If there is an articulation between the first and second metatarsal, then there is a small oval facet laterally.

On the base at the junction of the inferior and medial surfaces where the tibialis anterior tendon inserts is a small tubercle. On the opposite side of the base, at the junction of the inferior and lateral surfaces, there is a tuberosity for the insertion of the peroneus longus tendon. The remaining surfaces are rough for the attachment of ligaments.

The head of the first metatarsal is quadrilateral in shape and larger than the lesser metatarsals. It is also unique in that it presents with a ridge or crista that begins on the anterior aspect of the articular cartilage and continues plantarly (see Fig. 2-4). When viewed from above, the beginning of the crista is lateral to the midpoint between the medial and lateral borders of the head. A sagittal plane drawn through the crista is parallel to the lateral surface of the shaft of the metatarsal, but is everted by 13° when compared to the base of the bone.[8,12] During stance, the crista is angulated from the supporting surface by 78°; however, dur-

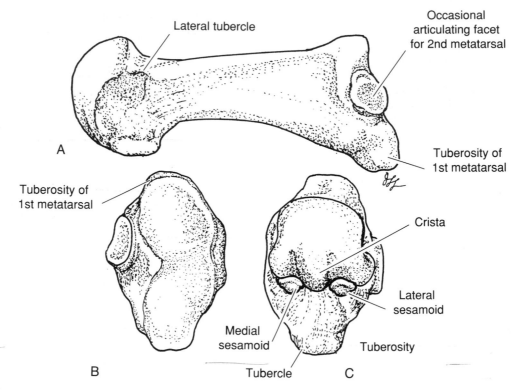

**Fig. 2-4.** Structural features of the first metatarsal. (**A**) Lateral view. (**B**) Posterior surface of the base. (**C**) Anterior surface of the head. Note sesamoids articulating with the grooves on the plantar condyles.

ing loading of the first metatarsophalangeal joint, the crista becomes perpendicular to the supporting surface such that each sesamoid carries roughly equal weight.[12,13]

On each of the plantar condyles there is a groove for the articulation with the sesamoids. Normally the groove on the medial plantar condyle is larger than the groove on the lateral plantar condyle.[12,13] According to Yoshioka, there are three areas of articulation: on the first metatarsal head; the grooves for articulation with the sesamoids; and the distal-dorsal aspect of the head for articulation with the base of the proximal phalanx.[12]

### The Second Metatarsal

The second metatarsal is the longest metatarsal in the foot. It regularly articulates with the proximal phalanx, distad; the second cuneiform, proximad; the first cuneiform, mediad; and the third cuneiform and third metatarsal, laterad. Occasionally there is an articulation with the first metatarsal medially. This bone has strong ligamentous attachments to the surrounding bones.

The base is wedge shaped with the base up and apex down. A facet covers the entire posterior surface of the base that is for articulation with the second cuneiform. The medial surface presents with an oval facet at the posterosuperior border for articulation with the medial cuneiform. If there is an articulation between the first and second metatarsal, then there is a small facet anterior to the facet for the cuneiform. The lateral surface has two facets that are separated by a roughened area. Both these facets are divided by a vertical ridge into an anterior and posterior facet. Both the posterior facets articulate with the third cuneiform, while the anterior facets articulate with the base of the third metatarsal. The remaining surfaces are roughened for the attachment of ligaments.

## The Third Metatarsal

The third metatarsal articulates with the third cuneiform, proximally; the second metatarsal, medially; the fourth metatarsal, laterally; and the base of the proximal phalanx, distally. The entire posterior surface is covered by a facet that articulates with the anterior surface of the third cuneiform. This surface is triangular in shape with the apex inferior. The medial surface has two facets at the posterior border for articulation with the base of the second metatarsal. These two facets are separated by a thin strip of rough bone. The lateral surface has a single oval facet at the posterosuperior border for articulation with the fourth metatarsal. The remainder of the surfaces are roughened for the attachment of ligaments.

## The Fourth Metatarsal

The fourth metatarsal articulates with five bones; the cuboid, proximally; the third cuneiform and metatarsal, medially; the fifth metatarsal, laterally; and the proximal phalanx, distally. This is the only metatarsal that has a rectangular base. The entire posterior surface of the base contains a rectangular facet for articulation with the cuboid. The medial surface presents with a single facet at the posterosuperior border, which is divided into an anterior and a very small posterior facet by a vertical ridge. The anterior facet articulates with the base of the third metatarsal; the small posteriod facet articulates with the third cuneiform; and the lateral surface of the fourth metatarsal has a single facet for the articulation with the fifth metatarsal base.

## The Fifth Metatarsal

The fifth metatarsal articulates with three bones: the base of the proximal phalanx, the cuboid, and the fourth metatarsal. The base is pyramidal to triangular in shape with the apex pointing inferolateral. The posterior surface is triangular in shape and is covered with a single articular facet. The apex points laterally and articulates with the cuboid. The distinguishing feature of this metatarsal is a large tuberosity (*styloid process*) found on the lateral surface. The tuberosity is subcutaneous and rough for the attachment of ligaments and muscles. The medial surface presents with a single oval facet for the articulation with the fourth

metatarsal base. The remaining surfaces are rough for the attachment of ligaments and muscles.

## The Phalanges

### General Characteristics

The phalanges are the bones that make up the toes. There are 14 phalanges in the foot: 2 in the hallux and 3 in each of the lesser digits. It is a common occurrence to find the middle and distal phalanges of the fifth digit fused to each other. The phalanges can be divided into rows: proximal, middle, and distal (see Fig. 2-2). Although very small, the phalanges are still long bones and consist of a base, body or shaft, and head.

### Development

All the phalanges develop from two centers of ossification. The primary centers found in the shafts of distal phalanges are first to appear (see Table 2-1). The proximal phalanges are next to appear, followed by the middle phalanges. The secondary centers or the epiphysis appear in the bases of the phalanges between the second and eighth years, with fusion occurring by 18 years of age. There is great deal of variability in the time and order of appearance of these centers.

### Proximal Phalanges

The base of the phalange is concave for articulation with the respective metatarsal head. The body is compressed from side to side, and longitudinally it is slightly convex. The head presents with a trochlear surface for articulation with the middle phalanx. Tubercles are present on the inferior side of the base and dorsal side of the head for the attachment of collateral ligaments.

### Middle Phalanges

The first digit or the hallux does not have a middle phalanx. The base of the middle phalanx has a corresponding surface for articulation with the head of the proximal phalanx. The body is broader that the proximal phalanx. The head of the middle phalanges has a trochlear surface for articulation with the base of the distal phalanx. Small tubercles are present on both sides of the head for the attachment of collateral ligaments.

### Distal Phalanges

These bones are at the level of the toe nails. The base and the shaft are similar in shape to the middle phalanges. The head of the distal phalanx is characterized by a flattened surface for the support of the toenail and a tuberosity plantarly.

## Sesamoids and Accessory Ossicles

Sesamoids are fibrous, cartilaginous, or osseous structures that are almost always contained with a tendon. Anomalous sesamoids frequently present in the joint capsules of the various metatarsophalangeal and interphalangeal joints of the foot. Although the precise functions of sesamoids are uncertain, it has been suggested that they (1) alter the pull of a tendon, (2) decrease friction at articular surfaces, and (3) decrease pressure within a tendon to allow circulation to the tendon.[14–16]

There are only two regular sesamoids in the foot, the *medial* (*tibial*) and *lateral* (*fibular*) *hallucal sesamoid*. Each sesamoid is oval, measuring approximately 10 mm in length and 8.5 mm in width, with the tibial sesamoid being larger and more elongated than the fibular sesamoid.[12,16] These sesamoids are located in the tendon of the flexor hallucis brevis muscle proximal to the metatarsophalangeal joint and articulate only with the head of the first metatarsal. The tibial sesamoid articulates more distal in the head than the fibular sesamoid.[13] It is rather common to see these two sesamoids present as bipartite sesamoids.[16]

Accessory bones differ from sesamoids in that they are not located within tendons.[8,9,15] These are developmental anomalies and represent aberrant ossification centers or an abnormal separation of an ossification center. Many of these bones will have a synovial membrane surrounding it and the adjacent bone, thus forming a regular synovial joint. Accessory bones in the foot are common findings. Located between the dorsal aspects of the bases of the metatarsals, near the tarsus, the *os intermetatarseum* is the third most frequently occurring accessory bone in the foot.[8] It is most commonly found between the first and second metatarsals.[8]

## ARTHROLOGY

An *anatomic synovial joint* is defined as a joint that is enclosed within a single synovial membrane.[15] An anatomic synovial joint may be simple, compound, or complex. A simple anatomic joint is the articulation between two bones. The best example of this type of joint is a metatarsophalangeal or an interphalangeal joint. A compound joint is defined as more than two bones enclosed within a single synovial membrane; the best example of this is the greater tarsal joint. In this joint, several of the tarsal bones articulate with one another and the metatarsals; however, because it is enclosed within a single synovial membrane it is considered a single anatomic joint. A complex joint is defined by the presence of a intrasynovial cartilaginous structure of which the knee joint is a good example.

Ligaments that support joints can be *intracapsular, capsular,* or *extracapsular.* Those ligaments that are intracapsular have either one or both of their attachments deep to the joint capsule. Although these ligaments are intracapsular they are still extrasynovial. Most of the ligaments in the forefoot are capsular ligaments; that is, the joint capsule has localized thickenings which are renamed. Extracapsular ligaments are ligaments that support a joint, but they are not typically attached to the joint capsule. The calcaneofibular ligament is an excellent example of an extracapsular ligament.

### The Tarsometatarsal Joint

The tarsometatarsal joint is a functional joint composed of three anatomic joints. The bones that form the functional tarsometatarsal joint are all the metatarsal bases, the three cuneiforms, and the cuboid. The tarsi are connected to the metatarsus by dorsal, plantar, and interosseus ligaments.

### Dorsal Tarsometatarsal Ligaments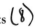

There are eight dorsal ligaments. One ligament attaches from each metatarsal to each of the respective cuneiforms and cuboid. The remaining three attach from the first cuneiform to the second metatarsal base; the second metatarsal base to the third cuneiform; and from the third cuneiform to the fourth metatarsal base, respectively.

### Plantar Tarsometatarsal Ligaments (9)

There are nine plantar ligaments, which attach exactly the same as do the dorsal ligaments with one exception: there is an additional ligament attaching from the first cuneiform to the third metatarsal base.

### Interosseus Tarsometatarsal Ligaments

There are only three interosseus ligaments attaching from the roughened areas of the first cuneiform to the second metatarsal base (LisFranc's ligament), from the second metatarsal base to the third cuneiform, and from the third cunciform to the fourth metatarsal base.[10]

*LisFranc lig = 1st cuneiform to 2nd met base*

### Synovial Membrane

Three different anatomic joints form the functional joint known as the synovial membrane. The *greater tarsal synovial membrane* encloses the cuneonavicular, intercuneiform, the cuneocuboid, the second cuneometatarsal, third cuncometatarsal, and the third cuneiform-fourth metatarsal joints. The *medial tarsometatarsal synovial membrane* encloses the first metatarsal and first cuneiform joint. The *lateral tarsometatarsal synovial membrane* encloses the fourth and fifth metatarsal bases to the cuboid.

## Intermetatarsal Joints

The bases of the second to fifth metatarsals are connected by dorsal, plantar, and interosseus intermetatarsal ligaments. The strongest ligaments are the interosseus ligaments, while the weakest ligaments in this group are the dorsal. If present, the first and second metatarsals have only a few weak interosseus fibers attaching to each other. These articulations are enclosed in the greater tarsal, the medial tarsometatarsal, or the lateral tarsometatarsal synovial membrane.

## Metatarsophalangeal Joints

The metatarsophalangeal joints are the articulations between the head of a metatarsal and the base of the proximal phalanx. Each metatarsophalangeal joint is a single anatomic joint. However, when all these joints act together they are considered a functional joint. The ligaments supporting the metatarsophalangeal joints are, in general, similar in all five joints (Fig. 2-5). The ligaments are mostly capsular and are best defined on the medial side of the joint. However, because of the hallucal sesamoids the ligaments around the first metatarsophalangeal joint have a slightly different structure.

### Lesser Metatarsophalangeal Joints

#### Fibrous Joint Capsule

The fibrous capsule surrounds the entire joint and is thin dorsally. The fibrous capsule is redundant, especially plantarly, to allow flexion and extension of the digits. An extensor expansion dorsal to the capsule provides additional support to the joint.

#### Medial and Lateral Collateral Metatarsophalangeal Ligaments

Proximally these capsular ligaments are attached to the tubercles on the dorsomedial and dorsolateral aspect of the head of the metatarsal. Distad, they become difficult to distinguish from the joint capsule and attach to the corresponding plantar tubercles on the base of the proximal phalanx.

#### Plantar Metatarsophalangeal Ligament

The plantar metatarsophalangeal ligament attaches proximally from the head of the metatarsal to the base of the phalanx distally. The ligament extends plantarly from the medial tubercle to the lateral tubercle along the plantar surface of the joint. Some authors describe a part of the ligament that extends from the tubercles to the plantar plate as the *medial* or *lateral metatarsophalangeal suspensory ligament;* in preserved cadaveric dissections, however, these ligaments are very difficult to observe.

#### Plantar Plate

The plantar plate is a thickening of the plantar metatarsophalangeal ligament. Attached to this structure is the deep transverse metatarsal ligament and the fibrous flexor sheath. The function of the plantar plate is believed to be similar to that of the hallucal sesamoids.

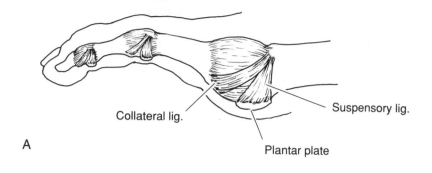

Collateral lig.

Suspensory lig.

Plantar plate

A

Collateral lig.

Suspensory lig.

Sesamoid bone

B

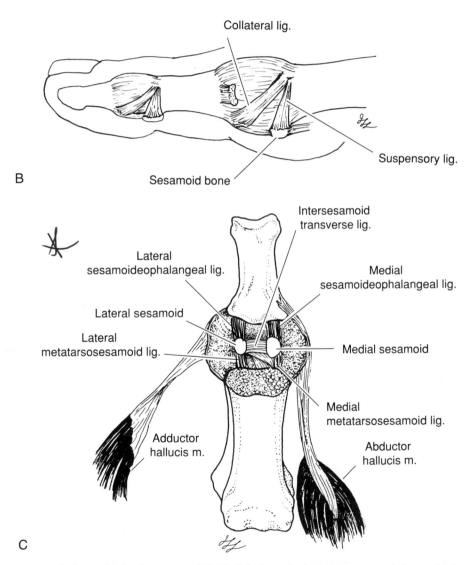

Intersesamoid
transverse lig.

Lateral
sesamoideophalangeal lig.

Medial
sesamoideophalangeal lig.

Lateral sesamoid

Medial sesamoid

Lateral
metatarsosesamoid lig.

Medial
metatarsosesamoid lig.

Adductor
hallucis m.

Abductor
hallucis m.

C

**Fig. 2-5.** Metatarsophalangeal joint ligaments. (**A**) Medial view of a lesser metatarsophalangeal joint. (**B**) Medial view of the first metatarsophalangeal joint. (**C**) Intracapsular view of the sesamoideal ligaments. The head of the first metatarsal has been removed.

## Synovial Membrane

Five synovial membranes enclose each metatarsophalangeal joint.

### First Metatarsophalangeal Joint

Many ligaments and tendons are described as attaching to the hallucal sesamoids. In dissection, however, it is very difficult to separate the various layers attaching to each sesamoid; all the ligaments and tendons blend into a single fibrous mass that is strongly adherent to each sesamoid.

## Fibrous Joint Capsule

Like the lesser metatarsophalangeal joints the fibrous joint capsule surrounds the entire joint, is thin dorsally, and is redundant, especially plantarly. The joint capsule is attached to the sesamoids plantarly.

## Plantar Metatarsophalangeal Ligament

This ligament attaches proximally from the head of the metatarsal to the base of the phalanx distally. The ligament extends plantarly from the medial tubercle to the lateral tubercle along the plantar surface of the joint.

## Medial and Lateral Metatarsosesamoideal Ligaments

These ligaments, which are actually a part of the plantar metatarsophalangeal ligament that has been renamed, are attached from the metatarsal proximally to the sesamoids distally (Fig. 2-5C).

## Medial and Lateral Sesamoideophalangeal Ligaments

These ligaments are also a part of the plantar metatarsophalangeal ligament that has been renamed; they attach from each sesamoid proximally to the plantar aspect of the base of the proximal phalanx (Fig. 2-5C).

## Intersesamoid Ligament

The intersesamoid ligament ia s small broad ligament; on intracapsular dissection of the joint, the ligamentous fibers are clearly seen extending from the medial to the lateral sesamoid (Fig. 2-5C).

## Medial and Lateral Metatarsophalangeal Suspensory Ligaments

This section of the plantar metatarsophalangeal ligament extends from the medial and lateral tubercles to the medial and lateral sesamoids. These ligaments, as compared to the suspensory ligaments of the lesser metatarsophalangeal joints, are easily observed.

## Medial and Lateral Collateral Metatarsophalangeal Ligaments

Proximally these ligaments are attached to the tubercles on the dorsomedial and dorsolateral aspect of the head of the metatarsal. The medial collateral metatarsophalangeal ligament at its proximal attachment, however, is clearly intracapsular. Distad, they become difficult to distinguish from the joint capsule, and attach to the corresponding plantar tubercles on the base of the proximal phalanx.

## Deep Transverse Metatarsal Ligament

This ligament is actually an intermetatarsal ligament, but it is considered here because of its role in metatarsophalangeal joint stability. This ligament is composed of four slips connecting the metatarsal heads to one another; thus, this ligament prevents splaying of the distal end on the metatarsals. The deep transverse metatarsal ligament is found plantarly attaching to the plantar plate. This proximal edge of the ligament is at the level of the most posterior part of the plantar condyles of the metatarsal. The distal edge usually does not extend past the distal end of the metatarsal.

The structure of the deep transverse metatarsal ligament between the first and second metatarsal heads is somewhat controversial. Most texts describe a single ligamentous slip connecting the two heads.[7,9,15] However, with careful dissection it is easily seen that the ligament connecting the two heads is actually bifurcated into dorsoproximal and plantodistal slips.[8,17] The plantar slip is the most distal part of the ligament and is attached from the plantar plate of the second metatarsophalangeal joint to the lateral sesamoid of the first metatarsophalangeal joint. The dorsal slip is somewhat posterior to the plantar slip and is attached from the plantar plate of the second metatarsophalangeal joint to the dorsolateral aspect of the joint capsule of the first metatarsophalangeal joint. The tendon of the ad-

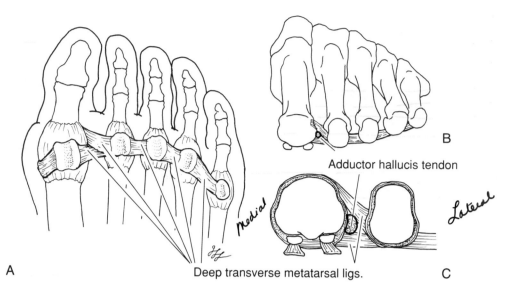

**Fig. 2-6.** (**A–C**) Anterior view of the first intermetatarsal space to illustrate the bifurcated nature of the first slip of the deep transverse metatarsal ligament.

ductor hallucis passes between these two slips (Fig. 2-6).

## Interphalangeal Joints

There are two groups of interphalangeal joints: the proximal interphalangeal joints, which are the articulations between the base of the middle and the head of the proximal phalanges; and the distal interphalangeal joints, which are the articulations between the head of the middle and the base of the distal phalanges. In the hallux there is only one interphalangeal joint. The ligaments of all the interphalangeal joints are similar to one another and are best observed in the proximal interphalangeal joints.

### Fibrous Joint Capsule

Like the metatarsophalangeal joints, the joint capsule is thin dorsally and thickened plantarly. The dorsal side of these joints receive additional support from tendons.

### Plantar Interphalangeal Ligaments

This is a thickening of the joint capsule from the medial tubercle to the lateral tubercle across the plantar aspect of the joint. Some authors describe a suspensory ligament appearing on either side of the joint. However, these ligaments can be extremely difficult to observe.

### Medial and Lateral Collateral Interphalangeal Ligaments

These capsular ligaments extend from the medial and lateral tubercles on the head of the phalanx to the base of the middle or distal phalanx.

### Synovial Cavities

There are nine synovial cavities enclosing the nine interphalangeal joints of the foot.

## MYOLOGY
### Fascia of the Foot

Over the foot and digits, the superficial fascia is very thin. In lean individuals, the fascia is more fibrous in nature. The cutaneous nerves and superficial veins pass in this layer of fascia. In the toes, the arterial supply is deeply located in this layer. Thick adipose

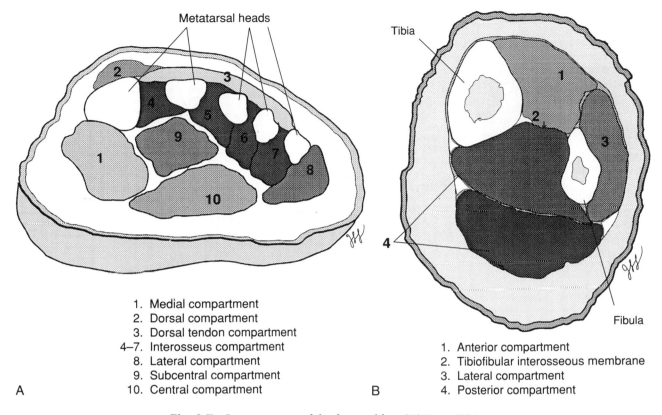

Metatarsal heads

1. Medial compartment
2. Dorsal compartment
3. Dorsal tendon compartment
4–7. Interosseus compartment
8. Lateral compartment
9. Subcentral compartment
10. Central compartment

A

Tibia

Fibula

1. Anterior compartment
2. Tibiofibular interosseous membrane
3. Lateral compartment
4. Posterior compartment

B

**Fig. 2-7.** Compartments of the foot and leg. (**A**) Foot. (**B**) Leg.

tissue is present under areas of extreme pressure and stress, such as the ball of the foot and the heel.

The deep fascia of the foot is continuous with the deep fascia of the leg. At the ankle, the fascia becomes thick and organized into transverse bands called retinacula. The *dorsal pedal fascia* is continuous with the plantar fascia and the fascia of the digits. Plantarly, the deep fascia is more complex. The *plantar fascia* is divided into medial, central, and lateral divisions. At the point where two of the divisions meet, the fascia sends thick septa deep into the foot to form compartments (Fig. 2-7A).

The central division of the plantar fascia is that part of the fascia referred to as the *plantar aponeurosis*. It is the thickest and strongest part of the deep fascia. Proximally, the fascia attaches to the calcaneal tuberosity and ends distally by dividing into a superficial and deep strata.[18] The superficial stratum attaches to the skin in the furrow behind the toes. At the level of the metatarsal heads, the deep side of the superficial stra-

tum passes transversely to form the *superficial transverse metatarsal ligament*. The deep stratum divides in five slips, which embrace the metatarsal at the level of the anatomic neck before blending with the deep transverse metatarsal ligament. Proximal to the metatarsal heads, the plantar aponeurosis forms *sagittal septa*, which compartmentalize the tendons and neurovascular bundle to each digit. At the level of the metatarsal heads, the deep fascia is attached to the skin by *vertical fibers*. These vertical fibers, along with the deep transverse metatarsal ligament, form a hollow through which the plantar neurovascular bundle passes (Fig. 2-8).[18,19] The neurovascular bundle is protected inferiorly by fat bodies that extend throughout the weight-bearing areas of the forefoot. These fat bodies act as cushions so that the plantar vessels and nerves are not compressed during weight-bearing.[18]

The deep fascia of the digits is continuous with the deep fascia of the foot. The deep fascia of each digit is specialized dorsal to the metatarsophalangeal joint

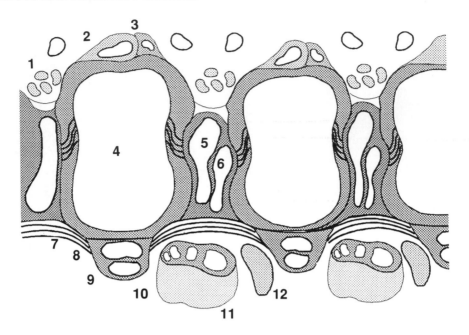

1. Neurovascular bundle
2. Long extensor tendon
3. Short extensor tendon
4. Metatarsal head
5. Dorsal interroseus m.
6. Plantar interroseus m.
7. Deep transverse metatarsal lig.
8. Long flexor tendon
9. Short flexor tendon
10. Neurovascular bundle
11. Adipose tissue
12. Lumbrical

**Fig. 2-8.** Anterior view of a lesser metatarsophalangeal joint showing the tendinous, neurovascular, and fascial structures.

and is known as the *extensor expansion*. Distally, the deep fascia covers the tendons and holds them against the phalanges. Plantarly, the deep fascia forms sheaths to tightly hold the flexor tendons against the phalanges. These *flexor sheaths* prevent what is commonly referred to as "bowstringing" of the long and short flexor tendons. In each of the flexor sheaths are short synovial sheaths that allow the tendons to move freely. Several parts of the flexor sheaths are easily identifiable. The thick *annual ligaments* surround the interphalangeal joints, while the thin *cruciate ligaments* help to hold the tendon against the shaft of the phalanx. The deep fascia attaches directly to the medial and lateral sides of the phalanges and the distal part of the distal phalanx.

## Extrinsic Muscles of the Foot

The muscles that control the forefoot include both extrinsic and intrinsic muscles. Most of the extrinsic muscles, from the three compartments of the leg, help to control the forefoot (Table 2-2; see also Fig. 2-7B).

### Tibialis Anterior Muscle

The tibialis anterior muscle originates from the lateral condyle of the tibia, the upper two-thirds of the lateral surface of the shaft of the tibia, and the adjacent area of the interosseus membrane. The muscle forms a tendon that crosses the ankle joint and is the most medial tendon on the dorsal foot. The tendon inserts into the medioplantar aspect of the first cuneiform and into the

**Table 2-2.** Vascular and Nerve Supply to the Extrinsic and Intrinsic Muscles of the Foot, Listed According to Their Insertions

| Muscle | Innervation | Vascular Supply |
|---|---|---|
| Tibialis anterior | Deep peroneal | Anterior tibial |
| Peroneus longus | Superficial peroneal | Peroneal |
| Extensor hallucis longus | Deep peroneal | Anterior tibial |
| Extensor digitorum brevis | Deep peroneal, lateral terminal br. | Dorsalis pedis, lateral tarsal |
| Flexor hallucis longus | Tibial, lower muscular br. | Peroneal and posterior tibial |
| Flexor hallucis brevis | Medial plantar, 1st plantar proper digital br. | Medial and lateral plantar[a] |
| Abductor hallucis | Medial plantar | Medial plantar |
| Adductor hallucis | Lateral plantar, deep terminal br. | Lateral plantar[a] |
| Extensor digitorum longus | Deep peroneal | Anterior tibial |
| Extensor digitorum brevis | Deep peroneal, lateral terminal br. | Dorsalis pedis, lateral tarsal |
| Flexor digitorum longus | Tibial, lower muscular branches | Posterior tibial |
| Flexor digitorum brevis | Lateral plantar | Medial and lateral plantar |
| 1st lumbricale | Medial plantar, 1st common digital br. | Medial plantar |
| 1st dorsal interosseus | Lateral plantar, deep terminal br. | 1st dorsal metatarsal |
|  | Deep peroneal, 1st interosseus br. | 1st plantar metatarsal |
| 2nd dorsal interosseus | Lateral plantar, deep terminal br. | 2nd dorsal metatarsal |
|  | Deep peroneal, 2nd interosseus br. | 2nd plantar metatarsal |
| Extensor digitorum longus | Deep peroneal | Anterior tibial |
| Extensor digitorum brevis | Deep peroneal, lateral terminal br. | Dorsalis pedis, lateral tarsal |
| Flexor digitorum longus | Tibial, lower muscular br. | Posterior tibial |
| Flexor digitorum brevis | Lateral plantar | Medial and lateral plantar |
| 2nd lumbricale | Lateral plantar, deep terminal br. | 2nd plantar metatarsal |
| 1st plantar interosseus | Lateral plantar, deep terminal br. | 2nd plantar metatarsal |
|  | Deep peroneal, 2nd interosseus br. |  |
| 3rd dorsal interosseus | Lateral plantar, deep terminal br. | 3rd dorsal metatarsal |
|  |  | 3rd plantar metatarsal |
| Extensor digitorum longus | Deep peroneal | Anterior tibial |
| Extensor digitorum brevis | Deep peroneal, lateral terminal br. | Dorsalis pedis, lateral tarsal |
| Flexor digitorum longus | Tibial, lower muscular br. | Posterior tibial |
| Flexor digitorum brevis | Lateral plantar | Medial and lateral plantar |
| 3rd lumbricale | Lateral plantar, deep terminal br. | 3rd plantar metatarsal |
| 2nd plantar interosseus | Lateral plantar, deep terminal br. | 3rd plantar metatarsal |
| 4th dorsal interosseus | Lateral plantar, superficial terminal br. | 4th dorsal metatarsal |
|  |  | 4th plantar metatarsal |
| Extensor digitorum longus | Deep peroneal | Anterior tibial |
| Peroneus tertius | Deep peroneal | Anterior tibial |
| Flexor digitorum longus | Tibial, lower muscular br. | Posterior tibial |
| Peroneus brevis | Superficial peroneal | Peroneal |
| Flexor digitorum brevis | Lateral plantar | Medial and lateral plantar |
| Abductor digit minimi | Lateral plantar | Lateral plantar |
| 4th lumbricale | Lateral plantar, deep terminal br. | 4th plantar metatarsal |
| Flexor digiti minimi brevis | Lateral plantar, superficial terminal br. | 4th plantar metatarsal |
|  |  | Plantar arch |
| 3rd plantar interosseus | Lateral plantar, superficial terminal br. | 4th plantar metatarsal |

*Abbreviation:* br, branch.

[a] Plantar arch, plantar metatarsal branches of the lateral plantar artery.

tubercle found on the medioplantar aspect of the base of the first metatarsal. Several small slips from the tendon may insert onto the talus or the deep fascia about the foot.

### Extensor Hallucis Longus Muscle (EHL)

The origin of the extensor hallucis longus muscle is deep to the extensor digitorum longus and tibialis anterior muscles. The extensor hallucis longus originates from the middle half of the anterior surface of the fibula and the adjacent interosseus membrane. The muscle ends in a tendon before crossing the ankle joint. It is situated lateral to the tibialis anterior tendon. As the tendon courses distad it crosses from the lateral side of the anterior tibial vessels to the medial side. The tendon inserts into the dorsal surface of the base of the distal phalanx of the hallux. At the level of the first metatarsophalangeal joint a small tendinous slip regularly inserts into the first metatarsophalangeal joint capsule. The tendinous slip is called the *extensor hallucis capsularis* and is present in more than 80% of all cases studied.[20–22]

### Extensor Digitorum Longus Muscle (EDL)

The extensor digitorum longus muscle originates from the lateral tibial condyle, the upper three-fourths of the anterior surface of the fibular shaft, and the adjacent interosseus membrane. This muscle forms a tendon before crossing the ankle joint. On the dorsal aspect of the foot, the tendon of extensor digitorum longus is lateral to the extensor hallucis longus tendon. The dorsalis pedis artery and the deep peroneal nerve are thus situated between these two tendons.

After passing through the inferior extensor retinaculum, the tendon splits into four slips, one to each of the lesser digits. Each tendon slip passes to the metatarsophalangeal joint of the lesser digits and is enclosed by the extensor expansion. Each of the four tendons follows the longitudinal axis of the digit, and at the head of the proximal phalanx each tendon trifurcates into a middle and two collateral slips.[23] The middle slip inserts into the dorsal surface of the base and shaft of the middle phalanx. The two collateral slips (medial and lateral) reunite at the head of the middle phalanx then insert into the dorsal surface of the base of the distal phalanx. At each of the insertions, the tendon splits to wrap around the phalanx. Variations of this muscle include missing tendinous slips or

tendons that have joined with the extensor digitorum brevis tendons.

### Peroneus Tertius Muscle

The peroneus tertius muscle originates from the distal one-third of the anterior surface of the shaft of the fibula and the adjacent interosseus membrane. The tendon crosses the ankle in the same synovial sheath as the extensor digitorum longus tendons. The peroneus tertius tendon is fan shaped at its insertion into the superior surface of the base and shaft of the fifth metatarsal. There may be an anomalous tendon that passes deep to the tendon of peroneus brevis to insert on the medial aspect of the shaft of the fifth metatarsal.[15]

### Peroneus Longus Muscle

The peroneus longus muscle originates from the lateral condyle of the tibia, the upper two-thirds of the lateral surface of the shaft and head of the fibula, and from the deep fascia. During its course at both the angle and the cuboid, the peroneus longus makes a sharp turn. The muscle ends in a tendon that passes posterior to the ankle joint (through the lateral malleolar sulcus just posterior to the peroneus brevis tendon). The tendon passes along the lateral surface of the calcaneus and enters the plantar foot by coursing through the peroneal canal on the plantar surface of the cuboid. Through its course in the plantar foot, the tendon is enclosed within a fibrous sheath. The tendon finally inserts into the lateroplantar surface of the first cuneiform and the tuberosity on the base of the first metatarsal. The tendon of this muscle may fuse to the tendon of the peroneus brevis or insert, in part, to the third or fifth metatarsal base.[15]

### Peroneus Brevis Muscle

The peroneus brevis muscle arises from the distal third of the lateral surface of the shaft of the fibula and adjacent deep fascia. The muscle ends in a tendon following the course of the peroneus longus, but is situated anterior to the peroneus longus tendon at the lateral malleolus. Along the lateral surface of the calcaneus, the peroneus brevis tendon courses superior to the peroneus longus tendon. The peroneus brevis tendon inserts onto the tuberosity of the fifth metatarsal base. The peroneus brevis tendon may be fused to the peroneus longus tendon, or there may be an accessory slip that inserts into the shaft of the fifth metatarsal or into the lateral aspect of the base of the fifth proximal phalanx.[8]

### Flexor Hallucis Longus Muscle

The flexor hallicus longus muscle originates from the lower two-thirds (except for the most distal) of the posteriolateral surface of the shaft of the fibula and adjacent interosseus membrane. On the most posterior aspect of the muscle belly, a tendon forms before crossing the ankle joint. The tendon passes through the sulcus on the posterior aspect of the tibia, through the sulcus on the posterior surface of the body of the talus, and beneath the sustentaculum tali. It lies deep to the flexor digitorum longus tendon and often shares a fibrous slip with the tendon called the *knot of Henry*. The tendon of flexor hallucis longus continues through the second layer of the plantar muscles, through a groove formed by the two hallucal sesamoids, and inserts into the plantar surface of the base of the distal phalanx of the hallux.

### Flexor Digitorum Longus Muscle

The flexor digitorum longus muscle originates from the posterior surface of the tibia, distal to the popliteal line, but medial to a vertical line. The muscle ends in a tendon that passes through the medial malleolar sulcus posterior to the tibialis posterior tendon. As the muscle continues on its course into the foot, it passes inferior to the sustentaculum tali and into the second layer of plantar muscle. At this point, the tendon is inferior to the tendon of the flexor hallucis longus and receives a fibrous slip from this tendon. Just distal to the knot of Henry, the tendon splits into four slips, one to each of the lesser digits. Each tendinous slip passes through the flexor digitorum brevis tendons and inserts onto the plantar surface of the base and shaft of the distal phalanx. At the level of the cuneonavicular articulations, the tendon of the flexor digitorum longus serves as the insertion and origin for the muscles in the second layer of the foot.

### Tibialis Posterior Muscle

The tibialis posterior muscle originates from two heads: a medial head originates from the posterior surface of the tibia lateral to the vertical line and distal to the popliteal line, and a lateral head originates from the medial surface of the fibular shaft. Just lateral to the origin of the muscle is the origin of the flexor hallucis longus. Between these two muscles, passing distal along the crista medialis, the peroneal artery is found. A tendon is formed before it crosses posterior to the ankle joint. The tendon passes deep to the flexor digitorum longus tendon, through the medial malleolar sulcus, and beneath the sustentaculum tali (hence the deltoid ligaments are deep) and the spring ligament. The tendon inserts onto the tuberosity of the navicular and then sends tendinous slips (or expansions) to the sustentaculum tali, all the cuneiforms, the cuboid, and metatarsal bases.[2-4]

## Intrinsic Muscles of the Foot

There are 19 intrinsic muscle of the foot. There is only 1 muscle in the dorsal foot, while the plantar foot contains 18 muscles. For ease of description the plantar muscles are divided into four layers, numbered one to four from superficial to deep, respectively. However, a more practical way to group the muscles of the foot is by the compartments formed by the deep fascia. The plantar fascia sends a *medial* and *lateral intermuscular septa* deep into the foot, thus dividing the foot into medial, central, lateral, and interosseus compartments (see Fig. 2-7A and Table 2-2).

### Extensor Digitorum Brevis Muscle (EDB)

The extensor digitorum brevis muscle is located deep to the tendons of the extensor digitorum longus. The nerves and vessels of the dorsal foot are located deep to the tendons of this muscle. The extensor digitorum brevis has an osseous origin from the superior and lateral surfaces of the calcaneus just anterolateral to the calcaneal sulcus. This muscle also originates from the interosseus talocalcaneal ligament and the deep surface of the inferior extensor retinaculum. The muscle forms four distinct muscle bellies, each ending in a tendon. The most medial muscle belly and tendon is often referred to as the *extensor hallucis brevis*. The extensor hallucis brevis tendon inserts into the dorsal aspect of the base of the proximal phalanx of the hallux. The remaining three tendons insert into the lateral side of the extensor digitorum longus tendons of digits two, three, and four. This muscle quite often varies from normal. It is common to find either additional myotendinous units or that tendon slips are absent.

## First Layer of Plantar Foot Muscles

### Abductor Hallucis Muscle

In a person who is standing the abductor hallucis muscle is seen as a bulge on the medial side of the foot. A tunnel is formed between this muscle and the medial surface of the calcaneus, called the *porta pedis.* This tunnel is continuous with the tarsal tunnel superiorly. The plantar vessels and nerves enter the foot by way of the porta pedis. The abductor hallucis muscle originates from the medial process of the calcaneal tuberosity and from the surrounding deep fascia. The origin from the flexor retinaculum is a strong attachment. The muscle courses distally along the medial side of the foot and ends in a tendon. Occasionally, a strong attachment is found onto the tuberosity of the navicular. The tendon of the abductor hallucis primarily inserts into the medioplantar aspect of the base of the proximal phalanx. Before passing across the medioplantar aspect of the first metatarsophalangeal joint, a tendinous slip attaches to the medial aspect of the medial hallucal sesamoid. Rarely, a second slip occurs that inserts in the second toe. The abductor hallucis muscle also may originate from the flexor hallucis longus.

### Flexor Digitorum Brevis Muscle

The flexor digitorum brevis muscle originates from the medial process of the calcaneal tuberosity and the surrounding deep fascia. The muscle passes distad in the center of the foot, dividing into four tendinous slips one to each of the lesser digits. At the level of the base of the proximal phalanx, each flexor digitorum brevis tendon splits in two and reunites at the head of the proximal phalanx. The tendon inserts into the plantar surface of the base and shaft of the middle phalanx. This split allows the flexor digitorum longus tendon to pass. Anomalies of this muscle are relatively infrequent; however, the most common variation occurs in the fifth digit where the tendon may be absent or originate from the flexor digitorum longus.

### Abductor Digiti Minimi Muscle

The abductor digiti minimi muscle originates from the lateral margin of the medial process and the entire lateral process of the calcaneal tuberosity and surrounding deep fascia. The muscle may originate, in part, from the tuberosity of the fifth metatarsal. The muscle passes along the plantar aspect of the tuberosity of the fifth metatarsal, then along the lateral side of the foot. The muscle ends in a tendon that inserts (along with the flexor digiti minimi brevis) on the lateral side of the base of the proximal phalanx. There are two variations of this muscle. A separate myotendinous unit, which is attached from the calcaneus to the tuberosity of the fifth metatarsal, is called the *abductor ossis metatarsi quinti muscle.*[8] A single myotendinous unit, separate from the abductor digiti minimi, extends from the calcaneal tuberosity to the fifth proximal phalanx and is called the *accessory abductor muscle.*[8]

## Second Layer of Plantar Foot Muscles

### Quadratus Plantae Muscle

The quadratus plantae muscle originates from two heads that are separated by the long plantar ligament. The larger medial head originates from the medial surface of the calcaneus, up to the groove for the flexor hallucis longus. The lateral head originates from the inferior surface of the calcaneus distal to the lateral process of the calcaneal tuberosity. Both heads unite and pass anteriorly to insert into the tendon of the flexor digitorum longus muscle. It is common that these two heads do not unite before insertion. As such, the medial head may insert into the second, third, and fourth digital tendon slips of the flexor digitorum longus muscle. Only rarely is the lateral head absent.[8,15]

### Lumbricale Muscles

The first lumbricale muscle is unipennate and originates from the medial side of the first tendon of the flexor digitorum longus. The second, third, and fourth lumbricales are bipennate in structure and originate from the adjacent sides of the long flexor tendons. Each muscle passes distad along the medial side of the metatarsal, but inferior to the deep transverse metatarsal ligament (Fig. 2-8). At the distal edge of the deep transverse metatarsal ligament, the lumbricale tendons make a sharp upward turn. The tendon then inserts into the medial side of the extensor wing part of the extensor expansion at the level of the base of the proximal phalanx. When an anomaly is present it is usually the absence of one of the muscles, most commonly the fourth lumbricale. *

## Third Layer of Plantar Foot Muscles

### Flexor Hallucis Brevis Muscle

The flexor hallucis brevis muscle has a Y-shaped tendinous origin. The lateral origin is from the cuboid (posterior to the peroneal sulcus) and adjacent area of the third cuneiform. The medial origin is from the tendon of the tibialis posterior and the medial intermuscular septum. Both heads of origin converge and pass anteromedial toward the plantar surface of the first metatarsal. The muscle forms a medial and lateral muscle belly. At the level of the anatomic neck of the first metatarsal, each muscle belly head forms a separate tendon containing a sesamoid. The medial tendon contains the tibial hallucal sesamoid and inserts into the medial side of the plantar surface of the base of the proximal phalanx. The lateral tendon contains the fibular hallucal sesamoid and inserts into the lateral aspect of the plantar surface of the base of the proximal phalanx. The two heads form a deep sulcus for the passage of the flexor hallucis longus tendon. A small triangular area is formed by the sesamoids and the muscle. In this space one finds the first plantar metatarsal artery and adipose tissue.[8,24]

### Adductor Hallucis Muscle

The adductor hallucis muscle originates from two heads, an oblique and a transverse head. It is the transverse head that is sometimes referred to as the *transverse pedis muscle*. The smaller transverse head originates from the plantar metatarsophalangeal ligaments of the third, fourth, and fifth digits and the deep transverse metatarsal ligament. The oblique head originates from the plantar surfaces of the second, third, and fourth metatarsal bases and the tendinous sheath of the peroneus longus. The oblique head courses anteromedially toward the first intermetatarsal space. At the anatomic neck of the first metatarsal, the oblique head divides into medial and lateral slips. The medial slip inserts directly on the lateral hallucal sesamoid while the lateral slip continues distal to join the transverse head. The conjoined tendon formed by the two heads passes through the bifurcated deep trans-

verse metatarsal ligament and inserts into the inferolateral aspect of the base of the proximal phalanx of the hallux (see Fig. 2-6). Infrequently a separate myotendinous unit, called the *oppenens hallucis muscle,* is sent to the first metatarsal from the oblique head.[15]

### Flexor Digiti Minimi Brevis Muscle

The flexor digiti minimi brevis muscle arises from the plantar surface of the base of the fifth metatarsal and from the sheath of the peroneus longus muscle. The muscle passes anteriorly along the lateral aspect of the fifth metatarsal. It inserts into the lateral and inferolateral aspect of the base of the proximal phalanx of the fifth digit, along with the abductor digiti minimi muscle. The oppens digiti quinti is a flat, triangular muscle that has an origin similar to the flexor digiti minimi brevis but an insertion that is on the lateral surface of the fifth metatarsal shaft.

## Fourth Layer of Plantar Foot Muscles

### Plantar Interossei Muscles (3)

Each of the three plantar interossei muscle originates from the plantar surface of the base and medial surface of a metatarsal shaft. The first plantar interosseus muscle arises from the plantar surface of the base and the medial surface of the shaft of the third metatarsal, the second interosseus muscle from the fourth metatarsal, and the third interosseus muscle from the fifth metatarsal. The muscle passes directly distad ending in a tendon. The tendon of each of the plantar interossei muscles passes superior to the deep transverse metatarsal ligament. Each tendon has an attachment to the extensor expansion and inserts into the medial side of the base of the proximal phalanx of its respective digit.

### Dorsal Interossei Muscles (4)

These four bipennate muscles originate from the adjacent sides of the metatarsal shafts. For example, the first dorsal interosseus muscle originates from the lateral side of the shaft of the first metatarsal and the medial side of the shaft of the second metatarsal, and the second dorsal interosseus muscle originates from the lateral side of the shaft of the second metatarsal and the medial side of the shaft of the third metatarsal.

Each muscle ends in a tendon that passes superior to the deep transverse metatarsal ligament. The first dorsal interosseus muscle inserts into the medial side of the base of the second proximal phalanx and extensor expansion. The second, third, and fourth muscles insert into the lateral side of the base of the proximal phalanx and the extensor expansion. There are numerous anomalies of these muscles. Most commonly, the dorsal and plantar interossei are one muscle, or the dorsal interossei muscles spring from only one side of the metatarsal.[8]

## Extensor Expansion

The extensor expansions are deep fascial structures encompassing the extensor tendons. There are four extensor expansions, one to each of the lesser digits. The extensor expansion over the fifth digit is not so defined as the other lesser digits. There are contributions to the extensor expansion from both the dorsal muscles and the plantar muscles.

The central structure of the extensor expansion is formed by the extensor digitorum longus tendons (Fig. 2-9). The extensor digitorum brevis, lumbricales, plantar, and dorsal interossei muscles all have an attachment to the expansion. Wrapping around the metatarsophalangeal joint are thick transversely directed fibers called the *extensor sling*. The interossei and extensor digitorum brevis have attachments to the sling before insertion. Thin obliquely directed fibers

called the *extensor wing* are attached to the distal edge of the deep transverse metatarsal ligament and to the extensor digitorum longus tendon. Because of the insertion of the lumbricale muscles, the medial side of the extensor wing is better defined than is the lateral side.[25]

## NERVE SUPPLY TO THE FOOT

### Saphenous Nerve

The saphenous nerve is the continuation of the femoral nerve and is the only nerve in the foot that is not derived from the sciatic nerve. In the leg, the saphenous nerve follows the course of the greater saphenous vein. At the ankle, this nerve divides into anterior and posterior divisions. The posterior division supplies the skin about the medial ankle. The anterior division crosses the ankle joint anterior to the medial malleolus and continues distad along the dorsomedial aspect side of the foot up to the first metatarsophalangeal joint (Fig. 2-10).

### Deep Peroneal Nerve

The deep peroneal nerve supplies the muscular innervation to the intrinsic muscles of the dorsal foot. It also contributes to the innervation of the first and second dorsal interossei muscles. The deep peroneal nerve passes into the foot adjacent to the dorsalis pedis ar-

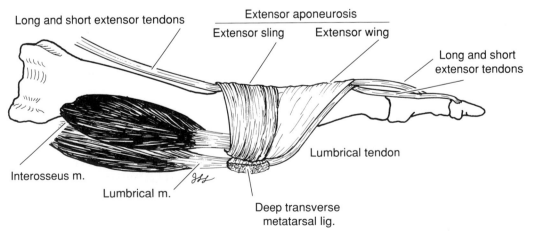

**Fig. 2-9.** Extensor expansion from the medial side of a lesser metatarsophalangeal joint.

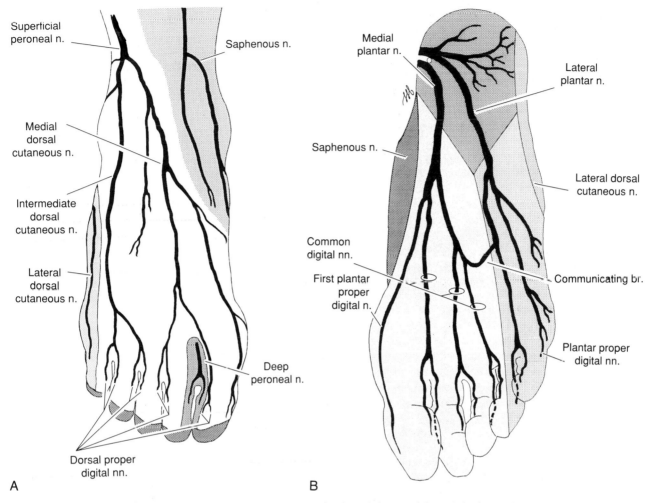

**Fig. 2-10.** Cutaneous innervation to the foot. (**A**) Dorsal foot. (**B**) Plantar foot.

tery and between the extensor hallucis longus and extensor digitorum longus tendons. The nerve terminates by dividing into a medial and lateral terminal branch.

### Medial Terminal Branch

The medial terminal branch follows the course of the dorsalis pedis artery distad. In the first intermetatarsal space, the nerve divides in two dorsal proper digital nerves. Before its termination, a small interosseus branch supplies the first dorsal interosseus muscle and the first metatarsophalangeal joint. The medial terminal branch also has a communicating branch that joins the medial dorsal cutaneous nerve. The dorsal

proper digital nerves are the terminal branches of the medial terminal division of the deep peroneal nerve. These nerves supply the adjacent dorsolateral side of the hallux and the dorsomedial side of the second digit (see Fig. 2-10).

### Lateral Terminal Branch

Directed anterolaterally, the lateral terminal branch follows the course of the lateral tarsal artery and passes deep to the extensor digitorum brevis muscle. This nerve flattens deep to the extensor digitorum brevis muscle. This enlargement is often referred to as a pseudoganglion. Arising from the pseudoganglion, there is a muscular branch to the extensor digitorum brevis muscle and three interosseus branches that terminate at the metatarsophalangeal joints of the second, third, and fourth digits. These branches supply articular innervation to the intertarsal and the second, third, and fourth metatarsophalangeal joints. Occasionally, the first of these interosseus branches gives a muscular branch to the second dorsal and first plantar interossei muscles (see Table 2-2).

## Superficial Peroneal Nerve

This nerve becomes superficial in the distal third of the leg. It terminates by dividing into the medial and intermediate dorsal cutaneous nerves (see Fig. 2-10).

### Medial Dorsal Cutaneous Nerve

The medial dorsal cutaneous nerve is directed anteromediad across the anterior aspect of the ankle joint and bifurcates into its terminal branches. The medial branch is directed to the dorsomedial border of the hallux and is called the *medial dorsal digital nerve*. This branch also communicates with the saphenous nerve and the medial terminal division of the deep peroneal nerve.

The lateral branch is directed to the second interosseus space. Just distal to the metatarsophalangeal joint, the dorsal digitial nerve splits into two *dorsal proper digital nerves* that supply the adjacent dorsal sides of the second and third digits.

### Intermediate Dorsal Cutaneous Nerve

This branch is smaller than the medial dorsal cutaneous nerve and passes along the dorsolateral aspect of the foot. Throughout its course in the foot, the intermediate dorsal cutaneous nerve is a visible, thin, cordlike structure. This nerve divides into a medial and lateral dorsal digital nerve. The medial dorsal digital nerve supplies dorsal proper digital nerves to the adjacent sides of the third and fourth digits. The lateral dorsal digital nerve supplies dorsal proper digital nerves to the adjacent sides of the fourth and fifth digits. The distribution of the intermediate dorsal cutaneous nerve varies greatly.[8,26] Common variations of this nerve include a branch supplying the dorsolateral aspect of the fifth toe instead of the lateral dorsal cutaneous nerve, or the lateral dorsal cutaneous nerve supplying the adjacent sides of the digits in the fourth

web space instead of the intermediate dorsal cutaneous nerve.[8,26]

## Lateral Dorsal Cutaneous Nerve

The lateral dorsal cutaneous nerve is the continuation of the *sural nerve* in the foot. The sural nerve courses posterior to the lateral malleolus along with the lesser saphenous vein. Once it passes inferior to a line formed by the medial and lateral malleolus, the sural nerve is renamed to the lateral dorsal cutaneous nerve. The nerve passes distally along the lateral margin of the foot along with the lateral marginal vein. The nerve ends by supplying the dorsolateral aspect of the fifth digit. This nerve communicates with the lateral dorsal digital nerve of the intermediate dorsal cutaneous nerve (see Fig. 2-10).

## Nerves to the Plantar Foot

The tibial nerve is the nerve that supplies the plantar foot. The tibial nerve bifurcates, just proximal to the medial malleolus, into the medial and lateral plantar nerves. These nerves course with the plantar vessels behind the medial malleolus between the calcaneus and the abductor hallucis muscle.

### Medial Plantar Nerve

The medial plantar nerve is the larger of the two terminal divisions of the tibial nerve. It accompanies the medial plantar vessels (the nerve being situated lateral). After entering the foot, the nerve is directed anteriorly between the flexor digitorum brevis and the abductor hallucis muscles. There are usually several small cutaneous branches that pierce the plantar aponeurosis to supply the skin on the medioplantar aspect of the foot. Two muscular branches supply the abductor hallucis and the flexor digitorum brevis muscles. There are several articular branches, which supply the tarsal joint. The *first plantar proper digital nerve* is the most medial branch and supplies a muscular branch to the flexor hallucis brevis muscle. This nerve ends by supplying cutaneous innervation to the medioplantar aspect of the hallux (see Fig. 2-10).

The medial plantar nerve terminates by dividing into three *common plantar digital branches*. These nerves arise at the level of the bases of the metatarsals.

At this point the nerves are situated deep to the flexor digitorum brevis muscle. Each common digital branch then passes distad to the plantar interosseus spaces one through three. As the branches pass distal they lie in a space between the adjacent flexor tendons, but deep to the plantar aponeurosis. Just before crossing the metatarsophalangeal joint, each common plantar digital nerve emerges from the deep side of the plantar aponeurosis to lie in the superficial fascia. Distal to the metatarsophalangeal joint, each of the common plantar digital nerves branch into two *plantar proper digital nerves* that supply the plantar aspect of the adjacent sides of the first to fourth digits. The first common digital nerve also gives a muscular branch to the first lumbricale. The third common digital nerve also receives a communicating branch from the fourth common plantar digital nerve (a branch from the lateral plantar nerve).

### Lateral Plantar Nerve

The lateral plantar nerve is the division of the tibial nerve that supplies most of the intrinsic muscles of the plantar foot (see Table 2-2). This nerve passes with the lateral plantar artery, but is situated medial to the vessels. The nerve courses between the flexor digitorum brevis and the abductor digiti minimi muscles and divides into deep and superficial terminal divisions at the base of the fifth metatarsal. Before its termination, the lateral plantar nerve has several cutaneous branches that pierce the plantar aponeurosis to supply the skin of the lateroplantar foot (see Fig. 2-10). Additional branches before its termination include muscular branches to the quadratus plantae and the abductor digiti minimi muscles and articular branches to the tarsus.

The deep terminal division accompanies the plantar arch and supplies muscular branches to the lumbricales (2, 3, 4), adductor hallucis, plantar interossei (1, 2), and the dorsal interossei (1, 2, 3) muscles.

The superficial terminal division divides into the fourth common digital nerve and a plantar proper digital nerve. The fourth common plantar digital branch passes into the fourth interosseus space and divides into two plantar proper digital nerves. This branch, like the other common plantar nerves, is at first situated deep to the plantar aponeurosis, then at the level of the metatarsophalangeal joint passes into the super-

ficial fascia of the foot. The fourth common digital nerve sends a communicating branch to the third common digital nerve deep to the plantar aponeurosis. The presence of this communicating branch is somewhat variable. For example, Nissen[19] states that the communicating branch is frequently absent, while Jones and Klenerman[27] claim that it was present in each of their specimens. The Jones and Klenerman study indicates that the communicating branch between the two nerves may occur more proximal than previously thought.[27] In general, the communicating branch joins to the third plantar common digital nerve somewhere between the point of bifurcation into its plantar proper digital nerves and midshaft of the fourth metatarsal.

The plantar proper digital branch passes obliquely anterolaterad, supplying the lateral plantar aspect of the fifth digit. Before entering the digit, muscular branches supply the flexor digiti minimi brevis, third plantar interosseus, and fourth dorsal interosseus muscles.

## Proper Digital Nerves

Each digit of the foot is supplied by four proper digital nerves: two plantar and two dorsal propers (see Fig. 2-10). These nerves are numbered from 1 to 10 in a medial to lateral fashion. The dorsal proper digital nerves pass along the dorsomedial or dorsolateral aspect of each digit, while the plantar proper digital nerves pass along the plantomedial or plantolateral aspect of each digit.

The level at which the proper digital nerves form varies from the dorsal to the plantar side of the foot. Although the plantar proper digital nerves consistently originate a few millimeters proximal to the web formed by the skin between the digits, the level at which the dorsal proper digital nerves originate varies considerably. The dorsal proper digital nerves can originate as far proximal as the ankle joint or as far distal as the web space. The dorsal proper digital nerves are smaller than the plantar nerve and terminate near the proximal nail fold. The plantar proper digital nerves course to the end of the digits, supplying branches to the lateral and medial borders of the digit and to the distal edge of the nail.[28]

Each dorsal proper digital nerve supplies cutaneous innervation to either the dorsolateral or dorsomedial

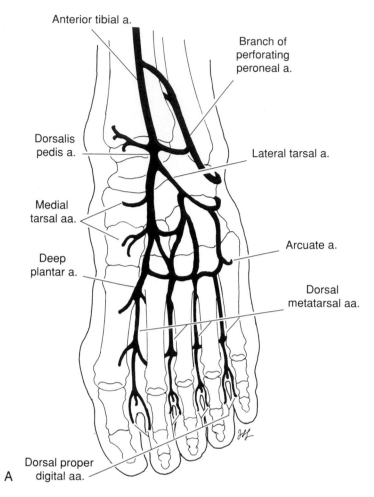

**Fig. 2-11.** General pattern of the arterial supply to the foot. (**A**) Dorsal foot. (*Figure continues.*)

aspect of the digits, distally to the proximal nail fold. The plantar proper digital nerves supply cutaneous innervation to either the plantomedial or plantolateral aspect of the digits. The plantar proper digital nerves also supply cutaneous innervation to the tips of the digit and the distal aspect of the nail. All proper digital nerves help to provide articular innervation to the interphalangeal joints.

Each proper digital nerve originates from one of the six nerves supplying the foot. Plantarly, the proper digital nerves originate from either the medial or lateral plantar nerve. Dorsally, there is considerable variation to the origin of the digital nerves off the intermediate dorsal cutaneous and the lateral dorsal

cutaneous nerve.[26] The two most common variations are that the tenth dorsal proper digital nerve arises from the intermediate dorsal cutaneous or that the eighth and ninth dorsal proper digital nerves arise from the lateral dorsal cutaneous nerve.

## VASCULAR SUPPLY

### Arterial Supply to the Dorsal Foot

In the now classic study by Huber,[29] the *dorsalis pedis artery* and its branches could be superimposed on a general arterial network pattern in 98% of the cases studied (Fig. 2-11). Specifically, there are numerous

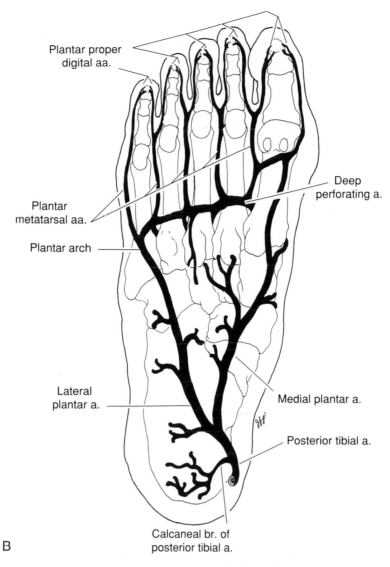

Plantar proper
digital aa.

Deep
perforating a.

Plantar
metatarsal aa.

Plantar arch

Lateral
plantar a.

Medial plantar a.

Posterior tibial a.

Calcaneal br. of
posterior tibial a.

B

**Fig. 2-11** (*Continued*). (**B**) Plantar foot.

variations of the course of the arteries in the foot; however, these variations can be explained as small-caliber or absent vessels or parts of vessels from the general pattern. In 78 percent of the cases studied, the dorsalis pedis artery continued from the anterior tibial artery and at the first metatarsal base, the dorsalis pedis artery bifurcated into its terminal divisions, the first *dorsal metatarsal artery* and the *deep plantar artery*.[29] In 12% of the cases, the dorsalis pedis artery was absent or so small as to be considered absent. In these

individuals the perforating branch of the peroneal artery supplied the dorsal foot. Only approximately 35 percent of the time does the normal arterial pattern of the foot occur.[8,29] The branches of the dorsalis pedis artery are the lateral tarsal, medial tarsal, arcuate, first dorsal metatarsal, and deep plantar arteries.

**Arcuate Artery**

The arcuate artery is present in only 54 percent of individuals and when present varies in its point of

**Table 2-3.** Principal Sources of the Dorsal Metatarsal Arteries[a]

| Author | First | | Second | | Third | | Fourth | |
|---|---|---|---|---|---|---|---|---|
| | Dorsal | Plantar | Dorsal | Plantar | Dorsal | Plantar | Dorsal | Plantar |
| Adachi | 80.9 | 19.3 | 36.1 | 56.5 | 35.7 | 57.0 | 33.9 | 63.5 |
| Huber | 76.5 | 8.5 | 55.0 | 33.5 | 59.0 | 23.0 | 40.5 | 37.5 |

[a] Data are percentages of arteries arising from dorsal or plantar arteries, respectively.
(Data from Huber[29] and Adachi.[30])

origin and size. This artery usually branches from the dorsalis pedis artery at the level of the first tarsometatarsal joint; however, it may branch more proximal near the first cuneonavicular articulation.[8,29] When present this artery courses lateral beneath the tendons of the extensor digitorum brevis and anastomoses with the lateral plantar and the lateral tarsal arteries.

### Dorsal Metatarsal Arteries

Although the arcuate artery is often described as being the only source of the second, third, and fourth dorsal metatarsal arteries, in fact the plantar arteries can be an important source for these arteries as well.[29] In those individuals in whom the arcuate artery is short or small, the lateral tarsal artery can also give rise to the dorsal metatarsal arteries. Although the medial, most dorsal, metatarsal arteries have their origin from the dorsal arterial network, it is quite common for the lateral, most dorsal, metatarsal arteries to originate from the plantar arteries. The termination of the dorsal metatarsal arteries is usually a bifurcation into the dorsal proper digital arteries; however, the dorsal metatarsal tarsal arteries often continue plantarly to contribute to the formation of the plantar proper digital arteries (see Fig. 2-11).

### *First Dorsal Metatarsal Artery*

This artery usually branches from the dorsalis pedis artery near the base of the first metatarsal. However, the first dorsal metatarsal artery may arise from a plantar artery (8.5 percent, Huber[29]; 19.1 percent, Adachi[30]) or it may be absent (24 percent, Huber[29]). The course of the first dorsal metatarsal artery is distal on the superior surface of the first dorsal interosseus muscle. At the web space the artery ends by bifurcating into two dorsal digital arteries. The two dorsal

digital branches supply the adjacent sides of the first and second toe. Before its termination, a dorsal digital branch passes beneath the extensor hallucis longus tendon to the dorsomedial side of the first toe.

The first dorsal metatarsal artery forms an anastomosis with the first plantar metatarsal artery just distal to the deep transverse metatarsal ligament but proximal to the bifurcation into the dorsal digital arteries. The artery forming this communication is the *anterior perforating artery*.

### *Lesser Dorsal Metatarsal Arteries*

The *second, third,* and *fourth dorsal metatarsal arteries* follows a similar course as the first dorsal metatarsal artery, except within their respective dorsal intermetatarsal spaces. Near the base of each metatarsal the lesser dorsal metatarsal arteries receive a *posterior perforating artery* that forms an anastomosis with the plantar arteries. The origin of the lesser metatarsal arteries differs among them. While the second dorsal metatarsal artery usually originates from the dorsal arterial network, the fourth dorsal metatarsal artery usually originates from the plantar arteries. The fourth dorsal metatarsal artery also differs in that before the bifurcation into the dorsal digital arteries, the fourth dorsal metatarsal artery gives off a dorsal digital branch to the dorsolateral aspect of the fifth digit.

## Arterial Supply to the Plantar Foot

The arterial supply to the plantar foot is from the terminal divisions of the posterior tibial artery. The posterior tibial artery bifurcates into the lateral and medial plantar arteries between the medial malleolus and the medial process of the calcaneal tuberosity (distal to the bifurcation of the plantar nerves). Both vessels enter the foot along with the plantar nerves.

## Medial Plantar Artery

The medial plantar artery is smaller than the lateral plantar artery. This artery courses between the abductor hallucis and the flexor digitorum brevis muscles, medial to the plantar nerve. It continues to pass distad to the base of the hallux, where it becomes smaller and divides into a superficial and deep branch. The deep branch passes deep to supply the bones in the midfoot. The superficial branch continues along the medioplantar aspect of the hallux. The superficial branch is often referred to as the *medial plantar marginal artery*. Only rarely do these arteries form a superficial plantar arch.[15,28,30] This artery anastomoses with the first dorsal metatarsal artery and the first, second, and third plantar metatarsal arteries.

This artery supplies blood to the following bones of the foot: most of the tarsal bones, the first metatarsal, and the sesamoids. This artery also supplies the abductor hallucis, flexor digitorum brevis, quadratus plantae, first lumbricale, and the flexor hallucis brevis muscles.

## Lateral Plantar Artery

The lateral plantar artery is larger than the medial plantar artery. It courses with, but lateral to, the lateral plantar nerve. The artery courses to the lateral side of the foot passing deep to the flexor digitorum brevis and superficial to the quadratus plantae muscles. The artery comes to rest in the septum between the flexor digitorum brevis and the abductor digiti minimi muscles. It rests on the medial side of the base of the metatarsal. As the artery courses anterolateral, it becomes superficial. At the base of the fifth metatarsal the artery turns sharply medial, coursing deep as the *plantar arch*. The plantar arch rests on the bases of the metatarsals and will form an anastomosis with the *deep plantar artery*. The deep plantar artery is situated deep to the oblique head of the adductor hallucis muscle and superficial to the interossei muscles. The artery supplies the flexor digitorum brevis, quadratus plantae, and the abductor digiti minimi muscles as well as some of the tarsal bones.

### *Plantar Proper Digital Branch*

This branch bifurcates from the lateral plantar artery at the base of the fifth metatarsal and crosses to the plantolateral aspect of the fifth metatarsal and digit.

### *Plantar Arch*

The plantar arch has two main groups of branches, the posterior perforating and the plantar metatarsal arteries. From the plantar arch, near the bases of the metatarsals three *posterior perforating arteries* arise that anastomose with the second, third, and fourth dorsal metatarsal arteries (Fig. 2-12). The plantar arch directly supplies the flexor hallucis brevis, flexor digiti

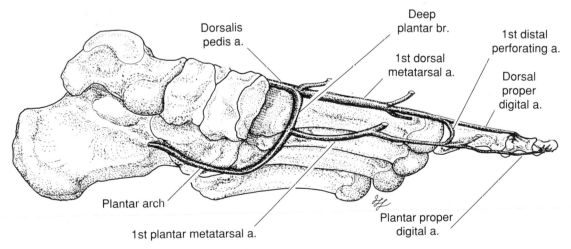

Dorsalis pedis a.

Deep plantar br.

1st dorsal metatarsal a.

1st distal perforating a.

Dorsal proper digital a.

Plantar arch

1st plantar metatarsal a.

Plantar proper digital a.

**Fig. 2-12.** Metatarsal arteries as viewed from the medial side of an intermetatarsal space. Note that the two arteries communicate by way of the anterior and posterior perforating arteries.

minimi brevis, and the oblique head of the adductor hallucis muscles.

There are a total of four plantar metatarsal arteries, each lying along the midline of the shaft of medial four metatarsals.[28] With the exception of the first, each of the plantar metatarsal arteries rests on the plantar surface of the plantar interossei muscles. The artery courses distally to the web space where it divides into two branches to supply the adjacent sides of the digits. These branches are called the plantar proper digital (plantar digital) branches. Before bifurcating, each plantar metatarsal artery anastomoses to the dorsal metatarsal artery via the anterior perforating artery (Fig. 2-12).

The first plantar metatarsal artery follows a different course than the other plantar metatarsal arteries. After branching from the plantar arch, the first plantar artery passes distal deep to the flexor hallucis brevis muscle. At the level of the anatomic neck of the metatarsal, the first plantar metatarsal artery forms a cruciate anastomosis with the medial plantar artery (superficial branch). The first plantar metatarsal artery then emerges from the deep aspect of the muscle in a triangular space formed by the sesamoids and the muscle bellies. The first plantar metatarsal artery then bifurcates (see Fig. 2-11). The branches of the bifurcation pass on either side of the hallucal sesamoids. The medial branch (medial plantar hallucal artery, medial plantar marginal artery) supplies the medioplantar aspect of the hallux. The lateral branch continues distal into the web space where it bifurcates into plantar proper digital arteries that supply the adjacent side of the hallux and second digit.

### Digital Arterial Network

The blood supply within the digits presents with little variation. Each of the digits is supplied by four proper digital arteries. The majority of the blood supply to the digit is by way of the plantar arterial vessels (see Fig. 2-12).[28] Among the plantar proper digital arteries there are numerous anastomoses, with the medial plantar proper digital artery being significantly larger in the hallux and fourth digits (see Fig. 2-11).[28] According to the study by Edwards, on the plantar surface of the shaft of the proximal phalanx in the hallux there is a regular, well-formed, transverse communicating artery between the two plantar proper digital arteries.

The terminal ends of the proper digital arteries arborize to form a rete around the tuft of the distal phalanx. Again, the plantar proper digital arteries are the major supply to this rete.[28]

## Blood Supply to the Bones of the Foot

Bone, like any other structure in the body, has a regular blood supply. The blood supply to a long bone usually enters the bone in several locations (Fig. 2-13). The vessels, after entering the bone, branch into a complicated network of vessels that supply discrete regions of the bone. The arterial supply then drains into venous channels that follow the course of the arteries and then exit the bone.

Typically a long bone is supplied by one or two principal nutrient arteries that enter the bone in the shaft.[15] After entering the bone, the principal nutrient artery bifurcates into descending and ascending branches. These arteries follow a spiraling course as they pass toward the ends of the bone. Each of these arteries sends *medullary arteries* that course to the center of the bone and *cortical arteries* which pass toward the surface of the bone. Finally the principal nutrient artery anastomoses with the arteries supplying the ends of the bone.

The ends of a long bone are covered by hyaline cartilage and are not penetrated by arteries. Therefore, the blood supply to the ends of a bone is by way of arteries that enter near the cartilage. There are usually numerous *epiphyseal (capital) arteries* that enter the bone just proximal to the articular surface. The epiphyseal arteries are branches from periarticular vascular networks, which also supply the joint capsule. *Metaphyseal arteries,* which are numerous, also supply the ends of a long bone. These arteries however usually branch from local systemic arteries, in much the same way that the principal nutrient artery branches from its parent artery. Both the epiphyseal and metaphyseal arteries form significant anastomoses with each other and with the principal nutrient artery.

The periosteum of bones contains a very fine network of vessels. This *periosteal capillary plexus* is formed from local systemic arteries. This plexus has an extensive anastomosis with cortical arteries. In areas where a muscle originates from a bone, the periosteal plexus forms an anastomosis not only with the

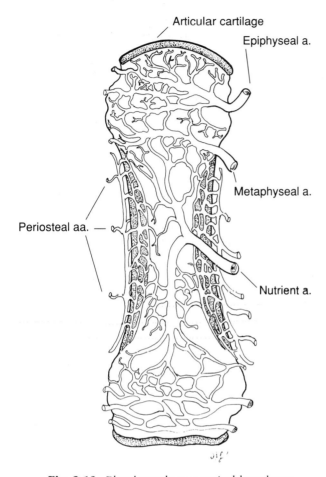

Articular cartilage

Epiphyseal a.

Metaphyseal a.

Periosteal aa. —

Nutrient a.

**Fig. 2-13.** Blood supply to a typical long bone.

cortical branches but with the capillaries of the muscle as well.

### First Metatarsal

The first dorsal metatarsal and first plantar metatarsal arteries supply most of the blood to this bone with an inconsistent source from the superficial branch of the medial plantar artery.[31–33] The single principal nutrient artery supplying this bone is most often a branch from the first dorsal metatarsal artery. There are four distal metaphyseal arteries that enter on the dorsal and plantar corners of the head. The dorsal arteries are typically larger than the plantar and supply the dorsal two-thirds of the head; the plantar metaphyseal arteries supply the inferior one-third of the head; and the

epiphyseal arteries supply the lateral and medial sides of the metatarsal head.

### Sesamoids

The hallucal sesamoids receive their blood from the first plantar metatarsal artery after the anastomosis with the superficial branch of the medial plantar artery. Each sesamoid receives one to three branches. These branches anastomose within the sesamoid.

### Lesser Metatarsals

The second through fifth metatarsals receive their blood from both the dorsal and the plantar metatarsal arteries. The principal nutrient artery enters on the lateral surface of the shaft of the lesser metatarsals, except in the fifth metatarsal where the principal nutrient artery enters on the medial surface of the shaft.[34]

### Phalanges

The phalanges receive their blood supply mainly from the proper digital arteries. The proximal phalanges receive their blood mostly from the dorsal proper digital arteries; the distal phalanges receive their blood supply predominantly from the plantar proper digital arteries; and the middle phalanges receive their blood supply from both the dorsal and plantar proper digital arteries. In general, the principal nutrient artery enters these bones on the lateral surface, with the exception of the distal phalanges, where it enters the bone plantarly.[9,32] Each bone has numerous tiny metaphyseal and epiphyseal arteries.

## Venous Return

### Superficial Veins of the Foot

The veins of the lower limb can be divided into a superficial and deep system. The deep veins carry most of the blood back to the heart. However, both the superficial and deep veins contain values that prevent the backflow of blood in the leg.[35]

On the dorsum of the foot, two dorsal digital veins drain each digit. The dorsal digital veins in turn drain into the superficial dorsal metatarsal veins rather than emptying into the deep metatarsal veins. The superficial metatarsal veins end in the *dorsal venous arch*. Proximal to the arch is an irregular venous network that drains into the marginal veins of the foot. On the dorsolateral border of the foot, the *lateral marginal vein* is formed by many small veins from the plantar and dorsal foot. This vein passes posterior to the lateral malleolus and is continuous with the *lesser (small) saphenous vein*. On the medial side of the foot, the *medial marginal vein* is formed by the veins draining the inferomedial and dorsomedial foot. This vein passes anterior to the medial malleolus and is continuous with the *greater saphenous vein*.

Plantarly, in the toe-furrow a small *plantar venous arch* is located in the superficial fascia. This vein joins the medial and lateral marginal veins. The venous arch contains intercapitular veins, which are veins connecting the dorsum of the foot to the plantar foot.

## Lymphatics

There are two locations in the lower limb where lymph nodes can be regularly found, the popliteal fossa and just inferior to the inguinal ligament. The popliteal group of lymph nodes receive both deep and superficial vessels. This group contains one to three nodes and is situated deep in the fossa around the politeal vein. On occasion, a lymph node is associated with the anterior tibial vessels just anterior to the interosseus crural membrane.

The second group of lymph nodes are the inguinal lymph nodes. This group has a deep and superficial set of nodes. The *superficial inguinal lymph nodes* are located in the superficial fascia of the anterior thigh inferior to the inguinal ligament. This set of 15 to 20 nodes is divided into two subgroups, an upper group that is parallel to the inguinal ligament and a lower group which is parallel to the femoral vein. It is the lower group of superficial inguinal lymph nodes that receives vessels mostly from the lower limb. These nodes send vessels (efferents) to the *iliac nodes,* which eventually empty into the cisterna chyli. A small group of *deep iliac lymph nodes* is located around the femoral vein (near the inguinal ligament) or in the femoral canal (*lymph node of Cloquet*). These nodes receive deep lymph vessels and have efferents to the iliac lymph nodes.

The lymphatic vessels in the foot consist of a superficial and deep set, corresponding to the superficial and deep veins. Like veins, the lymph vessels have valves, and the superficial system communicates with the deep. The *subcutaneous lymphatic capillary plexus* is most abundant in the plantar foot. This plexus drains into one of two collecting vessels, the medial or the lateral. The medial group is the larger of the two and follows the course of the greater saphenous vein. This group terminates in the lower group of inguinal lymph nodes. The lateral group forms vessels that pass both anterior and posterior to the lateral malleolus. Those vessels passing posterior follow the course of the lesser (small) saphenous vein to enter the popliteal lymph nodes. Those passing anterior join the medial group to end in the lower group of inguinal lymph nodes.

The deep lymphatic vessels accompany the deep vessels and drain into the popliteal lymph nodes or the anterior tibial lymph nodes, if present. The efferent vessels of the popliteal lymph nodes drain into the deep inguinal nodes.

## REFERENCES

1. Hootnick DR, Packard DS, Levinsohn EM, Factor DA: The anatomy of a human foot with missing toes and reduplicating of the hallux. J Anat 174:1, 1991
2. Chung CS, Myrianthopoulos NC: Racial and prenatal factors in major congenital malformations. Am J Hum Genet 20:44, 1968
3. Moore KL: The Developing Human. 3rd Ed. WB Saunders, Philadelphia, 1982
4. Zwilling E: Limb morphogenesis, p. 301. In Abercrombie M, Brachet J (eds): Advances in Morphogenesis. Vol. 1. Academic Press, New York, 1961
5. Mauro MA, Jaques PF, Moore MD: The popliteal artery and its branches: embryonic basic of normal and variant anatomy. AJR 150:435, 1988.
6. Netter FH: The Ciba Collection of Medical Illustrations. Vol. 8: Musculoskeletal System. Part 1: Anatomy, Physiology, and Metabolic Disorders. Ciba-Geigy Corp., Summit, 1987
7. Clemente CD: Gray's Anatomy. 30th American Ed. Lea & Febiger, Philadelphia, 1985
8. Sarrafian SK: Anatomy of the Foot and Ankle. JB Lippincott, Philadelphia, 1983
9. Draves DJ: Anatomy of the Lower Extremity. Williams & Wilkins, Baltimore, 1986
10. Edeiken J: Roentgen Diagnosis of Diseases of Bone. 3rd Ed. Williams & Wilkins, Baltimore, 1981
11. Straus WL: Growth of the human foot and its evolutionary significance. Contrib Embryol Carnegie Inst 19:93, 1927

12. Yoshoka Y, Siu DW, Cooke DV, Bryant JT, Wyss U: Geometry of the first metatarsophalangeal joint. J Orthop Res 6:878, 1988
13. David RD, Delagoutte JP, Renard MM: Anatomical study of the sesamoid bones of the first metatarsal. J Am Podiatr Assoc 79:536, 1989
14. Mottershead S: Sesamoid bones and cartilage: an inquiry into their function. Clin Anat 1:59, 1988
15. William PL, Warwick R, Dyson M, Bannister LH: Gray's Anatomy. 37th Ed. Churchill Livingston, New York, 1989
16. Aseyo D, Nathan H: Hallux sesamoid bones. Anatomical observations with special reference to osteoarthritis and hallux valgus. Int Orthop 8:67, 1984
17. Valvo P, Hochman D, Reilly C: Anatomic and clinical significance of the first and most medial deep transverse metatarsal ligament. J Foot Surg 26:194, 1987
18. Bojsen-Moller F, Flagstad KE: Plantar aponeurosis and internal architecture of the ball of the foot. J Anat 121:599, 1976
19. Nissen KI: Plantar digital neuritis, Morton's metatarsalgia. J Bone J Surg 30B:84, 1948
20. Sgarlotto TE, Sokoloff TH, Mosher M: Anomalous insertion of extensor hallucis longus tendon. J Am Podiatr Assoc 59:192, 1969
21. Lundeen RO, Latva D, Yant J: The secondary tendinous slip of the extensor hallucis longus (extensor ossis metatarsi hallucis). J Foot Surg 22:143, 1983
22. Tate R, Pachnik RL: The accessory tendon of extensor hallucis longus. J Am Podiatr Assoc 66:899, 1976
23. Rega R, Green DR: The extensor hallucis longus and the flexor hallucis longus tendons in hallux abducto valgus. J Am Podiatr Assoc 68:467, 1978
24. Ger R: Clinical anatomy of the flexor hallucis brevis muscle. Clin Anat 1:117, 1988
25. Sarrafian SK, Topouzian LK: Anatomy and physiology of the extensor apparatus of the toes. J Bone Joint Surg 51A:669, 1969
26. Lemont H, Hernandez A: Recalcitrant pain syndromes of the foot and ankle: evaluation of the lateral dorsal cutaneous nerve. J Am Podiatr Assoc 62:331, 1972
27. Jones JR, Klenerman L: A study of the communicating branch between the medial and lateral plantar nerves. Foot Ankle 4:313, 1984
28. Edwards EA: Anatomy of the small arteries of the foot and toes. Acta Anat 41:81, 1960
29. Huber JF: The arterial network supplying the dorsum of the foot. Anat Rec 80:373, 1941
30. Adachi B, Hasche K: Das Arteriensystem der Japaner. Vol. 1. Maruzen, Kyoto, 1928
31. Jaworek TE: The intrinsic vascular supply to the first metatarsal. J Am Podiatr Assoc 63:555, 1973
32. Crock HV: The blood supply of the lower limb bones in man. ES Livingston, Edinburgh, 1967
33. Shereff MJ, Yang QM, Kummer FJ: Extraosseous and intraosseous arterial supply to the first metatarsal and metatarsophalangeal joint. Foot Ankle 8:81, 1987
34. Shereff MJ, Yang QM, Kummer FJ, Frey CC, Greenidge N: Vascular anatomy of the fifth metatarsal. Foot Ankle 11:350, 1991
35. Styf J: The venous pump of the human foot. Clin Physiol 10:77, 1990

# 3
# Biomechanics

*DARYL PHILLIPS*

Hallux valgus seems to be the hallmark of forefoot deformities. Its occurrence in the modern society has been estimated to be between one-tenth,[1] one-sixth,[2] and one-third[3,4] of the population. It has also been noted to occur at least twice as often in women as in men.[5] It has on several occasions been referred to as the "hallux valgus complex",[3,6] meaning that when it occurs, it is associated with a multitude of other symptoms or deformities of the forefoot. These include calluses under the forefoot, metatarsalgia, splayfoot, flatfoot, plantar fascitis, and hammer toes. Thus, in the study of hallux valgus one often must discuss all these other deformities.

Hallux valgus seems to be a deformity that was uncommon until the wearing of fully enclosed shoes and boots. Early Greek and Roman sculptures are devoid of this deformity. Meyer,[7] in comparing skeletal remains, reported that early Pecos Indians, an unshod population, had a lower hallux abductus angle than shod Yugoslav peasants from a similar time period. The earliest mention of such deformity in the literature was in the eighteenth century. During the nineteenth century, its occurrence and etiology were discussed many times. During the nineteenth and twentieth centuries, several expeditions by scientists into the undeveloped areas of the world, notably Africa and the islands of the Pacific, noted that hallux valgus is only rarely seen in those who do not wear shoes. Hoffmann[8] reported that the foot is fan shaped, with the hallux in a straight line in natives of the Philippines and in central Africans, and that the digits become compressed toward one another when one starts wearing shoes (Fig. 3-1). Maclennan[9] noted 3.2 percent of the men and 8.3 percent women over the age of 30 years in New Guinea highlands had evidence of hallux valgus, while fewer of the lowland natives

had the deformity. Kalcev[10] reported 17 percent of males and 15 percent of females in Madagascar showed hallux abductus (by Meyer's line) greater than 10° versus 50 percent of European woman. James[11] reported on the very straight inner border of the feet in Solomon Island natives, seeing no cases of hallux valgus, and also noting the much stronger intrinsic foot muscles compared to Europeans. Haines and McDougall[12] reported that one adult Burmese woman started to develop bunions after wearing shoes only 3 months. Engle and Morton[13] reported very few foot problems exist in the shoeless African native population, and that the orthopedic surgeon would have very little work with these people. Jeliffe and Humphreys[14] reported that almost no orthopedic deformities were seen in the 464 barefoot Nigerian soldiers they examined.

Others also note that hallux valgus rarely occurs in those who only wear sandals and other types of shoe gear that keep the first and second digits separated. Sim-fook and Hodgson[4] reported that hallux valgus was almost 20 times more common in Chinese who wore shoes than in the barefooted population who lived on boats. Kato reported that the deformity is not present in any of the ancient Japanese footprints. Morioka[15] reported that it does not occur in the forestry workers who wear *jikatabi,* a rubber shoe that keeps the big toe separated from the other toes, but has become common in a new generation who wear western-style logging boots. Thus Japan has noted a great increase in the occurrence of this deformity during the last half of the twentieth century as its citizens have adopted western footwear over the traditional Japanese footwear.[16]

From the fact that the deformity occurs mostly in the shoe-wearing population, and that women tend to

39

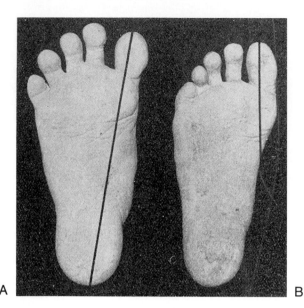

**Fig. 3-1.** (**A**) A foot that has never worn shoes. (**B**) A normal foot that has worn shoes. Feet that have never worn shoes are commonly found to have the digits in alignment with their respective metatarsals, giving the foot a fan shape. Normal feet that wear shoes are commonly found to have the digits in alignment with the longitudinal axis of the rearfoot, thus giving the foot a sarcophagus shape. (From Hoffman,[164] with permission.)

A                                                           B

wear pointed-toed, high-heeled shoes, the most obvious conclusion would be and has been that wearing misfitted, pointed-toed shoes is the primary etiology in initiating hallux valgus.[17–22] Porter[23] noted the importance of good shoes in treating people with hallux valgus and suggested that surgery not be performed if the patient is unwilling to wear the proper shoes. Knowles[24] argued that shoes alone could correct hallux valgus by having a special shoe constructed for a patient with hallux valgus that fanned out at the toes to allow space for the toe to adduct back to alignment with the first metatarsal. After 3.5 years the patient showed some improvement on one side and little improvement on the other. Barnett also performed a limited study on nine experimental subjects and eight controls over 2 to 3.5 years, showing that some feet did decrease the hallux abductus angle in special shoes with extra toe room, while some still showed a mild increase in the deformity even when wearing the special shoes; women were more prone to increase

the deformity and less likely to decrease it with the special shoes than men.[25] Shine also partly confirmed these conclusions by examining 88 percent of the feet in St. Helena, where approximately 50 percent of the population wears shoes on a voluntary basis but men and women wear very much the same types of shoes. He found that bunions were much more frequent in the shoe-wearers, and that the severity of the bunions increased with the increase in the number of years that the person had worn shoes. However, even when both sexes wore similar sensible, rounded shoes there was still a marked increase in the occurrence of hallux valgus in females compared to males.[26] Craigmile[27] did show, in 1953, that a group of children who were kept properly fit for shoes, with changes every 3 to 4 months, did have decreased incidence of hallux valgus than was observed in the general population of children. She also noted that hallux valgus incidence was higher in the group of children who wore shoes with pointed toes and/or no support in the arch.[27]

The facts are then that hallux valgus is a deformity seen almost exclusively in the shoe-wearing population. However, many other observations have been made to show that many other factors must be considered in deciding the exact etiology of hallux valgus. Ely,[28] for example, pointed out that if the wearing of ill-fitting, pointed-toed shoes alone were the cause of hallux valgus, it would mean that a direct correlation should be found between the degree of poor fit or the degree of the pointedness and the degree of hallux valgus. Mensor[29] noted that such cannot be shown, and in fact those in the lower working class, who wore less fashionable shoes, suffered more. Wilkins[30] also noted that the feet of poor men and women are more susceptible to deformity than the feet of those who are well off. Narrow, pointed, high-heeled shoes are worn by both classes of women while in neither class do men wear such shoes. The footwear of the poor, however, is of poorer quality with less variation in fitting and in poorer repair. Heath[31] reported that an examination of various shoe lasts showed that many of the pointed-toe shoe lasts actually gave more freedom for the toes than the rounded-toe shoe lasts. Many individuals who wear pointed-toed shoes do not develop hallux valgus, and there are also many who wear "sensible" shoes who do develop hallux valgus.[32] There are also those who develop hallux valgus on only one foot, although wearing the same type of shoe on both feet, and there are also those who develop hallux valgus who wear no shoes.[33,34] Barnicot and Hardy[35] showed a significant difference in the hallux abductus angles between European and Nigerian feet, but found no difference between Nigerians who wore shoes and those who did not. In addition, Gottschalk et al.[36] found that white feet developed hallux valgus twice as commonly as black feet in South Africa although both groups wore shoes. Others have found that the wearing of arch supports inside a shoe can give significant relief or even prevent surgery on bunions,[37,38] while others have proposed that arch supports should be worn postoperatively to prevent recurrence of the deformity.[39] Hawkins and Mitchell[40] thought that shoes could only produce bunions if a metatarsus primus (adductus) deformity was already present. Thus, in studying the etiology of hallux valgus, factors must be found that in themselves could produce hallux valgus but are much more likely to produce the deformity when shoes are worn.

Some individuals have considered heredity and the congenital nature of the disease.[41] There are a few isolated reports of babies being born with hallux abducto valgus[42]; however, none of these report large bunions accompanying the hallux deformity. More than 50 percent of those who do have bunions report that the deformity was noticed before the age of 20, usually during the pubescent years.[43] Hicks[44] concluded that if a woman can reach the age of 20 with a hallux abductus angle of less than 10° it is very unlikely that she would ever develop hallux valgus. Sandelin[45] noted that hereditary influence was manifested in 54 percent of hallux valgus cases, and Johnston,[46] in examining one family tree, concluded that hallux valgus was transmitted as an autosomal dominant trait with incomplete penetrance. Jordon and Brodsky[47] proposed that the role of foot wear was only secondary, serving to aggravate an already existing mild deformity. Wallace[48] reported in an examination of 224 nine-year-olds that all those with evidence of hallux valgus showed either a positive family history or had a mobile first metatarsal that was plantar-flexed below the level of the others. Metcalf[49] reported that 80 percent of those with hallux valgus had abnormal pronation in their feet and that anterior arch plates gave relief to a large percentage. Hardy and Clapham[50] also showed that there was a high correlation between hallux valgus and pronation of the foot, plantar calluses,

and limitation of mobility in the transverse tarsal joint. Pronation and broken arches, both the medial arch and/or the anterior metatarsal arch, has also been named by many others to be a major factor in the development of the deformity.[51-54] McNerney and Johnston,[55] as well as Carl et al.,[56] have demonstrated greater generalized ligamentous laxity in the joints in those with hallux valgus than those who did not have it. Other factors that have also been shown to be at least part of the etiology include rheumatoid arthritis,[57-59] amputation of the second toe, neurologic disorders, abnormal joint obliquity in the first metatarsocuneiform joint,[60] excessive transverse plane roundness of the first metatarsal head,[61] and the presence of accessory bones between the bases of the first and second metatarsal.[62,63]

Hallux valgus is combined with a medial or dorsomedial prominence of the first metatarsophalangeal joint that is commonly called a "bunion." The degree of hallux valgus was originally measured by the acute angle formed by Meyer's line, which is a line that is tangent to the medial side of the heel and to the medial side of the first metatarsal head, and a second line that is tangent to the two most medial points along the hallux. After the advent and widespread use of x-ray examinations in evaluating deformities, the hallux valgus angle has since become defined by a line that bisects the shaft of the first metatarsal and a line that bisects the shaft of the first proximal phalanx. Because there is a continuum of values in the population, various numbers have been used over the years to try to define the boundary between the normal hallux valgus and the abnormal hallux valgus value. Some have based this value on those who suffer from bunions and those who do not; however, there is considerable overlap in the hallux valgus angles between these two groups. Some have based this value on the average value seen in the unshod natives of the world, which is between 0° and 5°; however, this places most of those who wear shoes in the abnormal category. Others have tried to find the average value in the general population, but because of the number who do suffer from bunions, this shifts the normal curve to an increased value. Thus normal values have been considered to be at any point between 0° and 30° (Fig. 3-2). Although no absolute value can be established that unequivocally defines the boundary between normal and abnormal, it has generally become accepted

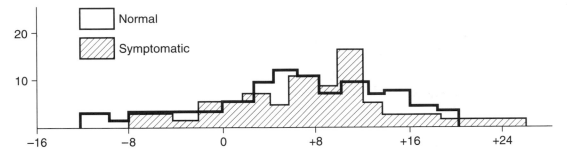

**Fig. 3-2.** Although the normal hallux valgus angle is considered to be about 15°, there are individuals who have a larger angle than this with no signs or symptoms of hallux valgus, and there are those with a smaller angle who do have symptomatic hallux valgus. This histogram by Barnicot and Hardy compares the hallux valgus angle of those with normal feet and those with symptomatic hallux valgus. (From Barnicot and Hardy,[35] with permission.)

that if the hallux angle becomes more than 15°,[60,64] the patient may be considered to have some degree of abnormality. The decision to treat any abnormality is then based on whether the patient is having symptoms or is likely to develop symptoms.

## ANATOMY AND FUNCTION OF THE NORMAL FIRST RAY

The basic functional anatomy must be first considered in discussing the development of hallux valgus deformity. The first metatarsophalangeal joint is actually two joints with a common joint capsule and interrelated muscles and ligaments (Fig. 3-3). The distal portion is a partial ball-and-socket type morphology between the first metatarsal and the proximal phalanx, while the second portion is a rounded groove between the plantar first metatarsal and the dorsal surface of two sesamoids. These sesamoids are connected by vertical fibers to the sides of the first metatarsal head and by horizontal fibers to the plantar base of the proximal phalanx. In addition, oblique fibers run from the epicondyles of the metatarsal head to the plantar sides of the base of the proximal phalanx. It is now considered that the sesamoids are ossification centers that develop within the plantar plate under the first metatarsal head.[65] They are connected by very dense fibers that are akin to the tissue found in the lesser plantar plates, forming what is commonly called the intersesamoidal ligament. The lateral sesamoid also is

connected by very strong fibers to the plantar plate under the second metatarsal head by the transverse intermetatarsal ligament. The strength of these connections, which is determined by both the strength of the fiber and the geometry between fibers, means that the distance between the sesamoids and the plantar plate of the second metatarsal head is almost always seen to remain constant.[66,67] Finally, there are attachments of the sesamoids to the deep vertical fibers of the plantar fascia that are pulled taut when the sesamoids are pulled forward. When the plantar fascia is tightened up, all the fibers of the forefoot are also tightened, which increases the resistance of the soft tissues to compression.

In addition to their ligamentous attachments, the sesamoids are also strongly attached to several tendons. The flexor hallucis brevis has origins from the cuboid, the lateral cuneiform, the medial septum, and the metatarsal extension of the posterior tibial tendon. It divides distally and invests both sesamoids. The abductor hallucis blends its lateral fibers with the medial tendon of the flexor brevis so that a portion of its fibers helps invest the medial sesamoid[68] (Fig. 3-4). The oblique head of the adductor hallucis is much smaller in man than in lower primates.[69] It arises from the peroneal sheath and the bases of the central three metatarsals, and blends its medial fibers with the lateral head of the flexor hallucis brevis, thus helping in the investment of the lateral sesamoid. Further distally its lateral fibers join those of the transverse head of the adductor hallucis to send their fibers directly to

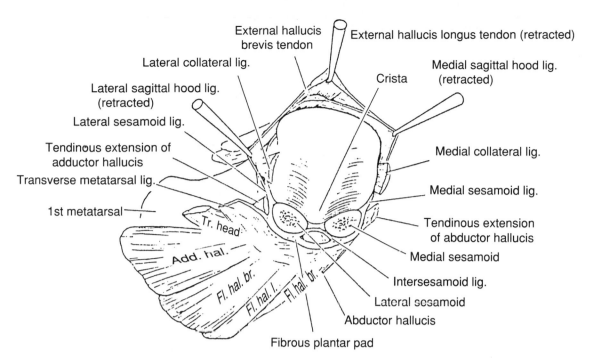

**Fig. 3-3.** Normal anatomy around the first metatarsophalangeal joint. The first metatarsophalangeal joint is a socket composed of the sesamoids, the base of the proximal phalanx, and the surrounding ligaments, with the first metatarsal only attached by ligaments inserting into the medial and lateral epicondyles of the first metatarsal. (From Alvarez et al.,[108] with permission.)

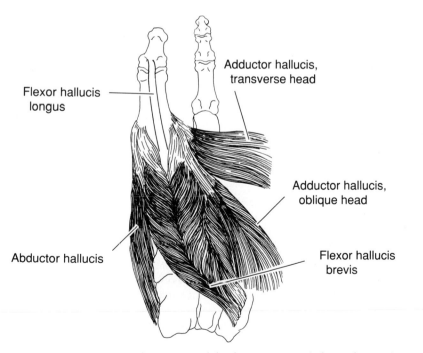

**Fig. 3-4.** Orientation of the normal musculature around the first metatarsophalangeal joint. (From McCarthy and Grode,[66] with permission.)

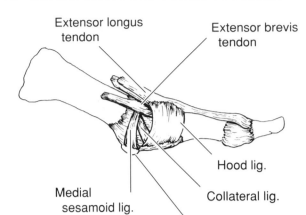

Extensor longus tendon

Extensor brevis tendon

Hood lig.

Collateral lig.

Medial sesamoid lig.

Medial sesamoid

**Fig. 3-5.** The extensor hood attaches to the plantar aspect of the first metatarsophalangeal joint capsule and anchors the extensor hallucis longus and brevis in place over the dorsal aspect. (From Haines and McDougall,[112] with permission.)

the plantar base of the proximal phalanx.[70] Thus, because of the ligamentous and tendinous attachments of the sesamoids to the proximal phalanx, the distance between the sesamoids and the proximal phalanx will also attempt to remain constant, and if one looks at the strength of the ligamentous and fibrous attachments of the sesamoids, one finds the weakest attachments of the sesamoids to be those with the metatarsal head.

Several other tendons pass the first metatarsophalangeal joint (Fig. 3-5). The transverse head of the adductor hallucis is a small muscle originating from the transverse intermetatarsal ligament segments and forming a conjoined tendon with the oblique head of the adductor hallucis to proceed directly to the lateral base of the proximal phalanx. It is commonly called the transversus pedis muscle. The flexor hallucis longus muscle runs in a groove just under the inter-sesamoidal ligament and is held firmly in place within this groove. It then proceeds forward to lie within a groove under the entire length of the proximal phalanx before attaching to the base of the distal phalanx. The extensor hallucis longus runs over the dorsal surface of the first metatarsophalangeal joint, and while it was commonly thought of as being free of the metatarsophalangeal joint such that it made a beeline to its attachment at the base of the distal phalanx, it is now realized that it is anchored by the fibers of the exten-

sor sling to the sesamoids and follows the longitudinal axis of the proximal phalanx. The extensor digitorum brevis inserts into the lateral side of the extensor digitorum longus at the level of the metatarsophalangeal joint.

The major motion of the first metatarsophalangeal joint is dorsiflexion in the sagittal plane. The distal metatarsal head is spherical from side to side and is mildly in spiral shape in the sagittal plane.[71] The radius of curvature of the articular surface from side to side is about the same as the width of the metatarsal head,[72] thus allowing the proximal phalanx not only dorsiflexion motion, but also abduction–adduction and inversion–eversion motion. These transverse and frontal plane motions are usually kept to a minimum by the collateral ligaments of the joint, and also by the sesamoids riding in their grooves. Thus, for the hallux to abduct, the sesamoids must be pulled laterally part way out of their grooves. If the sesamoids are well compressed in their grooves, then the joint is much harder to abduct than if there is no compression between the sesamoids and their grooves. When the hallux everts, the plantar-lateral sesamoid ligament tightens from compression of the lateral sesamoid in its groove, and the medial sesamoid ligament slackens. If the toe is in a maximally dorsiflexed position, both ligaments are already tightened and the range of eversion of the toe is decreased.

No one has fully studied the transverse plane motion in the first metatarsophalangeal joint; however, it is assumed to occur around the center of curvature of the metatarsal head when viewed on the transverse plane, which means that this vertical axis would pass directly between the sesamoids. If this is the case, then the pull of the abductor hallucis in a plantar-medial direction is combined with an equal pull of the adductor hallucis in a plantar-lateral direction (Fig. 3-6). A pull of both heads of the flexor hallucis brevis would produce a straight plantar flexion of the joint as would a pull of the flexor hallucis longus and a pull of the extensor hallucis longus; this occurs because all three produce a vector that passes directly through the vertical axis of motion. The more rounded the first metatarsal head is, the closer the vertical axis would lie to the joint surface. Thus, small displacements medially or laterally in the round first metatarsal head will produce greater angular changes than in the flatter first metatarsal head. It also means that greater transverse angular torque is more likely to develop with a

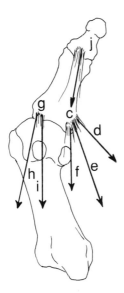

**Fig. 3-6.** The pull of the plantar instrinsic muscles on the proximal phalanx when the joint is in abducted position, showing that there is a significant overload of the muscles to the lateral side. c, insertion of lateral conjoined tendon; d, transverse head of adductor hallucis; e, oblique head of adductor hallucis; f, lateral tendon of flexor hallucis brevis; g, insertion of medial conjoined tendon; h, abductor hallucis; i, medial tendon of flexor hallucis brevis; j, flexor hallucis longus. (From Dykyj,[116] with permission.)

given amount of pull of either the adductor or abductor hallucis muscle in the rounded first metatarsal head.

The first metarsophalangeal joint, therefore, must be considered as a modified socket with the base of the proximal plalanx and the sesamoids, with their ligamentous attachments forming a cup that is well anchored together, and the first metatarsal floating within, very loosely attached to the cup structures. Because of the spiral shape of the first metatarsal head in the sagittal plane, the axis of dorsiflexion–plantar flexion does not stay fixed. When the first metatarsophalangeal joint dorsiflexes in a non-weight bearing situation, the axis of motion moves in a circular pattern from center to distal, then dorsal and finally distal-proximal, producing a sliding action of the joint surface.[73,74] However, when the foot is in a weight-bearing situation the hallux stays fixed and the entire metatarsal lifts and rotates around an axis that moves from the central surface in an arc proximally and superiorly[75] (Fig. 3-7). Because of the sliding action of the hallux on the phalanx, if the first metatarsal rotated solely around this axis it would also roll forward, thus producing an abnormal compression between the proxi-

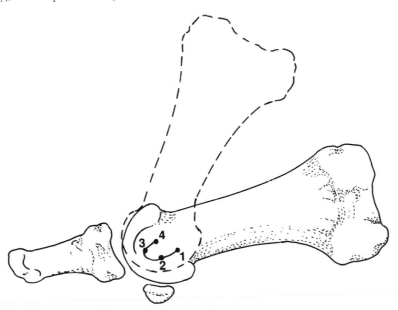

**Fig. 3-7.** The axis of the first metatarsophalangeal joint in open kinetic chain moves in a semicircular pattern as the proximal phalanx moves from full plantar flexion to full dorsiflexion. Note that if the first metatarsal moved around this axis in closed kinetic chain, the first metatarsal head would lose contact with the ground (dotted line). (From Shereff,[74] with permission.)

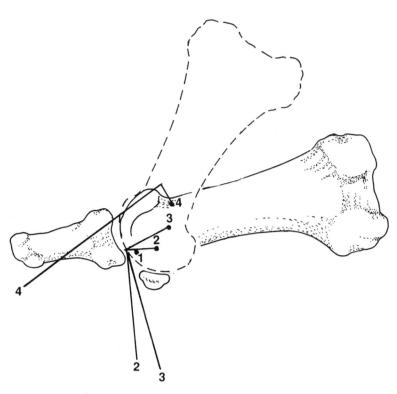

**Fig. 3-8.**  By combining a plantar flexion motion of the first metatarsal with the dorsiflexion of the first metatarso-phalangeal joint, the first metatarsal rotates around a moving axis, as determined by Hetherington et al. (From Hetherington et al.,[75] with permission.)

mal phalanx and the metatarsal head that would induce damage to the articular surfaces. This abnormal compression is avoided, however, by the metatarsal rotating around a proximal axis such that it moves proximally, in a plantar direction relative to the plantar plane of the foot (Fig. 3-8). In fact, if the forefoot is prevented from plantar-flexing, the first metatarsophalangeal joint will be prevented from dorsiflexing, even when it is non-weight-bearing.[76]

As was noted, closed kinetic chain dorsiflexion of all the metatarsophalangeal joints occurs during the propulsive phase of gait. This occurs by the heel lifting and the ankle joint plantar-flexing while all the foot bones rotate around the axes of motion in the metatarsal heads. If one looks at the metatarsal heads, however, a fairly straight line is noted that connects the central portions of the second, third, fourth, and fifth metatarsal heads. This line is almost parallel with the

ankle joint axis (Fig. 3-9). A line that connects the first and second metatarsal heads is oblique to the line connecting the lesser metatarsal heads and is essentially perpendicular to the direction of motion.[77] Because the ankle joint axis is externally directed to the direction of motion when the subtalar joint is neutral, when the ankle joint plantar-flexes, the lesser metatarsal heads would stay in contact with the ground and the first would rise off the ground unless the first also plantar flexed. Likewise if the first and second metatarsal heads dorsiflexed, the third, fourth, and fifth metatarsal heads would come off the ground unless the rearfoot inverted to keep the lateral heads on the ground. During propulsion, the metatarsophalangeal joints dorsiflex between 40° and 60°[78]; however the ankle joint only plantar-flexes about half as much. It would thus seem apparent that for all the metatarsophalangeal joints to stay on the ground through a nor-

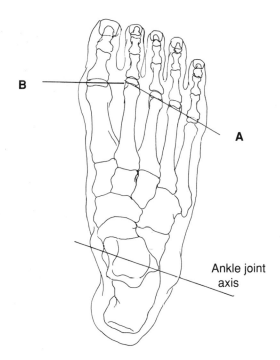

**Fig. 3-9.** During propulsion the lesser metatarsophalangeal joints rotate around an axis that lies along line. A, while the first metatarsophalangeal joint rotates around line B. To keep all five metatarsal heads against the ground, the ankle joint must plantar-flex around an axis that is almost parallel with line A while the subtalar joint supinates and the first metarsal plantar-flexes to keep the first metatarsal head on the ground. (From Bojsen-Møller,[133] with permission.)

mal degree of propulsion, both these mechanisms must occur; that is, the ankle joint must plantar flex, the first metatarsal must plantar flex, and the rearfoot must supinate.

It was noted by many early authors that one of the most obvious changes between the primate and human foot was in the shape and motion of the first metatarsal.[79] The evolutionary trend has been for the first metatarsal to become a major weight-bearing bone and the lesser metatarsals to become less significant for weight-bearing.[80] The primate has a first metatarsal that is much shorter than in the human, with the first metatarsocuneiform joint facing medially, approximately 30 degrees more than in humans,[81] so that its motion is very much like the thumb, being used in apposition with the lesser metatarsals.[82,83] The adduc-

tor hallucis is a very large fan-shaped muscle originating along the entire shaft of the second metatarsal, while in man it has shrunk to two small heads.[69] In man the first metatarsal has become much longer, about the same length as the second metatarsal, and the first metatarsocuneiform is directed much more anteriorly. Its range of motion has become much smaller, and it does not function as an opposer of the second metatarsal. The adductor hullucis has become much reduced in size, while the flexor hallucis brevis and the abductor hallucis have increased.

The motion of the first metatarsal proximally was described first by Hicks[84]; he described the combined motion of the first metatarsal and first cuneiform around one single axis that was called the axis of the first ray. This axis proceeded from the navicular tuberosity, slightly inferior to the base of the third metatarsal and slightly superior. This would mean that the axis would be approximately 45° angulated laterally with the frontal plane and slightly angulated upward (Fig. 3-10). Motion around this type of axis would pro-

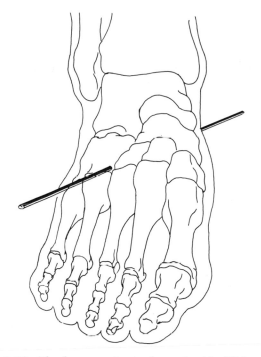

**Fig. 3-10.** The first-ray axis was determined by Hicks to be almost 45° to the frontal and sagittal planes and slightly tilted downward as it proceeded from proximal to distal. (From Hicks,[84] with permission.)

duce an equal number of degrees in the sagittal and frontal planes and just a slight angular motion on the transverse plane. Because of the length of the head from the axis, motion in the sagittal and transverse planes would exhibit relatively large excursions, while frontal plane motion would exhibit a relatively small excursion. Ebisui[85] divided the motion of the first into a motion that was first mainly a sagittal plane motion of the first metatarsocuneiform joint, followed by a rolling motion at the first naviculcuneiform and the first–second intercuneiform joint such that the first metatarsal would first dorsiflex and then the first cuneiform would invert. Kelso et al.[86] further studied the motion of the first ray relative to the fixed second ray and noted that the dorsiflexion of the first ray relative to the second ray also produced an inversion motion, while plantar flexion produced an eversion motion. The average sagittal plane motion was 12.4 mm with the average frontal plane motion of 8.2°. Although Kelso et al. did not compare degree motions, the ratio of frontal to sagittal plane motion did vary significantly, from 0.27 to 1.41. This indicates that there is significant variance between individuals in the angular deviation of the first-ray axis from the sagittal plane. If such interindividual variety exists in the deviation of the axis from the sagittal plane, it would also be logical to assume that significant interindividual variety exists in the deviation of the axis from the transverse plane. If the axis is deviated from posterodorsal to anterior-plantar, then the first ray when it dorsiflexes and inverts will also abduct toward the second metatarsal (Fig. 3-11A). However if it is deviated from postero-plantar to anterodorsal, then when the first ray dorsiflexes and inverts, it will also adduct away from the second metatarsal (Fig. 3-11B). No studies have been performed to determine what type of variation in the axis orientation exists in the population.

Because of the multiplane effect of the first metatarsal motion dorsiflexion of the first metatarsal relative to the second will result in the first metatarsal also inverting and either adducting or abducting according to the direction of the axis. Likewise, as the first metatarsophalangeal joint dorsiflexes during gait and the first metatarsal plantar-flexes relative to the second, to allow the ankle joint to plantar-flex the first metatarsal everts relative to the second and will move closer or further away from the second according to the direction of the axis. Thus, closed kinetic chain dorsiflexion

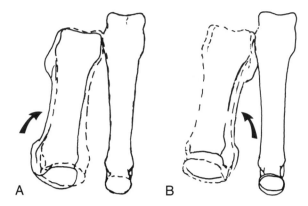

**Fig. 3-11.** (**A**) If the axis of the first ray is directed distal-plantar, as Hicks described, when the first metatarsal dorsiflexes and inverts it moves closer to the second metatarsal. (**B**) If the axis is directed distal-dorsal, as would happen when the lesser tarsus everts, then when the first metatarsal dorsiflexes and everts, it would move away from the second metatarsal, thus increasing the intermetatarsal spacing.

of the joint in which the hallux is held stable produces a frontal plane rotation within the joint such that there is a relative inversion of the first proximal phalanx on the metatarsal head[87] as well as possibly some degree of transverse plane motion.

A further study of the transverse and frontal plane motion within the first metatarsophalangeal joint can be attained by studying the effect of the rearfoot motions on the forefoot. D'Amico and Schuster[88] and Oldenbrook and Smith[89] both demonstrated that as the rearfoot pronates and the calcaneus becomes everted to the ground the metatarsals also will evert relative to the ground, and when the calcaneus becomes inverted to the ground all the metatarsals will invert to the ground. It is logical then to assume that when the forefoot is everted to the ground, the axis of the first ray will become more everted causing it to point in a more dorsal direction, and when the forefoot is inverted to the ground, the axis of the first ray will become more inverted causing it to point in a more plantar direction.

With eversion of the forefoot, the first and second metatarsals experience greater pressure against the ground, which places a supination force on the longitudinal axis of the midtarsal joint and a dorsiflexion force on the first and second metatarsals. Because the midtarsal joint is further from the forefoot than the axis of the first ray, it may be assumed upward force against the plantar surface of the first metatarsal will place a stronger supination torque around the midtarsal joint than around the first-ray axis and thus the midtarsal joint will tend to supinate until the forefoot is on the ground.[85] Hicks demonstrated the small range of motion that is present around the longitudinal axis of the midtarsal joint compared to the other tarsal joints. Phillips and Phillips[90] also demonstrated that to keep the midtarsal joint fully pronated the forefoot would have to exponentially evert more than the rearfoot as the subtalar joint pronated. Thus with every degree that the rearfoot everts and pronates, the midtarsal joint must invert a greater amount to compensate. In the average foot, the end of midtarsal joint supination around the long axis can be expected when the calcaneus everts more than 4°–6°, although there are great variances in the population. Once the midtarsal joint has reached the end of its range of motion to compensate for rearfoot eversion, therefore, additional eversion of the rearfoot will be compensated by dorsiflexion of the first ray. As the first ray dorsiflexes it also inverts relative to the second metatarsal, although it may remain somewhat everted to the floor.

As was noted previously, when the metatarsophalangeal joint dorsiflexes in closed kinetic chain, the rearfoot inverts as do all the metatarsals; however, because the first metatarsal is plantar-flexing, it is everting relative to the second metatarsal and thus the first metatarsal inverts less than the other metatarsals during propulsion. The purpose of propulsion is to generate force against the ground to propel the center of mass forward and onto the opposite leg. Thus, ground reaction forces not only must exceed body weight to lift the body mass upward before it begins its descent down for the opposite foot, but they must also generate a forward shear to push the body mass forward, and a slight medial shear to allow the smooth transfer of weight onto the opposite limb.

The normal action of the muscles around the first metatarsophalangeal joint must also be noted. During static standing, little to no muscle activity is required except in the triceps surae.[91,92] During walking, the extensor hallucis longus is mainly a swing-phase muscle, beginning its contraction in the last portion of propulsion and ending its contraction before the entire forefoot has contacted the ground. Its basic function is to produce a straight open kinetic chain dorsi-

flexion of the metatarsophalangeal joint. The other muscles that cross the metatarsophalangeal joint are all stance-phase muscles. The flexor digitorum longus begins firing during contact period and the flexor hallucis brevis with the abductor and adductor begin firing before the heel comes off the ground.[93,94] It is the firing of all these plantar muscles that stabilizes the hallux against the ground so that the metatarsal may roll forward without the hallux also rolling forward. When the peak of backward force against the ground is reached, the long plantar muscles relax and the extensor hallucis longus contracts, allowing the metatarsal head to lift from the ground and the foot to start rolling forward onto the end of the toe. When the anterior tibial starts firing then the entire foot dorsiflexes at the ankle joint, clearing the toe from the ground.[95]

## DEVELOPMENT OF HALLUX ABDUCTO VALGUS

A contraction of the abductor normally places a plantar flexion, adduction, and inversion torque on the proximal phalanx, while a contraction of the adductor hallucis will place a plantar flexion, abduction, and eversion torque on the proximal phalanx. When these fire together, the frontal and transverse plane torques are neutralized such that a straight plantar flexion force is produced. Robinson proposed that the problem with hallux valgus was in the sesmaoid apparatus, and that removal of both sesamoids would prevent the occurrence of the deformity.[96] Nayfa and Sorto[97] showed that the hallux valgus angle quickly increased within 29 months of removal of the tibial sesamoid, thus showing the importance of the tibial sesamoid in balancing the force coming from the fibular sesamoid. Cralley et al.[98] found that there was a high positive correlation between hallux valgus, the mass of the flexor hallucis brevis, and the mass of the oblique head of the adductor hallucis, which could overpower the pull of the abductor hallucis. McBride[99] proposed that if the toe was even slightly everted, which would shift the sesamoids laterally such that the vertical axis around which transverse plane motion occurs would not pass directly between the sesamoids, then a transverse plane torque would be produced when their corresponding muscles both contract with equal force, which would allow the hallux to move to the lateral side of the first metatarsal. The relationship of the longitudinal axis around which frontal plane motion occurs has never been investigated, but it has been hypothesized that if the tibial sesamoid moves directly plantar to the first metatarsal that the abductor hallucis loses all its inversion and adduction torque and cannot counteract any eversion and abduction torque produced by the adductor hallucis. Hallux valgus would thus ensue whether or not the patient wore shoes.[100]

Schubert[101] attributed the abnormal pull of the abductor hallucis when learning to walk—when pronation was present—as the greatest contributing factor in the development of hallux valgus. As was noted, the abductor and adductor hallucis contract during late midstance and through propulsion. However, in the highly pronated foot these muscles begin contracting almost from the beginning of heel contact.[102,103] (Fig. 3-12). This means that these muscles begin contracting before the first metatarsal can contact the ground, while it is still dorsiflexed and inverted relative to the second metatarsal, and abduction and adduction balance around the first metatarsal is lost in the early stages of contact.

All cases of hallux valgus demonstrate a sesamoid apparatus that has moved laterally under the first metatarsophalangeal joint (Fig. 3-13). In moving laterally, the medial sesamoidal and medial collateral ligaments become stretched; microtears develop that subsequently heal in a thickened but more disorganized manner, thus making the medial ligaments weaker than the lateral ones.[104] The medial sesamoid moves closer to the vertical axis while the lateral sesamoid

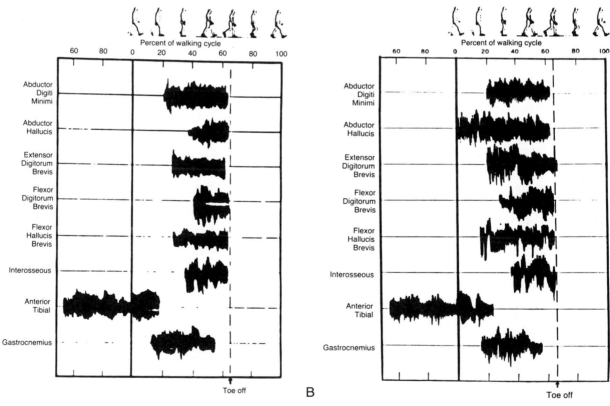

A

B

**Fig. 3-12.** (**A**) Electromyograph (EMG) activity of foot muscles in the normal foot. (**B**) EMG activity of foot muscles in the highly pronated foot. In the highly pronated foot, there is significantly greater EMG activity in the abductor hallucis and the flexor hallucis brevis muscles. This study by Mann and Inman did not observe the adductor hallucis as did Shimazaki. (From Mann and Inman,[102] with permission.)

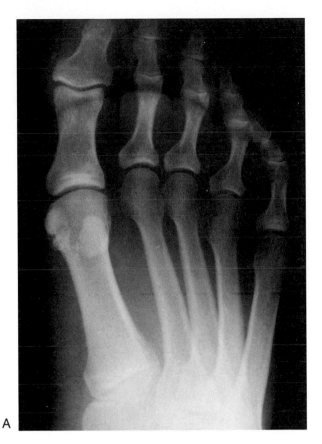
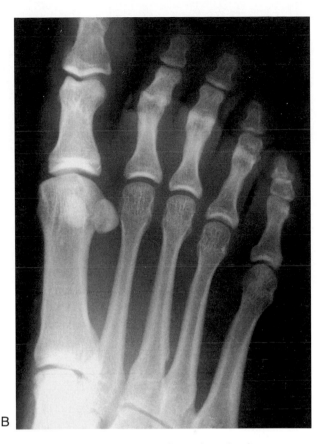

A                                    B

**Fig. 3-13.** (**A**) Radiograph of normal foot that is supinated. (**B**) Radiograph of the same foot when the foot is pronated. Note the appearance of "lateral displacement" of the sesamoids and the hallux, which is actually caused by the first metatarsal dorsiflexing and inverting. (From Inman,[165] with permission.)

has moved further away, such that if the adductor hallucis, the flexor hallucis brevis, and the abductor hallucis would all contract with equal force there would be a net lateral motion of the joint. In viewing the lateral sesamoid movement on the frontal plane, it is noted that the medial sesamoid has also moved in a plantar direction to lie under the crista of the first metatarsal head, while the lateral sesamoid has also moved in a dorsal direction, around the side of the head of the first metatarsal (Fig. 3-14). Erosions appear in the tibial sesamoid, and degeneration of the plantar metatarsal crista also begins. Iida and Basmajuian[105] have demonstrated that once the hallux is in an abducted position, when the abductor and adductor hallucis muscles contract, there is a decreased force ex-

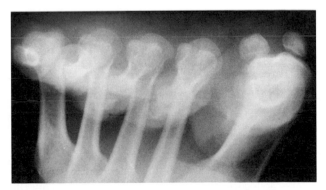

**Fig. 3-14.** As the hallux becomes displaced laterally, the tibial sesamoid encroaches and compresses the plantar crista of the first metatarsal head. (From Maldin,[119] with permission.)

erted by both but the abductor hallucis force is decreased more than the adductor hallucis force.

As the medial sesamoid moves laterally, it impinges upon the intersesamoidal ridge on the plantar aspect of the first metatarsal head. Chondromalacia and then erosions first appear, followed by an erosion of the crista altogether.[106,107] In addition, new cartilage forms for the lateral sesamoid on the plantar lateral side of the first metatarsal head.[108] With the hallux in this laterally deviated position, compression forces are decreased in the center of the metatarsophalangeal articulation and increased around the periphery of the

phalangeal articulation.[109] Thus, the medial rim of the phalanx increases its pressure into the metatarsal head as it goes through its dorsiflexion motion, creating articular cartilage disorganization, degeneration, and atrophy[10] and forming a groove into the medial side of the metatarsal head.[111] Once this groove has been formed, the articular cartilage medial to it begins a disuse atrophy and eventually disappears altogether. This gives the appearance of a hypertrophy of the medial head of the first metatarsal, but if the medial prominence of the first metatarsal head relative to the shaft of the bone is measured it will be found to be the

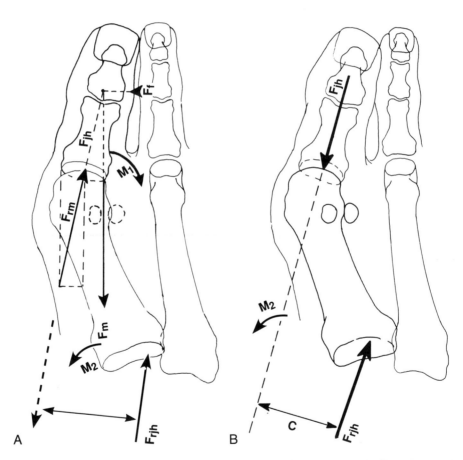

**Fig. 3-15.** (**A**) When the hallux is in an abducted position, the pull of the flexor hallucis longus ($F_m$) creates an abduction moment around the vertical axis of the first metatarsophalangeal joint ($M_1$). It also produces a compressive force within the first metatarsophalangeal joint ($F_{rm}$) and a friction force against the ground ($F_f$). (**B**) The equal and opposite force of $F_{rm}$ (labeled $F_{jh}$) and the compressive force in the first metatarsocuneiform joint ($F_{rjh}$) combine to create an adduction moment of the first metatarsal ($M_2$), which would increase the first intermetatarsal angle. (From Snijders et al.,[134] with permission.)

same size in both the normal and the hallux valgus foot. The medial eminence is thus the original medial epicondyle of the first metatarsal.[112]

The flexor hallucis longus proceeds forward, lying directly plantar to the intersesamoidal ligament. In a normal foot, the vertical axis of the metatarsophalangeal joint passes directly through the flexor hallucis longus tendon such that when the muscle contracts a straight compression is produced on the plantar aspect of the joint, causing the joint to move straight down (Fig. 3-15). In hallux valgus, however, with the sesamoids displaced laterally, the vertical axis lies medial to the tendon. There is therefore a lever arm between the flexor hallucis longus and the vertical axis,

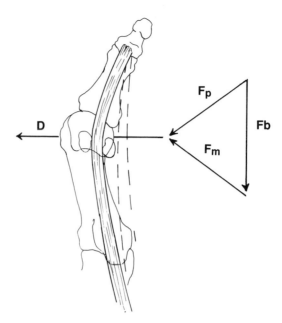

**Fig. 3-17.** The extensor hallucis longus does not actually bowstring the first metatarsophalangeal joint as was often drawn (dotted line), but is held in place by the extensor hood. However the pulley action around the first metatarsophalangeal joint does create a resultant buckling force (D →) to push the first metatarsal medially. (From Rega and Green,[113] with permission.)

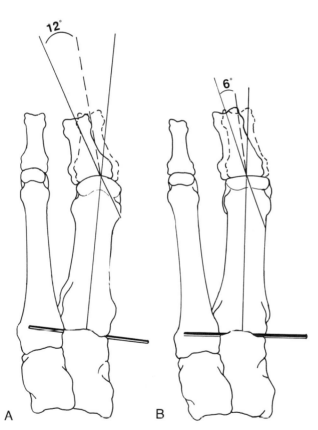

**Fig. 3-16.** A comparison of (**A**) a round first metatarsal head and (**B**) a flat first metatarsal head shows that the same linear displacement laterally of the base of the first proximal phalanx results in twice the angular displacement on the round head as that on the flat head. (From Mann and Coughlin,[166] with permission.)

which means that when the flexor hallucis longus contracts, it places a torque to pull the hallux into an abducted position (Fig. 3-16).

Some individuals have implicated the extensor hallucis longus in the formation of hallux valgus, noting that it bowstrings laterally to the metatarsal head in patients showing the deformity thus when it contracts would create an abduction of the hallux. Rega and Green,[113] and also Schuberth et al.,[114] however, have shown that the extensor hallucis longus does not shift to any great extent laterally over the center of the head of the metatarsal, but instead remains anchored over the metatarsophalangeal joint by the extensor sling mechanism, functioning very much like a pulley (Fig. 3-17). Brahm[115] has shown that the more rounded the head of the first metatarsal in the transverse plane, the greater is the likelihood of the hallux buckling lateralward. If the toe becomes very much abducted, then the extensor hallucis longus would pull the base of the hallux in a proximal medial direction putting a medially directed push against the first metatarsal head, which would increase the distance of the first metatarsal away from the second.[116] It should also be noted that all the plantar muscles contract during the stance phase of gait, whereas the extensor hallucis longus is basically a swing-phase muscle. If it was an important direct contributor of hallux valgus, the great toe would become more dorsiflexed, without the valgus rotation, with increasing deformity. The extensor hallucis longus is more likely to contribute to the development only after the hallux abductus is already well developed.

# THE DEVELOPMENT OF METATARSUS PRIMUS ADDUCTUS

Truslow[117] is given credit for coining the term *metatarsus primus varus* although others had recognized the deformity and recommended treating it before him. Many of the treatment failures have been ascribed to failure to fully treat the first metatarsal deformity.[118] In reality, the deformity is mainly a transverse plane deformity and therefore should properly be called metatarsus primus adductus or metatarsus

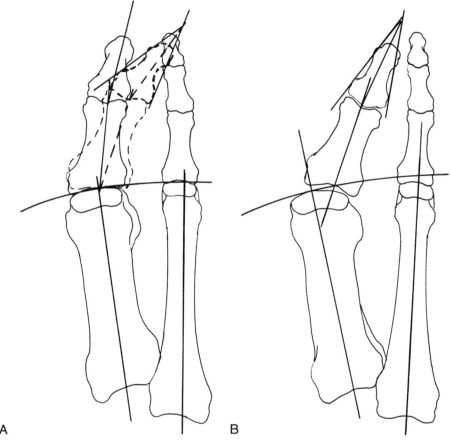

A                     B

**Fig. 3-18.** The relationship between hallux abductus interphalangeus angle and the ability of the second digit to stop the development of hallux valgus. (**A**) The interphalangeal angle is high, which means that the metatarsophalangeal joint can abduct very little before the hallux makes contact with the second digit. (**B**) The interphalangeal angle is low, which means that the metatarsophalangeal joint can abduct much more before the hallux makes contact with the second digit. Thus, greater moments are present in Fig. B than in Fig. A, to adduct the first metatarsal, increasing the intermetatarsal angle. (From Duke et al.,[127] with permission.)

primus adducto varus. It is recognized by an increased angle and distance between the first and second metatarsal heads (Fig. 3-18). Many individuals have found a correlation between the degree of hallux abductus and the first–second intermetatarsal angle, although it has not been a perfect linear correlation.[119] The exact degree of the distance or angle between the first and second metatarsal that demarcates normal from abnormal has been discussed numerous times. It has been usually proposed that a 5°–9° angle between the first and second metatarsals be considered to be the normal value.[120] However, it has also been proposed that if the angle between the first and fifth metatarsals is greater than 29° then an abnormal intermetatarsal angle may be less than a pathologic 10°.[121] Many have also observed that a general splaying of the entire forefoot often occurs, although the increased spread of the lesser metatarsals is quite small compared to that in the first intermetatarsal space. It is now well accepted that any treatment of bunions without the treatment of the concomitant metatarsus primus adducto varus will produce very little benefit to the patient, because the hallux valgus deformity will usually reoccur in a short period of time. There have been many explanations given for the development of the increased space between the first and second metatarsals, and they all probably contribute to this important aspect of the deformity.

It is now accepted that hallux valgus complex is a progressive disorder in which the hallux begins to deviate and then proceeds to subluxation.[122] It has been noted that there is a relationship between the degree of hallux abductus and the first intermetatarsal angle, in that as the degree of hallux abductus increases so does the degree of the first intermetatarsal angle. Girdlestone and Spooner[123] explained that so long as the proximal phalanx created compression directly proximal, that the first metatarsal would be stable, and that the increase in the first intermetatarsal angle would result from the first metatarsal escaping from the stabilizing effect of the proximal phalanx. Hardy and Clapham[124] noted in children with hallux valgus that the displacement of the great toe occurred usually before the age of 14 while the intermetatarsal angle did not show much increase until after the age of 15, thus arguing against the metatarus primus adductus being the primary deformity. Robbins[125] noted that the degree of intermetatarsal angle increase is very slow until the combined angle of the proximal phalanx abductus with the first metatarsal plus the distal phalanx abductus with the proximal phalanx reaches about 30° of abduction. After this, the slope of the relationship line between hallux abductus and first intermetatarsal angle increases approximately 10 fold, such that there are relatively larger increases in the degree of the first intermetatarsal angle for increases in the hallux abductus angle.[125] Viladot[126] noted that feet in which the great toe was shorter than the second showed fewer abnormalities than those in which the great toe was longer than the second. Duke et al.[127,128] showed that the greater the length of the first metatarsal, or the greater the abductus angle between the proximal and distal phalanges of the hallux, the greater the likelihood of bunions and the less the hallux abductus angle increase for the degree of intermetatarsal angle increase (Fig. 3-18). The demonstration by Hewitt[129] that hallux valgus and hammer toe of the second digit occurred eight times more frequently than either deformity separately reinforces the implication that the second toe acts as a buttress to prevent excessive lateral motion of the hallux. Thus the hallux may be fairly free to move laterally until it abuts against the second toe, and if the hallux is to move further laterally, either the second toe will have to move out of the way or the hallux must move on top of or under the second toe. Heden and Sorto[130] confirmed that the average patient with hallux valgus showed a mildly longer first metatarsal and also a longer proximal phalanx. Thus the greater the degree of interphalangeal joint abductus, or the longer the digit, the less the great toe will be able to adduct before it comes into contact with the second digit. Levick argued that as long as the second digit was fully stable, that the second digit would act as the origin for the first dorsal interosseous muscle, which would be the major force that would prevent the first metatarsal from moving medially away from the second metatarsal.[131] Stein[132] also attributed stability of the first metatarsal on the transverse plane to muscle action, but argued that it was the abductor hallucis that compressed the metatarsophalangeal joint on the medial side, which prevented the first metatarsal from moving medialward.

It has been noted that with the lateral movement of the hallux the net muscular pull by all the plantar muscles produces a lateral torque around the vertical metatarsophalangeal joint axis. After the hallux has contacted the second digit, which approximates the critical angle that Robbins discussed, the resistance of the second digit to being abducted increases the medial force against the first metatarsal head with muscular contraction. When the hallux is pulled laterally and is compressed against the first metatarsal head, there is also a direct medial force effected against the first metatarsal head, which would push the first metatarsal away from the second metatarsal. Bojsen-Möller[133] calculated that the medial force against the first metatarsal head was equal to the posterior shear force that the hallux placed against the ground times the tangent of the hallux abductus angle. Snijders et al.[134] developed a more complete model, showing that, as the hallux abductus angle increases, there is an exponential increase in the abducting moment around the metatarsophalangeal joint and the adducting moment at the metatarsocuneiform joint when the flexor muscles contract. Thus the marked increased in the intermetatarsal angle is observed with increasing degrees of hallux abductus.

When one first starts looking at radiographs of feet with hallux valgus, the intermetatarsal angle is reminiscent of the skeletal shape of the primates, with the marked first intermetatarsal angle. It has been hypothesized that the increased first intermetatarsal angle is an atavistic trait.[135] Many have stated that those with metatarsus primus adducto varus have a first metatarsocuneiform joint surface that is deviated medially from being perpendicular to the second metatarsal (Fig. 3-19), and that correction of the bunion involves correction of this angle by either joint fusion or first cuneiform osteotomy.[136] Although this deviation appears in many cases of increased intermetatarsal angle, there have been no studies on the potential association of the increase deviation with the first intermetatarsal angle. It may be that if the joint surface angle is increased medially, then the first metatarsal is more likely to move medially,[137,138] or it may be that this increase in the angle is an optical illusion caused by other malalignment of the foot. Elftman and Manter noted that the relationship between the forefoot and the rearfoot in man resembled that of the foot in the chimp when the midtarsal joint was supinated,[139] or the corollary to this could be that when the forefoot is pronated against the rearfoot in humans that it begins to resemble the shape of the chimpanzee foot.

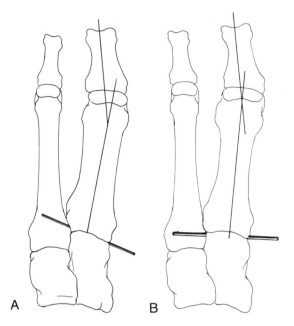

**Fig. 3-19.** (**A & B**) It has been hypothesized that an atavistic metatarsocuneiform joint that is oriented medially as in Fig. A is more likely to develop metatarsus primus adductus than a metatarsocuneiform joint that is oriented to face more anteriorly as in Fig. B. (From Mann and Coughlin,[166] with permission.)

As noted previously, Kelso et al. confirmed the Hicks model of the first metatarsal motion as being a dorsiflexion–inversion or a plantar flexion–eversion motion relative to the second metatarsal. Jones[140] and then Manter[141] demonstrated that normally the first metatarsal bears approximately twice the load of the other metatarsals. Although Mayo[142] and Nilsonne[143] have noted that a majority of hallux valgus cases show the first metatarsal longer than the second metatarsal, which would normally throw increased weight-bearing onto the first metatarsal head, Stokes et al.[144,145] and Hutton and Dhanendran[146] have shown, in patients with hallux valgus, a decrease in weight-bearing under the first metatarsal and a transfer of weight laterally under the lesser metatarsals. Wyss et al.[147] showed that there is normally a force of approximately 350 newtons between the sesamoids and the metatarsal head. This amount of force would normally prevent the medial sesamoid from being able to ride over the central crista, so the first metatarsal head must become unweighted for the medial sesamoid to displace laterally.

Metatarsalgia is commonly a reported symptom in the hallux valgus complex, and it may be explained by decreased weight-bearing of the first metatarsal. Morton[148] first referred to this condition as hypermobility of the first metatarsal. Decreased weight-bearing of the first metatarsal could be seen in a patient who walks on the lateral side of the foot, or it may be seen if the first metatarsal moves in a dorsal direction relative to the second. It can also been seen if there is lack of muscular activity that would stabilize it against the ground. Because almost all patients with hallux valgus show the sesamoids everted laterally under the first metatarsal, it has been argued because of the strong ligamentous support between the sesamoids and the second ray that it is not the sesamoids that have everted against the first metatarsal but instead the first metatarsal has inverted relative to the sesamoids. It should be noted that, for the medial sesamoid to move laterally under the plantar crista, some loss of compression must occur between the sesamoid and the metatarsal head. Thus the first metatarsal head would have to decrease its weight-bearing load, then invert to produce the change in the sesamoid position. Galland and Jordan[149] first supported this view that the increase in the intermetatarsal angle was caused by the first metatarsal dorsiflexing and adducting, which gave the impression that the transverse metatarsal arch had fallen.

The reason for decrease in the weight-bearing load and inversion of the first metatarsal has been hypothesized to result from two factors: an eversion of the midfoot and rearfoot, and a loss of plantar-flexing force by the peroneus longus. The relationship between the pronation of the rearfoot and the development of hallux valgus has long been noted; seldom has hallux valgus been observed to develop with a high arch or supinated foot.[150] Lundberg and Sulja[151] argued that the increased length of the first metatarsal seen in patients with hallux valgus is caused by the dorsiflexion of the first metatarsal that occurs when the foot pronates. Inman[152] demonstrated that when a normal foot is radiographed in a pronated position, the sesamoids are seen to move laterally from being centered under the first metatarsal. Greenberg[153] showed a positive correlation between the combined transverse plane pronation in the subtalar and midtarsal joints and the degree of hallux valgus, Ross[154] showed a positive correlation between the fall of the arch in weight-bearing and the degree of hallux valgus, and Stevenson[155] has shown more certainly a positive correlation between the eversion of the rearfoot and the development of hallux valgus. The possible relationship between pronation of the rearfoot and the development of hallux valgus has been explained with many types of models.

The first explanation is that when the rearfoot everts, the foot becomes more abducted to the line of progression. As the foot becomes abducted to the line of progression, the toe will no longer tend to dorsiflex during propulsion in a line perpendicular to the articular surface of the metatarsal; instead, the foot will lift off, and move in a medial direction to the toe during propulsion. In other words the toe will dorsiflex and abduct to the metatarsal during propulsion (Fig. 3-20).

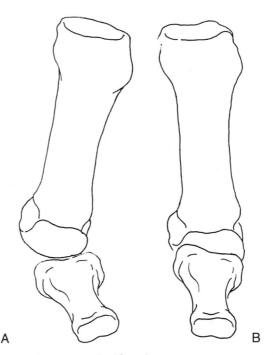

Fig. 3-20. (A) When the foot is pointed straight ahead, there is a straight dorsiflexion force in the metatarsophalangeal joint during propulsion. (B) If the foot is abducted, then the hallux will also abduct against the metatarsal head as it dorsiflexes during propulsion.

It is noted that when the rearfoot everts all the metatarsals evert to the surface, which would transfer the weight onto the medial three metatarsals. The natural inclination is for all the metatarsals to seek equal weight-bearing. This can be accomplished by two mechanisms: inversion of the midfoot at the midtarsal joint, or dorsiflexion of the medial metatarsals, starting at the first. If the first metatarsal remained in its neutral position, it would still be plantar to the second metatarsal, which is also everted. Thus the first metatarsal must dorsiflex above its neutral position to be at the same. level. This dorsiflexion would also be accompanied by an inversion motion relative to the second metatarsal. It is also noted that an eversion of the midfoot would also cause the first-ray axis to project in a more dorsal-distal direction, which would mean that there would be more relative adduction of the first metatarsal away from the second metatarsal as it dorsiflexed and inverted. It is noted that the second metatarsal has a much smaller range of motion than the first metatarsal; thus, although the first metatarsal may be able to seek a level at the same height as the second metatarsal, the second metatarsal is still below the level of the third and thus weight may be borne by the second metatarsal that the lateral forefoot may have borne previously (Fig. 3-21). Thus it is not uncommon for a callous to develop under the metatarsal head with hallux valgus.

The fact that the first metatarsal may dorsiflex and invert relative to the second metatarsal does not answer the question as to why the first metatarsal weight-bearing may be less than the weight-bearing under the second. Even though the first metatarsal may dorsiflex to the level of the second, the lateral three metatarsals are still off the ground, and thus the midtarsal joint would have to accept the function of placing these metatarsals onto the ground. Hicks proposed a midtarsal joint that allows almost pure frontal plane motion around a longitudinal axis that places the first two metatarsals medial to it and the other three lateral to it. Thus an upward pressure of the ground under the first two metatarsals would place an inversion force against the longitudinal axis of the midtarsal joint until force against the lateral three metatarsal heads is equalized. As the forefoot inverts around the longitudinal axis of the midtarsal joint to place the lateral three metatarsal heads onto the ground, the first metatarsal will tend to rise off the ground, decreasing its weight-bearing load.

A common finding then is to have not only a callus under the second metatarsal but also one under the third metatarsal, meaning that equilibrium has been achieved around the longitudinal axis of the midtarsal joint but without achieving full weight-bearing across all the metatarsal heads. This phenomenon of callous buildup, which was commonly attributed to a collapse of the metatarsal arch, is now easily explained by the combined actions of the subtalar, midtarsal, and first-ray axes when the foot pronates.

The determination of whether the longitudinal axis of the midtarsal joint completely accounts for the pronated rearfoot, or whether the first ray dorsiflexes–inverts, and to what degree each occurs, must be determined by a study of the location of the axis of each. When force is placed upward against the first metatarsal, a dorsiflexion force is placed against the first ray and also a supination force is placed against the longitudinal axis of the midtarsal joint. The joint that moves first then is dependent on which joint has the stronger torque being placed upon it. Because torque is equal to the force (both of which are equal) multiplied by the lever arm multiplied by the sine of the angle between the force and the axis of motion, whichever joint has the longer lever arm and the axis that is closer to being parallel with the ground will move first to the end of its range of motion. Thus if the foot moves first around the longitudinal axis of midtarsal joint, and if there is adequate motion in the joint for it to fully compensate for the rearfoot pronation, then there would be no need for the first ray to dorsiflex and invert relative to the second. Thus a pronated rearfoot may never show any signs of a hallux abducto valgus or metatarsus primus adductus deformity. Unfortunately no clinical methods have been proposed for determining the location of the midtarsal joint or first-ray axes nor of quantifying the degree of motion around the midtarsal joint axis. Once these methods have been developed then a multifactorial analysis may indeed prove these hypotheses.

The question may be asked as to why the first metatarsal does not plantar flex as the longitudinal axis of the midtarsal joint supinates. The answer may be that it passively does because gravity pulls the first ray downward; however, it still fails to develop a force underneath. The most common explanation for this phenomenon has been that force underneath the first metatarsal head is generated by the peroneus longus

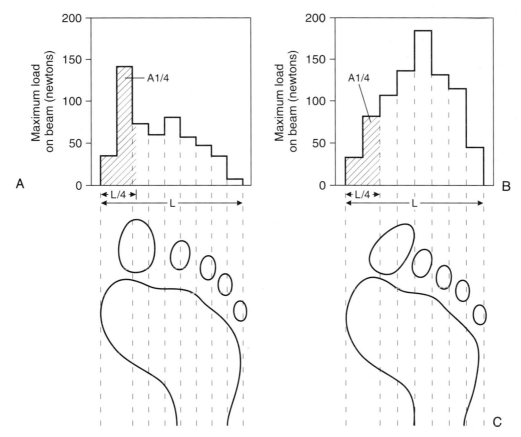

**Fig. 3-21.** Peak loads recorded across the forefoot in a typical normal and a typical hallux valgus foot. (**A**) In the normal foot the first metatarsal bears approximately twice the peak load as any of the other metatarsals. (**B**) In the foot with hallux valgus, there is a loss of weight-bearing load by the first metatarsal and a transference of peak loads to the second and third metatarsals. This produces a callus formation under the second and third metatarsal heads because of the increased weight transferrence. (**C**) A Harris Beath Mat records clinically the transference of weight from the first metatarsal head to the lesser metatarsals. This transference of weight was described by Dudley Morton as hypermobility of the first ray. (Figs. A and B from Stokes et al.,[145] and Fig. C from Harris and Beath,[167] with permission.)

as it pulls the first metatarsal–first cuneiform in a plantar-lateral eversion direction (Fig. 3-22). Hicks[156] noted that the peroneus longus has a strong arch-raising function because of its strong plantarflexion force on the first metatarsal. The amount of plantar pulling is directly proportional to the height change between the lateral side of the cuboid and the base of the first metatarsal, and also on the stability of the cuboid on the calcaneus. The greater the height change between the medial and lateral sides of the foot, the greater the proportion of the pull of the peroneus longus that can be converted into pulling the first metatarsal down

against the ground. As the rearfoot everts, which causes the height of the arch to drop, the less proportion of the peroneus longus pull that can be converted into a plantar force of the first metatarsal against the ground. It should also be noted that the peroneus longus also pulls the cuboid laterally and in an eversion manner, and that to exert all its force into the first metatarsal the cuboid must be stabilized firmly against the calcaneus. This is usually accomplished by the midtarsal joint passively reaching the end of its pronation motion around the longitudinal axis before heel lift. However in the pronated foot, the peroneus

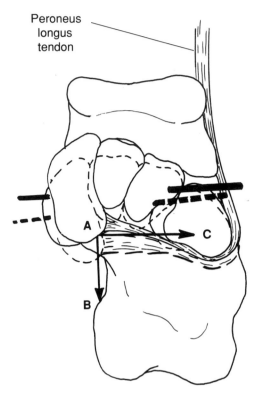

Peroneus
longus
tendon

**Fig. 3-22.** When the foot pronates the axis of the first ray moves from the position indicated by the solid line to the position indicated by the dotted line. The insertion of the peroneus longus to the plantar first metatarsal also moves downward, which decreases the plantar component of its force vector.

longus is also attempting to actively evert the cuboid, which would then force the first metatarsal into a more dorsiflexed-inverted position. Thus normal stabilization of the first ray against the ground by the peroneus longus is aided by the active inversion of the rearfoot, which is passively everting the cuboid against the calcaneus. The final consideration of the action of the peroneus longus has to do with its length. In the normal foot, the supination of the rearfoot increases the length of the peroneus longus. This lengthening of the muscle increases its plantar pull and the velocity with which it can contract. In the pronated foot, with the calcaneus everted and the midtarsal joint more abducted to the rearfoot than in the neutral foot, the peroneus longus is in a shortened position. The force with which it can contract in this shortened position,

as well as its velocity of contraction, is thus decreased making it a much poorer plantar flexor-evertor of the first metatarsal than it would be if the rearfoot was undergoing its normal motions.

The question must finally come full turn again as to how shoe wear increases the incidence of the development of hallux valgus. Again, it must be emphasized that the phenomenon cannot be argued even though very little scientific evidence has been presented that actually explains the mechanism of why it happens. The explanation that it is the pointed toes that abnormally abduct the hallux does not explain why two-thirds of the population who do wear pointed toes do not develop hallux valgus, nor why it develops in those wearing shoes with very round toes. The fact is that the western shoe, no matter its style, does hold the hallux mildly abducted relative to the first metatarsal, which would prevent the incidence of hallux varus; however most shoes, even fashion ones, are constructed on lasts that do not abduct the proximal phalanx more than 15 degrees, which has been established as a normal degree of abduction. Thus additional aspects of shoe design must promote abnormal hallux motion, first-ray motion, or even midtarsal and subtalar joint motion. Some of the possibilities are listed here.

Henderson[157] stated that the failure in the strength of the arch is the cause of most of the ills of the human foot. He noted that foot ills, including weak painful feet, are practically unknown in aboriginal feet. He hypothesized that shoes inhibit the development of the important arch-supporting muscles within the foot.

Ceeney[158] noted that shoes must not only fit the foot by size, but that the shape of the shoe must also fit the foot. Many shoes that are well fit by size requirements still do not match the shape of the foot, and thus will not make the foot comfortable. Root et al.[159] stated that hallux abductus only occurred in feet with an adducted forefoot type. Because most shoes seem to hold the long axis of the digits parallel with the long axis of the rearfoot,[160] they hypothesized that the more the forefoot is adducted to the rearfoot, the more the shoewear will hold the hallux abducted to the first metatarsal, which would tend to move the sesamoids into a more lateral position to initiate the hallux abductus (Fig. 3-23). Lindsay[161] also argued that most

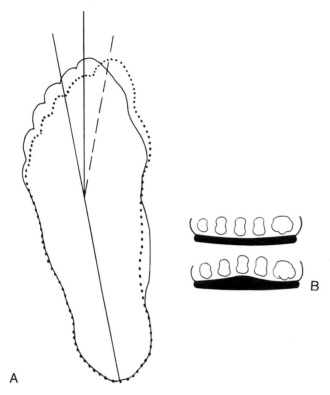

A

B

**Fig. 3-23.** (**A**) An adducted forefoot type (solid line) that is placed in a straight last shoe will pronate in the rearfoot to place the forefoot in a more rectus position (dotted line). (**B**) It is also noted that most shoes are built on the inside with the area under the central metatarsal heads lower than the surface under the first metatarsal head. It has been hypothesized that this may also contribute to abnormal dorsiflexion of the first metatarsal inside the shoe. (From Lindsay,[161] with permission.)

shoes are not built with adequate forefoot adductus. In relationship to this is the fact that few, if any, persons when they buy shoes try to find a shoe built on a last with the same degree of forefoot adductus that exists in their foot when the subtalar joint is in its neutral position. Emslie[162] pointed out that if a foot with an adducted forefoot morphology is placed into a shoe that has less forefoot adductus than the foot, then the subtalar joint will be forced to pronate to allow the forefoot to abduct to the rearfoot to fit into the shoe; the midtarsal joint, by being unable to supinate, will prevent adequate propulsion. Thus many people with

a forefoot adductus morphology may be fitting their feet into shows with a last that is too straight and which is inducing hallux valgus because of these the pronation mechanisms.

Lindsay also argued that shoes are built with the bottom of the sole convex, which would cause the third metatarsal to seek the lowest level. This would cause the first and fifth metatarsals to tend to dorsiflex above the level of the other metatarsals, which may also initiate a relative lateral movement of the hallux, especially in a new shoe. While the frontal plane convexity of the sole is necessary for manufacturing processes, some shoe companies have responded by placing a metatarsal "cookie" just behind the central metatarsal heads to allow the first and fifth metatarsals to plantar-flex to or slightly below the level of the central three.

Early writers often blamed a high heel for the cause of bunions, describing the shoe as being too short, too long, too narrow, etc. Raising the heel height does increase the weight that is pushed forward and cause the metatarsophalangeal joints to function in a more dorsiflexed position and the plantar fat pad to be pulled forward. It might be possible that the dorsiflexed position of the hallux could induce a plantar movement of the first metatarsal and cause the foot to function as if the patient had an everted forefoot condition. Such everted forefoot conditions do induce a pronatory motion during propulsion in an attempt to move body weight onto the opposite foot. Phillips et al.[163] hypothesized that it was not a high-heeled shoe in and of itself that induced hallux valgus, but that possibly most high heels have a very small heel area and that pronation of the foot occurs just before propulsion, which was concluded to occur because the small heel surface prevented the foot from supinating. They demonstrated that if the heel of the shoe was moved medially approximately 3–4 mm that the pronation of the foot decreased before it entered propulsion.

There may be other factors in the shoe that could also cause the foot to pronate more than it would if the patient did not wear shoes. This question has not been satisfactorily answered by any researcher, nor do shoe companies produce data on new shoes that are introduced to show that the shoes increase or decrease the ability of the foot to function close to the ideal.

# REFERENCES

1. Craigmile DA: Results of a surgery of children's feet in the borough of Ealing. Med Officer 83:229, 1950
2. Gould N, Schneider W, Ashikaka T: Epidemiological surgery of foot problems in the continental United States 1978–1979. Foot Ankle 1:8, 1980
3. Dykes RM, Grundy F, Lee HB: Foot ailments in the general population. Med Officer 87:223, 1952
4. Sim-Fook L, Hodgson AR: A comparison of foot forms among the non-shoe and shoe-wearing Chinese population. J Bone Joint Surg 40A:1058, 1958
5. Plaster HM: Hallux valgus as related to first metatarsal length pattern. J Natl Assoc Chiropodists 47:176, 1957
6. Creer WS, Sayle W: Common foot ailments. Br Med J 2:5, 1938
7. Meyer M: A comparison of hallux abducto valgus in two ancient populations. J Am Podiatry Assoc 69:65, 1979
8. Hoffmann P: Conclusions drawn from a comparative study of the feet of barefooted and shoe-wearing peoples. Am J Orthop Surg 3:105, 1905
9. Maclennan R: Prevalence of hallux valgus in a Neolithic New Guinea population. Lancet i:1398, 1966
10. Kalcev B: The hallux position in natives of Madagascar. East Afr Med J 40:47, 1963
11. James CS: Footprints and feet of natives of the Solomon Islands. Lancet ii:1390, 1939
12. Haines RW, McDougall A: Shoe design and the great toe (letter). Lancet 1:678, 1954
13. Engle ET, Morton DJ: Notes on foot disorders among natives of the Belgian Congo. J Bone Joint Surg 13:311, 1931
14. Jelliffe DB, Humphreys J: Lesions of the feet in African soldiers (a clinical surgery of 464 Nigerian troops). J Trop Med Hyg 55:1, 1952
15. Morioka M, Kumura K: Morphologica and functional changes of feet and toes of Japanese forestry workers. J Hum Ergol 3:87, 1974
16. Kato T, Watanabe S: The etiology of hallux valgus in Japan. Clin Orthop Relat Res 157:78, 1981
17. Goldthwait JE: The treatment of hallux valgus. Boston Med Surg J 129:533, 1893
18. Wilson HA: An analysis of 152 cases of hallux valgus in 77 patients with a report upon an operation for its relief. Am J Orthop Surg 3:214, 1905–1906
19. Buka AJ: Bunion and hallux valgus. Am J Surg 8:332, 1930
20. Kreuscher PH, Kelikian H: Hallux valgus (bunions). Ill Med J 67:453, 1935
21. McMurray TP: Treatment of hallux valgus and rigidus. Br Med J 1:218, 1936
22. Allan FG: Hallux valgus and rigidus. Br Med J 1:579, 1940
23. Porter JL: Why operations for bunion fail with a description of one that does not. Surg Gynecol Obstet 8:89, 1909
24. Knowles FW: Effects of shoes on foot form: an anatomical experiment. Med J Aust 1:579, 1953
25. Barnett CH: The normal orientation of the human hallux and the effect of footwear. J Anat 96:489, 1962
26. Shine IB: Incidence of hallux valgus in a partially shoe wearing community. Br Med J 1:1648, 1965
27. Craigmile DA: Incidence, origin and prevention of certain foot defects. Br Med J 2:749, 1953
28. Ely LW: Hallux valgus. Surg Clin North Am 6:425, 1926
29. Mensor MC: Hallux valgus: report of cases. Calif West Med 28:341, 1928
30. Wilkins EH: Feet, with particular reference to school children. Med Officer 66:5, 1941
31. Heath AL: Why most shoes don't fit correctly. Boot and Shoe Recorder 168:54, 1965
32. Robinson HA: Bunion: its cause and cure. Surg Gynecol Obstetrics 27:343, 1918
33. Anderson W: Lectures on contractions of the fingers and toes: their varieties, pathology and treatment. Lecture III. Contraction of the toes. Lancet ii:213, 1891
34. Bankart ABS, Blundell AS: The pathology and treatment of hallux valgus. Med Press Circ 96:33, 1913
35. Barnicot NA, Hardy RH: The position of the hallux in West Africans. J Anat 89:355, 1955
36. Gottschalk FAB, Sallis JG, Beighton PH, Solomon L: A comparison of hallux valgus in three South African populations. South Afr Med J 57:355, 1980
37. Hamsa WR: Hallux valgus, a study of end results of 339 bunionectomies. Nebr Med J 22:225, 1937
38. Hauser EDW: Hallux valgus—prophylactic measures and operative techniques. Surg Clin North Am 21:169, 1941
39. Anderson RL: Hallux valgus, report of end results. South Med Surg 91:74, 1929
40. Hawkins FB, Mitchell CL, Hedrick DW: Correction of hallux valgus by metatarsal osteotomy. J Bone Joint Surg 27:387, 1945
41. Ellis VH: A method of correcting metatarsus primus varus. J Bone Joint Surg 33B:415, 1951
42. Heller EP: Congenital bilateral hallux valgus. Ann Surg 33:798, 1928
43. Piggott H; The natural history of hallux valgus in adolescence and early life. J Bone Joint Surg 42B:749, 1960
44. Hicks JF: The health of children's feet. The manufacturer's problem—how to compromise. Chiropodist 20:213, 1965

45. Sandelin T: Hallux valgus and its operative treatment. JAMA 80:736, 1923

46. Johnston O: Further studies of the inheritance of hand and foot anomalies. Clin Orthop 8:146, 1956

47. Jordan HH, Brodsky AE: Keller operation of hallux valgus and hallux rigidus: an end result study. AMA Arch Surg 62:586, 1951

48. Wallace WA: Predicting hallux abducto valgus. J Am Podistr Med Assoc 80:509, 1990

49. Metcalf CR: Acquired hallux valgus: late results from operative and non-operative treatment. Boston Med Surg J 167:271, 1912

50. Hardy RH, Clapham JCR: Observations on hallux valgus. J Bone Joint Surg 33B:376, 1951

51. Cleveland M: Hallux valgus—final results in 200 operations. Arch Surg 14:1125, 1927

52. Hiss JM: Hallux valgus, its cause and simplified treatment. Am J Surg 11:51, 1931

53. Howorth B: Dynamic posture in relation to the feet. Clin Orthop Relat Res 16.74, 1960

54. Mann RA: Hallux valgus. AAOS Instruct Course Lect 31:180, 1982

55. McNerney JE, Johnston WB: Generalized ligamentous laxity, hallux abducto valgus and the first metatarsophalangeal joint. J Am Podiatr Med Assoc 69:69, 1979

56. Carl A, Ross S, Evanski P, Waugh T: Hypermobility in hallux valgus. Foot Ankle 8:264, 1988

57. Rubin LM: Rheumatoid arthritis with hallux valgus. J Am Podiatry Assoc 58:481, 1968

58. Kirkup JR, Vidigal E, Jacoby RK: The hallux and rheumatoid arthritis. Acta Orthop Scand 48:527, 1977

59. Vidigal EC, Kirkup JR, Jacoby RK: The rheumatoid foot: pathomechanics of hallux deformities. Rev Assoc Med Bras 26:23, 1980 (Engl abstr.)

60. Kleinburg S: The operative cure of hallux valgus and bunions. Am J Surg 15:75, 1932

61. Donick II, Berlin SJ, Block LD, Costa AJ, Fox JS, Martorana VJ: An approach for hallux valgus surgery—fifteen-year review: part I. J Foot Surg 19:113, 1980

62. Young JK: The etiology of hallux valgus of the intermetatarseum. Am J Orthop Surg 7:336, 1909

63. Henderson RS: Os intermetatarseum and a possible relationship to hallux valgus. J Bone Joint Surg 45A:117, 1963

64. LaPorta G, Melillo T, Olinsky D: X-ray evaluation of hallux abducto valgus deformity. J Am Podiatry Assoc 64:544, 1974

65. Haines RW: The mechanism of the metatarsals in spread foot. Chiropodist 2:197, 1947

66. McCarthy DJ, Grode SE: The anatomical relationships of the first metatarsophalangeal joint. J Am Podiatry Med Assoc 70:493, 1980

67. Jahss MH: The sesamoids of the hallux. Clin Orthop Relat Res 147:88, 1981

68. Thomas SA: Hallux varus and metatarsus varus, a five-year study (1954–1958). Clin Orthop 16:109, 1960

69. Keith A: The history of the human foot and its bearing on orthopaedic practice. J Bone Joint Surg 11:10, 1929

70. Martin BF: Observations on the muscles and tendons of the medical aspect of the sole of the foot. J Anat 98:437, 1964

71. Yoshioka Y, Siu DW, Derek T, Cooke V, Bryant JT, Wyss U: Geometry of the first metatarsophalangeal joint. J Orthop Res 6:878, 1988

72. Brahm SM: Shape of the first metatarsal head in hallux rigidus and hallux valgus. J Am Podiatr Med Assoc 78:300, 1988

73. Shereff MJ, Bejjani FJ, Kummer FJ: Kinematics of the first metatarsophalangeal joint. J Bone Joint Surg 68A:392, 1986

74. Shereff MJ: Pathology, anatomy and biomechanics of hallux valgus. Orthopaedics 13:939, 1990

75. Hetherington VJ, Carnett J, Patterson BA: Motion of the first metatarsophalangeal joint. J Foot Surg 28:13, 1989

76. Mygind HB: Some views on the treatment of hallux valgus. Acta Orthop Scand 23:152, 1953

77. Bojsen-Möller F, Lamoreux L: Significance of free dorsiflexion of the toes in walking. Acta Orthop Scand 50:471, 1979

78. Hetherington VJ, Johnson RE, Albritton JS: Necessary dorsiflexion of the first metatarsophalangeal joint during gait. J Foot Surg 29:218, 1990

79. Morton DJ: Evolution of the human foot. Am J Phys Anthropol 7:1, 1924

80. Morton DJ: Significant characteristics of the Neanderthal foot. Nat Hist 26:310, 1926

81. Latimer B, Lovejoy CO: Hallucal tarsometatarsal joint in Australopithecus afarensis. Am J Phys Anthropol 82:125, 1990

82. Morton DJ: Mechanism of the normal foot and of flat foot. J Bone Joint Surg 6:368, 1924

83. Elftman H, Manter J: The evolution of the human foot with special reference to the joints. J Anat 70:56, 1935

84. Hicks JH: The mechanics of the foot. I. The joints. J Anat 87:345, 1953

85. Ebisui JM: The first ray axis and the first metatarsophalangeal joint. An anatomical and pathomechanical study. J Am Podiatry Assoc 58:160, 1968

86. Kelso SF, Richie DH Jr, Cohen IR, et al: Direction and range of motion of the first ray. J Am Podiatry Assoc 72:600, 1982

87. David RD, Delagoutte JP, Renard MM: Anatomical study

of the sesamoid bones of the first metatarsal. J Am Podiatry Assoc 79:536, 1989

88. D'Amico JC, Schuster RO: Motion of the first ray: clarification through investigation. J Am Podiatry Assoc 69:17, 1979

89. Oldenbrook LL, Smith CE: Metatarsal head motion secondary to rearfoot pronation and supination. J Am Podiatry Assoc 69:24, 1979

90. Phillips RD, Phillips RL: Quantitative analysis of the locking position of the midtarsal joint. J Am Podiatry Assoc 73:518, 1983

91. Smith JW: Muscular control of the arches of the foot in standing: an electromyographic assessment. J Anat 88:152, 1954

92. Basmajian JV, Stecko G: The role of muscles in arch support of the foot. J Bone Joint Surg 45A:1184, 1963

93. Sheeifeld FJ, Gersten JW, Mastellone AF: Electromyographic study of the muscles of the foot in normal walking. Am J Phys Med 35:223, 1956

94. Gray EG, Basmajian JV: Electromyography and cinemetography of the leg and foot ('normal' and flat) during walking. Anat Rec 161:1, 1968

95. Fujita M: Role of the metatarsophalangeal joints of the foot in level walking. J Jpn Orthop Assoc 59:985, 1985

96. Robinson HA: The etiology of bunion. Mil Surgeon 62:807, 1928

97. Nayfa TM, Sorto LA Jr: The incidence of hallux abductus following tibial sesamoidectomy. J Am Podiatry Assoc 72:617, 1982

98. Cralley JC, McGonagle W, Fitch K: The role of adductor hallucis in bunion deformity, part II. J Am Podiatry Assoc 68:473, 1978

99. McBridge ED: A conservative operation for bunions. J Bone Joint Surg 10:735, 1928

100. McGlamry ED: Hallucal sesamoids. J Am Podiatry Assoc 55:693, 1965

101. Schubert DA: The role of the abductor hallucis in metatarsus primus varus associated with hallux valgus. J Am Podiatry Assoc 53:752, 1963

102. Mann R, Inman VT: Phasic activity of intrinsic muscles of the foot. J Bone Joint Surg 46A:469, 1964

103. Shimazaki K, Takebe K: Investigations on the origin of hallux valgus by electromyographic analysis. Kobe J Med Sci 27:139, 1981

104. Grode SE, McCarthy DJ: The anatomical implications of hallux abductor valgus. J Am Podiatry Assoc 70:539, 1980

105. Iida M, Basmajian JV: Electromyography of hallux valgus. Clin Orthop Relat Res 101:220, 1974

106. Sutro CJ: The big toe. Comparative anatomic and radiographic study of the metatarsophalangeal articulation. Bull Hosp Joint Dis 26:141, 1965

107. Scranton PE, Rutkowski: Anatomic variation of the first ray. part II. disorders of the sesamoids. Clin Orthop Relat Res 151:256, 1980

108. Alvarez R, Haddad RJ, Gould N, Trevino, S: The simple bunion: anatomy at the metatarsophalangeal joint of the great toe. Foot Ankle 4:229, 1984

109. Miller F, Arenson D, Weil LS: Incongruity of the first metatarsophalangeal joint. The effect of cartilage contact surface area. J Am Podiatry Assoc 67:328, 1977

110. Jaworek TE: The histologic patterns in functional boney adaptation as applied to congruous and subluxed joints. J Am Podiatry Assoc 65:953, 1975

111. Clark JJ: Hallux valgus and hallux varus. Lancet i:609, 1900

112. Haines RW, McDougall A: The anatomy of halux valgus. J Bone Joint Surg 36B:272, 1954

113. Rega R, Green DR: The extensor hallucis longus and flexor hallucis longus tendons in hallux abductor valgus. J Am Podiatr Med Assoc 68:467, 1978

114. Schuberth JM, Cralley JC, Wingfield EJ: Extensor hallucis tendons of normal and hallux abductor valgus feet. J Am Podiatry Assoc 72:125, 1982

115. Brahm SM: Shape of the first metatarsal head in hallux rigidus and hallux valgus. J Am Podiatr Med Assoc 78:300, 1988

116. Dykyj D: Pathologic anatomy of hallux abductor valgus. Clin Podiatr Med Surg 6:1, 1989

117. Truslow W: Metatarsus primus varus or hallux valgus? J Bone Joint Surg 7:98, 1925

118. Mitchell CL, Fleming JL, Allen R, Gleeney C, Sanford GA: Osteotomy-bunionectomy for hallux valgus. J Bone Joint Surg 40A:41, 1958

119. Maldin RA: Axial rotation of the first metatarsal as a factor in hallux valgus. J Am Podiatr Med Assoc 62:85, 1972

120. Carr CR, Boyd BM: Correctional osteotomy for metatarsus primus varus and hallux valgus. J Bone Joint Surg 50A:1353, 1968

121. Price GFW: Metatarsus primus varus: including various clinicoradiologic features of the female foot. Clin Orthop Relat Res 145:217, 1979

122. Piggott H: The natural history of hallux valgus in adolescence and early adult life. J Bone Joint Surg 42B:749, 1960

123. Girdlestone GR, Spooner HJ: A new operation of hallux valgus and hallux rigidus. J Bone Joint Surg 19:30, 1937

124. Hardy RH, Clapham JCR: Hallux valgus, predisposing anatomical causes. Lancet i:1180, 1952

125. Robbins HM: The unified forefoot. II. The relationship between hallux valgus and metatarsus primus adductus. J Foot Surg 22:320, 1983

126. Viladot A: Metatarsalgia due to biomechanical alternation of the forefoot. Orthop Clin North Am 4:165, 1973

127. Duke H, Newman LM, Bruskoff BL, Daniels R: Relative metatarsal length patterns in hallux abducto valgus. J Am Podiatry Assoc 72:1, 1982

128. Duke H, Newman LM, Bruskoff BL, Daniels R: Hallux abductus interphalangeus and its relationship to hallux abducto valgus. J Am Podiatry Assoc 72:625, 1982

129. Hewitt D, Stewart AM, Webb JW: The prevalence of foot defects among wartime recruits. Br Med J 2:745, 1953

130. Heden RI, Sorto LA Jr: The buckle point and metatarsal protrusion's relationship to hallux valgus. J Am Podiatry Assoc 71:200, 1981

131. Levick GM: On the arch-raising role of certain intrinsic muscles of the foot. J Anat 56:196, 1933

132. Stein HC: Hallux valgus. Surg Gynecol Obstet 66:889, 1938

133. Bojsen-Møller F: Anatomy of the forefoot, normal and pathologic. Clin Orthop Relat Res 142:11, 1979

134. Snijders CJ, Snijder JGN, Philippens MMGM: Biomechanics of hallux valgus and spreadfoot. Foot Ankle 7:26, 1986

135. Lapidus PW: Operative correction of the metatarsus varsus primus in hallux valgus. Surg Gynecol Obstet 58:183, 1934

136. Lapidus PW: The author's bunion operation from 1931 to 1959. Clin Orthop Relat Res 16:119, 1960

137. Jones AR: Hallux valgus in the adolescent. Proc R Soc Medicine (Sect Ortho) 41:392, 1948

138. Durman DC: Metatarsus primus varus and hallux valgus. AMA Arch Surg 74:128, 1957

139. Elftman H, Manter J: The evolution of the human foot with special reference to the joints. J Anat 70:56, 1935

140. Jones RL: The human foot. An experimental study of its mechanics and the role of its muscles and ligaments in the support of the arch. Am J Anat 68:1, 1941

141. Manter JT: Distribution of compression forces in the joints of the human foot. Anat Rec 96:313, 1946

142. Mayo CH: The surgical treatment of bunion. Ann Surg 48:300, 1908

143. Nilsonne H: Hallux rigidus and its treatment. Acta Orthop Scand 1:295, 1930

144. Stokes IAF, Hutton WC, Evans MJ: The effects of hallux valgus and Keller's operation on the load-bearing function of the foot during walking. Acta Orthop Belg 41:695, 1975

145. Stokes IAF, Hutton WC, Stott JRR, Lowe LW: Forces under the hallux valgus foot before and after surgery. Clin Orthop Relat Res 142:64, 1979

146. Hutton WC, Dhanendran M: The mechanics of normal and hallux valgus feet—a quantitative study. Clin Orthop Relat Res 157:7, 1981

147. Wyss UP, McBride I, Murphy L, Cooke TDV, Olney SJ: Joint reaction forces at the first MTP joint in a normal elderly population. J Biomech 23:977, 1990

148. Morton DJ: Hypermobility of the first metatarsal bone, the interlinking factor between metatarsalgia and longitudinal arch strains. J Bone Joint Surg 10:187, 1928

149. Galland WI, Jordan H: Hallux valgus. Surg Gynecol Obstet 66:95, 1938

150. Goldner JL, Gaines RW: Adult and juvenile hallux valgus: analysis and treatment. Orthop Clin North Am 7:863, 1976

151. Lundberg BJ, Sulja T: Skeletal parameters in the hallux valgus foot. Acta Orthop Scand 43:576, 1972

152. Inman VT: Hallux valgus, a review of etiological factors. Orthop Clinics North Am 5:59, 1974

153. Greenberg GS: Relationship of hallux abductus angle and first metatarsal angle to severity of pronation. J Am Podiatry Assoc 69:29, 1979

154. Ross FD: The relationship of abnormal foot pronation to hallux abducto valgus, a pilot study. Prosthet Orthotics Int 10:72, 1986

155. Stevenson MR: A study of the correlation between neutral calcaneal stance position and relaxed calcaneal stance position in the development of hallux abducto valgus. Master's thesis, Curtin University of Technology, Perth, Western Australia, 1991

156. Hicks JH: The mechanics of the foot. IV. The action of the muscles on the foot in standing. Acta Anat 27:180, 1955

157. Henderson MS: The human foot: functional development and weaknesses. Minn Med 16:323, 1933

158. Ceeney E: Form of the foot in relation to footwear. Chiropodist 8:304, 1953

159. Root ML, Orien WP, Weed JH: Normal and Abnormal Function of the Foot. Clinical Biomechanics Corporation, Los Angeles, 1977

160. Mennell J: Footgear and common sense. Br Med J 2:1107, 1939

161. Lindsay EA: The tragedy of footwear. Lancet 2:1209, 1939

162. Emslie M: Prevention of foot deformities in children. Lancet ii:1260, 1939

163. Phillips RD, Reczek DM, Fountain D, Renner J, Park DB: Modification of high-heeled shoes to decrease pronation during gait. J Am Podiatr Med Assoc 81:215, 1991

164. Hoffman P: Conclusions drawn from a comparative study of the feet of barefooted and shoe-wearing peoples. Am J Orthop Surg 3:115, 1905
165. Inman VT (ed): DuVries' Surgery of the Foot. 3rd Ed. CV Mosby, St. Louis, 1973
166. Mann RA, Coughlin MJ: Hallux valgus: etiology, anatomy, treatment and surgical considerations. Clin Orthop Rel Res 157:32, 1981
167. Harris RI, Beath T: The short first metatarsal: its incidence and clinical significance. J Bone Joint Surg Am 31:553, 1949

# 4

# Review of Adult Foot Radiology

*LAWRENCE OSHER*

In the workup of a hallux valgus deformity the practitioner is often faced with unexpected radiographic findings. Usually, the first course of action is to order additional pedal studies, which may provide the additional detail needed to help resolve or localize the apparent pathology. If the problem is within the purview of conventional radiography, a library text, if available, is often hurriedly consulted.

It is clearly not possible to encompass all of pedal radiology within the confines of a single chapter of this volume. Designed for the physician already familiar with basic musculoskeletal radiographic terminology, the following information will serve as a handy outline of foot pathology that may be encountered in the routine workup of the patient with hallux valgus deformity. Particular effort has been given to simplify the process of generating basic differential diagnoses. Pictorial examples are provided throughout this chapter.

## RECOMMENDED APPROACH TO THE PEDAL RADIOGRAPH

Basic radiographic findings are not necessarily commonly seen. Their correct description, utilizing objective radiologic terminology and subsequent categorization, is vital to the generation of an appropriate differential. Traditional radiographic approaches often prescribe that, for every bone lesion, the following disease categories must be routinely considered:

Developmental anomalies
Trauma
Dysplasias and dysostoses

Metabolic disease (dystrophies included)
Infections and inflammatory processes
Tumor and tumor-like conditions
Degenerative disease and ischemic necrosis

However, this approach is presumptive; not only is an understanding of these basic bone radiographic changes clearly required, but one is expected to identify and then classify any lesion(s). Many radiographic bony abnormalities simply cannot be categorized at first glance by the average physician, despite the ability to correctly describe the basic pathologic changes. For these practitioners, a more intuitive approach utilizing clinical and laboratory data is required (studies clearly show improved accuracy in the reading of radiographs when appropriate clinical and laboratory data are provided). The following steps are recommended:

1. Identify the given views.
2. Discern *normal* from *abnormal* by describing any pathology in standard objective radiographic terminology.
3. Note available clinical and laboratory data.
4. Synthesize objective radiographic findings (item 2, above) with the significant clinical and laboratory data (3) to designate a spectrum of possible disease states in which both the radiographic and the clinical data could occur.
5. Rank individual diseases of this spectrum (4) as to their probability of occurrence, that is, most likely to least probable. This is the essence of differential diagnosis.
6. Suggest additional radiographic or other studies that might assist further in the differential diagnosis.

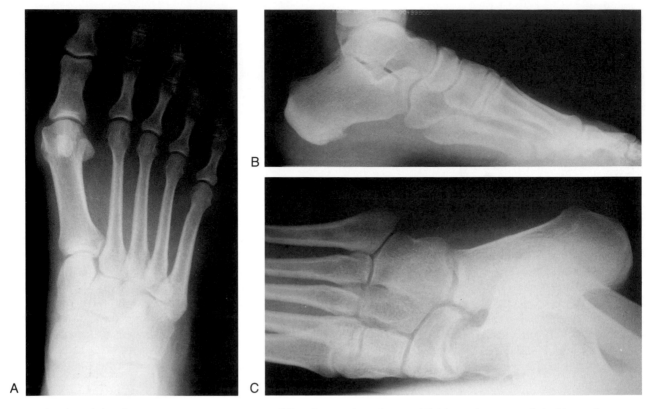

**Fig. 4-1.** (**A**) Reference anteroposterior view. (**B**) Reference lateral view. (**C**) Thirty-degree medial oblique foot view demonstrating incomplete calcaneonavicular coalition. Note separation between second and third cuneiforms.

A standard bone survey should be ordered whenever there is suspicion of multiple areas of involvement other than the foot. The standard bone survey comprises these radiographs:

Two views of skull
Two views of lumbar or thoracic spine
Anteroposterior view of pelvis
Anteroposterior views of arms and thighs

## REVIEW OF INDICATIONS FOR THE BASIC ADJUNCT PEDAL VIEWS

It will be helped to first study the reference anteroposterior (Fig. 4-1A) and reference lateral views (Fig. 4-1B) before reviewing the following lists.

1. Medial oblique (−15° to 30°) (Fig. 4-1C)
     Jone's fracture/base of fifth metatarsal
     Lateral digits
     Posterolateral talar process
     Most accessory bones *except* os tibial externum
     Lesser metatarsal head and base pathology
     Lateral plantar calcaneus/foraminae
     Subungual exostosis
     Fibular sesamoid (10° study)
2. Isherwood medial oblique 45°–60°. This view will not visualize middle subtalar joint detail (Fig. 4-2).
     Anterior facet of talocalcaneal joint
     Anterior process os calcis
     Calcaneonavicular coalition
     Steidas process of talus
3. Lateral oblique (15°–30°) (Fig. 4-3)
     Accessory navicular (os tibial externum)
     Haglund's disease/navicular pathology
     Cornuate/"gorilloid" navicular

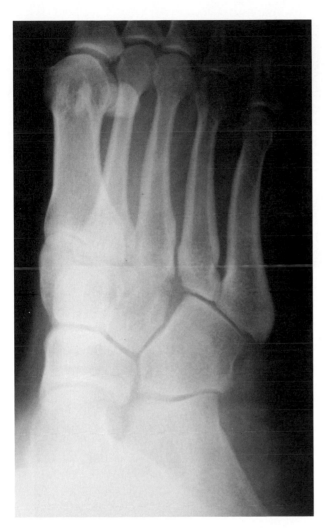

**Fig. 4-2.** Isherwood medial oblique demonstrating normal shape of anterior calcaneal process. Note separation between third cuneiform and cuboid bones.

Fracture medial cuneiform
First metatarsophalangeal joint (MPJ) and medial
  hallux detail
Possible talonavicular coalition
Subungual exostosis/osteochondroma distal
  phalanx
Tibial sesamoid bone (45°–60°)
4. Hallux lateral
  Skyline hallux
  Distraction, sesamoid fracture at MPJ

Interphalangeal sesamoid
Subungual exostoses and osteochondroma
Plantar cortex of distal phalanx
5. Harris–Beath (Fig. 4-4A)
  T-C coalitions (Fig. 4-4B), posterior and middle
  facet evaluation. (The anterior facet *cannot* be
  visualized adequately.)
  Coronoaxial skyline of the sustentaculum tali.
  Fractures of the os calcis, to evaluate posterior
  facet for longitudinal split as well as calcaneal
  foreshortening. These may be combined with
  various oblique axial views (Broden, Anthon-
  sen, etc.).
  Arthritic changes of the subtalar joint.
6. Calcaneal axial
  Skyline of os calcis, which images cortical loss,
  protrusions, or promontories. The subtalar
  joint is not imaged.
  True space occupying lesions of the calcaneal
  body should be discriminated from a pseudo-
  cystic foramen calcaneum.
  Varus deformity of os calcis.
  Post trauma to rearfoot.
7. Forefoot (sesamoid) axial (Fig. 4-5A)
  Hypertrophic plantar metatarsal condyles
  Structural abnormalities of metatarsals, best visu-
    alized in coronal plane
    Changes to cristae
    Differentiation of symmetrically placed medial
      first metatarsal head erosions from cysts
      (Fig. 4-5B)
  Sesamoid detail
    Fractures
    Arthritic changes (cysts, erosions, bony prolif-
      erations, fusions)
  Sesamoid position (preoperative evaluation)
  Foreign bodies in plantar forefoot
  Base of metatarsal bones

## THE BASIC PEDAL RADIOGRAPHIC DIFFERENTIALS

The following section is intended as a summation of commonly encountered pathologic conditions in pedal radiology. Topics such as bone tumors and con-

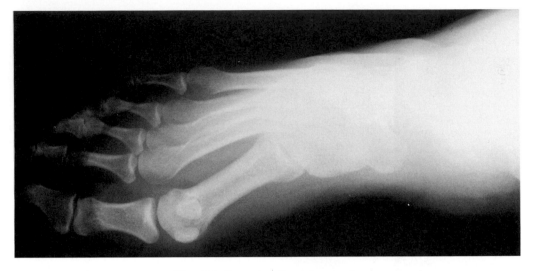

**Fig. 4-3.** Lateral oblique foot study.

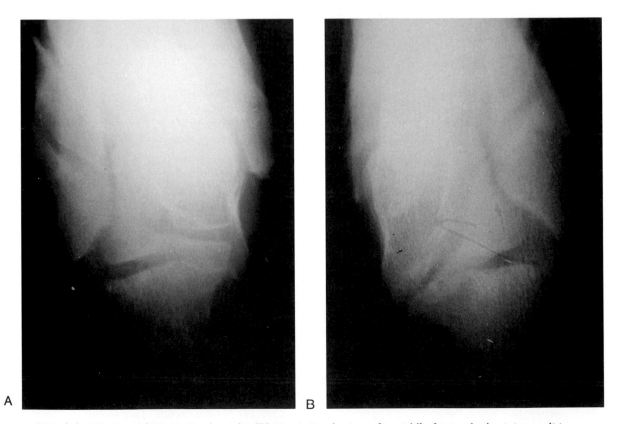

**Fig. 4-4.** (**A**) Normal Harris-Beath study. (**B**) Harris-Beath view of a middle facet subtalar joint coalition.

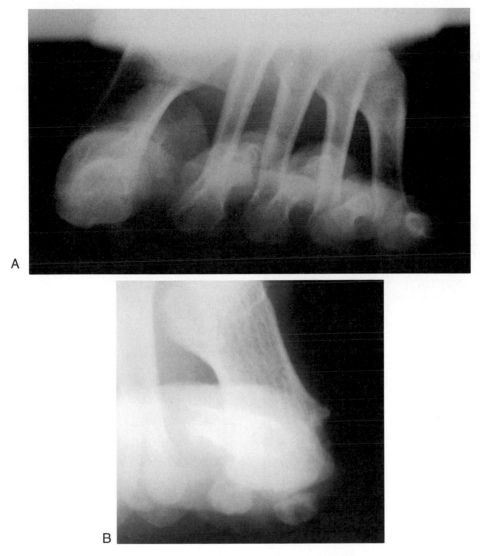

**Fig. 4-5.** (**A**) Normal forefoot axial study. (**B**) Magnification of forefoot axial study showing large (10.0-mm) medial first metatarsal head erosion in a patient with chronic gouty arthritis. Note cystic/erosive change tibial sesamoid bone.

genital disorders are beyond the scope of this chapter and are not included.

## The Common Arthropathies

### Adult Rheumatoid Arthritis

1. General features
   Articular complaints of the small joints of hands and feet; initial pedal onset occurs in approxi-mately 15 percent of patients. These may be asymmetric initially, but eventually are bilaterally and symmetrically distributed in the joints.
   Remissions and exacerbations may occur, with the remission period not exceeding 3 months.
   Occurrence is bilateral and symmetrical.
   Typical forefoot target zones
      Fifth MPJ, most common medically and later-ally

Medial interphalangeal joint (IPJ) hallux
Medial aspects of first through fourth metatarsal heads
2. Early radiographic features (predominantly MPJs (metatarsal heads) and medial IPJ hallux)
   Fusiform soft tissue swelling
   Juxta-articular osteopenia
   Concentric joint space narrowing
   Small para-articular cystic erosions (<5 mm)
3. Progressive forefoot radiographic findings (Fig. 4-6)

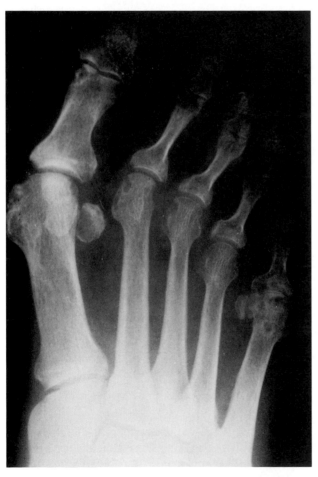

**Fig. 4-6.** Progressive forefoot radiographic changes. Extensive erosive changes are noted of the first, second, third, and fifth metatarsal heads. In addition, the medial aspect of the hallux IP joint is involved. Note the absence of PIP and DIP joint involvement and presence of cyst formation on fifth metatarsal head.

Cysts/pseudocysts
Erosive involvement of base of proximal phalanges
Osseous "island" formation (fifth metatarsal head)
Digital deformities; deviations and subluxations
Nonosseous (fibrous) ankylosis (exceptions; carpus and tarsus)
4. Midfoot and rearfoot radiographic findings (forefoot involvement typically precedes rearfoot by many years)
   Rigid flatfoot deformity common
   Bony ankylosis of tarsal joints
   Concentric narrowing of tarsal/intertarsal joints, which may lack juxta-articular osteoporosis and typically lack periarticular erosive changes
   Secondary osteoarthritis, especially talonavicular joint and posterior facet of subtalar joint
   "Bywater's" retrocalcaneal bursal lytic lesions

### Spondyloarthropathies (Seronegative Arthritides)

1. Clinical characteristics of the seronegative arthritides
   Familial tendency
   Sacroiliitis
   Mucocutaneous affectations
   Major types (considerable clinical overlap exists)
      Psoriatic arthritis
      Reiter's disease
      Enteropathic arthritis
      Ankylosing spondylitis
   Target sites
      Early digital and heel involvement with enthesopathic findings
      MPJs, proximal interphalangeal joints (PIPJs), and distal interphalangeal joints (DIPJs)
      Hallucal sesamoids
      Calcaneus, ankle and knee joints
2. Pedal radiographic changes of seronegative arthritis (Figs. 4-7 to 4-10)
   Early changes soft tissues are nonspecific.
   Asymmetric dactylitis (Fig. 4-7) exhibits profound fusiform digital soft tissue swelling secondary to joint effusions, and flexor tenosynovitis with or without periostitis.

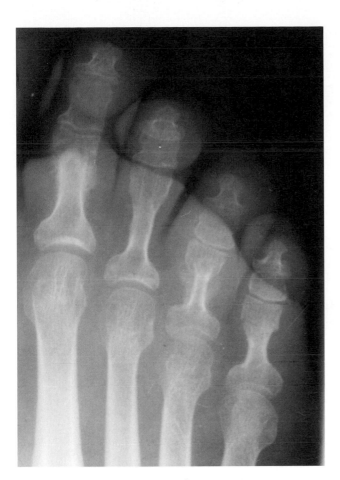

**Fig. 4-7.** Asymmetric dactylitis with periostitis of second and fourth toes in a patient with Reiter's disease.

Underlying osseous changes may be present in approximately 50 percent of patients.

Periosteal apposition adjacent to symptomatic joints and tendoligamentous attachments occurs during symptomatic periods.

Osteosclerosis is common but osteoporosis is lacking.

Poorly defined juxta-articular erosions are common with marginal "whiskering periostitis."

Intra-articular bony ankylosis is also common, especially psoriatic arthritis (Fig. 4-8).

Joint space narrowing is uniform.

Acrolysis is present (Fig. 4-9).

Minimal cyst formation occurs.

Erosive and proliferative bony calcaneal changes occur (Fig. 4-10).

3. General comparison of adult rheumatoid arthritis versus seronegative arthritis

Seronegative arthritis lacks nodules.

Bilateral asymmetric presentation is common in seronegative arthritis (oligoarticular).

These following joints are uncommonly involved in adult rheumatoid arthritis:

DIPJs

PIPJs (in foot only)

Sacroiliac (SI) joints (symmetric)

Thoracolumbar joint

Dactylitis and enthesopathies are common (initial) complaints in seronegative arthritis; early heel complaints occur in seronegative arthropathies.

Seronegative arthritis often lacks profound osteopenia.

Seronegative arthritis lacks significant cystic degeneration.

Rheumatoid arthritis lacks periostitis and acrolysis.

Medial, lateral, and central erosive changes to IP hallux occur in rheumatoid arthritis.

## Psoriatic Arthritis

1. Correlative clinical data of psoriatic arthritis

Good correlation between nail changes and arthritis (not skin)

Bilateral asymmetric oligoarthritis

Five patterns of arthritic attack

Asymmetric oligoarthritis (70 percent)

Symmetric polyarthritis (15 percent)

DIP joint only (5 percent)

Arthritis mutilans (5 percent)

Ankylosing spondylitis (5 percent)

Target sites

IP hallux (considered the most destructive arthropathy of the hallucal IP joint)

PIPs, DIPs, and MPs

Sesamoids

Calcaneus (Resnick's sites 2–5)

Ankle joint

2. Radiographic changes of psoriatic arthritis in foot

Normodensity or osteopenia seen during acute phases (typically ephemeral)

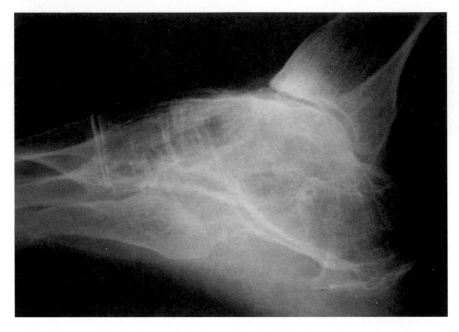

**Fig. 4-8.** Generalized bony ankylosis along with a large "fluffy" infracalcaneal spur in a patient with mutilating psoriatic arthritis.

Bony ankylosis of DIPJs, PIPJs, and MPJs as well as tarsal bones (Note: As many as 30 percent of joints in psoriatic arthritis fuse) (Fig. 4-8)

Joint space widening and narrowing

Subchondral sclerosis

Localized osteosclerosis

Marginal joint "mouse-ear" erosions that may be obscured by periosteal reaction

Resorption and proliferative osseous changes that may lead to arthritis mutilans with typical "pencil-and-cup" deformities or to digital contractions/subluxations

"Ivory phalanx syndrome," or profound osteosclerosis of hallucal distal phalanx secondary to condensation of bone on periosteal and endosteal surfaces (Fig. 4-9)

Generalized sclerosis of os calcis and large, poorly defined "fluffy" spurs during symptomatic periods

Asymmetric digital dactylitis (Fig. 4-7)

Distal phalangeal tuft resorption (acro-osteolysis) (Fig. 4-9)

## Reiter's Disease

1. Correlative clinical data of Reiter's disease
     Young males
     Urethritis (typically nongonococcal) or enteritis
     Conjunctivitis
     Mucocutaneous lesions
         Keratodermia blennorrhagicum
         Balanitis
         Mouth
     Arthritis
         Not common in upper extremities
         Dactylitis or heel pain a common initial complaint
         Joint deformity not as severe as in psoriatic arthritis
         Forefoot joint involvement typically monoarticular
         End-stage arthritis mutilans rare (Launois' deformity)
   Pedal target sites
     MTP joints

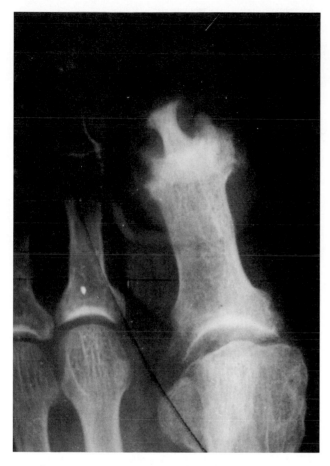

**Fig. 4-9.** Psoriatic arthritis. Visible is an "ivory" osteosclerotic distal phalanx of hallux. Note the acrolysis as well as intra-articular bony ankylosis of the IP joint.

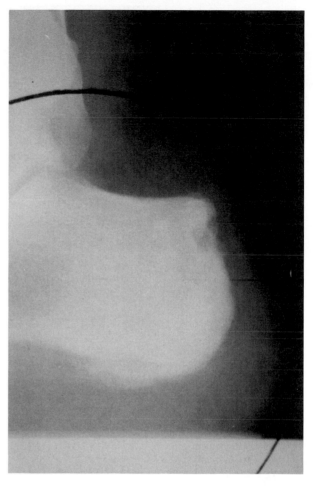

**Fig. 4-10.** Seronegative heel showing typical erosive finding of retrocalcaneal bursal area and also large "fluffy" heel spur at infracalcaneal attachment of plantar fascia/intrinsics. Note generalized sclerosis of os calcis.

   First IP joint, medial and lateral
   Calcaneus
   Achilles tendon
   Ankle joint
2. Radiographic features of Reiter's disease versus psoriatic arthritis
   Except for the hallux IP joint, DIP and PIP joint involvement is not as common as in psoriatic arthritis.
   There is a greater tendency for osteopenic changes in Reiter's, particularly during acute phases (which last longer). Normal mineralization then returns.
   There is also a lesser tendency for bony ankylosis in Reiter's disease.

   Early loss of retrocalcaneal recess along with achilles tendon swelling is common; subjacent erosive and proliferative calcaneal lesions (sites 1, 2, & 4) occur in Reiter's disease (Fig. 4-10).
   Joint space widening is not uncommon in psoriatic arthritis.

**Osteoarthritis (Degenerative Joint Disease)**

1. Correlative clinical data of pedal osteoarthritis
   This is typically a secondary osteoarthritis. It is commonly accepted that an association exists with pathomechanics/altered stress patterns

across joint(s) associated with the following:
First MPJ axis of motion/instant center altera-
tion
Angle of metatarsus adductus
First ray pathomechanics with pronation
Sagittal plane elevation of first metatarsal/ray
Other typical forms of secondary pedal osteoar-
thritis
Trauma: osteochondritis dissecans, Freiberg's
infraction, post sprains and fractures
Congenital: tarsal coalitions, hereditary multi-
ple exostosis, multiple epiphyseal dysplasia
Arthritides: rheumatoid arthritis, calcium pyro-
phosphate dihydrate deposition disease
(CPPD).
Iatrogenic: after hallux abducto valgus surgery
Common pedal target sites
First MP joint(s)
Medial column joints (greater mobility with
pronation)
Joints previously traumatized
2. Radiographic changes in osteoarthritis (Fig. 4-11)
Unilaterally or bilaterally asymmetric
Minimal soft tissue signs
Asymmetric/focal (symmetric narrowing late)
joint space narrowing
Subchondral sclerosis/eburnation
Subchondral cysts
Marginal osteophytes
Paucity of periarticular fragmentation
Absent erosions

### Erosive Osteoarthritis

1. Key clinical data of erosive osteoarthritis
Occur predominantly in postmenopausal
women
Pedal target sites most often IP joints
2. Radiographic changes in erosive osteoarthritis
Soft tissue swelling
Marginal osteophyte formation
Central joint space erosive changes producing a
typical "seagull" appearance
Bony ankylosis common and may dominate ra-
diographic picture

### Gouty Arthritis

1. Correlative clinical data of gouty arthritis
Pedal target sites may involve any site in the foot.

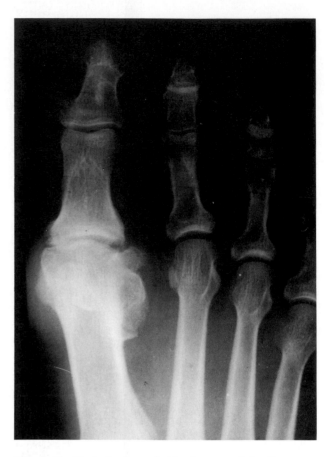

**Fig. 4-11.** Typical osteoarthritic changes of the first metatarsophalangeal joint include focal narrowing, subchondral
sclerosis, and marginal osteophytosis/proliferative changes
including sesamoids.

First MPJ arthritis (65 percent initially, 90 per-
cent at some time)
Hallux IP joint
Tarsometatarsal joint (see Fig. 4-13)
Ankle joint
2. Early radiographic changes (Fig. 4-12A)
Extreme periarticular soft tissue swelling
Significant osseous changes absent
Typically monoarticular
3. Late (chronic) changes
Joint space preserved until late
Asymmetric polyarticular (chronic)
Erosions (Fig. 4-12B and C)
Juxta-articular/para-articular
May be extra-articular

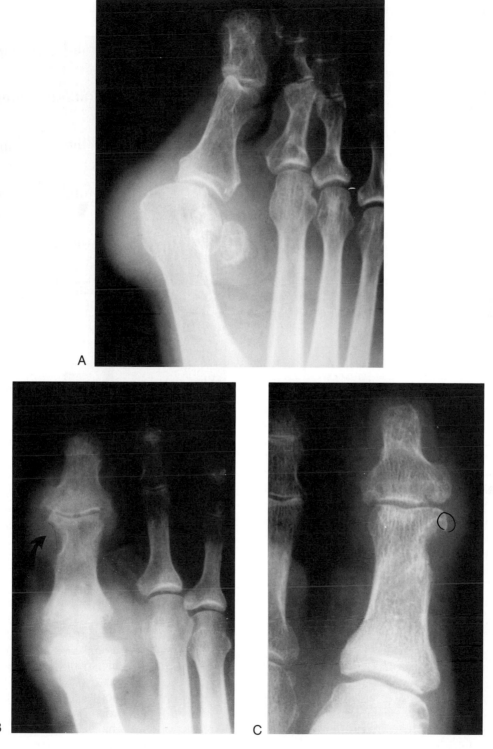

**Fig. 4-12.** (**A**) Acute gouty arthritis of the first metatarsophalangeal joint. (**B**) Chronic gouty arthritis. Visible is a large erosive change of hallucal proximal phalanx (10.0 mm) that is clearly both extra-articular as well as periarticular. Note eccentric soft tissue tophae of IPJ and MPJ. (**C**) Large erosive change of medial hallucal proximal phalanx along with lateral erosive change at IP joint margin. These changes are unusual in adult rheumatoid arthritis. Note the subchondral density is normal.

Large size (often >5.0 mm) with "punched-out" appearance

Overhanging, proliferative margins (Martel's sign)

Sclerotic lining

Tophi (Fig. 4-12B)

Eccentric focal soft tissue masses typically with subjacent erosions (versus rheumatoid arthritis nodules)

May rarely become calcified

Subchondral bony density typically unchanged (normodensity)

Bony ankylosis and periostitis not overall prominent features

Osseous infarcts

End-stage osteolysis may mimic malignancy or somewhat resemble Charcot joint disease (especially when midfoot is involved) (Fig. 4-13)

### Systemic Lupus Erythermatosus

1. Correlative clinical data of systemic lupus erythermatosus (SLE)

    Young females, increased incidence in blacks

    Deforming, nonerosive arthritis of two or more joints

    Multisystem, including central nervous system (CNS) (seizures, etc.), pulmonary (effusions, pleuritis, etc.), renal (to 50 percent glomerulonephritis), cardiac, and skin (malar butterfly or discoid plaquelike scaling

    Pedal target sites

    MPJs

    Terminal phalangeal tufts (occasionally)

2. Radiographic changes in SLE

    Bilateral and symmetrical joint involvement

    Soft tissue swelling

    Juxta-articular osteopenia

    Minimal/absent joint space narrowing

    Deforming, nonerosive arthropathy involving MPJs (reversible) with subluxations and dislocations

    Symmetric polyarthritis

    Osteonecrosis/Freiberg-like deformities

    Soft tissue calcifications

    Occasional acrolysis of distal phalanges

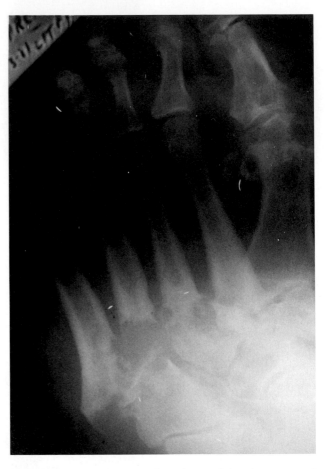

**Fig. 4-13.** Extensive osteolysis base of fourth metatarsal bone in a patient with chronic gouty arthritis. The changes may otherwise resemble charcot joint arthropathy.

### Septic Arthritis

1. Correlative clinical data of septic arthritis

    This is an acute, red, hot monoarticular arthritis.

    It may occur secondary to hematogenous osteomyelitis in adults and infants or otherwise in certain joints in children where the metaphysis is intra-articular (e.g., hip).

    Associated signs and conditions in adult patients

    Debilitation

    I.V. drug user

    Prosthetic joint

    Direct trauma

    Contiguous osteomyelitis

    Post gonorrheal infection

2. Radiographic changes in suppurative (pyogenic) arthritis

    Soft tissue swelling about joint

    Poorly marginated osseous erosions (peripheral periarticular "bare" areas and/or central involvement)

    Central joint space erosions

    Rapid (1–3 weeks) concentric chondrolysis/joint space narrowing

    Reactive sclerosis (lacks osteopenia)

    Eventual intra-articular bony ankylosis

    Involvement of adjacent bony structures producing classic picture of osteomyelitis

3. Radiographic changes in nonsuppurative, tuberculous arthritis

    Phemister's triad

        Gradual (slow) loss of joint space

        Juxta-articular osteoporosis

        Peripheral osseous erosions

    Subchondral osseous erosions, central and peripheral (peripheral are seen more often in hip/knee/ankle)

    Tendency toward fibrous ankylosis

    Late joint space loss

    Less periostitis than pyogenic and gonorrheal

4. Correlative clinical data of gonococcal arthritis

    Male > female

    Onset sudden or insidious

    Days 1 to 3

        Systemic signs/symptoms

        Rash and fever/chills

    Days 4 to 6

        Pauciarticular or polyarticular

        Small joints of foot

        Enthesopathy, calcaneous

        Knee > ankle > wrist > shoulder > foot > spine

        Lower extremities > upper extremities

    Associated with multiple joints and tenosynovitis

5. Radiographic findings in gonococcal arthritis

    As with pyogenic if untreated

    Osteoporosis and soft tissue swelling if treated

### Charcot Joint Arthropathy

1. Differential diagnosis of disorders that may produce a radiographic picture of neuropathic joint disease

    Diabetes mellitus

    Tertiary syphilis

    Congenital indifference to pain

    Other neuropathic etiologies

        Syringomyelia

        Spina bifida

        Charcot-Marie-Tooth disease (rare)

        Post-trauma

    Pyrophosphate arthropathy (talonavicular joint)

    Idiopathic osteonecrosis of navicular

    Avascular necrosis of talus

    Hemophilia

    Primary amyloidosis

    Post sympathectomy

2. Correlative clinical data of diabetic Charcot joint arthropathy

    About 1 percent incidence among diabetic patients

    Signs typically worse than symptoms

    Soft tissue swelling with increased range of motion (ROM) and subsequent decreased ROM often with crepitus

    Associated with long-standing diabetes, poor control, and diabetic neuropathy

    Pedal target sites

    Weight-bearing "hypertrophic":

        Ankle joint (Fig. 4-14)

        Lisfranc's joint (Fig. 4-15.)

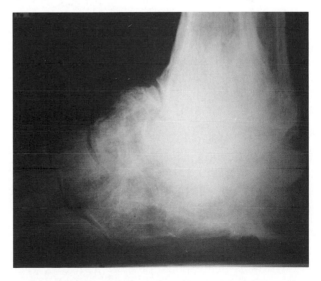

**Fig. 4-14.** "Hypertrophic" Charcot joint deformity of the ankle in a patient with underlying neuropathy.

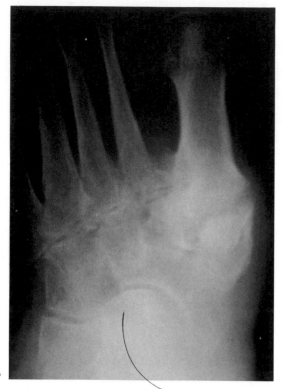

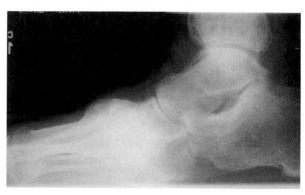

**Fig. 4-15.** (**A**) Anteroposterior view of hypertrophic Charcot joint deformity of Lisfranc's joint with resultant cube-foot deformity. (**B**) Lateral view of cube-foot deformity (same patient as in Fig. 4-15A).

Chopart's joint
Subtalar joints (rarer)
Non-weight-bearing atrophic:
  IP and MP joints
  Ankle joint (rare)
3. Radiographic findings in diabetic neuroarthropathy (Charcot joints)
  Early
    Soft tissue swelling
    Digital subluxation
    Well-defined metaphyseal cortical defects
    Circumscribed zone of osteopenia
    Subchondral "picture-framing" osteopenia
    Possible underlying fracture
  Progressive
    Poorly defined metaphyseal cortical defects
    Periosteal reaction
    Extensive osseous erosion and lysis (Fig. 4-16A)
    Fragmentation

*Note:* The radiographic changes in this stage mimic acute, direct-extension osteomyelitis. However, the presence of osteopenia and lysis suggests an intact vascular supply, and should not be misconstrued as a criterion to amputate.
Late, with significant weight-bearing (see Figs. 4-14 and 4-15)
  Generalized sclerosis adjacent to site
  Variable joint space narrowing
  Extensive osseous fragmentation
  Hypertrophic "bulky" osteophytes
  Severe destruction/disorganization
  "Cube foot" forefoot abduction (Fig. 4-15A and B)
  Occasional bony ankylosis
Late, without significant weight-bearing (Fig. 4-16B)
  Sclerotic "pointed tubular bone" deformity with diaphyseal sparing

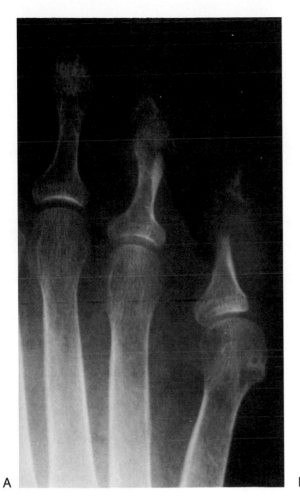
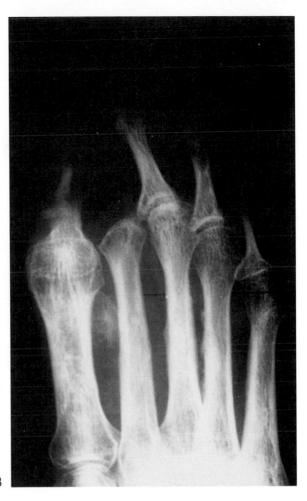

A

B

**Fig. 4-16.** (**A**) Progressive stage of diabetic osteolysis of the fifth toe. These changes are radiographically indistinguishable from acute osteomyelitis (direct-extension type). (**B**) End-stage pointed tubular bone deformities in a patient with underlying neuropathy.

Overt osteolysis
Restitution of integrity (forefoot)
Arthritis mutilans
Ankylosis not uncommon

### Diffuse Idiopathic Skeletal Hyperostosis

1. Correlative clinical data for diffuse idiopathic skeletal hyperostosis (DISH)
   Older than 50 years
   Common axial syndesmophyte disease with appendicular manifestations
   Males > females

Benign nature of complaints; back stiffness with mild pain, talalgia, "tennis elbow," dysphagia
Not a true arthropathy
Pedal target areas, attachments of major soft tissue tendons and ligaments into bone (pure enthesopathy)
2. Pedal radiographic findings (Fig. 4-17), enthesopathic osseous spurring
   Common in dorsal midfoot
   Calcaneus: large, poorly defined osseous appositions frequent at all major attachment sites
   Base of fifth metatarsal
   Anteriomedial navicular

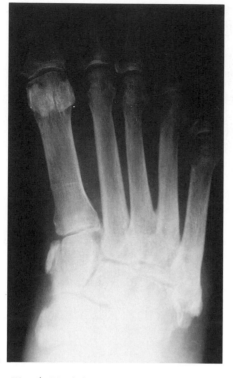

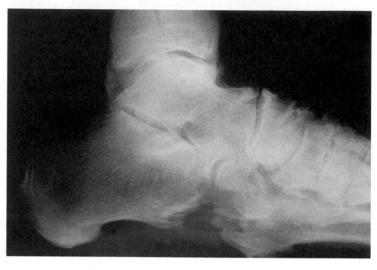

**Fig. 4-17.** (**A**) Anteroposterior view of midfoot of 91-year-old woman with underlying diffuse idiopathic skeletal hyperostosis. Extensive osseous apposition is noted at attachments sites of the flexor hallucis brevis (sesamoids), peroneus brevis, and anterior tibial tendons. (**B**) DISH. This lateral view of same patient in Fig. 4-15A shows extensive dorsal midfoot spurring as well as calcaneal and deltoid ligamentous involvements.

Medial first cuneiform
Hallucal sesamoids
Forefoot joint capsular ossific spurring late (>75 years)
Metatarsal shafts (inconsistent)
Soft tissue ossification/calcifications not uncommon
3. Postoperative new bone formation of implants

## Basic Differentials of "Solid" Periostitis

Solid periostitis is basically a reaction to some subperiosteal or extraperiosteal irritant. Common causes include the following:

Osteomyelitis
Arthritis (seronegative, etc)
Bone tumor

Reaction to chronic soft tissue inflammation
Reaction to trauma/hematoma subperiosteal space
Healing fracture.

## Basic Differentials of Generalized (Symmetric) Solid Periostitis of Adults

1. Primary (familial, idiopathic) hypertrophic osteoarthropathy
   *Radiographic*
   Tarsals, metatarsals, and phalanges
   Diaphyseal/metaphyseal/epiphyseal
   "Shaggy" irregular periostitis (spiculated)
   Ligamentous ossification
2. Secondary hypertrophic osteoarthropathy (HOA) (Fig. 4-18)
   Underlying primary lesion (often bronchogenic cancer)

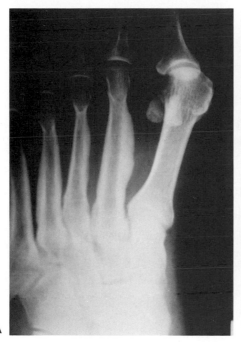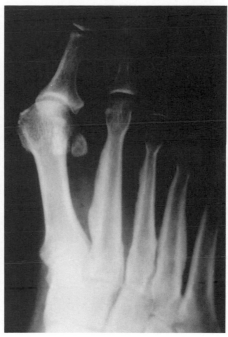

**Fig. 4-18.** **(A & B)** Secondary HOA. "Solid," linear periosteal new bone formation of metatarsal shafts 2, 3, and 4 bilaterally are seen in a patient with underlying oat cell lung carcinoma.

Joint symptoms and signs worse in 30 to 40 percent
*Radiographic*
Metatarsals and phalanges
Diaphyseal/metaphyseal
Often linear or laminated, regular or irregular periostitis
Periarticular osteoporosis and swelling
Differential diagnosis, DISH and juvenile rheumatoid arthritis

3. Thyroid acropachy
    Hyperthyroidism
    Clubbing
    Periostitis
    Exopthalmos
    Soft tissue swelling/myxedema
    *Radiographic*
    Diaphyseal
    Shaggy, spiculated periostitis

4. Hypervitaminosis A (may be residual in adults)
    *Radiographic*
    Metatarsals
    Diaphyseal only, periostitis

Wavy or undulating cortical hyperostosis
Other findings
    Epiphyseal, invagination and hypertrophy
    Metaphyseal widening, cupping, and shortening
    Premature closure of growth plates
5. Vascular insufficiency
6. Chronic venous stasis (tibial periostitis)
7. Polyarteritis nodosum
8. Tuberous sclerosis
9. Fluorosis
10. DISH (occasional)

## Selected Disorders of Increased Tubular Bony Diameters (and also Acropachy)

1. Diaphyseal
    Acromegaly
    Paget's disease
2. Metaphyseal
    Osteopetrosis (osteosclerotic)
    Pyle's disease (no osteosclerosis)
    Gaucher's disease (no osteosclerosis)

## Shortened Tubular Bone Deformities (Brachydactyly)

1. Hallux
   Diabetic neurotrophic osteoarthropathy
2. Phalanges and metatarsals
   Diabetic neurotrophic osteoarthropathy
   Idiopathic, isolated anomaly
   Rheumatoid arthritis
   Pseudohypoparathyroidism (especially first and fourth metatarsals)
   Pseudopseudohypoparathyroidism
   Turner syndrome (especially fourth metatarsal)
   Basal cell nevus syndrome
   Hereditary multiple exostoses
   Juvenile rheumatoid arthritis
   Infarction
   Trauma (fracture, burn, etc.)
   Sickle cell disease
3. Flattened metatarsal heads
   Freiberg's infraction
   Diabetic neurotrophic osteoarthropathy

## Some Disorders of Decreased Tubular Bony Diameters

1. Acromegaly
2. Diabetic neuro-osteoarthropathy (DNOAP)
3. Juvenile rheumatoid arthritis
4. Congenital syphilis

## Selected Pointed Tubular Bone Deformities

1. DNOAP
2. Psoriatic arthritis
3. Alcoholic neuroarthropathy
4. Scleroderma, dermatomyositis
5. Seronegative arthropathies
6. Buerger's disease (TAO)
7. Arteriosclerosis obliterans
8. Raynaud's disease

## Acrolysis

1. Idiopathic
2. Scleroderma
3. Psoriasis (see Fig. 4-9)

4. Neuroarthropathy
   Diabetes
   Tabes dorsales
   Syringomyelia
5. Hyperparathyroidism
6. Vascular
   TAO
   Raynaud's disease
7. Leprosy
8. Post Injury
   Frostbite
   Burns
9. Polyvinylchloride (PVC) workers
10. Dilantin and ergot therapy
11. Chronic gout (asymmetric)
12. Epidermolysis bullosa

## "Bone Within a Bone" Appearance

1. Osteopetrosis
2. Sickle cell disease
3. Sickle cell–$\beta$-thalassemia disease
4. Some heavy metal intoxications (e.g., phosphorus)
5. Chronic osteomyelitis
6. Congenital syphilis

## Selected Sclerotic Disorders (Internal Osseous Disorders)

1. Transverse metaphyseal banding
   Heavy metal (lead) poisoning
   Osteopetrosis
   Phosphorus osteopathy
   Scurvy
   Congenital syphilis (metaphysitis)
   Hypervitaminosis A and D
   Leukemia (acute)
   Reinforcement lines of osteoporosis
2. Solitary circumscribed foci of osteosclerosis
   Enostoses (bone islands)
   Osteoid osteoma (medullary)
   Osteoma
   Focal infarct (Fig. 4-19)
   Old nutrient foraminae (especially calcaneus)
   Healed fibrous bone lesion
3. Multiple circumscribed foci of osteosclerosis
   Osteopoikilosis
   Gardner syndrome (osteomata)
   Medullary fat necrosis/infarction

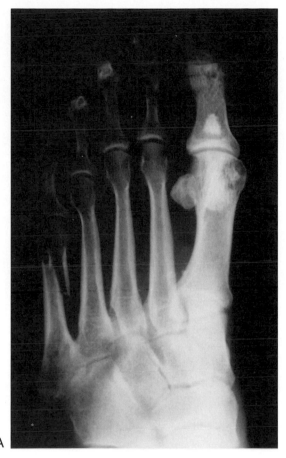

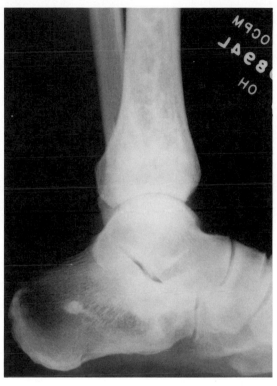

**Fig. 4-19.** (**A**) Base of hallucal proximal focal osteosclerotic infarct in a patient with alcoholic pancreatitis. (**B**) Focal osteosclerotic lesion of os calcis (same patient as in Fig. 4-19A). Considering the nonhealing fifth metatarsal fracture, sickle cell disease remained a primary disorder to rule out.

4. Patchy-diffuse osteosclerosis/sclerotic foci
   Previous infarct (may have serpiginous qualities)
   Endosteal fracture "callus"
   Fibrous dysplasia
   Sclerosing osteitis in infection
   Chronic osteomyelitis
   Osteoblastic metastases (breast, prostate)
   Idiopathic osteonecrosis (navicular)
   Paget's disease
   Secondary hyperparathyroidism
   Primary osteogenic bone tumors
   Fairbank disease
   Epiphyseal bone infarction:
      Osteochondroses
      Post-traumatic
      Systemic lupus erythematosus

   Metaphyseal bone infarction:
      Sickle cell disease
      Infiltrated collagen vasculitides diagnosis
      Infections in juxtametaphyses
      Pancreatitis (Fig. 4 20).
      Steroids (pheochromocytoma)
      Rheumatoid arthritis
   Granuloma
5. Diffuse sclerosis of bones
   Osteopetrosis/pycnodysostosis
   Paget's disease
   Hematopoietic disorders: mastocystosis, anemias, myelofibrosis, leukemias
   Metastases
   Hypervitaminosis A and D

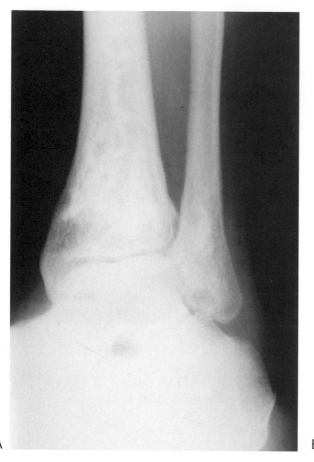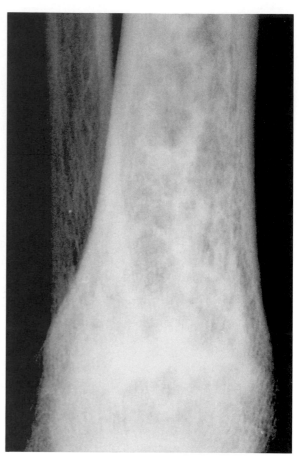

**Fig. 4-20.** (**A**) Patchy-diffuse intramedullary osteosclerosis of the distal tibia. Osteoslcerotic metatases must be ruled out. (**B**) Distal tibia (same patient as in Fig. 4-20A).

Hypo/pseudohypo- and pseudopseudohypo-parathyroidism
Fluorosis
Melorheostosis
Chronic osteomyelitis

## Selected Osteopenic Disorders

1. Subperiosteal resorption (rapid)
   Hyperparathyroidism
   Reflex sympathetic dystrophy syndrome (RSDS)
   Tendon avulsion (e.g., cortical desmoid)
2. Spotted deossification (rapid)
   Reflex sympathetic dystrophy syndrome (RSDS) (Fig. 4-21)
   Disuse osteoporosis (occasionally)

3. Generalized/nonregional (*, pediatric)
   Senile osteoporosis
   Osteomalacia (osteoporosis with bending)
   Rickets (osteoporosis with bending)*
   Chronic alcoholism
   Malabsorption/malnutrition
   Vitamin C (scurvy) deficiency*
   Neuromuscular diseases/cerebral palsy
   Osteogenesis imperfecta*
   Endocrine:
      Hyperparathyroidism/Renal Osteodystrophy*
      Hypogonadism
      Diabetes mellitus (long-standing, poor control)
      Cushing's disease
      Hyperthyroidism

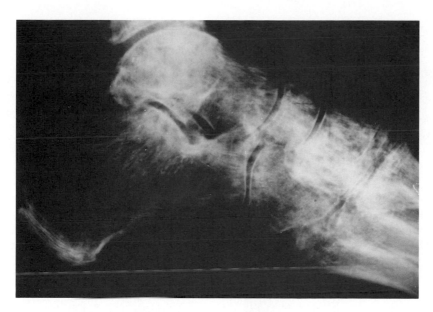

**Fig. 4-21.** "Spotty" juxta-articular or cancellous bony deossification in a patient with underlying reflex sympathetic dystrophy syndrome.

Hypothyroidism
Collagen diseases
Chronic anemias (e.g., iron deficiency)*
Multiple myeloma
Metastatic disease
Iatrogenic (steroids, heparin therapy)
4. Localized osteopenia
RSDS (may be seen as early as 3–4 weeks)
Post-traumatic disuse/immobilization atrophy (seen at about 8–10 weeks)
*Note:* Hawkin's sign, a favorable radiographic sign suggesting the potential to heal, is merely the presence of a thin zone of *subchondral* lucency of the talar dome at a time (usually 8–10 weeks post trauma) when disuse osteoporosis is radiographically apparent elsewhere.
Paget's disease (lytic phase I)
Regional migratory osteopenia
Tumor
Juvenile rheumatoid arthritis
Early osteomyelitis (Fig. 4-22)
5. Multiple radiolucencies, primarily in multiple metaphyses (modulation of normal growth pattern at the epiphyseal plate and metaphyseal junction)
Congenital syphilis

Hypervitaminosis A, excess osteoclastic activity in metaphysis with active new bone proliferation in diaphysis
Hypovitaminosis C, scurvy (Barlow's disease)
6. Reticular areas of radiolucency
Sickle cell anemia
Anemias, thalessemia
7. Regional osteopenic disorders/speckled or patchy multiple radiolucencies (may mimic "moth-eaten" destruction; typically involve cancellous bone)
Reflex sympathetic dystrophy syndrome (RSDS)
Rapidly forming osteoporoses
8. Focal osteopenia
Internal lysis
Acute osteomyelitis (see Fig. 4-22)

## Calcifications

Calcifications are typically classified into three categories. The first is metastatic, a disturbance of Ca and $PO_4$ metabolism (Ca × $PO_4$ >60–70); the second is calcinosis, in which Ca and $PO_4$ metabolism is normal; and third, dystrophic, wherein calcium is deposited in devitalized tissues.

1. Associated pathologies with metastatic calcification
Widespread bone resorption

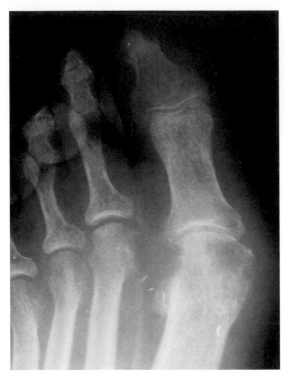

**Fig. 4-22.** Focal osteopenia of the medial first metatarsal head in acute osteomyelitis. An erosion of the terminal phalangeal tuft is also apparent.

Primary and secondary hyperparathyroidism
Hypoparathyroidism
Pseudohypoparathyroidism
Massive bone destructive processes
    Metastatic tumors
    Multiple myeloma
    Leukemia
Miscellaneous, such as gut absorption
    Sarcoidosis
    Hypervitaminosis D
    Idiopathic hypercalcemia
    Immobilization/paralysis
    Milk-alkali syndrome
    Cystic fibrosis
    Hyperphosphatemia
2. Idiopathic calcinosis
    Calcinosis interstialis universalis
    Tumoral calcinosis
    Calcific peritendinitis and bursitis
3. Dystrophic calcification associations

Postinfection, infestation
Ehlers–Danlos syndrome
Neoplasms/tumor necrosis
Trauma
Connective tissue diseases
Vascular disease
Neuropathy
Hematoma
Injection sites
Blunt trauma
4. Generalized calcinosis
    Calcinosis interstitialis universalis
        Longitudinal direction, plaque-like
        Skin and subcutaneous; occasionally tendons and muscles suggesting myositis, but no true bone formation occurs
    Tumoral calcinosis
        Often periarticular
        Large, solid, lobulated
    Collagen vascular diseases
        Dermatomyositis
            Fine, often reticular
            Associated with malignancies
            Often circumscribed (calcinosis circumscripta)
        Scleroderma with calcinosis (Thibierge–Weissenbach syndrome)
            Achilles tendon
            Forefoot
            Tuftal
            Leg; streaky or diffuse linear
            Circumscribed, lobulated or flocculent
5. Periarticular calcification(s)
    Synovial osteochondromatoses
    Calcific tendinitis
    Collagen vascular diseases
    Systemic lupus erythematosis
    Hyperparathyroidism and renal osteodystrophy
    Hypoparathyroidism
    Hypervitaminosis D
    Milk-alkali syndrome
    Tumoral calcinosis
    Calcinosis universalis
    Articular disorders
        CPPD
        Calcium hydroxyapatite deposition
        Gout
        Infection

6. Bursal, tendinous, or ligamentous calcifications
   Calcific bursitis
   Gout and pseudogout (Fig. 4-23)
   Hypervitaminosis D
   Calcium hydroxyappetite deposition disease
   Ochronosis, Wilson's disease
   Secondary hyperparathyroidism (occasionally primary)
7. Acral calcification
   Raynaud's disease
   Systemic lupus
   Scleroderma/CREST syndrome
   Dermatomyositis
   Calcinosis circumscripta universalis

## Vascular Calcifications

1. Monckeberg's medial sclerosis
2. Calcific arteriosclerosis
3. Intravascular phleboliths (rare in forefoot)
   Calcifications in veins
   Maffucci syndrome when pedal involvement is extensive (hemangiomas)
   Hemangioma

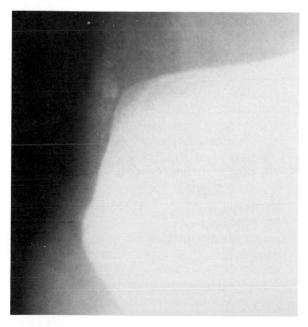

**Fig. 4-23.** CPPD. Note the fine, linear calcification in the achilles tendon.

4. Underlying calcifying disorder (especially secondary hyperparathyroidism in younger patients)
5. Premature atherosclerosis
   Nephrotic syndrome
   Hypothyroidism
   Diabetes
   Cushing syndrome

## Soft Tissue Ossification

1. Neoplasm (e.g., parosteal osteosarcoma)
2. Post-traumatic ossification
3. Ossifying hematoma
4. Surgical scar
5. Severe burns
6. Paralysis
7. Myositis ossificans
   Heterotopic ossification of soft tissue with metaplasia of the intermuscular connective tissue (not secondary to muscle inflammation)
8. Radiographic findings
   Soft tissue mass, early (possible association with periostitis, 7–10 days)
   Peripheral osteoid (lacy new bone) formation 4–6 weeks post injury
   Lucent, cystic central changes
   Maturity, 5–6 months; trabeculation apparent
   Radiolucent band (zone) between myositic mass and subjacent bone cortex
   Ectopic bone, usually lying along axis of involved muscle

## Appearance of Loose Intra-Articular Ossific Bodies

1. Avulsion fracture
2. Synovial osteochondromatoses
3. Osteochondral fracture
4. Degenerative joint disease
5. Freiberg's infraction
6. CPPD
7. DISH

## Dactylitis

1. Seronegative arthritis (with enthesopathy)
2. Sickle cell anemia
3. Spina ventosa/tuberculosis

4. Syphilis
5. Sarcoidosis (occasionally)
6. Traumatic periostitis

## Coarsened Trabecular Pattern

1. Paget's disease
2. Hemoglobinopathies
3. Gaucher's disease

## Heel Pad Thickening

This anomaly is defined with a non-weight-bearing lateral pedal view; in women, it is greater than 21 mm, and in men, greater than 23 mm.

1. Acromegaly
2. Dilantin therapy
3. Obesity
4. Peripheral edema
5. Myxedema
6. Infection

# OVERVIEW OF PEDAL APPLICATIONS FOR THE NEWER, "STATE-OF-THE-ART" ANCILLARY IMAGING MODALITIES

## Tomography: Overview and Advantages

Tomography is primarily indicated for imaging planar detail in areas of complex osseous anatomy. The tomographic principle allows for the "focusing-in" of a cross-sectioned anatomic plane by blurring all superimposed image detail outside of a predetermined focal plane. This focal plane lies at the system fulcrum, around which the x-ray tube head and film move in opposite directions. Those factors that increase the width of the blur (increasing angular arc, distance from film or focal plane), as well as the efficiency of blurring motion, improve the quality of the resultant studies.

Effective pedal imaging can usually be attained with either linear or circular tomography. However, the resolving power of complex or pleuridirectional (trispiral and hypocycloidal) tomography is superior to

that of plain film radiography in that it is able to "efface" the overlying bony cortex to allow for visualization of internal medullary osseous lesions. With respect to image quality, the orientation of x-ray tube travel can be significant in that maximum blurring occurs when the longitudinal axis of the part to be studied is perpendicular to the direction of tube travel.

Most pedal techniques employ 0.5-cm-slice thickness with wide-angle tomography (30°–50°). Wide-angle tomography is best for tissues with high inherent contrast (bone) but result in unacceptable soft tissue detail. In the foot, the true extent of geographic destruction within cancellous bone(s) may not be appreciated with plain film radiography. Tomography can often elucidate the extent of this involvement. However, prolonged exposure times to ionizing radiation are typically required. Largely replaced by computed tomography (CT) scanning, tomography of the foot still has one great advantage over modern CT scans, that is, the ability to directly image sagittal plane detail in all patients.

### Primary Disadvantages of Tomography

1. Radiation dosage
2. Ghost images
3. Availability (particularly pleuridirectional units)
4. Poor soft tissue visualization
5. Superimposed blurring

### Major Pedal Indications

1. Orthogonal plane imaging of the tarsal bones (especially sagittal plane)
2. Infection (bony involvement)
   Determination of the limits/extent of destruction, particularly when cancellous bone is involved
   Periosteal reactions
   Sequestrum
3. Tarsal coalitions
4. Imaging of destruction/tumors/internal margination of bone
   Small caliber, lacking significant osteosclerosis (e.g., medullary osteoid osteoma
   Geographic and/or moth-eaten destruction in cancellous bony areas
   Cortical erosion
   Matrix details inferior to CT scans

5. Postoperative complications
    Bone graft incorporation
    Metallic implant problems
6. Trauma
    General evaluation of tarsal bony fracture(s)
    Talar stiedas process fractures
    Ankle joint pathology, e.g., osteochondral fractures
    Evaluation of fracture healing or nonunions
7. Joints
    Locate/identify juxta-articular and periarticular calcific and ossific bodies.
    Evaluate joint space integrity of tarsal joints (complex anatomy).

## Magnetic Resonance Imaging: Brief Overview

Magnetic resonance is the phenomenon of resonating interaction between magnets (magnetic materials or atoms) and magnetic fields. In essence, certain substances can undergo the absorption of energy from externally applied electromagnetic field waves when the frequency is properly "tuned." When properly tuned, just like sound waves resonating within a wine glass, all the atomic nuclei of a given species act in concert (spin coherently in "phase"). They simultaneously start to "tip" (perturb) in a different direction with an angle determined by the duration of application. The law of entropy dictates that these excited substances must release electromagnetic radiation of a similar frequency in returning to their original energy states when the radiofrequency field waves are no longer applied.

In applying this concept to the imaging of living tissues, the nuclei of certain atoms can behave like small magnets and develop "poles." These nuclei typically have unpaired protons or neutrons and therefore possess spinning electrical charges that generate a magnetic field. In selecting atoms to optimally image living tissues, one might intuitively look for atoms that emit the best (strongest) signals and are found throughout all body tissues; hydrogen, a component of water, proves to be the best choice.

When the patient is placed within the strong magnetic field gantry of the magnetic resonance image (MRI) scanner, hydrogen atoms tend to align and oscillate with the external magnetic field. Their oscillating frequencies (about 42.5 million cycles per second in a 1.0-tesla (T) magnet and 64 megahertz in 1.5 T), known as the Larmor frequency, fall into the radio wavelength bands of the electromagnetic spectrum. These nuclei are then stimulated (perturbed, tipped) by a series of short radio wave burst/pulse cycles to various tip angles; the hydrogen atoms then "relax" to their previous, unexcited alignments, concurrently emitting magnetic radiance signals. These data are then used to reconstruct an image.

The microenvironment of hydrogen may change from tissue to tissue throughout the body. This affects the behavior of the hydrogen atom during imaging and therefore the emitted signals after excitation. These effects can be observed through the measurement of T1 and T2 relaxation time constants of hydrogen for certain tissues. Simply put, one T1 interval represents an exponential regrowth constant in the original magnetic field direction and is the time it takes for hydrogen nuclei to emit 63 percent of the energy absorbed from the stimulating pulse. T1 time constant values are dependent on the external magnetic field strengths. One T2 interval represents the exponential decay of phase coherence in a plane perpendicular to the main magnetic field and is the time required for 63 percent of the signal to be lost by dephasing. T2 time constants are largely independent of the applied external magnetic field strength.

It is important to realize T1 and T2 relaxation times form the basis of tissue characterization and contrast. The values of T1 and T2 are approximately the same in pure water (e.g., urine and cerebrospinal fluid). In the complex microenvironments of living body tissues, water may be impure; it is often in solution, it can be in motion or tightly bound in a crystal lattice, or it may be attached to macromolecules, compartmentalized, subjected to thermal effects, viscosity, and so on. In contradistinction to pure water values, both T1 and T2 are greatly shortened and the signal fades correspondingly faster. The effects of flow are variable. Paramagnetic substances such as methemoglobin formation (old hematoma) or intravenous gadolinium injection shorten T1 and greatly shorten T2 relaxation times of tissues.

It is, however, impossible to discriminate between T1 and T2 effects with a single stimulating pulse because only regional hydrogen concentration would be measured. Discrimination is accomplished largely through the employment of various radiofrequency pulsing techniques or the injection of paramagnetic contrast agents. With respect to pulse sequences, to evince these differences and therefore maximally contrast tissue signals, two or more pulses are applied in rapid succession. Employing such pulse sequences, images can be "weighted" to maximize either their T1 or T2 signal characteristics. The time interval between repetitive pulses is the "time to repeat" (TR) and the user-determined time interval between pulse and signal measurement or echo return from the patient is the "time to echo" (TE). In standard spin-echo pulse sequences, a short TR and TE will yield a T1-weighted images whereas a long TR and TE interval will yield T2-weighted images. Long TR and short TE times produce the "balanced," proton density image.

In general, a TR greater than 1.5 seconds (1,500 msec) and a TE greater than 0.4 seconds (40 msec) are considered long. T1-weighted images are often acquired with 500/20 (millisecond) TR/TE combinations, respectively, and T2-weighted images with 2,000/80 TR/TE combinations, respectively.

Pathology often alters the normal relaxation time of a given tissue, and thus allows for this delineation from normal tissues. In general, shortened T1 and lengthened T2 relaxation times produce brighter signal intensities and vice versa. Although absolute signal intensities can change considerably with changes in both TR and TE, the relative intensities do not change significantly between many tissues.

It is standard procedure to employ spin-echo pulse cycle imaging in the foot to provide proton density (balanced), T1- and T2-weighted images. Newer pulse-sequence methods are yielding exciting results while reducing MRI patient scanning times:

a. Short-tau inversion recovery techniques (STIR) are now performed along with T1-weighted and T2 fat saturation images to improve the contrast between normal and pathologic tissues. Occasionally, in the workup of infection, STIR images along with only T1 images are acquired. In these instances, the addition of T2-weighted images may contribute useful information and eliminate some false-positive readings (e.g., septic arthritis with possible osteomyelitis).

b. Gradient-echo techniques (FLASH, GRASS) employ a single partial flip angle (usually from 5° to 30°) RF pulse along with two opposing magnetic gradients that first dephase and then ultimately rephase nuclei ("gradient reversal"). This yields a free induction decay (FID) echo. Depending on the technique, gradient-echo methods can substantially reduce MRI scan times (1 sec per scan is not uncommon). The signal intensities of tissues may vary in that marrow signals are typically darker and hyaline cartilage can be substantially brighter (from afar, these images may mimic T2-weighted spin-echo images). Soft tissue contrast is poor when compared to standard spin-echo imaging, although gradient-echo techniques can often improve imaging of hematoma and calcifications.

c. Saturation pulse sequence (e.g., CHESS) techniques can effectively cancel the signals emanating from protons bound to either fat or water in a given voxel. Additionally, post-contrast T1 with gadolinium-DTPA fat saturation often improves the T1 tissue (marrow) contrast.

Surface coils are commonly used to yield a small field of view (FOV) and maximize detail (maximize signal-to-noise ratio). The smallest coil possible should be employed to fit the body part in foot and ankle imaging. Two knee coils, and occasionally head coils, are used. Flat surface coils are often best for achilles tendon imaging. Even though MR imaging of the foot and ankle is now commonplace in podiatric medical practice, the practitioner must be wary of sending patients for scanning to hospitals or imaging centers that do not routinely perform pedal MR scans or to institutions that prefer not to do them. Studies are often suboptimal under these circumstances.

### The MRI Gray Scale: Normal Signal Intensities

1. High intensity:
   Fat
   Marrow
2. Low to intermediate intensity:
   Muscle
   Hyaline cartilage
3. Very low intensity:
   Cortical bone
   Air
   Ligaments and tendons
   Fibrocartilage

4. Variable intensity (low-intensity T1; high with T2):
   Inflammatory or edematous tissue
   Neoplastic tissue
   Hemorrhage (interstitial)
   Hematoma (intensity varies with age of hematoma)
   Increased initial T1 and T2
   Progressive decrease of T1 greater than T2 (effect seen with field strengths >1.0 T)
   Fluid-filled structures

### General Advantages of MRI

1. Superior soft tissue contrast
2. Safety (nonionizing)
3. Sensitivity to blood flow
4. Multiplanar/triplanar pedal imaging; true orthogonal planes can be acquired, any plane can be imaged
5. Contrast enhancement with minimal risk; contrast agents can be employed
6. Highly sensitive to many pathologies; however, not specific

### Limitations of MRI

1. MRI has longer scanning times than CT. Newer pulse sequencing may soon minimize this problem.
2. Although the sensitivity for pathology often approaches 100 percent (e.g., osteomyelitis), the specificity is considerably less for many osseous abnormalities, particularly those involving abnormal marrow signals. In these instances, the morphologic appearance may be more reliable than the marrow signal.
3. Large metallic objects in the vicinity of the scanner, particularly ferromagnetic objects, can cause significant image disruption/distortion. In addition, a significant health hazard to the patient may occur with smaller ferromagnetic objects (orthopedic hardware, pellets) secondary to either dislodgment or heating during the actual scanning procedure.
4. Imaging of calcifications (except gradient echo/FLASH) is provided.
5. Negative imaging of the bony cortex is available.
6. Tissue heating occurs with MRI, although it is mild.
7. MRI is contraindicated with cardiac pacemakers.
8. MRI has a high cost.
9. MRI must be interpreted in the clinical context.

### Common MRI Overlap (Look-Alike) Pathologies

1. Healed osteomyelitis
2. Fracture
3. Infarct
4. Diabetic neuropathic bone disease (noninfective bone disease; osteolysis)
5. Septic arthritis (may evoke abnormal signal intensities in adjacent bone marrow)

### General Pedal Applications of MRI

1. Infection (osteomyelitis, cellulitis, abscesses)
2. Avascular necrosis
3. Reflex sympathetic dystrophy syndrome
4. Neoplasms (bony and soft tissue, including metastases and true neuroma from Morton's neuroma)
5. Hematoma
   Fluid collections
   Postoperative dead space
6. Joint Evaluation
   Arthritis (low-signal synovial hypertrophy, cartilaginous narrowing)
   Subchondral cysts
   Internal derangements
   Ligament (ankle) and tendon pathology
   Tenosyovitis
   Chronic tendinitis
   Tendon rupture, total and partial
   Effusion, bursitis
   Fibrosis
7. Post-trauma
   Stress fracture/insufficiency fracture
   Osteochondritis dessicans (acute and old)
8. Marrow pathology
9. Nonmetallic foreign bodies; nonferromagnetic metallic foreign bodies

## Computed Tomographic Imaging

The basic principle employed in computed tomographic (CT) scanning is that the internal structure of the body may be reconstructed in orthogonal planes by gathering attenuation data from multiple x-ray projections in many different directions. These x-ray beam scanning projections course through a fairly thin body plane, and the transmitted radiation registers with highly sensitive scintillation crystal detectors or xenon gas ionization chamber detection systems. Since the inception of CT, each newer generation of CT scanners has resulted in dramatic decreases in overall scanning time over the previous generation. Concurrently, image quality has improved with advances in computers as well as their image reconstruction algorithms. "Pencil-thin" x-ray beams have been replaced with fan-shaped beams, and rotating detector systems have largely been supplanted by stationary rings of detectors lining the scanning gantry.

In CT image reconstruction, a body plane is subdivided into many smaller blocks of tissue (voxel; volume element) and then each block face (pixel on a picture screen readout) is assigned a number (linear attenuation coefficient) correlated to its x-ray beam attenuating power in that projection. These numbers, so-called "CT numbers," are based on the Hounsfield scale and allow the computer to assign gray-scale values to the image. Basically, the image may be centered around a given tissue's Hounsfield unit (either osseous or soft tissue) with a range of gray tones extending a variable, user-determined width (window width) above and below this numeric center point (window level). At the extremes of this range of gray tones are pure black and pure white. In common practice, bone and/or soft tissue windows are acquired.

Although MRI has largely replaced CT scanning for soft tissue and marrow imaging, CT scanning is superior in visualization of calcific and bony cortical lesions. Additionally, soft tissue–osseous interface pathology (e.g., tendinous impingement) may be accurately imaged with CT. Other pedal applications include diagnosing pathology not clearly delineated with plain film radiographs (usually occult around tarsal bones and ankle joint) and also surgical planning (e.g., osteochondritis dessicans, tumor, complex fractures, rearfoot surgery).

## Overall Advantages of CT Scanning

Despite the following list of advantages, plain film radiographs should always be obtained before ordering CT scans.

1. Short scan times range between 1 and 5 seconds per slice.
2. Precise imaging of regional density differences. Newer CT scanners can measure tissue density to

1.0 Hounsfield units (1.0 H.U. = 0.1 percent of the density of water).
3. In comparison to conventional tomography, CT scanning offers the great advantage of producing cross-sectional images of superior contrast and detail without the superimposed blur or ghost image distortion.
4. In comparison with both conventional radiography and tomography, CT scans yield superior soft tissue contrast/delineation (through windowing) combined with the added capability of assigning Houndsfield (CT) attenuation values to pathologic tissue (Table 4-1). This can often help characterize the basic tissue makeup.
5. Three-dimensional CT imaging holds promise in the construction of preoperative models in areas of complex anatomy.
6. Although ancillary MRI has largely supplanted CT scanning of the soft tissue anatomy/pathology, in most aspects CT imaging remains a superior imaging modality for imaging of the skeletal system and soft tissue calcifications/ossifications.
7. CT can be used with cardiac pacemakers.
8. CT can be used with ferromagnetic materials.
9. CT may also be used with contrast studies such as arthrography.

## Overall Limitations of CT Scanning

1. X-ray image has limitations; image is generally inferior to MR imaging soft tissue contrast.
2. CT scans produce ionizing radiation with potential long-term effects.
3. Pregnant female patients should not be scanned unless absolutely necessary.
4. Invasive contrast studies are often routinely employed.

**Table 4-1.** Hounsfield Units (quantized attenuation values)

| |
|---|
| Heavy metal, >>>1,000 |
| Compact/cortical bone, 1,000 |
| Calcification, 200–800 (600–1,000) |
| Clotted blood, 40–60 |
| Blood, 25–40 |
| Muscle, 20–40 |
| Water, 0 |
| Fat, 50––100 |
| Air, −1,000 |

5. Physical constraints of the scanning gantry limits imaging to predominantly the transverse plane.
6. *Sagittal plane imaging of the foot cannot generally be obtained directly.* Basic CT scanner design precludes direct sagittal plane imaging of the foot in most patients. Although the computer is capable of reformatting (reconstructing) those anatomic planes not directly imaged, such images suffer from significant degradation of image quality. However, in about 30 to 40 percent of patients, direct sagittal plane imaging can be accomplished via internal (occasionally external) leg rotation with the knees flexed.
7. CT scanning is not devoid of some significant reconstruction artifacts; some of the more important ones include motion artifacts, streak artifacts, and beam-hardening artifacts. Note: Although the presence of a ferrometallic object(s) does not preclude scanning, streak artifacts of many metallic objects may significantly distort or totally obscure image detail (even more than MRI) when the object is large and lies within the image plane.

## Common Pedal Applications for CT Scanning

1. Bony cortex/cortical pathology
2. Calcifications
3. Evaluation of neoplasms (H.U. assignments) (particularly bone tumors)
   Internal margination/destructive typing
   Matrix
   Periosteal reaction
4. Trauma/nonunion
   Tarsal bony fractures
   Fractures of the os calcis (tendinous impingement)
   Osteochondritis dessicans
   Lisfranc fracture evaluation (image fracture pattern/elucidate osseous fragments)
5. Infection (especially chronic)
   Involucrum
   Cortex/sequestrum
   Abscesses/plantar space infections
6. Joints
   Subtalar joint arthritis
   Evaluation of tarsal coalitions
   Prosthesis (may be limited by artifacts)

Charcot joints (to ascertain degree of lysis, elucidate loose bodies, etc.)
7. Infarction
   Osteonecrosis of navicular
   Distal tibia
8. Muscles (pyomyositis)

## BRIEF REVIEW OF RADIOGRAPHIC BIOMECHANICAL EVALUATION

The biomechanical evaluation is performed from the anteroposterior and lateral pedal radiographs. Standardization of foot position is essential for biomechanical radiographic evaluation. The accepted standard in podiatric medicine is proper placement of the patient in their midstance angle and base of gait. Inasmuch as first and fifth ray angles, indices, and bunion criteria are reviewed elsewhere in this text, they are not covered in this section. The succeeding axis descriptions should not be construed as axes of motion.

## Anteroposterior View

1. Metatarsus adductus angle (Fig. 4-24)
   Usual upper limit: 14°–17°
   Normal adult range: 5°–17°
   Pathologic: >20°
   Values increase slightly with supination and decrease moderately with pronation.
   Method (Fig. 4-24)
      The angle is formed by the longitudinal axis of the lesser tarsus and the second metatarsal longitudinal axis. A transection to the lesser tarsal bones must first be constructed by identifying the four corners of a trapezoid that approximates these bones. Care must be taken not to utilize the lateral fourth metatarsocuboid joint margin or the styloid process of the fifth metatarsal base.
   Alternate method (Engel et al.; not depicted)
      The four corners of the second cuneiform are defined by points, and a longitudinal bisection to this cuneiform is then constructed. The intersection of this bisection with the bisection of the second metatarsal bone defines the metatarsus adductus angle. This

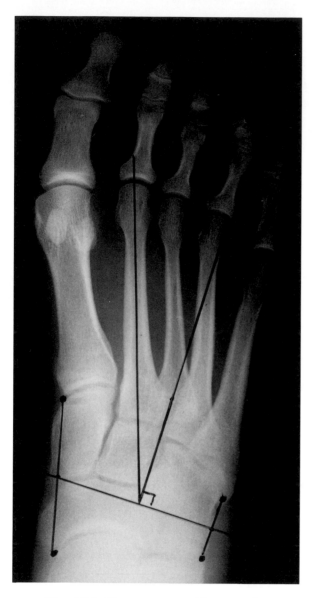

**Fig. 4-24.** The metatarsus adductus angle.

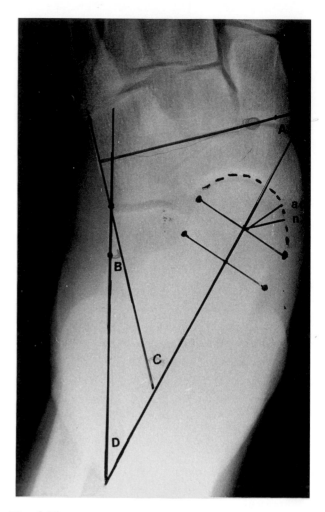

**Fig. 4-25.** Line AC is drawn to actual point of talonavicular articulation; line N is drawn to the average normal point spanning 75 percent of the articular surface of the taler head. Angle A is the talonavicular angle; B, the cuboid abduction angle; C, the talocuboid angle; D, the talocalcaneal angle.

method is much faster and reliably produces angular values about 3° higher than method (a).

2. Talocalcaneal angle (Fig. 4-25) (angle of Kite; Harris–Beath angle)

Normal ranges

    Infants, 30°–50°

    Age 1–10, about 30°

    Adolescents >5 years, 20°–35°

    Adults, 17°–21°

Decreased in subtalar joint supination

The angle is formed by the intersection of the longitudinal bisection of the talar neck (column tali) and longitudinal axis of the rearfoot. The longitudinal calcaneal axis (column calcanei) is typically substituted for the longitudinal rearfoot axis. This axis can be constructed with either a line parallel to the anteriolateral surface of the calcaneus or perpendicular to the plane of the inferior calcaneocuboid articulation

3. Cuboid abduction angle (calcaneocuboid angle) (see Fig. 4-25)

   Normal range: 0°–5°

   Increased with midtarsal joint pronation

   Decreased with midtarsal joint supination

   The angle is formed by the intersection of the column calcanei and the longitudinal axis of the cuboid. A line drawn parallel to the lateral surfaces of each of these bones usually suffices (in lieu of geometric bisection).

4. Talonavicular angle (see Fig. 4-25)

   Normal range: 70° ± 10°

   Increased in supination

   Decreased in pronation

   The angle is formed by the column tali and the transection of the lesser tarsal bones.

   *Alternate method*

   The angle is formed by the bisection of the talar neck and a tangent to the proximal effective articular surface of the navicular. Inasmuch as the concave portion of any convex–concave articulation typically displays a thin subchondral sclerotic line spanning the joint, this easily delineates the effective articular surface. Although this method is faster, it is less commonly employed.

5. Talonavicular articulation (percent articulation of talus)

   Normal range: 75 percent of talar head articulates with navicular

   Decreases in pronation

   Increases in supination

   Inasmuch as the articulating surface limits of the talar head must be defined to form the distal bisecting segment of the column tali, the percent of talonavicular articulation can be accurately approximately by creating 45° angles to the midpoint of this segment (see Fig. 4-25).

6. Talocuboid angle (see Fig. 4-25)

   Normal range: 31° ± 2°

   Increases in pronation

   Decreases in supination

   Possible associations (36° moderate increase in IM)

   The angle is formed by the intersection of the longitudinal bisection of the talus and a line drawn parallel to the lateral surface of the cuboid.

7. Forefoot adductus angle (Fig. 4-26)

   Normal range: 0°–10°

   The angle is formed by the intersection of the column calcanei (or longitudinal axis of rearfoot,

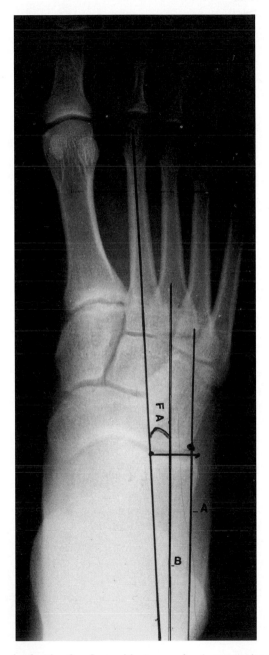

**Fig. 4-26.** The forefoot adductus angle. A comparison of two different methods of forming the longitudinal rearfoot axis yields two parallel lines in this case.

when obtainable) and the longitudinal axis of the second metatarsal.

## Lateral View

1. Lateral cyma line (Fig. 4-27)

   Normal range: Two continuous/conjoined hyperbolic curves

   Anterior break: Pronation

   Posterior break: Supination

   An ideally continuous **S**-shaped line formed by a tracing through the talonavicular and calcaneocuboid articular surfaces. Disruption is suggestive of abnormal rearfoot/subtalar joint mechanics. When a discontinuity occurs, the relative position of the talonavicular joint surface with respect to the calcaneocuboid joint surface determines the naming of the "break" (anterior or posterior). Invariably, when the arc formed by the talonavicular surface transects the calcaneocuboid joint, the cyma line is anterioinferiorly displaced. With a posterior cyma line, the two joint surface tracings do not intersect.

2. Talar declination angle (Fig. 4-28)

   Normal range: 21° ± 4°

   Increases in pronation

Decreases in supination

   The angle is formed by the intersection of the lateral talar axis (column tali) and the weight-bearing reference line. The talar declination angle equals the lateral talocalcaneal angle minus the calcaneal inclination angle.

3. Calcaneal inclination angle (see Fig. 4-28)

   Normal range: 18°–23°

   0°–10°, very low (flatfoot)

   10°–20°, low to medium

   20°–30° medium

   >30°, high (posterior pes cavus)

   The angle is formed by the intersection of the weight-bearing reference line and a line connecting the most posterior inferior point of the os calcis with the anterior inferior osseous limit of the os calcis at the calcaneocuboid joint. Older methods suggest this line connect the posterior inferior and the anterior inferior osseous landmarks of the calcaneus.

4. Lateral talocalcaneal angle (see Fig. 4-28)

   Normal range: 45° ± 3°

   Increases in pronation

   Decreases in supination

   The angle is formed by the intersection of the column tali and the column calcanei. This be-

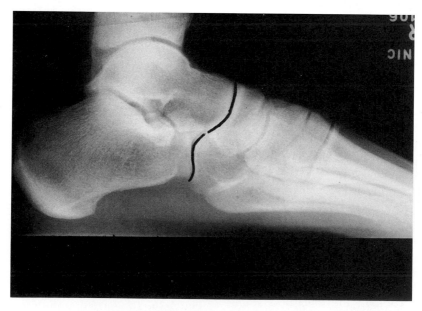

**Fig. 4-27.** A normal cyma line.

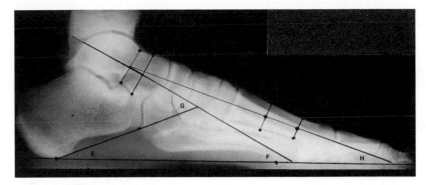

**Fig. 4-28.** Angle E is the calcaneal inclination angle; F, the talar declination angle; G, the lateral talocalcaneal angle; H, the metatarsal (first) declination angle.

comes the external angle of a triangle with opposite angles of talar declination and calcaneal inclination angle. The lateral talocalcaneal angle therefore equals talar declination plus calcaneal inclination angles.

5. Metatarsal declination angle(s) (see Fig. 4-28)
   Normal ranges (from S. Fuson and S. Smith)
   23° ± 8°, first metatarsal
   25° ± 4°, second metatarsal
   15° ± 4°, fifth metatarsal
   Increases in supination/pes cavus
   Decreases in pronation/flatfoot
   The angle is formed by the intersection of the longitudinal axis of the respective metatarsal and the weight-bearing reference line.

6. Lateral talometatarsal angle (not depicted) (talo-first metatarsal angle; Meary's angle)
   Normal range: 0°–14°
   15° or greater: cavus foot
   Age 5 years or less: negative angle
   Adult negative angle: pronation/flatfoot
   The angle is formed by the intersection of the lateral talar axis and the longitudinal bisection of the first metatarsal. The intersection of these two lines suggests the apex of deformity, particularly in cavus foot deformities. In a rectus foot, the column tali typically passes through the first metatarsal. In a pronated foot (or metatarsus primus elevatus), the column tali passes inferior to the first metatarsal head and vice versa with anterior cavus/supination.

7. Posterior Facet (declination) angle (not depicted)
   Normal range Approximately 45°
   Increases in pronation
   Decreases in supination
   The posterior facet angle, which is formed by the intersection of a line tracing through the posterior facet and the weight-bearing surface, is a gross indicator of pathology.

## SUGGESTED READINGS

### General

Aegerter E, Kirkpatrick JA Jr: Orthopedic Diseases. WB Saunders, Philadelphia, 1975

Berquist TH: Radiology of the Foot and Ankle. Raven Press, New York, 1989

Brower A: Arthritis in Black and White. WB Saunders, Philadelphia, 1988

Chapman S, Nakielny R: Aids to Radiological Differential Diagnosis. Bailliere Tindall, London, 1990

Dahnert W: Radiology Review Manual. Williams & Wilkens, Baltimore, 1991

Edeiken J: Roentgen Diagnosis of Diseases of Bone. Williams & Wilkins, Baltimore, 1989

Felson B, Reeder M: Gamuts in Radiology. Audiovisual Radiology of Cincinnati, Cincinnati 1987

Forrester DM, Kricun ME: Imaging of the Foot and Ankle. Aspen. 1988

Greenfield G: Radiology of Bone Disease. JB Lippincott, New York, 1990

Keats T: An Atlas of Normal Roentgen Variants That May Simulate Disease. Year Book Medical Publishers, Chicago, 1984

Kinsman S, Kroeker R: Leg–Podiatry Radiography. California State Dept. of Health, Sacramento, California, 1973

McCarty DJ: Arthritis & Allied Conditions. Lea & Febiger, Philadelphia, 1985

Meschan I: Roentgen Signs in Diagnostic Imaging. Vol. 2. Appendicular Skeleton. WB Saunders, Philadelphia, 1985

Montagne J, Chevrot A, Galmiche JM: Atlas of Foot Radiology. Masson, New York, 1981

Ravin CE, Cooper C: Review of Radiology. WB Saunders, Philadelphia, 1990

Resnick D: Common disorders of synovium-lined joints: pathogenesis, imaging abnormalities, and complications. AJR 151:1079, 1988

Resnick D, Niwayama G: Diagnosis of Bone and Joint Disorders. Vols. 1–6. WB Saunders, Philadelphia 1988

Sartoris DJ, Resnick D: Radiological evaluation of patients with arthritis. Pathol Annu 86:293, 1986

Silverman FN: Caffey's Pediatric x-ray diagnosis. Yearbook Medical, Chicago, 1985

Weissman S: Radiology of the Foot. Williams & Wilkins, Baltimore, 1989

### Ancillary Imaging Modalities

Berquist TH: Magnetic Resonance of the Musculoskeletal System. Raven Press, New York, 1987

Curry TS, Dowdey JE, Murry RC Jr: Christensen's Physics of Diagnostic Radiology, Lea & Febiger Philadelphia, 1990

Edelman R, Hesselink JR: Clinical Magnetic Resonance Imaging. WB Saunders, Philadelphia, 1990

Horowitz AL: MRI Physics for Radiologists. A visual Approach. Springer-Verlag, New York, 1992

Hounsfield GN: Computerized transverse axial scanning (tomography). Br J Radiol 46:1016, 1973

Oloff-Solomon J, Solomon MA: Computed tomographic scanning of the foot and ankle. Clin Podiat Med Surg 5:931, 1988

Oloff-Solomon J, Solomon MA: Magnetic Resonance Imaging in the Foot and Ankle. Clin Podiatr Med Surg 5:945, 1988

Resnick D: Bone and Joint Imaging. WB Saunders, Philadelphia, 1989

Wolf GL, Popp C: NMR—A Primer for Medical Imaging. Slack, Thorofare, NJ, 1984

### Biomechanics

Altman MI: Sagittal plane angles of the talus and calcaneus in the developing foot. J Am Podiatry Assoc 58:191, 1968

Coleman SS: Complex Foot Deformities in Children. Lea & Febiger, Philadephia, 1983

DiGiovanni JE, Smith SD: Normal biomechanics of the adult rearfoot. J Am Podiatry Assoc 66:812, 1976

Engel E, Erlick N, Krems I: A simplified metatarsus adductus angle. J Am Podiatry Assoc 73:620, 1983

Fuson SM, Smith SD: Angular relationships of the metatarsal, talus, and calcaneus. J Am Podiatry Assoc 68:463, 1978

Gamble FO, Yale I: Clinical Foot Roentgenology. Kreiger, Huntington, NY, 1975

Giannestras JJ: Foot Disorders: Medical and Surgical Management. Lea & Febiger, Philadelphia, 1973

Greenberg GS: Relationship of Hallux Abductus Angle and First Metatarsal Angle to Severity of Pronation. J Am Podiatry Assoc 69:29, 1979

Kaschak TJ, Laine W: Surgical radiology. Clin Podiatr Med Surg 5:797, 1988

LaPorta GA, Scarlet J: Radiographic changes in the pronated and supinated foot. J Am Podiatry Assoc 67:334, 1977

Meary R: On the measurement of the angle between the talus and the first metatarsal. Symposium sur le pied creux essentiel. Rev Chir Orthop 53:389, 1967

Montagne J, Chevrot A, Galmiche JM: Atlas of Foot Radiology. Masson, New York, 1981

Root ML, Orien WP, Weed JH: Clinical Biomechanics. Vol. II. Normal and Abnormal Function of the Foot. Clinical Biomechanics, Los Angeles, 1977

Sgarlato TE: A Compendium of Podiatric Biomechanics. California College of Podiatric Medicine, 1971

Solomon M: Roentgenographic Biomechanical Evaluation of the Foot. Johnathan Douglass, 1973

Templeton AW, McAlister WH, Zim ID: Standardization of terminology and evaluation of osseous relationships in congenitally abnormal feet. AJR 93:374, 1965

Whitney AK: Radiographic Charting Technique. 1976

# 5
# Clinical Evaluation of Hallux Abducto Valgus

*RONALD E. JOHNSON*

The clinical evaluation of the hallux abducto valgus deformity is extremely important. It is imperative that the nature and type of deformity are identified and documented to understand the presenting problem unique to each patient. Of equal importance is the fact that many patients presenting with hallux abducto valgus and associated symptoms will require surgical intervention to adequately treat the pathologic condition. In view of this fact the physician is required to not only evaluate the local complaint, but also must determine the patient's status with respect to surgery and postoperative recovery.

## PATIENT HISTORY

Obtaining the patient's medical history is an important aspect of the evaluation of any patient, but is of particular importance in the patient presenting with hallux abducto valgus. Many clinicians believe that 95 percent of diagnoses can be made through obtaining a careful patient history.[1] Information obtained from the patient history will provide valuable data that can be used in making decisions with regard to the extent of the patients symptoms and development of a rational treatment plan, and in evaluating the patient's ability to undergo surgical procedures if required.

The medical history should focus on the areas of the chief complaint, with emphasis on the history of the present illness and past medical history with respect to the chief complaint. A record should be made of the onset of the symptoms, progression of the symptoms, and any aggravating factors as well as elements that provide relief of the local symptoms. The type of pain as well as the location and duration of pain symptoms should be noted and documented in addition to any significant changes with regard to swelling or sensory changes. Difficulties experienced by the patient, such as problems associated with ambulation, wearing of shoes, or limitation of activities, remain a significant part of the history of the present illness.

The past medical history is important for eliciting important information with respect to previous type of treatment for hallux abducto valgus and bunion complaints. This is especially important if previous surgical treatment has been utilized. The surgical results and the patient's perception of this treatment should be elicited and documented. If surgical intervention has been previously employed, it is important to record the type of anesthesia used, the patient's reaction to anesthesia, and the patient's history with respect to the postoperative recovery period.

If a conservative approach to treatment has been used previously in the treatment of hallux abducto valgus, important information can be obtained relating to those treatment plans that have been effective or ineffective, and those plans that may have resulted in the exacerbation of the patient's symptoms. Only through a thorough approach to the patient's history of the present problem and past medical history can an accurate picture be obtained to assist the physician in the assessment as to the extent of the deformity and the disability experienced by the patient, and to provide insight necessary for the development of a sound treatment plan, whether a conservative or surgical approach.

Obtaining a good medical history is an essential part of any evaluation, but is again of utmost importance in the patient for whom a surgical treatment plan might be considered. In light of the fact that many patients with hallux abducto valgus require surgical intervention, it appears logical that the history include information that might be necessary in the preoperative evaluation so that all potential risks can be weighed before proposing or beginning any type of treatment plan.

The past medical history is specifically vital to obtaining information regarding any current medications or medications the patient has been using recently. One should not overlook over-the-counter medications (e.g., nonsteroidal anti-inflammatory drugs, aspirin, antacids, cold preparations), recreational drugs, caffeine, nicotine, and alcohol use.

Allergies are of special significance. The specific allergy (e.g., food, drug, metals) and nature of the allergic response (e.g., syncope, respiratory, dermatologic) should be documented thoroughly. A review of previous medical records or communication with the patient's medical physician may be necessary to obtain accurate and reliable information.

The patient's status with respect to past surgical history should be explored. One should bear in mind that the patient may not consider that minor or outpatient procedures are true surgical experiences, and this perception may need to be specifically elicited during the history-taking process. Again, associated with the history of past surgical procedures should be information related to previous anesthesia used and, of special significance, the patient's response to the anesthetic agent.

The review of systems is possibly the most important aspect of the past medical history. This portion of the past medical history involves an in-depth history review of each organ system in an organized manner. The questions should be designed so as to reveal any possible historical data that may not have been previously uncovered and that may present as a factor in determining the patient's risk with respect to surgical consideration. Of specific significance is asking female patients of child-bearing age about the possibility of pregnancy if medications, surgery, or anesthesia are a part of the treatment consideration.

The final area of required historical information is information relating to the patient's family history and social history. Important considerations would be obvious diseases that may have a bearing on the patient's current problem or postoperative recovery or present a risk of morbidity and mortality.

The social history or patient profile, as it is sometimes referred to, will present valuable information regarding the patient's current work status, family or support system, geographic living situation, and possibly activity level and interests. This information may prove invaluable in communicating with the patient with respect to possible surgical treatment as well as providing the physician with insight into the patient's expectations, requirements of treatment, and ability to successfully carry out a proposed treatment plan.

# PHYSICAL EXAMINATION

When a thorough clinical history has been obtained, a well-performed and well-documented physical examination must be completed. All patients for whom surgical treatment is proposed or who have medical history factors that may complicate even conservative treatment (e.g., diabetes, neuropathy, vascular disease) should receive a comprehensive and thorough medical physical examination. This examination should include an evaluation of the vital signs, cranial nerves, head and neck, cardiopulmonary system, gastrointestinal and genitourinary systems, and dermatologic and neurologic systems as well as the musculoskeletal system. The patient who has not had a complete medical physical examination or medical evaluation recently should also have a complete medical examination before the proposal of treatment for hallux abducto valgus.

The evaluation of the podiatric components of hallux abducto valgus is of prime importance to the decision-making process in patients with hallux abducto valgus and related conditions. The podiatric medical examination should be thorough and complete so that accurate and valid information can be acquired.

## Podiatric Vascular Examination

The evaluation of the patient's vascular status is always relevant and must be accessed before initiating any type of treatment, particularly because surgical considerations might be included in the treatment of hallux abducto valgus.

One of the most important skills of the examiner is the ability to determine the state of pulsations in the peripheral arteries of the foot and leg. The primary peripheral arteries that are usually evaluated are the dorsalis pedis, the posterior tibial, and possibly the femoral and popliteal arteries. A useful practice is to grade arterial pulsations on the basis of 0 to 4 in such a manner that 0 indicates a complete absence of pulsations; 1, marked impairment of arterial pulsations; 2, moderate impairment; 3, slight impairment, and 4, normal pulsations.[2]

Following examination of the pulses, the hair pattern on the legs is noted and especially any difference in temperature of the legs and the level at which this difference might occur. Color, temperature, and sensation of the foot and lower leg are evaluated and compared one foot to the other. Capillary filling is assessed by firmly pressing the finger over the distal aspect of the digits of the foot and observing the time required for normal color to return after release of the pressure. A finding of a time longer than 3–5 seconds could indicate vascular disease.

The legs should be elevated, noting undue pallor of the feet, and then the legs should be dangled over the edge of the examination table with the patient in the sitting position to evaluate any delay in venous or capillary filling time. In this position, a finding of dependent rubor, indicating reactive hyperemia, may be a sign of capillary ischemia.[3]

## Podiatric Neurologic Evaluation

Evaluation of the deep tendon reflexes should include the patellar and achilles reflexes as well as examination for ankle clonus and pathologic reflexes. Both lower extremities should be examined for sensory findings, which should include the patient's ability to distinguish between sharp and dull stimulants, proprioceptive stimulants, and vibratory testing. Muscle testing of the major muscle groups of the lower extremity should be performed bilaterally with comparison of one extremity one to the other. The muscle testing should include evaluation and documentation with respect to the strength and bulk of the muscles being evaluated.

## Podiatric Dermatologic Examination

Both feet should be inspected for any skin lesions, tumors, or ulcerations. The texture and turgor of the skin should be observed and recorded. Of significance in the patient presenting with hallux abducto valgus is the presence and location of any hyperkeratotic lesions on the plantar surface of the foot or areas of the hallux. These lesions should be noted along with their type, size, and location and whether the lesions are symptomatic.

The position and extent of hyperkeratotic lesions if present can be valuable in evaluating the function of the foot and associated hallux deformity. These hyperkeratotic lesions should be closely correlated with the findings of the biomechanical evaluation in each patient before proposing and initiating treatment of hallux abducto valgus.

## Podiatric Evaluation of Hallux Abducto Valgus

The usual presentation of symptoms of a patient with hallux abducto valgus is pain over the medial or dorsal medial aspect of the first metatarsal head region of the foot. A thorough evaluation of the area of palpable tenderness should be employed during the initial phase of the examination of the local deformity. Swelling or inflammation from an adventitious bursa about the area should be noted and documented (Fig. 5-1). Occasionally pain can present on the plantar aspect of the metatarsal phalangeal joint region as a result of degenerative changes at the sesamoid-metatarsal articulation. Numbness may also be encountered along the medial side of the hallux secondary to pressure over the sensory nerve in the area producing symptomatic paresthesias.[4]

Evaluation of the hallux abducto valgus deformity should be carried out with the patient weight-bearing as well as non-weight-bearing. Usually the hallux abducto valgus deformity is accentuated when the patient is standing or bearing weight on the foot. Equally important to this examination is an evaluation of the associated deformities (i.e., hammer toes, digital subluxation, hyperkeratotic lesions) present on weight-bearing.

Lateral deviation of the great toe may be a result of luxation within the metatarsal phalangeal joint or in-

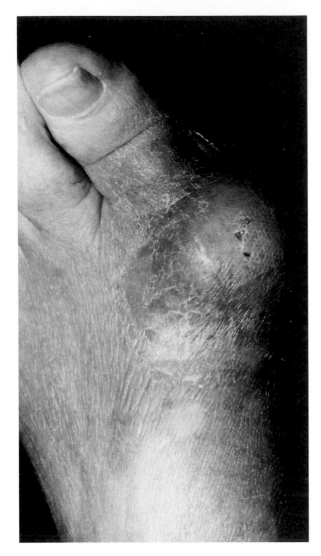

**Fig. 5-1.** Chronic bursitis associated with long-standing hallux valgus.

volve the structure of the hallux itself. Hallux abduction may be caused by positional or structural changes within the metatarsal phalangeal joint. This hallux abduction may also be caused by the structural shape of the proximal phalanx.[5] It is important to clinically differentiate the level and etiology of this lateral deviation so that the appropriate corrective procedure or procedures are selected.

The generally accepted normal range of motion of the first metatarsal phalangeal joint is approximately 70°–90° of dorsiflexion and approximately 30° of plantar flexion. Any limitation in either dorsiflexion or plantar flexion should be noted and compared to that of the contralateral extremity. Limitation might be an indication of intra-articular degeneration with osteophytic lipping or a result of contractures of the periarticular structures of the first metatarsal phalangeal joint.

The quality of the range of motion of the first metatarsal phalangeal joint should be evaluated. In the normal motion, there is no medial or lateral deviation from the sagittal plane, and the movement causes no pain when the hallux is moved through its full range of motion. Limitation of motion, pain on motion, or crepitation may indicate deterioration or degeneration of the articular surfaces of the joint.

The range of motion of first metatarsophalangeal joint should be evaluated with the joint in the natural or deviated position and in the corrected or rectus position by reducing the transverse plane deformity of the hallux adduction and moving the base of the proximal phalanx through a full range of motion on the metatarsal head. If lateral luxation of the fibular sesamoid and associated contracture of the plantar lateral structures is present, a significant lateral deviation of the hallux as it moves through the dorsiflexion portion of this range of motion is usually noted. The degree of this deviation will provide valuable insight into the extent of the contracture and the deforming forces present on the plantar lateral structures of the first metatarsophalangeal joint.

In some instances it will be observed that the hallux has no range of dorsiflexion if held in the corrected or rectus position and has its usual range of dorsiflexion when evaluated in its natural or deviation position. This is described by many clinicians as being track-bound or of joint tracking and is thought to be a result of adaptive changes of the joint producing a lateral deviation of the articular surface of the first metatarsal head. If this is present, careful radiographic and clinical intraoperative evaluation is necessary to determine if an osteotomy might be indicated to reduce this lateral joint surface deviation to render appropriate correction and minimize the incidence of recurrence of the deformity.

While much effort is spent evaluating the transverse plane aspect of the hallux abducto valgus deformity, minimal effort and documentation of the frontal plane

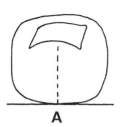
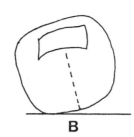
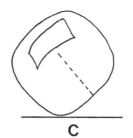
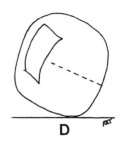

**A**          **B**          **C**          **D**

**Fig. 5-2.** Valgus rotation of the hallux. (**A**) Grade 0, no rotation. (**B**) Grade 1, rotation less than 25°. (**C**) Grade 2, rotation greater than 25°. (**D**) Grade 3, rotation greater than 45°.

of valgus component of the deformity is usually the rule. An attempt to evaluate and document the valgus position of the hallux has been suggested and would appear to be warranted.

The recommended classification used to describe this valgus component of the deformity is as follows; no rotation, grade 0; rotation less than 25°, grade 1; rotation greater than 25°, grade 2; and rotation greater than 45°, grade 3. Assessment is made with the patient standing. The 45° point is represented as one-half of a right angle; the 25° point is an approximation of one-quarter of a right angle (Fig. 5-2).[6]

Evaluation of the first ray and its range of motion is essential to selecting appropriate treatment of hallux abducto valgus and is of particular importance when evaluating for potential surgical procedures. The first ray dorsiflexion and plantar flexion should be evaluated with the subtalar joint and midtarsal joint in their neutral positions. One hand should be placed with the thumb and index finger located dorsal and plantar to the first metatarsal head and the thumb and index finger of the opposite hand placed over the approximate region of the second metatarsal head dorsally and plantarly in a similar fashion. The relationship of the thumbs and index fingers of both hands should be noted in this neutral position.

The first ray should then be dorsiflexed to the end of its range of motion and the interval between the level of the thumb or index fingers of both hands should be noted, measured, and recorded (Fig. 5-3). Similarly, the first ray should be plantar-flexed to the end of its plantar-flexory range of motion and the distance or interval between the thumb and index finger of both hands should again be noted (Fig. 5-4).

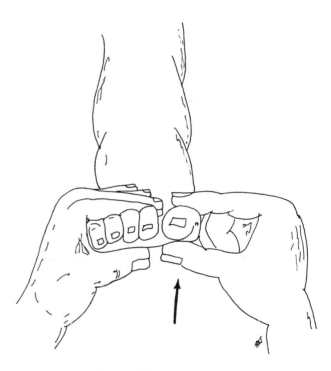

**Fig. 5-3.** Dorsiflexion of first ray to end of range of motion.

When dorsiflexion distance exceeds plantar flexion distance, the finding is consistent with dorsiflexed first ray. Conversely, when the plantar flexion distance exceeds the dorsiflexion distance, the finding is consistent with plantar-flexed first ray.[7] These findings are of significance in treatment considerations associated with hypermobile first ray and when contemplating surgical procedures that involve osteotomies of the first ray.

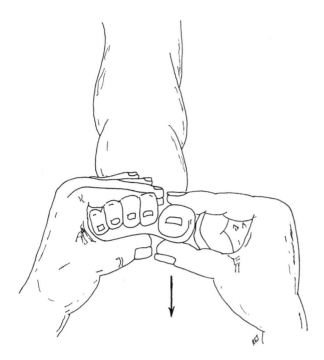

**Fig. 5-4.** Plantar flexion of first ray to end of range of motion.

Clinical evaluation of hallux abducto valgus should always include a complete biomechanical examination of the lower extremity. Hallux abducto valgus is considered by many clinicians to be a result of underlying biomechanical abnormalities. Therefore, related conditions such as the presence of ankle equines, metatarsus adductus, pes planes conditions, hypermobile first ray, forefoot varus, and calcaneal valgus, to name a few, must be clearly identified and considered if successful treatment of hallux abducto valgus is to be accomplished. The extent of these deformities must be fully understood if treatment is to be effective.

The history and physical examination, while an important entity in evaluation of hallux abducto valgus, must be combined with a complete radiologic evaluation of the deformity. These elements, along with a thorough understanding of the biomechanics and function of the first metatarsolphalangeal joint, will assist in the formulation and institution of an appropriate and well-designed treatment plan for the relief of symptoms associated with hallux abducto valgus.

## REFERENCES

1. Zier BG: Essentials of Internal Medicine in Clinical Podiatry. WB Saunders, Philadelphia, 1990
2. Fairbairn JF, Juergens JL, Spittell JS: Peripheral Vascular Diseases. 4th Ed. WB Saunders, Philadelphia, 1972
3. McCarthy ST (ed): Peripheral Vascular Disease in the Elderly. Churchill Livingstone, Edinburgh, 1983
4. Coughlin MJ: Hallux Valgus: causes, evaluation, and treatment. Postgrad Med 75:174, 1984
5. McGlamry ED (ed): Comprehensive Textbook of Foot Surgery. Williams & Wilkins, Baltimore, 1987
6. Smith RW, Reynolds JC, Stewart MJ, et al: Hallux valgus assessment. Report of the Research Committee of the American Orthopaedic Foot and Ankle Society. Foot Ankle 5:92, 1984
7. Root ML, Orien WP, Weed JH, et al: Biomechanical Exam of the Foot. Vol. 1. Clinical Biomechanics Corporation, Los Angeles, 1971

# 6

# Preoperative Assessment in Hallux Valgus

*DAVID M. LaPORTA*
*THOMAS V. MELILLO*
*VINCENT J. HETHERINGTON*

The goal of any bunion surgery is the elimination of pain, restoration of a congruous metatarsophalangeal joint, realignment of the hallux into a rectus position, and preservation of joint motion. The best method for predicting a successful surgical result in hallux valgus reconstruction is thorough preoperative planning. This helps ensure selection of the appropriate procedure to attain these goals. Preoperative planning should include a thorough history as to the progression of the deformity and an adequate clinical and radiographic examination. In addition, addressing the deformity by the choice of surgical procedures requires identifying its etiology and pathomechanics. This chapter reviews and details pertinent features of the preoperative clinical and radiographic examination.

## ETIOLOGY

The hallux abducto valgus deformity may result from a variety of contributing factors. Proper historical and clinical assessment of the patient in both a non-weight-bearing and weight-bearing manner and a thorough biomechanical evaluation, as well as an understanding of the microscopic pathologies occurring in and around the first metatarsophalangeal joint, will ensure a more predictable surgical result by selection of the appropriate procedure or procedures.

An historical review of the various etiologies shows that some still believe that shoe choice, excessive ac-tivity, and external environmental factors play a significant role in the development of hallux abducto valgus deformities. This belief persists despite historical studies that demonstrate these are aggravating factors, not primary pathologies. Hereditary factors are known to be causative only in that it is the foot type with its associated biomechanical abnormalities that is inherited, not necessarily the resulting pathologic condition known as hallux abducto valgus.

## Biomechanical Etiology

The biomechanical etiology of hallux abducto valgus has its origin in the rearfoot. The subtalar joint range of motion when excessive will most often lead to a pronated foot. External factors such as limb rotations and equinus conditions tend to accelerate the patho logic processes associated with hallux abducto valgus. The sequence of events usually commences when the calcaneus everts beyond the vertical in an excessively pronated foot. The resultant eversion unlocks the midtarsal joint, allowing the axes of the talonavicular and calcaneocuboid joints to become parallel to each other and resulting in an unstable midtarsal joint. This instability, which persists during stance, allows for hypermobility of the first ray at the time it should be most stable for propulsion.[1-3]

At the same time, the soft tissue musculature around the rearfoot and first ray become altered in the pronated foot. With calcaneal eversion, the pull of the flexor hallucis brevis and longus are altered. In addition, with an unstable midtarsal joint the route of the peroneus longus muscle tendon is altered, thereby affecting the motion about the first ray. The peroneus longus muscle, coursing around the cuboid, normally inserts into the base of the first metatarsal and the medial cuneiform and stabilizes the complex at toe-off. In a pronated foot, the peroneus longus cannot perform this function, and the resultant muscular and biomechanical alteration results in a hypermobile first ray.[4–9]

With the preceding definition and an understanding of the mechanics of hypermobility of the first ray as an etiology in hallux abducto valgus deformity, the first-ray axis and biomechanics of the subtalar and midtarsal joints can be discussed. The first ray possesses a triplane axis that courses in an anterior, lateral, and dorsal direction.[3,10] Therefore, dorsiflexion of the first metatarsal will be accompanied by adduction and plantar flexion will be accompanied by abduction.

Motion about the first ray is dependent on the peroneus longus muscle. As was previously discussed, the peroneus longus muscle in turn is dependent on the stability of the midtarsal joint because it uses the cuboid as its fulcrum. From the cuboid this muscle courses anterior and dorsal to exert its stability on the first ray. The triplane stability exerted on the first ray in normal biomechanics is one of plantarflexion, abduction, and a posterior pull. In normal gait therefore as the foot progresses from midstance into propulsion, the supinating subtalar joint also locks the midtarsal joint; this ensures a stable lateral column of the foot and provides the peroneus longus muscle with an efficient fulcrum at the cuboid to exert a plantar, lateral, and posterior pull on the first ray. Consequently, any pronatory influence that causes an unlocking of the midtarsal joint may result in metatarsus primus adductus over a period of time.[3,5]

Finally, it should be remembered that the first metatarsal head is firmly bound to the sesamoids by the tibial and fibular sesamoidal ligaments.[11,12] In the early stage of hallux abducto valgus deformity, these two ligaments firmly hold the sesamoids to the metatarsal head. Therefore, the early radiographic view of the deformity is actually dorsiflexion, adduction, and inversion of the first metatarsal. As the deformity progresses over time, the tibial sesamoidal ligament becomes functionally elongated as it adapts to stress placed on the medial side of the first metatarsophalangeal joint. The fibular sesamoidal ligament, conversely, functionally shortens along with the other lateral soft tissue structures. The first metatarsal rotates slightly at the metatarsal cuneiform articulation. In a pronated foot, this slight rotation of the metatarsal allows for an inversion or varus rotation of the first metatarsal head relative to the sesamoids. The hallux now moves in the opposite direction of the first metatarsal head, which accounts for the valgus or rotational component of the deformity. As the amount of hallux eversion increases over time, the tibial, intersesamoidal, and fibular sesamoidal ligaments continue to adapt functionally to the deformity. The surgical importance of the soft tissue adaptation lies in the fact that if valgus rotation of the hallux is a component of the deformity and if transection of the fibular sesamoidal ligament is not accomplished, there will still be some degree of valgus rotation left in the great toe.

With the advent of biomechanics and a more detailed radiographic evaluation of the deformity, the etiology in hallux abducto valgus deformity has become more refined and may be categorized as follows[3]:

1. Hypermobility of the first ray
2. Instability of the midtarsal joint
3. Calcaneal eversion beyond vertical
4. Instability of the peroneus longus

## Metatarsus Primus Varus

The first metatarsal articulates proximally with the first cuneiform via their articular surfaces and strong ligamentous support. As a result, any deviation or abnormality in this articulation can give rise to deformity. Some of the terms used to describe this relationship between the first metatarsal and the cuneiform, as well as the relationship between the first metatarsal and the second metatarsal, are *metatarsus primus varus, metatarsus primus adductus*, and an *increased intermetatarsal angle*. Quite often, and erroneously, these terms are used interchangeably. In reality, the term *metatarsus primus varus* classically is used to describe a condition in which both medial and lateral cortices of the metatarsal are of equal length, but there is an increase in the measurable angle between the first and second metatarsal that is secondary to a deviation at the first metatarsocuneiform joint.

Additionally, there exists a difference in the margins or sides of the cuneiform such that the lateral margin as compared to the medial margin of the first cuneiform is longer, causing an oblique angulation of the first metatarsocuneiform joint.[13,14] The clinical and radiographic effect is an increased intermetatarsal angle measurement on radiographs, and a pronounced first metatarsal medially on palpation. This type of cuneiform has often been termed *atavistic* and was originally discussed by Lapidus[15] in the surgical correction of hallux abductor valgus deformity. Klienberg in 1932[16] believed that such obliquity at the first metatarsophalangeal joint represented a medial cuneiform that was an atavistic remnant of a period when the hallux had a prehensile thumblike function.

The alternative concept of an os intermetatarsum as the proximate cause of a true metatarsus primus varus was a poor attempt to explain its occurrence. Objective studies by Wheeler[17] failed to demonstrate the correlation between the presence or absence of an os intermetatarsum and the development of metatarsus primus varus.

The radiographic diagnosis of metatarsus primus varus may be demonstrated by comparing the longitudinal bisection of the first metatarsal with the longitudinal bisection of the medial cuneiform. If the angle formed between this intersection is greater than 25°, a metatarsus primus varus deformity is said to exist within the first ray.[18] However, it should be emphasized that the obliquity seen on radiographic images may quite possibly represent a positional alteration produced by the imaging technique. In short, metatarsal primus varus is a true structural deformity that lies within the first metatarsal cuneiform relationship. Metatarsus primus adductus or increased intermetatarsal angle are indeed the same entity, and represent a deformity characterized by an increased angulation from a long axis bisection of the first and second metatarsals. The presence of metatarsus primus adductus is an important consideration in understanding the osseous pathologies associated with hallux abducto valgus. This change may be the result of long-standing biomechanical pathologies as opposed to inherent structural deformity, but in either event if any of the deformities of metatarsus primus varus or metatarsus primus adductus are pathologic, they must be corrected. In fact,

Hardy and Clapman[9] were the first to demonstrate that in younger patients it is an increase in the metatarsus primus adductus of the first ray that initiates the transverse plane rotation of the great toe. Of 78 patients who developed adult hallux valgus deformity, it was a consistent finding that the initiating factor in the osseous structure was an increased intermetatarsal angle, which was later followed by the hallux moving away from the midline of the body.

# CLINICAL EVALUATION

The podiatric surgeon should never base the selection of a surgical procedure solely on any one set of findings or evaluations. It is only after a thorough history and clinical examination in conjunction with assessment of standardized radiographs that one may consider the appropriate surgical procedure that will yield the best long-term result. All too often the preoperative clinical examination of the deformity is limited to the patient seated in the chair. It should be remembered that hallux abducto valgus is a dynamic propulsive phase deformity that obligates both non-weightbearing and weight-bearing examination, as well as palpation and gait analysis.

The practitioner should first obtain a thorough history of the patient's chief complaint. One should note the exact location of the pain as being deep within the first metatarsophalangeal joint or solely confined at the medial eminence, and if there is coexisting second metatarsal pain. One should inquire as to the duration of the pain. A long-standing deformity that has only recently worsened may be indicative of erosion of the plantar crista, which has now allowed the sesamoids to drift laterally unimpeded. It is equally important to establish any functional limitations resulting from the deformity. The practitioner should inquire if there is pain at rest, only in shoe gear, or on vigorous activity.

Another important consideration in the preoperative assessment in hallux abducto valgus reconstruction is the age of the patient. The practitioner should select the procedure that will yield a functional and cosmetic long-lasting result. In addition, associated deformities such as ankle joint equinus may also be addressed at this time in the younger patient. Finally, the podiatric history is no different from the standard format utilized in the medical arena. A thorough systemic history should be obtained on every patient contemplating any surgical procedure.

As mentioned previously, the clinical examination should be performed in both the non-weight-bearing and weight-bearing attitudes. It should be remembered that the physical examination should include a thorough assessment of vascular, dermatologic, neurologic, and musculoskeletal systems.

The examination of the bunion deformity should begin with thorough palpation of the bunion and first metatarsophalangeal joint to localize the exact area of tenderness. This preferably is done while placing the joint through an entire range of motion. Pain throughout range of motion at extreme dorsiflexion or plantar flexion may indicate synovial or cartilaginous changes. Although there is often a dorsomedial prominence, the presence of a bursal swelling should be noted. In addition, many patients exhibiting hallux valgus deformity may actually present with a chief complaint of a paronychia of the fibular nail border, which results from the abutment of the hallux against the second toe. The sesamoids and plantar crista should also be palpated for localized tenderness.

Examination of the first metatarsophalangeal joint range of motion is vital for a successful surgical outcome. First, the quantity of the range of motion should be noted. The normal first metatarsophalangeal joint should exhibit at least 65° of dorsiflexion and 15° of plantar flexion. Any decrease in the quantity of motion may be indicative of arthritic changes predisposing the joint to a hallux limitus deformity. Severe arthritic changes with cartilaginous erosions would make any attempt at osseous and soft tissue realignment futile in hallux valgus reconstruction.

The quality of motion within the first metatarsophalangeal joint should likewise be carefully evaluated. This evaluation should be performed with the joint in both the deviated and rectus position. Again, it should be noted if pain is elicited at the endpoint of the range of motion or throughout range of motion. Any crepitation should be noted as this may indicate articular damage or structural adaptation within the joint.

In addition to the first metatarsophalangeal joint, the entire first-ray range of motion should be evaluated. The first ray normally has an axis of motion approximately 5 mm toward dorsiflexion and plantar flexion. An increase in motion around the first-ray axis may indicate hypermobility, which may affect the selection of the appropriate surgical procedure.

Any callous formation should be noted as to its location around the bunion deformity. The callous pattern should be noted as plantar first metatarsal, plantar medial interphalangeal joint, or underneath the second metatarsal.[18–20]

# RADIOGRAPHIC EVALUATION

Proper radiographic evaluation of the hallux abducto valgus deformity requires standard preoperative weight-bearing views taken in the angle and base of gait.[21] It cannot be overemphasized that hallux valgus represents a dynamic deformity on which ground reactive forces exert a direct pronounced effect.

Standard preoperative views should consist of weight-bearing dorsiplantar, lateral, forefoot axial, and medial oblique projections. Dorsiplantar and lateral views together will allow the practitioner to accurately measure traditional relationships and identify positional and structural components of the deformity. A 45° medial oblique projection demonstrates hypermobility from lack of parallelity between the first and second metatarsals. The medial oblique projection will also act as a standard for assessment of pre- and postoperative correction of the deformity. The forefoot axial projection will aid in evaluating degenerative changes noted within the sesamoid apparatus. The plantar crista of the first metatarsal head may also be viewed and evaluated for erosive changes that may accelerate the deformity. We do not recommend evaluating the tibial sesamoid position on the forefoot axial view, because it should be remembered that activation of the "windless mechanism" will cause the deformity to appear less severe than it actually is.[3]

Finally, the preoperative radiographic evaluation must be combined with a thorough history of the patient's chief complaint and proper clinical examination in both the non-weight-bearing and weight-bearing stance.

## Intermetatarsal Angle

The intermetatarsal angle is formed by the angle produced at the intersection of the longitudinal bisection of the shafts of the first and second metatarsal (Fig. 6-1). A normal range for the intermetatarsal angle in the rectus foot is considered to be 0°–14°. In the adducted foot type, 0°–12° may be considered normal. An abnormally increased intermetatarsal angle may be termed *metatarsus primus adductus*.[22] This transverse plane relationship is one of the most important in selecting the appropriate surgical procedure. As the intermetatarsal angle approaches values greater than 15°, one may wish to consider a more proximally based osteotomy for greater correction. A metatarsal head or neck osteotomy may be considered when the intermetatarsal angle is mild to moderately increased.[23] Scott et al.[24] reported that when comparing the intermetatarsal angle, metatarsus primus varus, the metatarsal cuneiform angle, and the metatarsus omnis angle in patients with hallux valgus, medial deviation of the first metatarsal was measured differently by all four angles. Therefore, it appears the best measure of deviation of the first metatarsal is the intermetatarsal angle.[24]

## Hallus Abductus Angle

The hallux abductus angle or hallux valgus angle is formed by the intersection of a line drawn through the long axis of the first metatarsal and the long axis of the proximal phalanx (see Fig. 6-1). A normal hallux abductus angle is one that measures less than 16° in the rectus foot type. Mild deformity is present when this angle measures between 17° and 25°. The deformity is categorized as severe when the angle measures up to 35°. Finally, a subluxed joint is usually apparent when this relationship measures more than 35°.[24]

## Proximal Articulator Set Angle

The proximal articular set angle (PASA) is another valuable measurement of structural deformity within the metatarsal head. This angle is formed by a line representing the effective articular cartilage of the first metatarsal head and a perpendicular line to the bisection of the shaft of the first metatarsal[18] (Fig. 6-2A). An abnormal increase in PASA may demonstrate the loca-

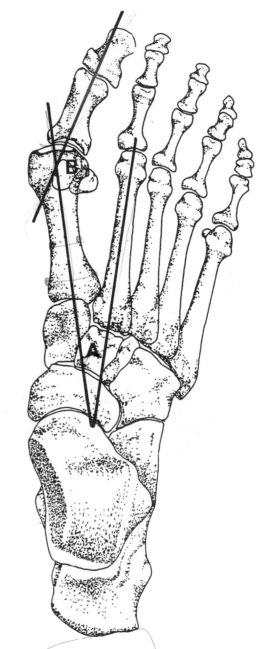

**Fig. 6-1.** A, Intermetatarsal angle; B, hallux abductus angle.

tion of a structural deformity in the head of the metatarsal, and it may progressively increase secondarily to structural adaptation of the articular cartilage surface as the deformity progresses. A normal PASA is one that measures less than 8° in the rectus foot. However, our

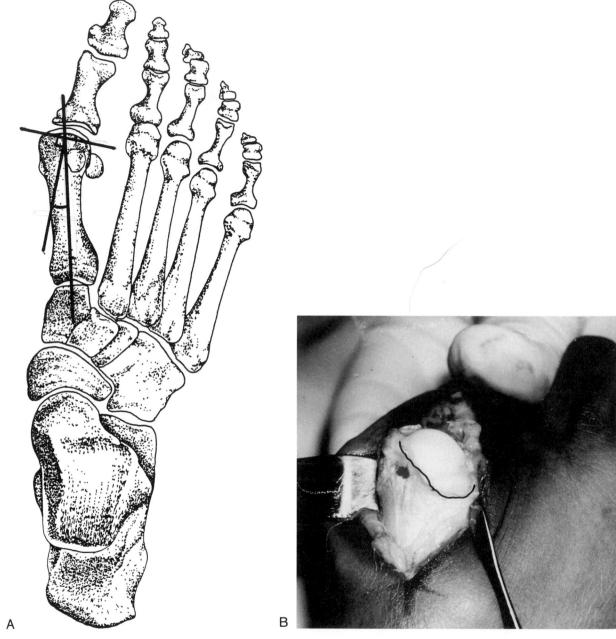

**Fig. 6-2. (A)** Proximal articular set angle. **(B)** Intraoperative photograph shows deviation of effective articular cartilage in a patient with hallux abducto valgus.

experience has led to the belief that the most reliable indicator of an abnormal PASA is to visualize the articular cartilage of the first metatarsal intraoperatively (Fig. 6-2B). Also, one should recognize that when performing an osteotomy at the base of the first metatarsal to correct an abnormal intermetatarsal angle, the PASA may be relatively increased to a point that the first metatarsal phalangeal joint is no longer congruous, necessitating a second distal osteotomy to connect for the relative increase in the PASA.

## Tangential Angle to the Second Axis

The tangential angle to the second metatarsal axis (TASA) is formed by the bisection of the effective articular surface of the first metatarsal and its perpendicular to the longitudinal axis of the second metatarsal[25] (Fig. 6-3). TASA is helpful in determining the angulation of a transverse V osteotomy when performing an Austin-type procedure. In fact, TASA actually redefines a rectus hallus because it compares the position of the hallux to the second toe angle and not to the shaft of the first metatarsal. Ideally, TASA should equal 0°, but an acceptable range is ±5°. A useful equation that may be employed preoperatively when assessing TASA is TASA = PASA − IM angle. Therefore, the only time it is indicated to reduce PASA to 0° is when the intermetatarsal angle is 0°. Utilizing this formula, one can see that TASA concomitantly reflects changes that occur in both the proximal articular set and the intermetatarsal angle in any given foot.[25]

## Distal Articular Set Angle

The distal articular set angle (DASA) represents the angle formed by the bisection of the shaft of the proximal phalanx and the line representing the effective articular cartilage of the base of the proximal phalanx (Fig. 6-4). A normal DASA is considered to be less than 8°. Historically, an abnormal DASA may be corrected by employing a proximal osteotomy near the base of the proximal phalanx. It should be remembered, however, that whenever hallux valgus deformity is present clinically and radiographically the proximal phalanx will also present with some degree of rotation on x-ray examination. This means that one is not viewing the true structural medial and lateral borders of the proximal phalanx. Therefore, preoperative assessment of DASA should be fully compared with the clinical amount of valgus deformity if correction at the base of the proximal phalanx via osteotomy is to be addressed.[26,27] Another factor to consider in measuring the DASA is the length of the proximal phalanx, or the presence of a distal angulational abnormality.

## Hallux Abductus Interphalangeus

The hallux abductus interphalangeus (HAI) angle is a comparison of the longitudinal bisection of the proxi-

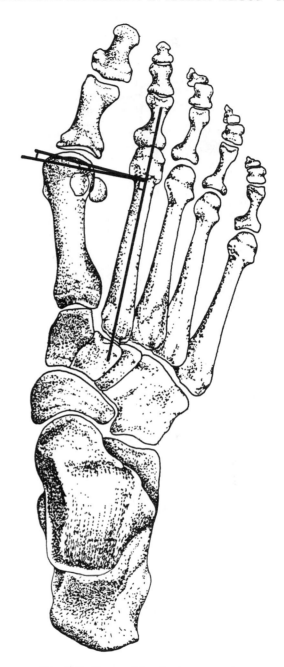

**Fig. 6-3.** Tangential articular set angle.

mal phalanx with the longitudinal bisection of the distal phalanx (Fig. 6-5). The HAI angle is usually considered normal when it measures within a range of 0°–10°. An increase is in this angle indicates that the level of deformity is present at the interphalangeal

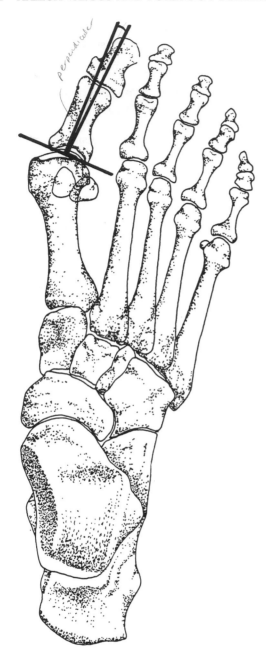

**Fig. 6-4.** Distal articular set angle.

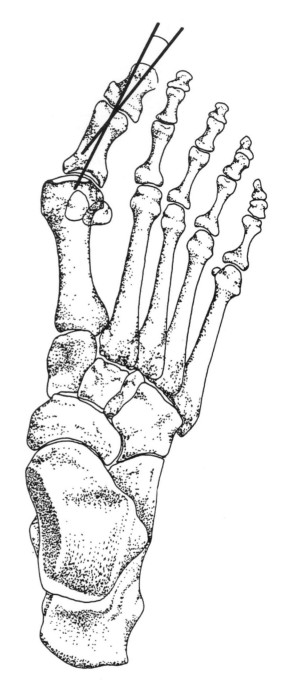

**Fig. 6-5.** Hallux abductus interphalangeus angle.

joint of the hallux. Correction of this deformity is usually addressed at the head of the proximal phalanx.[28]

Although osteotomies at the base of the proximal phalanx to correct for an abnormal DASA or hallux interphalangeus angle (HIA) have long been used as an adjunct procedure in the surgical management of

hallux abducto valgus deformity, it is our experience that the surgeon will get a more satisfactory functional and cosmetic result when performing an osteotomy at the head of the proximal phalanx if the HIA angle is abnormal.

## Tibial Sesamoid Position

The tibial sesamoid position describes the relationship of the tibial sesamoid to the bisection of the first metatarsal shaft on a weight-bearing dorsiplantar view. A numerical sequence of one to seven is described with increasing deformity[18] (Fig. 6-6). A tibial sesamoid position of four or greater represents a significant contraction of the fibular sesamoidal ligament and corresponding sesamoid apparatus. Many practitioners have advocated a fibular sesamoidectomy when the tibial sesamoid position is four or greater.[29] However, with adequate soft tissue release it is often possible to realign the fibular sesamoid under the head of the first metatarsal. Therefore our criteria for performing a fibular sesamoidectomy is when the sesamoid presents with severe arthritic changes or is fused to the lateral aspect of the first metatarsal head. Also, a fibular sesamoidectomy should be considered when one simply cannot relocate the tibial sesamoid under the metatarsal head.

Smith et al.[30] have recommended a simplified method of measuring the tibial sesamoid position us-

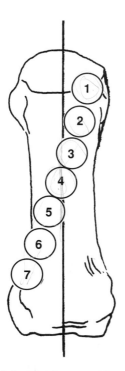

**Fig. 6-6.** Tibial sesamoid position.

ing gradations 0, 1, 2, and 3 rather than the traditional seven. They found the four-grade system was adequate and easier to apply than the seven-grade system in the literature.

Finally, as mentioned previously, one should not use a forefoot axial radiograph to assess the tibial sesamoid position. It should be remembered that when the metatarsal phalangeal joint is dorsiflexed to obtain the forefoot axial view, the windlass mechanism is activated, which allows the position to appear less severe than the deformity actually is.

## Relative Lengths of the First and Second Metatarsal

Metatarsal protrusion is the comparison of the first and second metatarsal lengths. A normal protrusion is +2 to −2 mm. The first and second metatarsal shafts are first bisected and extended proximally to their point of intersection. From this point a compass may be used to construct an arc to the most distal point of the first and second metatarsals. The distance between the arcs is now measured in millimeters (Fig. 6-7). If the first metatarsal is longer, a positive value is assigned; if shorter, a negative value.[18] There exists a strong correlation between a long first metatarsal and a hallux valgus or hallux limitus deformity. Therefore, the practitioner may wish to employ an osteotomy that will shorten the first metatarsal as well as correct for valgus deformity. In the case of a short first metatarsal, we do not recommend a lengthening procedure, because jamming may occur at the first metatarsal phalangeal joint and thus cause a limitus deformity.

## Metatarsus Adductus Angle

An accurate measurement of the metatarsus adductus angle should be made, especially in the preoperative planning of correction of juvenile hallux abducto valgus deformity. The midway point of both the medial aspect of the metatarsocuneiform joint and the talonavicular joint is first found. Similarly, the midway point of the lateral aspect of both the calcaneocuboid joint and fourth metatarsocuboid joint is found. These medial and lateral midway points when connected represent the perpendicular to the long axis of the lesser tarsus. A line perpendicular to the long axis of the lesser metatarsus is now drawn and compared to its bisection of the longitudinal axis of the second

mula is quite useful to assess the true intermetatarsal angle (IMAP):

$$IMAt = IM \ 1 - 2 + (MAA - 15°)$$

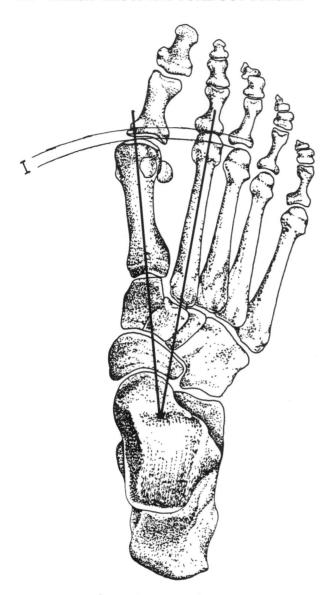

**Fig. 6-7.** Relative metatarsal protrusion.

metatarsal. The angle formed represents the metatarsus abductus angle[18] (Fig. 6-8).

The metatarsus adductus angle is considered normal when it is less than 15° in the rectus foot type. It has great clinical implications in the selection of a bunion procedure. As a general rule, it should be remembered that the greater the metatarsus adductus angle, the greater the hallux abductus angle and the smaller the intermetatarsal angle.[31] The following for-

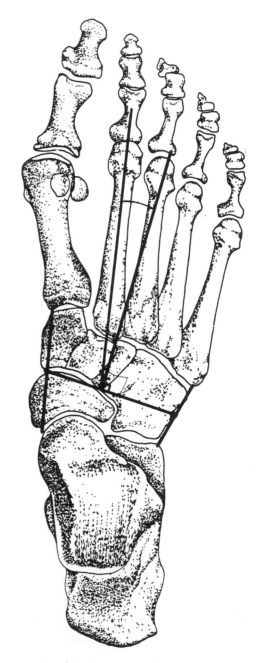

**Fig. 6-8.** Metatarsus adductus angle.

## First Metatarsophalangeal Joint Articulations

The articulating surface between the head of the first metatarsal and base of the proximal phalanx in hallux abducto valgus deformity may be described as congruous, deviated, or subluxed. A congruous joint is one in which lines representing the effective articular surfaces of the metatarsal head and base of the proximal phalanx are parallel; to 3° divergence is considered normal. The normal first metatarsal phalangeal joint should be congruous. However, a congruous joint can be found in hallux abducto valgus deformity and may represent a structurally adapted articulation (Fig. 6-9A).

The metatarsophalangeal joint is deviated when the lines representing the effective articular surface of the head of the first metatarsal and base of the proximal phalanx intersect at a point outside the joint (Fig. 6-9B). A normal range of deviated first metatarsophalangeal articulation is 4 percent to 25 percent. In the subluxed joint, effective articular lines of the first metatarsophalangeal joint intersect within the joint itself (Fig. 6-9C). The angle formed is usually greater than 25 percent. The subluxed first metatarsophalangeal articulation represents either a stage of deformity

with rapid progression. A common example would be in the patient with rheumatoid arthritis.

## Shape of the First Metatarsal Head

The shape of the first metatarsal head when viewed on a anteroposterior (AP) radiograph may be described as round, square, or square with a central ridge. A normal first metatarsal head demonstrates a smooth, continuous, circular pattern (Fig. 6-10A). It is often considered as the least stable of first metatarsophalangeal joint articulations. In the younger patient with a flexible deformity, the round first metatarsal head is the most amenable to soft tissue procedures.[32]

The square first metatarsal head is rarely found in hallux abducto valgus deformity (Fig. 6-10B). It is visually indicative of a hallux limitus or hallux rigidus deformity. The metatarsal head that is square with a central ridge is perhaps the most stable of the metatarsal head shapes (Fig. 6-10C). The central ridge is probably the plantar crista, which becomes more important when the first metatarsal is dorsiflexed (Fig. 6-10B). In a study of 6,000 school children, Kilmartin and Wallace[33] did not find statistical evidence to validate these beliefs. They concluded that "while the shape of the

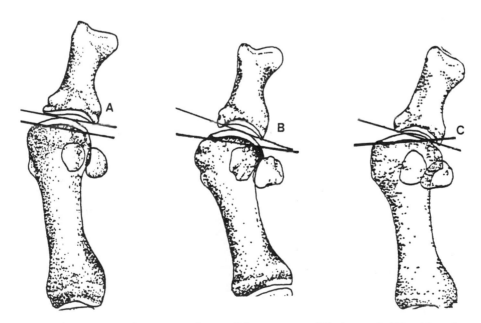

**Fig. 6-9.** Metatarsal joint articulation. **(A)** Congruous; **(B)** deviated; **(C)** subluxed.

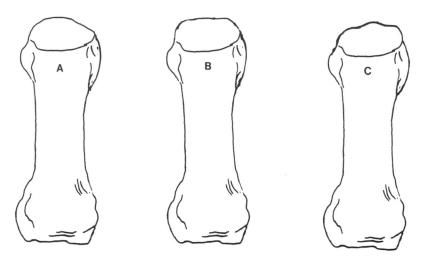

**Fig. 6-10.** Metatarsal head shape. **(A)** Round; **(B)** square; **(C)** square with central ridge.

metatarsal head may be an interesting radiological observation, it has little to contribute to the scientific assessment of first metatarsophalangeal joint pathology."[33]

## Metatarsocuneiform Joint

The metatarsocuneiform joint should also be assessed in hallux abducto valgus deformity. This articulation may be described as square, oblique, or round. As with the first metatarsal head, a rounded first metatarsocuneiform joint may be considered the most flexible and it is also most amenable to soft tissue correction. The most commonly observed shape in hallux abducto valgus deformity. A flat articulation is probably most clinically significant in the preoperative assessment of the deformity. An oblique metatarsocuneiform joint may represent an etiologic factor in the metatarsus primus varus deformity of the first metatarsal. In this instance, the practitioner may wish to select a basal osteotomy to reduce the intermetatarsal angle. An articulation between the first and second metatarsals may also exist blocking reduction of the intermetatarsal angle without metatarsal ostoetomy (Fig. 6-11).

## Radiographic Angular Relationships

After the practitioner has assessed all the pertinent traditional angular values, certain angular relationships may be gathered to aid one in the selection of the surgical procedures.

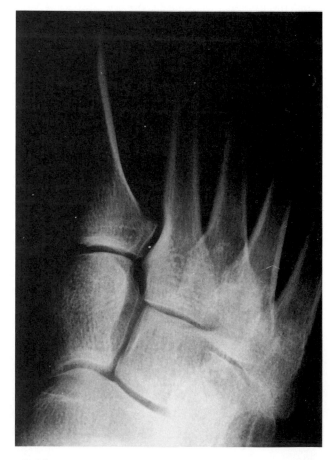

**Fig. 6-11.** Articulation between the first and second metatarsals that would resist a positional change in the intermetatarsal angle by soft tissue procedure alone.

A structural deformity is present when PASA + DASA = HA with PASA or DASA exhibiting an abnormal value. Joint evaluation will reveal a congruent joint. It should be remembered that it is not the absolute numbers that are important but their relationship to each other. In this situation, an osteotomy is indicated as part of the corrective procedure.

A positional deformity exists when PASA + DASA < HA with PASA and PASA both being normal. This is a soft tissue deformity and the joint position will be deviated or subluxed. Finally, a combined deformity is present when elements of both soft tissue and osseous structure contribute to the deformity.

# JUVENILE HALLUX VALGUS

Hallux valgus as it occurs in the juvenile is a deformity of the first metatarsophalangeal joint that may present with pain, is progressive in nature, and may lead to future degenerative changes and serve as source of embarrassment to the older child and young adult. The incidence of juvenile hallux valgus has been addressed by several authors. Craigmile[1] in 1953 studied children in the 12- to 15-year-old group; 22 percent of female and 4 percent of male children exhibited some degree of bunion deformity. Cole[34] in 1959 found that 39 percent of female and 21 percent of male school children between the ages of 8 and 18 displayed mild to severe hallux valgus. Gould and others[35] reported in 1980 the incidence of bunions in the 4- to 14-year-old group to be rare; however, they found it to be five times more frequent in blacks. The male to female ratio was reported as approximately 1:1. Hardy and Clapman[36] in 1951 and Piggott[37] in 1960 reported a history of onset of the deformity before the age of 20 in adult patients with hallux valgus. Johnston[38] reported on a family with a seven-generation pedigree of hallux valgus and felt that it was attributable to an autosomal dominant trait with incomplete penetrance of the gene.

The etiology of juvenile hallux valgus is multifactorial with both genetic and environmental components. There is no doubt that the biomechanics of the child's foot contribute to the development of hallux valgus. The pathomechanical problems most often associated with juvenile hallux valgus are abnormal pronation associated with flexible flatfoot deformity. Juvenile hallux valgus may also be the presenting complaint of a child or adolescent with metatarsus adductus.[15] In this situation, the intermetatarsal angle will not be as large when compared with a juvenile hallux valgus, but will present with a prominent bunion deformity. In this deformity, there is an increase in adduction of all the metatarsals as opposed only to the first in juvenile hallux valgus. Serious consideration must be given to the management of the metatarsus adductus deformity in conjunction with the hallux valgus deformity.

Neurologic disorders such as cerebral palsy and Down syndrome have also been associated with the development of hallux valgus in the juvenile. In Down syndrome, the primary foot deformity has been reported to be hypermobile flatfoot with laxity of the soft tissues, which readily leads to the development of the juvenile hallux valgus deformity.

Inflammatory arthritis, of which juvenile rheumatoid arthritis is an example, may also result in this deformity. Goldner and Gaines[39] described a congenital hallux valgus with a short first ray, skin contracture, and severe deviation of the toe. They considered that this should be treated early, and that soft tissue releases and skin grafting may be necessary as well as osteotomy and bone graft to elongate the first ray.

First-ray deformity in juvenile hallux valgus may be considered as dynamic or static. Dynamic hallux valgus is a result of first-ray hypermobility with development of metatarsus primus abductus secondary to deviation of the great toe. It may also be associated with an abnormally long first metatarsal and hallux interphalangeus. Hardy and Clapman[36] suggested that some factors caused a lateral displacement of the distal phalanx of the great toe. They proposed that the pull of the extensor hallucis longus tendon is transferred laterally to the axis of the great toe in a bowstring effect, and that once this process has started lateral displacement of the first digit must increase. They stressed that the deformity was caused primarily by displacement of the great toe and widening of the intermetatarsal angle secondarily. Lundberg and Sulja[40] found increased relative protrusion of the first metatarsal was positively correlated with the development of hallux valgus.

Hardy and Clapman[9] in 1951 found the first metatarsal, in cases of hallux valgus, to have a greater relative metatarsal protrusion than that of the controls. They noted that with a high degree of valgus of the hallux and a low intermetatarsal angle, the first metatarsal tended to have a greater protrusion relative to the second metatarsal as opposed to cases with a low degree of valgus and a high intermetatarsal angle in which the second had the greater relative protrusion. Static hallux valgus is associated with deformity of the medial cuneiform, possibly a congenital defect that results in metatarsus primus varus as the primary deformity. It may also be caused by a metatarsal deviation or widening of the epiphysis of the first metatarsal proximally on its lateral aspect.

Jones[41] though the primary deforming force in adolescent hallux valgus is adduction of the first metatarsal. He stated that a deformity of considerable severity may develop concurrently with the quick growth of the foot, and is associated with an adducted first metatarsal that was present at birth. He suggested that the metatarsal adduction was atavistic and related to evolutionary development. Bohm[42] described the early stages of embryologic development of the first metatarsal. Early in normal development, the first metatarsal is at the medial border of the first cuneiform and forms an angle of 50° with the long axis of the foot, obviously being in marked adduction. This adduction is seen in the fetus and up to fourth month of gestation, gradually reducing until birth.

Hawkins and Mitchell[43] believed that there was a tendency to underestimate the significance of a congenital metatarsus primus varus in the development of a juvenile hallux valgus deformity. Shoe deformity forces were felt to be secondary to the congenital metatarsus primus varus. Simmonds and Menelaus[44] also associated metatarsus primus varus with juvenile hallux valgus. They noted, as did Bonney and MacNab,[45] that metatarsus primus varus was the most important aspect needing correction in the adolescent if recurrence of the deformity was to be avoided, and believed it was a major factor contributing to the breakdown of the forefoot. Lapidus[15] classified hallux valgus into three groups with the most predominant group showing a congenital predisposition to metatarsus primus varus. Truslow[46] thought the primary deformity was a wedging of the medial cuneiform or the proximal end of the metatarsal. The outward deviation of the toe was secondary to this primary deformity.

As alluded to earlier, Piggott[37] in his studies on adolescent hallux valgus classified the metatarsophalangeal joint into three groups. These classes were con-

gruous, deviated, or subluxed. In his study he could produce little or no evidence that metatarsus primus varus was the underlying cause of hallux valgus. He concluded that the structural prognosis of hallux valgus in the adolescent is as follows: Congruity of the joint surfaces can be considered as normal and indicates that a progressive deformity will not occur, but subluxation indicates that deterioration is likely; the deviation may or may not progress to subluxation. He noted subluxation of the first metatarsophalangeal joint was seen before closure of the metatarsal and phalangeal epiphysis. However, in support of metatarsus primus varus, Durman[14] found a significant variation in shape of the first cuneiform. In his study, cuneiform deformity was present in 47 percent of patients with hallux valgus.

Thus we see that juvenile hallux valgus can be dynamic in nature, with deviation of the great toe resulting in a increase in the intermetatarsal angle or metatarsus primus abductus, or a static deformity in which the primary etiology is more proximal is a congenital effect, such as deformity of the medial cuneiform or base of the metatarsal. It is interesting to note that Luba and Rossman[47] show that preoperative compression and tension forces may act to perpetuate or stimulate active deformity by applying compression force to the epiphyseal plate medially and a tension force laterally, which may result in a asymmetric growth of the first metatarsal (Fig. 6-12). One could only speculate how this relationship interplays with the development of a structural metatarsus primus varus. In a study of 6,000 school children, Kilmartin et al.[48] failed to provide significant correlations between adduction of the first metatarsocuneiform joint, intercuneiform angle (an estimation of the alignment of the medial and intermediate cuneiforms), metatarsus adductus angle, or differentiation of growth patterns of the first metatarsal.[34]

Clinical evaluation of the juvenile patient with hallux valgus deformity should be complete and thorough, including integrity of the soft tissue, examination for liagmentous laxity, joint status, and mobility, complete neuromuscular evaluation, and biomechanical evaluation.

When considering surgery in the child with juvenile hallux valgus, several areas are important. As with the adult hallux abducto valgus deformity, the correct procedure is chosen after careful examination, both clini-

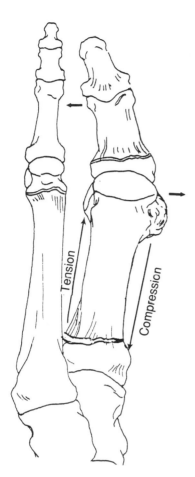

**Fig. 6-12.** Compressive and tension forces applied to the first metatarsal epiphysis as theorized by Luba and Rossman.

cally and radiographically. The growing foot, however, adds another dimension to this surgical correction. It appears that a slightly elevated intermetatarsal angle, at the time of examination in the child, may need greater reduction because of its tendency to increase with age. The timing of surgery should be related to the severity of symptoms, the estimation of progression of deformity based on radiographic criteria, and the skeletal age of the child. Estimation of skeletal age is important especially with regards to procedures around or involving the epiphyseal plate.

The goals of surgery in juvenile hallux valgus are primarily to correct the deformity, to reduce the intermetatarsal angle, to reduce the hallux abductus angle, to obtain and maintain a congruous metatarsophalangeal joint with realignment of the sesamoids, and to

have a pain-free range of motion. All this is predicated on the choice of the correct procedure.

A number of surgical procedures that may be used in the management of juvenile hallux valgus include soft tissue tendon-balancing procedures, whose main aim is to realign the osseous structures by correcting abnormality of soft tissue ligamentous and capsular structures. However, these procedures are infrequently done in the patient with juvenile hallux valgus as the primary procedure but are often used in conjunction with distal or proximal osteotomies that correct structural deformities. Distal metatarsal osteotomies can decrease the intermetatarsal angle and realign structural abnormalities in the transverse plane such as abnormal proximal articular set angles. They can shorten or maintain the length of the metatarsal. Distal osteotomies of use in juvenile hallux valgus include the Mitchell, Wilson, Austin, Reverdin, or Hohman types. Reduction of the intermetatarsal angle is accomplished by lateral displacement of those osteotomies. The degree of reduction will be less than that obtained with proximal osteotomies, and therefore lateral displacement osteotomy is used with intermetatarsal angles ranging from 12° to 16°. Proximal osteotomies include osteotomies of the metatarsal base, of the metatarsocuneiform joint in combination with a fusion, or cuneiform osteotomies. These osteotomies are used to correct hallus valgus deformities with increased intermetatarsal angles greater than 16°. Phalangeal osteotomy is limited to those cases in which structural deformity of the phalanx exist such as a transverse plane clinodactyly. Epiphysiodesis has been reported to be successful in the management of juvenile hallux valgus, and is best used in the child that is approaching skeletal maturity.[49]

Complications following surgery for juvenile hallux valgus include recurrence of the deformity. Scranton and Zuckerman[50] reported a failure rate of 50 percent in patients with long first metatarsals and a 56 percent failure rate associated with collapsing pes valgo planus. Drennan,[51] at an American Academy of Orthopedic Surgeons meeting in 1990, reported 30 to 50 percent recurrence of deformity after an initial procedure requiring secondary intervention. Metatarsalgia may occur postoperatively with excessive elevation or shortening of distal or proximal osteotomies. Excessive dorsiflexion may also lead to joint stiffness and secondary hallux rigidus. Total or partial premature epiphyseal plate closure may occur and result in shortening or angular deformity of the metatarsal, undercorrection, or overcorrection. Epiphyseal plate closure may result secondary to osteotomy or arthrodesis of the metatarsal cuneiform articulation.

Juvenile hallux valgus is a complex deformity that needs careful preoperative clinical and radiographic evaluation. Consideration should be given to the appropriate timing of the procedure relative to the skeletal growth of the child. It is important to remember that no one procedure is appropriate for all juvenile or adolescent hallux valgus deformities.

# REFERENCES

1. Craigmile DA: Incidence, origin and prevention of certain foot defects. Br Med J 2:749, 1953
2. Clough JG, Marshall HJ: The etiology of hallux abducto valgus. A review of the literature. J Am Podiatr Med Assoc 75:238, 1985
3. Root ML, Orien WP, Weed JH: Normal and Abnormal Function of the Foot. Los Angeles, Clinical Biomechanics Corp., 1977
4. Duke H, Newman LM, Bruskoff BL, et al: Relative metatarsal length patterns in hallux abducto valgus. J Am Podiatr Assoc 72:1, 1982
5. Gerbert J: Textbook of Bunion Surgery. 2nd Ed. Futura Publishing, New York, 1991
6. Harris RI, Beath T: The short first metatarsal: its incidence and clinical significance. J Bone Joint Surg Am 31:553, 1949
7. Robinson HA: Bunion: its cause and cure. J Surg Gynecol Obstet 27:343, 1918
8. Kalen V, Brecher A: Relationship between adolescent bunions and flatfeet. Foot Ankle 8:331, 1988
9. Hardy RH, Clapham JCR: Observations on hallux valgus. J Bone Joint Surg 33B:376, 1951
10. D'Amico JC, Schuster RO: Motion of the first ray. J Am Podiatr Assoc 69:17, 1979
11. DeBritto SR: The first metatarso-sesamoid joint. Int Orthop 6:67, 1984
12. Jahss MH (ed): The sesamoids of the hallux. Clin Orthop 157:88, 1981
13. Durman DC: Metatarsus primus varus and hallux valgus. Arch Surg 74:128, 1957
14. Durman DC: Metatarsus primus varus and hallux valgus. J Bone Joint Surg 39A:221, 1957
15. Lapidus PW: Operative correction of metatarsus primus varus in hallux valgus. Surg Gynecol Obstet 58:183, 1934
16. Kleinberg S: Operative care of hallux valgus and bunions. Am J Surg 15, 1932
17. Wheeler PH: Os intermetatarseum and hallux valgus. Am J Surg 18:341, 1932
18. LaPorta G, Melillo T, Olinsky D: X-ray evaluations of hallux abducto valgus deformity. J Am Podiatr Assoc 64:544, 1974
19. Jiminez AJ, Corey SV: Hallux valgus, intractable plantar keraotsis sub second metatarsal, hammertoe. In McGlamry ED (ed): Reconstructive Surgery of the Foot and Leg, Update '87. Podiatry Institute Publishing, Tucker, GA, 1987
20. Sage RA, Jugar DW: Hallux pinch calluses: some etiologic considerations. J Foot Surg 19:148, 1980
21. McCrea JD, Lichty TK: The first metatarsocuneiform articulation and its relationship to metatarsus primus varus. J Am Podiatr Assoc 69:700, 1979
22. Steel MW, Johnson KA, De Witz MA, et al: Radiographic measurements of the normal foot. Foot Ankle 1:151, 1980
23. Southerland C, Spinner SM: Preoperative criteria for hallux valgus surgery and use of convergent angled base wedge osteotomy. J Foot Surg 26:475, 1987
24. Scott G, Wilson DW, Bently G: Roentgenographic assessment in hallux valgus. Clin Orthop Relat Res 267:143, 1991
25. Schechter DZ, Doll PJ: Tangential angle to the second axis. J Am Podiatr Med Assoc 75:505, 1985
26. Balding MG, Sorto LA: Distal articular set angle. Etiology and x-ray evaluation. J Am Podiatr Med Assoc 75:648, 1985
27. Barnett CH: Valgus deviation of the distal phalanx of the great toe. J Anat 96:171, 1962
28. Duke H, Newman LM, Bruskoff BL, et al: Hallux abductus interphalangeus and its relationship to hallux valgus surgery. J Am Podiatr Med Assoc 72:625, 1982
29. McGlamry ED: Hallucal sesamoids. J Am Podiatry Assoc 55:693, 1965
30. Smith RW, Reynolds JC, Stewart MJ: Hallux valgus assessment: report of research committee of the American Orthopedic Foot and Ankle Society. Foot Ankle 5:92, 1984
31. Yu GV, DiNapoli R: Surgical management of hallux abducto valgus with concomitant metatarsus adductus. In McGlamry ED (ed): Reconstructive surgery of the foot and leg, Update '87. Podiatry Institute Publishing, Tucker, GA, 1987
32. Jahss MH: Hallux valgus: further considerations, the first metatarsal head. Foot Ankle 2:1, 1981
33. Kilmartin TE, Wallace WA: First metatarsal head shape in juvenile hallux abducto valgus. J Foot Surg 30:506, 1991

34. Cole AE: Foot inspection of the school child. J Am Podiatr Med Assoc 49:446, 1959
35. Gould N, Schneider W, Ashikaga T: Epidemiological survey of foot problems in the continental United States. 1978–1979. Foot Ankle 1:8, 1980
36. Hardy RH, Clapman JCR: Hallux valgus; predisposing anatomical causes. Lancet ii:1180, 1952
37. Piggott H: The natural history of hallux valgus in adolescence and early adult life. J Bone Joint Surg 42:749, 1960
38. Johnston O: Further studies on the inheritence of hand and foot anomalies. Clin Orthop Relat Res
39. Goldner JL, Gaines RW: Adult and juvenile hallux valgus: analysis and treatment. Orthop Clin North Am 7:863, 1976
40. Lundberg BJ, Sulja T: Skeletal parameters on the hallux valgus foot. Acta Orthop Scand 43:749, 1960
41. Jones RA: Hallux valgus in the adolescent. Proc R Soc Med 41:391, 1948
42. Bohm M: The embryonic origin of clubfoot. J Bone Joint Surg 27:229, 1945
43. Hawkins FB, Mitchell CL, Hedrick DW: Correction of hallux valgus by metatarsal osteotomy. J Bone Joint Surg 27:387, 1945
44. Simmonds FA, Menelaus MB: Hallux valgus in adolescent. J Bone Joint Surg 42B:761, 1960
45. Bonney G, McNab, L: Hallux valgus and hallux rigidus—a critical survey. J Bone Joint Surg 34B:366, 1952
46. Truslow W: Metatarsus primus varus or hallux valgus. J Bone Joint Surg 7:98, 1925
47. Luba R, Rosman M: Bunions treatment with a modified Mitchell osteotomy. J Pediatr Orthop 4:44, 1984
48. Kilmartin TE, Barrington RL, Wallace WA: Metatarsus primus varus. J Bone Joint Surg 73B:937, 1991
49. Fox IM, Smith SD: Juvenile bunion correction by epiphysiodesis of the first metatarsal. J Am Podiatr Med Assoc 73(9):448, 1983
50. Scranton PE, Zuckerman JD: Bunion surgery in adolescents: results of surgical treatment. J Pediatr Orthop 4:39, 1984
51. Drennan JC: Instructional Course Lectures, The Childs Foot I. In Proceedings, Annual Meeting AAOS, New Orleans, LA, February 1990

# 7

# Soft Tissue Procedures for Hallux Abducto Valgus

## GEORGE F. WALLACE

More than 100 procedures for the removal of a bunion (medial eminence) and correction of hallux abducto valgus deformity have been described.[1] In a rather simplistic classification, these procedures are either soft tissue corrections principally around the first metatarsophalangeal joint or those procedures that employ an osteotomy to correct a structural component of the deformity.

Although soft tissue procedures have been described as the sole means for the removal of a bunion or correction of hallux abducto valgus, in most instances they are now used when very strict preoperative criteria have been met.[2-8] However, it is imperative to remember that whenever an osseous procedure is performed, the deforming forces and pathology around the first metatarsophalangeal joint have been addressed and corrected using a "soft tissue procedure," usually in some modification from the original authors' descriptions.

## HISTORICAL PERSPECTIVE

The three most important procedures and those that serve as a foundation for any modifications are the Silver, Hiss, and McBride bunionectomies.

In 1923 Silver described his procedure, which consisted of removal of the medial eminence coplanar with the medial cortex, a lateral capsulotomy, adductor release, and reinforcement of the medial capsule via a V to Y capsulotomy.[9] He astutely realized this procedure should never be attempted when degenerative joint disease is present. In 49 surgeries on 31 patients, there were only 2 recurrences and 2 hallux varuses during a 2-year follow-up. The methodology by which these numbers were obtained was not reported.

Hiss in 1931 described hallux abducto valgus as a "buckle joint" whereby a tendon imbalance was caused by the altered and diminished pull of the abductor hallucis and the increased advantage of the adductor hallucis. His observation of the pathology elucidated the fact that the medial capsule was stretched while the lateral capsule was contracted. His insight brought about the concept of capsule tendon balance as a surgical goal. This could be accomplished by resection of the medial eminence, an adductor hallucis tenotomy, a medial elliptical capsulotomy, and the repositioning of the abductor hallucis more dorsally via sutures into the medial periosteum and capsule of the first metatarsal.[10] The latter would create fibrosis, periarticularly in hopes of preventing elongation and relaxation of the medial structures. Fibular sesamoidectomy was performed as needed.

The evolution of surgical procedures for bunion correction next addressed the fibular sesamoid and its significance in the formation of a bunion deformity. This concept was popularized by McBride.[11-13] In his original work of 1928, the medial eminence was removed coplanar with the first metatarsal, the adductor hallucis was released and transplanted into the lateral head of the first metatarsal, and the fibular sesamoid was removed if eroded, abnormal in shape, or displaced. The amount of displacement never was addressed. Two incisions were utilized: one dorsomedially and another through the first interspace. The

125

final position after closure was 10° of varus, but no mention was made of the long-term consequences of this overcorrection.[11]

In 1954, McBride further elucidated his surgical approach by staging the development of a bunion deformity.[12] In stage 1, the bunion is just beginning to form. No articular changes would be evident, and correction could be achieved by a closed tenotomy of the adductor hallucis. Stage 2 represents a moderate deformity; a rather large medial eminence with an adventitious bursa is found. In this instance the eminence is removed, the adductor hallucis is cut and a $\frac{1}{8}$- to $\frac{1}{4}$-in. wedge-shaped part of the medial capsule is removed. Stage 3 is a severe deformity characterized by a moderate amount of cartilage degeneration of the first metatarsophalangeal joint. For these cases, the fibular sesamoid is removed, the tenotomized adductor hallucis is resutured into the lateral aspect of the first metatarsal neck, and the first and second metatarsals are reapproximated using sutures through the capsules of each. Severe degenerative joint disease exists in stage 4. Both sesamoids may have to be removed if diseased. Again, no objective studies are contained in the paper to substantiate the claims proposed.

Finally, in 1967 McBride called the conjoined adductor hallucis the culprit of the bunion deformity.[13] A simple test determined if the adductor and lateral capsule were to blame and whether the fibular sesamoid should be excised. If the hallux corrected while the adductor was at rest but not weight-bearing, then just the adductor was contracted. Such a finding did not warrant the removal of the fibular sesamoid. Conversely, if the hallux was unable to correct while weight-bearing then the capsule was contracted and the sesamoid should then be excised.

Table 7-1 lists some of the lesser known authors of soft tissue procedures or those who for various reasons have not been given the proper credit for their work over the course of time. From the Silver, Hiss, and McBride papers, foot surgeons performed varied parts of these procedures. Their importance is paramount to adequate and long-term success of any hallucal procedure.

## OBJECTIVES OF SOFT TISSUE PROCEDURES

Pathology around the first metatarsophalangeal joint may present as a bunion (medial eminence) with or without adventitious bursa formation or as a hallux abducto valgus deformity whereby the hallux is abducted with or without valgus rotation. In the latter case, the intermetatarsal and hallux abductus angles can be significantly increased.

Such deformities alter the anatomy and thereby the mechanics of the structures of the first metatarsophalangeal joint. The medial structures are stretched while the lateral are contracted (Fig. 7-1). Mechanical advantage of the adductor hallucis over the abductor hallucis perpetuates the deformity. The abductor hallucis then becomes merely a plantar-flexor. In long-standing cases, cartilaginous changes occur at the articular surfaces as the hallux drifts laterally, thus depriving the medial cartilage of proper articulation by the proximal phalangeal base. In protracted cases, the hallux rotates in a valgus direction.

The main objectives of any procedure in hallux abducto valgus surgery are to correct the deformity, prevent recurrence, and maintain as nearly normal motion as possible.[14,15] Used as the entire procedure in rather mild cases and combined with procedures that realign deformed osseous structures im more severe cases, the Silver, Hiss, and McBride techniques can accomplish these stated objectives. Soft tissue procedures are never performed on congruent joints; the objective is to create one. If a soft tissue procedure is done alone on a congruent joint, the joint will ulti-

**Table 7-1.** Lesser Known Authors and Their Procedures

| Author | Date | Procedure |
|--------|------|-----------|
| Lothrop | 1873 | Adductor tenotomy and lateral capsulotomy |
| Fowler | 1887 | Remove head through interdigital incision |
| Syms | 1897 | Remove as much of medial eminence as needed to flatten |
| Schede | 1904 | "Simple exostectomy"—remove bone not in contact with proximal phalanx |
| Porter | 1909 | Remove two-thirds to three-fourths of metatarsal head |
| Mauclaire | 1924 | EHL and adductor into first metatarsal head |
| Balog | 1928 | Adductor into medial aspect of first metatarsal head. Abductor into EHL |
| Stein | 1938 | Two incisions; adductor release and abductor dorsally sutured into capsule |

*Abbreviation:* EHL, extensor hallucis longus.

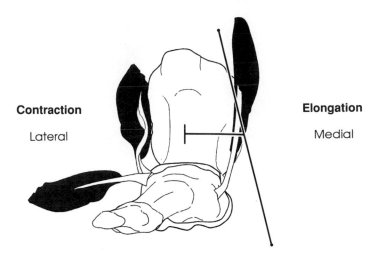

**Contraction**

Lateral

**Elongation**

Medial

**Fig. 7-1.** With the first metatarsophalangeal joint as the fulcrum, the medial structures are stretched (the elevated part of the see-saw) and the lateral structures are contracted.

mately become deviated and jam medially, leading to premature degenerative joint disease.

Whenever the first metatarsophalangeal joint undergoes surgery, the malaligned structures should be repositioned as anatomically as possible. The contracted tissues need to be relaxed (laterally) and the elongated tissues secured (medially) more tightly. In essence, a capsule tendon balance (actually a rebalancing) must be created.[10] Failure results in undercorrection, recurrence, or, if overcorrected, hallux varus.

## SURGICAL TECHNIQUES

Anyone who has attempted repair of a hallux abducto valgus realizes that the objectives are not so easily realized. For the purpose of this chapter, the following discussion presents the steps employed in the capsule tendon balance attempt.

A capsulotomy will open the medial or dorsimedial aspect of the first metatarsophalangeal joint, thus exposing the medial eminence. Any type may be used (e.g., U, T, inverted L, dorsolinear, semielliptical, etc.). The dorsal linear and T can easily overcorrect when tightened.[16] Although redundant capsule can be removed, there is no hard-and-fast rule to determine the amount. Suture placement in an oblique fashion can be effective in derotating the hallux when a semiellip-

tical capsulotomy is performed. The abductor hallucis can also be pulled more dorsally when oblique sutures are used. One should never, however, rely on the capsular closure to hold the ultimate position of correction.

Resection of the medial eminence depends on the procedures performed. In some instances no medial eminence need be removed, especially in the juvenile deformity. When a simple bunionectomy is warranted, the medial eminence can be resected almost flush with the first metatarsal medial shaft. Whether with an osteotome or power saw, the cut is made medial to the sagittal groove. This technique should be reserved for those patients who need the medial eminence resected for reason of a chronic bursal formation or a lesion over the eminence, or when complete correction is contraindicated (Fig. 7-2).

For those patients who need total correction of the deformity, the medial eminence should be removed medial to the sagittal groove, but the osseous blade should be angled to remove more bone from the dorsal surface than from the plantar (Fig. 7-3). When the correction is performed in this manner, the plantar articular tibial sesamoid surface is preserved. Hallux varus formation as a result of medially staking the head and tibial sesamoid peaking is prevented. Naturally, rough edges are always rasped smooth in motions away from the articular cartilage.

The lateral release should consist of completely

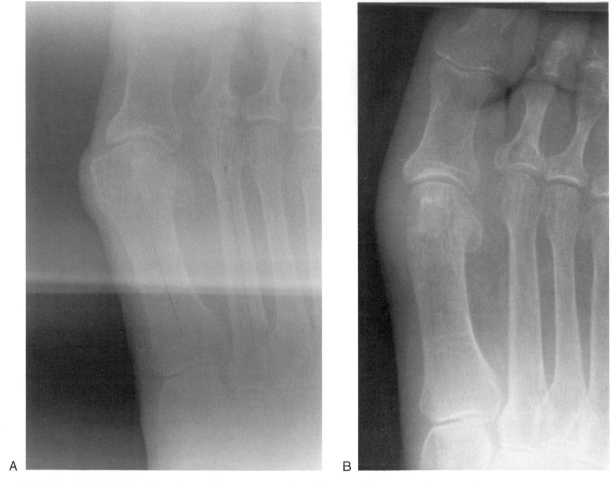

**Fig. 7-2.** **(A)** A 75-year-old patient with symptomatic hyperkeratotic lesion over the medial eminence. This patient is a poor candidate for osteotomy. **(B)** Postoperative radiograph with medial eminence removed. This eliminated the lesion.

tenotomizing the conjoined tendons (oblique and transverse) of the adductor hallucis, severing the deep transverse metatarsal ligament, and performing a lateral vertical capsulotomy and fibular sesamoid release. Completion will enable the hallux to move without restriction medially and repositions the sesamoids under the metatarsal head.

Historically, a separate incision of the first interspace was done to complete the lateral release. We now know that the interspace can be addressed through the initial dorsimedial incision when the superficial and deep fascial fibers are severed.

Retraction of the skin and extensor tendons exposes the most dorsal aspect of the first interspace. The back of a scalpel handle is used to bluntly dissect the interspace. The adductor tendons will be palpated, but the handle is able to proceed to the plantar surface proximal and distal to the adductor.

A successful and relatively quick technique for severing the tendons and ligament is to insert an opened curved hemostat from distal to proximal under the adductor and transverse ligament. Sharp dissection is then performed through the opened hemostat. No structures should impede the placement of the scalpel

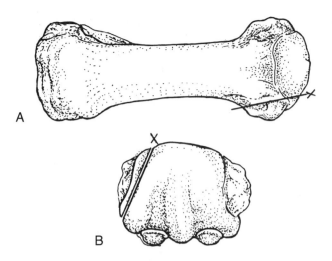

**Fig. 7-3. (A)** Angle of cut to preserve tibial sesamoid articulation. **(B)** Angle of cut when viewed dorsally. "X" indicates the sagittal groove.

handle when it is reinserted throughout the interspace. Complete release of the adductor tendons is the most important step of the lateral release.[6] Numerous veins are located in the interspace at this level, and thus hemostasis is critical. A release that is too proximal can jeopardize the deep plantar artery.

The fibular sesamoid is next addressed to be released. The capsule dorsal to the sesamoid is initially punctured, and the knife blade is moved distally then plantarly around the sesamoid. This incises the attachments of the adductor hallucis and flexor hallucis brevis to the proximal phalanx. A similar maneuver is performed around the sesamoid, proximally, then plantarly. A periosteal elevator may have to be inserted

superficial to the sesamoidal cartilage to aid in the sesamoid release (Fig. 7-4). The fibular sesamoid should appear in a more plantar position and is easily movable, adhering only by the intersesamoidal ligament. Degenerative joint changes of the metatarsosesamoidal joint may hinder the sesamoid from dropping.

If upon its release there is no mobility whatsoever, then the fibular sesamoid may be removed. Also, with a very high intermetatarsal angle, and if the patient is a poor candidate for an osseous procedure, fibular sesamoid removal can decrease the intermetatarsal angle by a few degrees via the concept of reverse buckling.[17–19]

Removing this sesamoid can tilt the balance of the joint to the medial side, especially if too much eminence is removed and the tibial sesamoid begins to drift medially and peaks from beneath the metatarsal head. A hallux varus can result, and this will be even more predictable if the medial capsule is tightened excessively and the intermetatarsal angle approaches 0 or negative degrees (Fig. 7-5).

Fibular sesamoid removal is not easy, especially when the sesamoids are completely articulating with the metatarsal or have just begun to move within the first interspace. Ease of removal can be accomplished when a tag of capsule is created laterally so the surgeon can hold onto the bone via the tag and manipulate it around the knife's cutting surface. At no time is it more critical to incise tissue next to bone. Failure to follow this rule can lead to severance of the long flexor.

A vertical lateral capsulotomy is created from just below the extensor tendons to the plantar aspect of

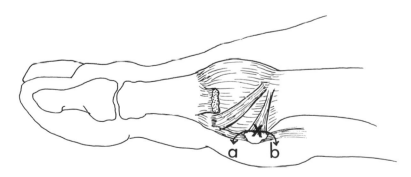

**Fig. 7-4.** Releasing fibular sesamoid. "X" is where blade is first inserted and is advanced to meet points a and b.

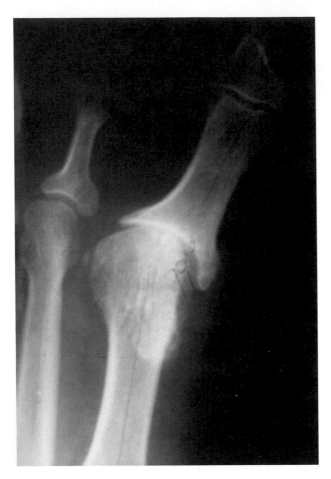

**Fig. 7-5.** Hallux varus. Note tibial sesamoid "peaking" from excessive resection of the medial eminence. Fibular sesamoid has been removed.

the joint. By distracting the joint distally and observing the puckering of the capsule, the joint is identified and the knife is inserted into the puckered area and moved plantarward.

After all the foregoing steps are completed, the hallux should be able to be manually placed in a corrected or slightly overcorrected position. Any hint of tightness laterally should warrant an inspection of the first interspace and determination of the structures that were incompletely released initially. Any found at this time are now released, as complete lateral release is paramount.

Capsulorraphy or reefing the medial capsule after all the prior steps have been performed can maintain the correction and balancing around the metatarsophalangeal joint. However, if too much redundant cap-

sule is removed, or the capsulotomy sutures are placed too tightly, the joint may be overcorrected and have a propensity to tilt medially. After capsular closure, the final position of the hallux can be visualized by loading the foot. Joint stiffness and jamming increase if too much capsule is removed.[6,20] Inadequate repair of the capsulotomy can predispose to a loss of correction.[21]

A few important concepts to remember: (a) Before capsular closure, the lateral structures should be completely loose. Manual adduction of the hallux should be easily accomplished. No springing back to the deforming position should occur. If it does, the lateral release is reevaluated. (b) After closure of the capsule, the foot should be moved into a simulated weightbearing position. The hallux and first metatarsal should now be in proper and physiologic alignment, and thus all preoperative angles must be corrected. If reliance is placed on the capsular sutures or dressings to maintain the correction, it will not stand the test of time.

The literature contains diverse opinions as to whether the extensor hallucis brevis be tenotomized to complete the rebalancing of the first metatarsophalangeal joint.[8,17,22] No studies have been formulated as to whether tenotomizing the extensor hallucis brevis leads to a diminished recurrence rate.

Intraoperatively, while the tourniquet is inflated, is not the time to determine if the long extensor is contracted. Tourniquet elevation will lead to many false positives. Should the tendon be taut per preoperative determination, then a slide lengthening can be done. This is performed before closure of the capsule.[8] Lengthening the tendon in the presence of a hypermobile first ray may increase the hypermobility.[18] Currently the extensor hallucis longus tendon is rarely lengthened during hallux abducto valgus surgery.

Extensive bowstringing of the long extensor ultimately decreases with reduction of the intermetatarsal angle. In very severe deformities, a residual bowstringing may exist. With these cases, the most medial part of the extensor hood may be incorporated into the capsular closure at the metatarsal neck.[17] At no time is the tendon itself punctured.

Transfer of the adductor hallucis has been advocated to aid in the correction of the soft tissue procedures. The theory is that when the adductor hallucis is transferred to the medial capsule, the fibular sesamoid is rotated into a more anatomic position via the torque of the medial capsule, which is transferred to the medial sesamoid via the tibial sesamoid ligament and on through the fibular sesamoid via the intersesamoidal ligament.[23] Forefoot splay is decreased as well as the intermetatarsal angle.

Adductor hallucis transfers are not performed in any patients with fibular sesamoid degenerative joint disease or atrophy of the tendon (which occurs frequently in older patients), or in those feet in which a structural intermetatarsal angle exists.[24]

Available length of the adductor tendon may preclude the transfer traversing all the way to the medial capsule via a route deep to the extensor hallucis longus at the metatarsal neck. In such cases, the tendon can be passed medially through a drill hole in the metatarsal or simply sutured to the lateral capsule.[5,8,11,18,25,26]

Adjunct soft tissue procedures when combined with an osseous procedure can be enhanced by suturing the capsules of the first and second metatarsals together with incorporation of the adductor hallucis.[27]

Extensive lateral releases have been implicated in the development of aseptic necrosis of the first metatarsal head when combined with distal osteotomies. Reports of 20 percent occurrence appear to be rather high.[28] Failure of a complete lateral release may lead to recurrence. Both aforementioned scenarios must be weighed carefully when performing this surgery.

# CRITERIA FOR SOFT TISSUE PROCEDURES

Patients presenting to the physician's office for surgical correction of a bunion or hallux abducto valgus deformity not only want the pathology removed but also desire a "new foot."[29] The agreement between their expectations and the final outcome may be less than ideal. Therefore, each case must be properly evaluated both clinically and radiographically to determine the proper procedure for not only the pathology but also for the patient's life-style, age, bone composition, and medical history.

Soft tissue procedures, namely the Silver and McBride procedures, may be used alone or in combination with osseous procedures (Fig. 7-6). As previously mentioned, the goal is to restore the balance around the first metatarsophalangeal joint. In the absence of any osteotomies (when used alone), patients undergoing the Silver and McBride procedures will heal more rapidly and be afforded quicker return to shoe gear. Obviously there is no need to await bone healing. Therefore, the procedures can prove to be very attractive to those who desire a quick, easy fix. However, if certain criteria are not met, then the chance of deformity recurrence increases.

Proper evaluation of any patient with hallux abducto valgus, in addition to pertinent history and neurovascular examination, consists of the following:

1. Presence or absence of medial eminence and lesions overlying the eminence. Is an adventitious bursa present?
2. Amount of hallux drift laterally and position of second toe. Amount, if any, of valgus rotation of hallux.
3. Evaluation of joint to include presence or absence of any crepitus, effusions, pain, or restricted range of motion. Is the joint track bound?
4. When in corrected position, is there pain at the most medial aspect of the cartilage on the first metatarsal or is the range of motion decreased?
5. Evaluation of ligamentous laxity.[30]
6. General foot type.

Radiographic evaluation in the angle and base of gait will consist of the following:

1. Measurement of intermetatarsal, hallux abductus, metatarsus adductus, hallux abductus interphalangus, proximal articular set, and distal articular set angles
2. Evaluation of metatarsal protrusion
3. Evaluation of the tibial sesamoid position
4. Evaluation of the shape of first metatarsal head (round, ridged, square)
5. Determination of the presence or absence of degenerative joint disease within the first metatarsophalangeal joint
6. Determination of whether a deviated, congruous, or subluxed joint is present
7. Evaluation of structural deformity: Proximal articular set angle (PASA) + distal articular set angle (DASA) = hallux abductus angle (HAA)
8. Evaluation of positional deformity: PASA + DASA < HAA[31]

When all the foregoing are determined, the decision process begins. The soft tissue procedures when

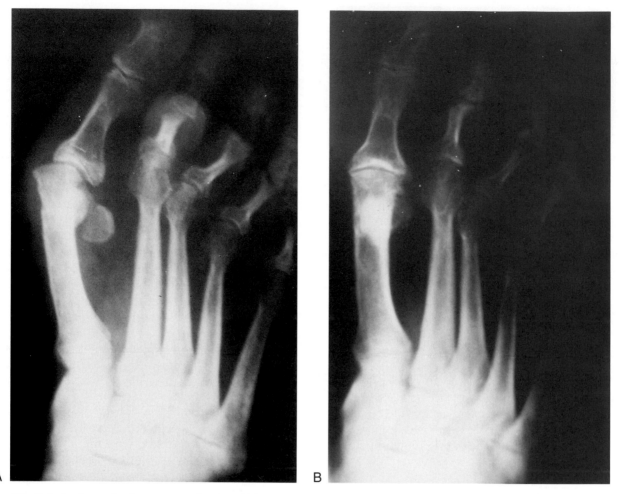

**Fig. 7-6.** Radiographs demonstrate the potential for correction of the adducto hallucis tendon after transfer on the intermetatarsal angle. **(A)** Preoperative radiograph of a patient who underwent previous forefoot surgery including bunionectomy of the first metatarsophalangeal joint; recurrence of the deformity is evident. **(B)** Postoperative radiograph after adductor hallucis transfer and fibular sesamoidectomy.

used alone should be performed only on positional deformities. Obviously, osseous correction would be necessary if structural deformities exist.[32]

When soft tissue procedures are used alone, there should also be no evidence of degenerative joint disease or restricted range of motion. No pain in the corrected or uncorrected position should be produced when the joint is stressed. A track-bound joint would be a contraindication. However, the first metatarsophalangeal joint should be deviated or subluxed, and preferably with a central ridge or squared. If it is congruous, the capsule tendon balance will more than

likely jam the joint medially and precipitate early degenerative joint disease. A rounded head can be unstable in the transverse plane and more easily disrupted if the capsule tendon balance is not adequate.

In general, the intermetatarsal angle should be less than 12°, and the hallux abductus angle less than 40°. Metatarsus adductus is not evident, and the metatarsal protrusion is negative.[20] Only mild pronatory changes are noted (Fig. 7-7).

The Silver bunionectomy, whereby just the medial eminence is removed, can be performed in the elderly especially when a lesion, bursa, or only bump pain are

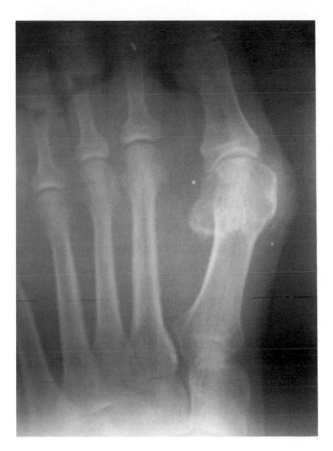

**Fig. 7-7.** Large intermetatarsal and hallux abductus angles would preclude performing only a soft tissue procedure.

the complaints. In these cases there should be limited expectations. Other more complex procedures may be contraindicated because of poor bone composition or healing capabilities. The long-term prognosis is rather poor. One can see that the indications are limited and the procedure thus is rarely used.[7,33]

For this chapter, the modified McBride bunionectomy consists of medial eminence resection and extensive lateral release with the fibular sesamoid remaining in vivo. The angle measurements as just listed would be sufficient criteria for the selection of this procedure.

In the "true" McBride bunionectomy the fibular sesamoid is removed. Care must be taken to prevent hallux varus by means of judicious resection of the medial eminence. More is removed dorsally than plantarly. The capsular repair is not tight, thus never

placing the hallux in an overcorrected position. The fibular sesamoid can be removed[34] if the tibial sesamoid position is greater than 4 although others[6] advocated only removing the sesamoid if 6 or greater. Even though a fibular sesamoidectomy can reduce mild rotary component of the hallux, its use today is somewhat infrequent.

Another method to determine whether a soft tissue procedure would be appropriate is to wrap a 3-in. Ace bandage around the forefoot and take a dorsiplantar weight-bearing film. If the first metatarsocuneiform joint gapped medially then these procedures would not adequately correct the deformity[35]; osseous work would be required.

The modified McBride bunionectomy is used with osseous procedures when the deformity is moderate to severe. The osteotomies, whether distal or proximal on the first metatarsal, will structurally alter the intermetatarsal angle. Because of the consequences of the hallux abducto valgus around the joint, the capsule tendon complex must be balanced; therefore, the modified McBride bunionectomy is used as previously described. Completion of both these procedures should produce a foot without deformity postoperatively.

Adductor transfers broaden the criteria for soft tissue procedures. If the intermetatarsal angle is positional, the metatarsocuneiform angle less than 24°, the metatarsal split distance greater than 2 mm, and the first metatarsal deformation angle less than 8°, then the adductor transfer can be performed with a satisfactory reduction of the stated parameters.[24]

Assuming a soft tissue procedure seems the logical choice on the basis of all the preoperative data, one can analyze the final outcome intraoperatively. The steps of the soft tissue procedure are completed. If on reduction of the intermetatarsal angle manually the first metatarsal springs back into adduction, then an osteotomy also should be performed.[33] Careful preoperative analysis should lessen the need to use this test.

## POSTOPERATIVE ANALYSES AND COMPLICATIONS

Surgical correction of hallux abducto valgus requires rigorous attention to anatomic dissection and surgical technique, and the capability preoperatively to analyze the foot and then select the appropriate procedure for that deformity and the patient's medical status and lifestyle. Soft tissue procedures prove to be very attractive to the patient because they are relatively easy to perform, require a minimal amount of healing, and permit the patient to return to wearing shoes quickly. However, if criteria are stretched to produce a quick and easy solution to a complex pathology, then the long-term results are suspect.

Recurrence of the deformity is the number one complication whenever a soft tissue procedure is used alone. Usually the procedure is inadequate to correct the existing pathology.[2,36] Failure to adequately repair the medial capsule can also increase the probability for recurrence.[21] Attempting a soft tissue procedure on a joint that was congruous preoperatively will only jam the medial side when the capsule is tightened. Failure to adequately complete the lateral release also leads to recurrences.

The high recurrence rate in juvenile patients (reported to be as high as 75 percent) indicates that soft tissue procedures should not be performed on this type of deformity.[37,39] Osseous correction is necessary; they will maintain the correction over time.

Removal of the fibular sesamoid can lead to hallux varus. This is especially true if the medial eminence has been removed too aggressively, the intermetatarsal angle is 0° or a negative value, and the tibial sesamoid moves medial to the first metatarsal (peaks). More than 13 percent of hallux varuses have been reported after fibular sesamoidectomy.[3,4,40–42] Overly zealous tightening of the medial capsule after removal of the fibular sesamoid can also result in a hallux varus developing either immediately postoperatively or over time as the capsule tendon balance falters and pulls excessively medially.

DuVries' modified McBride procedure has been performed in more than 2,700 cases with good to excellent results being reported in 90 percent.[43] Of significance was the plication of the first and second metatarsal heads together.

Using soft tissue procedures alone can decrease the intermetatarsal and hallux abductus angles by as much as 5° and 14°, respectively.[3] Reverse buckling applies retrograde forces to the first metatarsal and allows the intermetatarsal angle to reduce.[19] This will be more easily accomplished if the first metatarsocuneiform joint is round.[44]

Any time an osseous procedure is performed, whether distal or proximal on the first metatarsal, a modification of the soft tissue procedures is performed to balance the structures around the first metatarsophalangeal joint. Reduction of the intermetatarsal angle to normalcy combined with an incomplete lateral release predisposes the patient to a recurrence of the deformity.

Therefore, whenever an osseous procedure is performed the medial capsule is sutured and the foot is placed in simulated weight-bearing. A timid lateral release can be evident as a laterally drifting hallux. Conversely, excessive medial capsule tightening can tilt the hallux into varus.

Assuming that the medial capsular sutures or the postoperative dressing will hold the correction is naive. The capsule tendon balance and any osseous correction inadequately performed cannot rely on a dressing or a few medial sutures in the capsule to maintain satisfactory long-term results.

## POSTOPERATIVE COURSE

Soft tissue procedures have the shortest postoperative time periods for healing and returning to wearing shoes. This time period will be predicated on the amount of persistent edema. It is not always possible for the patient to alter shoe styles after one of these procedures.

As with any arthrotomy, the first metatarsophalangeal joint must be actively and passively exercised postoperatively.[45] Adhesions can render the joint stiff and lower the success rate. Exercises can be coupled with other physical therapy modalities to enhance the range of motion at the first metatarsophalangeal joint.

## REFERENCES

1. Kelikian H: Hallux Valgus, Allied Deformities of the Forefoot and Metatarsalgia. WB Saunders, Philadelphia, 1965
2. Bargman J, Corless J, Gross AE, Langer F: A review of surgical procedures for hallux valgus. Foot Ankle 1:39, 1980
3. Mann RA, Coughlin MJ: Hallux valgus—etiology, anatomy, treatment and surgical considerations. Clin Orthop 157:31, 1981

4. Johnson KA: Surgery of the Foot and Ankle. Raven Press, New York, 1989

5. Lawton JH: Forefoot surgery. p. 163. In Marcus SA (ed): Complications in Foot Surgery. 2nd Ed. Williams & Wilkins, Baltimore, 1984

6. Donick I, Berlin SJ, Block LD, et al: An approach for hallux valgus surgery—fifteen year review: part II. J Foot Surg 19:171, 1980

7. Baxter DE, Clain MR: Complications of exostectomy/Akin procedure. Contemp Orthop 23:103, 1991

8. Dobbs BM: Partial ostectomy of the first metatarsal head (Silver bunionectomy). p. 111. In Gerbert J (ed): Textbook of Bunion Surgery. 2nd Ed. Futura Publishing, Mount Kisco, NY, 1991

9. Silver D: The operative treatment of hallux valgus. J Bone Joint Surg 5:225, 1923

10. Hiss JM: Hallux valgus. Am J Surg 9:51, 1931

11. McBride ED: A conservative operation for bunions. J Bone Joint Surg 10.735, 1928

12. McBride ED: Hallux valgus, bunion deformity: its treatment in mild, moderate and severe stages. J Int Coll Surg 21:99, 1954

13. McBride ED: The McBride bunion hallux valgus operation. J Bone Joint Surg 49A:1675, 1967

14. Giannestras NJ: Foot Disorders: Medical and Surgical Management. 2nd Ed. Lea & Febiger, Philadelphia, 1976

15. Fuld JE: Surgical treatment of hallux valgus and its complications. Am Med 1:536, 1919

16. Gerbert J, Mercado OA, Sokoloff TH: The Surgical Treatment of the Hallux Abducto Valgus and Allied Deformities. Futura Publishing, Mount Kisco, NY, 1973

17. Ruch JA, Merrill TJ, Banks AS: First ray, hallux abducto valgus and related deformities. p. 133. In McGlamry ED (ed): Comprehensive Textbook of Foot Surgery. Williams & Wilkins, Baltimore, 1987

18. McGlamry ED, Feldman MH: A treatise on the McBride procedure. J Am Podiatry Assoc 61:161, 1971

19. Fenton CF, McGlamry ED: Reverse buckling to reduce metatarsus primus varus. J Am Podiatry Assoc 72:342, 1982

20. Jolly GP: Hallux abducto valgus and surgery of the first ray. p. 823. Levy LA, Hetherington VJ (eds): Principles and Practice of Podiatric Medicine. Churchill Livingstone, New York, 1990

21. Mann RA, Coughlin MJ: Hallux valgus and complications of hallux valgus. p. 65. In Mann RA (ed): Surgery of the Foot. 5th Ed. CV Mosby, St. Louis, 1986

22. Horn LM, Subotnick SI: Surgical intervention. p. 461. In Subotnick SI (ed): Sports Medicine of the Lower Extremity. Churchill Livingstone, New York, 1989

23. Kempe SA, Singer RH: The modified McBride bunionectomy utilizing the adductor tendon transfer. J Foot Surg 24:24, 1985

24. Pressman MM, Stano GW, Krantz MK, Novicki DC: Correction of hallux valgus with positionally increased intermetatarsal angle. J Am Podiatry Assoc 76:611, 1986

25. Brindly HH: Mobilization and transfer of the intrinsics of the great toe for hallux valgus. Clin Orthop 165:144, 1982

26. Joplin RJ: Correction of splay-foot and metatarsus primus varus. J Bone Joint Surg 4:779, 1950

27. Mann RA: Hallux valgus correction using a distal soft tissue procedure with a proximal crescentic osteotomy. Contemp Orthop 23:61, 1991

28. Jahss MH: Disorders of the hallux and the first ray. p. 943. In Jahss MH (ed): Disorders of the Foot and Ankle. 2nd Ed. WB Saunders, Philadelphia, 1991

29. Mann RA: The great toe. Clin Orthop 20:519, 1989

30. McNerney JE, Johnston WB: Generalized ligamentous laxity, hallux abducto valgus and the first metatarsocuneiform joint. J Am Podiatry Assoc 69:69, 1979

31. Donick I, Berlin SJ, Block LD, et al: An approach for hallux valgus surgery—fifteen year review: part I. J Foot Surg 19:113, 1980

32. Frankel JP: Structural or positional hallux abductus? J Am Podiatry Assoc 63:647, 1973

33. Coughlin MJ: Why bunion surgery fails. Contemp Orthop 23:27, 1991

34. Lipsman S, Frankel JP: Criteria for fibular sesamoidectomy in hallux abducto valgus correction. J Foot Surg 16:43, 1977

35. Romash MM, Fugate D, Yanklowit B: Passive motion of the first metatarsal cuneiform joint: preoperative assessment. Foot Ankle 10:293, 1990

36. Butlin WE: Modifications of the McBride procedure for correction of hallux abducto valgus. J Am Podiatry Assoc 64:585, 1974

37. Helal B: Surgery for adolescent hallux valgus. Clin Orthop 157:50, 1981

38. Scanton PE, Zuckerman JD: Bunion surgery in adolescents: results of surgical treatment. J Pediatr Orthop 4:39, 1984

39. Coughlin MJ, Bordelon RL, Johnson K, Mann RA: Presidents' forum–evaluation and treatment of juvenile hallux valgus. Contemp Orthop 21:169, 1990

40. Curda GA, Sorto LA: The McBride bunionectomy with closing wedge osteotomy. J Am Podiatry Assoc 71:349, 1981

41. Hansen LE: Hallux valgus treated by the McBride operation. Acta Orthop Scand 45:778, 1974

42. Jones RO, Harkless LB, Baer MS, Wilkinson SV: Retrospective statistical analysis of factors influencing the for-

mation of long-term complications following hallux abducto valgus surgery. J Foot Surg 30:345, 1991

43. Mann RA, DuVries HL: Major surgical procedures for
disorders of the forefoot. p. 563. In Mann RA (ed).
DuVries' Surgery of the Foot. 4th Ed. CV Mosby, St.
Louis, 1978

44. LaPorta G, Melillo T, Olinsky D: X-Ray evaluation of hallux abducto valgus deformity. J Am Podiatry Assoc
64:544, 1974

45. Donnery J, DiBacco RD: Postsurgical rehabilitation exercises for hallux abducto valgus repair. J Am Podiatr Med
Assoc 80:410, 1990

# 8

# Phalangeal Osteotomy for Hallux Valgus

## JOHN H. BONK

Adequate correction of hallux valgus may be attempted at various levels of the first ray complex, depending on appropriate determination of the apex of the deformity. Methods of correction may include first metatarsal base osteotomy and first metatarsal head osteotomy as well as uncomplicated first metatarsophalangeal joint soft tissue realignment. In those instances in which the major deformity lies distal to the first metatarsophalangeal joint, however, phalangeal osteotomy is well suited as the procedure or choice. The purpose of this chapter is to outline the role of osteotomy of the proximal phalanx of the hallux, the Akin-type procedure, in the correction of hallux valgus.

## HISTORICAL BACKGROUND

In 1925, Dr. O.F. Akin[1] described a procedure that included resection of the medial exostosis of the first metatarsal head and a portion of the base of the proximal phalanx. This was followed by a "cuneiform-shaped osteotomy" into the proximal phalangeal base, with inward rotation of the toe to straighten the hallux (Fig. 8-1). More than 40 years later, Colloff and Weitz[2] suggested that a major benefit of the Akin-type procedure is the ability to correct a mild to moderate deformity without disturbing the congruity and soft tissue relationships of the first metatarsophalangeal joint. Preoperative range of motion is then easily preserved. It was also suggested that this procedure would be inappropriate in cases involving "severe metatarsus primus varus, hallux rigidus and rheumatoid arthritis".[2]

A plethora of articles have subsequently described with various aspects of the Akin procedure. Most of these have addressed the indications for the procedure, as well as variations on placement, shape, and fixation of the actual osteotomy. For instance, osteotomy of the proximal phalangeal base, the original procedure presented by Dr. Akin, has been proposed as a correction for an abnormal distal articular set angle (DASA) (Fig. 8-2) while osteotomy in the distal metaphysis will predictably correct for an abnormal hallux abductus interphalangeus (HAI)[3–5] (Fig. 8-3). An excessively long proximal phalanx may be shortened quite nicely using a cylindrical variation of the Akin osteotomy.[6] Additionally, use of the Akin procedure as an adjunctive procedure has been given considerable discussion, most recently as combined with the Chevron-type osteotomy of the first metatarsal head.[7,8]

Discussions regarding fixation of the osteotomy have included descriptions of splinting, Kirschner wire utilization, and monofilament wire and internal screw fixation[9,10] (Fig. 8-4). It becomes readily apparent from a review of the literature, however, that utilization of the Akin-type procedure as primary and sole correction of hallux valgus deformity is rarely appropriate. Phalangeal osteotomy appears to be most useful as an adjunctive procedure that can complement toe correction provided by a closing base wedge osteotomy, distal metaphyseal osteotomy, or McBride-type bunionectomy, when such a procedure is used to correct a more proximal deformity.[2,7,11] Figure 8-5 demonstrates several applications of the Akin osteotomy of the hallux.

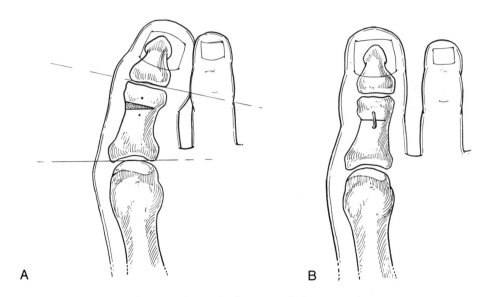

**Fig. 8-1.** (**A & B**) The original Akin procedure.

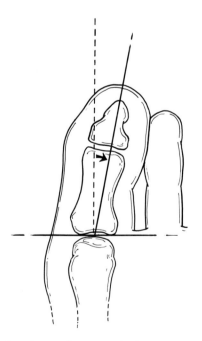

**Fig. 8-2.** Distal articular set angle (now greater than 8°).

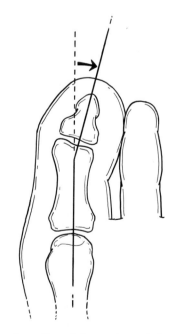

**Fig. 8-3.** Hallux abductus interphalangeus.

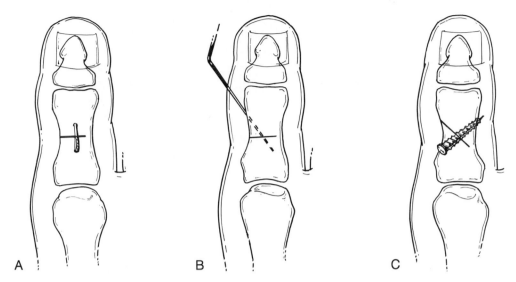

**Fig. 8-4.** Types of fixation. (**A**) Wire; (**B**) Kirschner wire; (**C**) screw.

## PROXIMAL AKIN PROCEDURE

The traditional Akin osteotomy is described as a transverse closing wedge osteotomy, performed approximately 5 mm distal to the articular surface of the base of the proximal phalanx (Fig. 8-6).

The first osteotomy is performed parallel to the phalangeal base and the second osteotomy is positioned parallel to the articular surface of the phalangeal head. On removal of the intervening osseous wedge and reduction of the osteotomy, symmetry of the medial and lateral aspects of the phalangeal shaft has been achieved.[1–5,12–14]

Although a painful hallux, often with accompanying pressure against the second digit, is usually the chief complaint, certain preoperative criteria will lead the practitioner to selection of the phalangeal osteotomy. According to Gerbert,[14] these criteria would include hallux abductus (with or without bunion deformity), a minimum valgus rotation of the hallux, and adequate first metatarsophalangeal joint range of motion without crepitus.

Radiographic examination should also be carried out. The following findings may signal the need for phalangeal correction: an incongruous first metatarsophalangeal joint must first be corrected by an additional procedure; adequate phalangeal length must be present; the metatarsus primus adductus angle must be normal; an abnormal DASA (usually greater than 8°) is present; and the HAI should be normal.[14]

It should be noted, however, that radiographic evaluation of the hallux may be somewhat deceiving and may erroneously suggest the need for an Akin procedure. For example, evaluation of a standard weight-bearing dorsoplantar radiograph may demonstrate an excessively high DASA, hinting that the deformity should be corrected at the phalangeal base. However, care must be taken to ensure that excessive valgus rotation of the hallux is not present, causing the illusion of an asymmetric proximal phalanx. Soft tissue realignment at the metatarsophalangeal joint may very likely derotate the frontal plane deformity and eliminate the need for phalangeal osteotomy.

Preoperative planning is helpful in predicting the amount of bone to be removed. Gerbert[14] has vigorously advocated the use of templates fashioned to preoperative radiographs, and this topic was given further consideration by Gohil and Cavolo.[15] Frey et al.[11] have published an elaborate mathematical analysis for the prediction of correction necessary. Regardless of the method employed, rectus, pain-free hallux with no impingement on the second digit is the goal.

Appropriate postoperative management is critical to avoid complications. Although ambulation may be al-

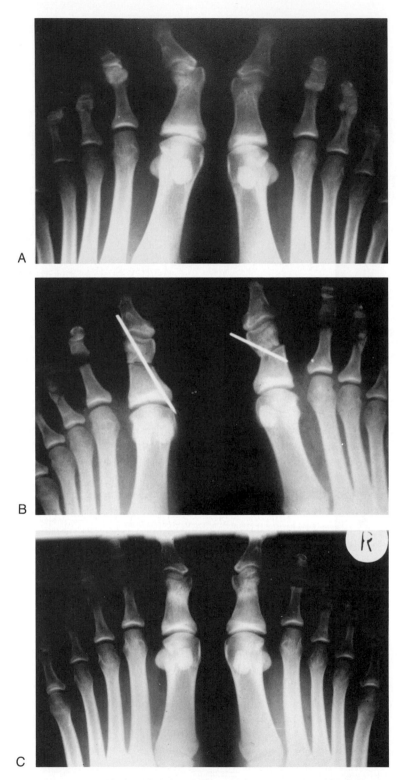

**Fig. 8-5.** (**A**) Preoperative congenital clinodyctyly of the great toes. Abnormal hallux interphalangeal angle is apparent. Deformity of the interphalangeal joint is also demonstrated. (**B**) Postoperative distal Akin osteotomy with Kirschner-wire fixation. (**C**) Postoperative result. (*Figure continues.*)

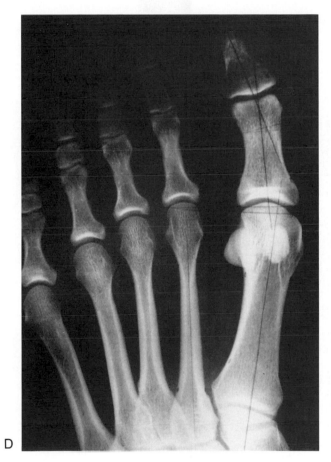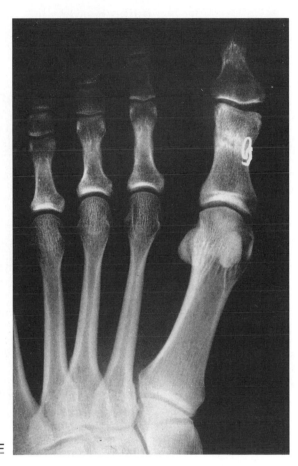

D                                                      E

**Fig. 8-5** (*Continued*).  (**D**) Preoperative hallux interphalangeus. (**E**) Postoperative distal Akin osteotomy with wire fixation. (*Figure continues.*)

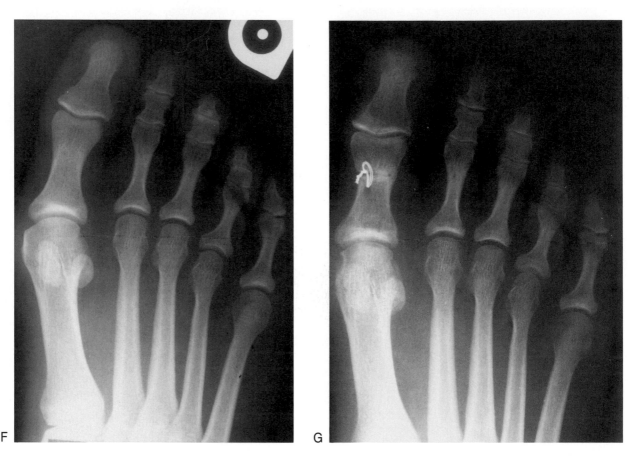

**Fig. 8-5** (*Continued*).  (**F**) Preoperative hallux valgus with interphalangeus. (**G**) Postoperative distal Akin osteotomy with wire fixation and intact lateral cortex. (*Figure continues.*)

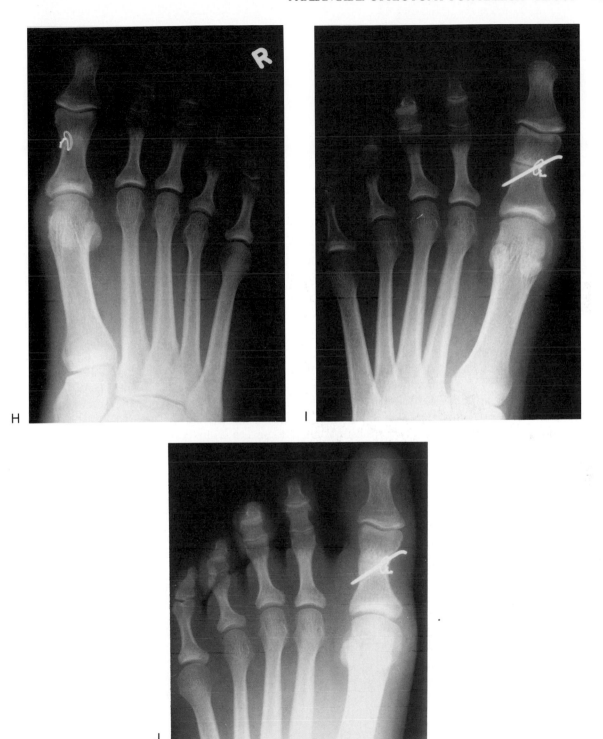

**Fig. 8-5** (*Continued*). (**H**) Postoperative radiograph demonstrating final result with complete bone healing. (**I**) Postoperative distal Akin osteotomy with fracture of the lateral cortex intraoperatively fixated by use of additional K-wire fixation. (**J**) Postoperative result.

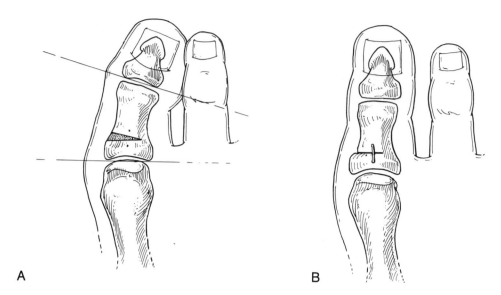

**Fig. 8-6.** (**A & B**) Proximal Akin procedure.

lowed immediately after surgery, use of a compressive dressing and a surgical shoe that eliminates the propulsive phase of gait are imperative. Athletic-type shoes may be worn at about the fourth week, with gradual return to normal shoe gear.[14]

In summary, use of the Akin osteotomy should be considered with realistic expectations. Indiscriminate use of the so-called bump-Akin bunionectomy with little regard for preoperative criteria will likely result in recurrence and dissatisfaction for both the practitioner and patient. Expectations that implementation of a proximal Akin procedure will correct a moderate to severe hallux valgus deformity will likely be met with disappointing results. The proximal Akin proce-

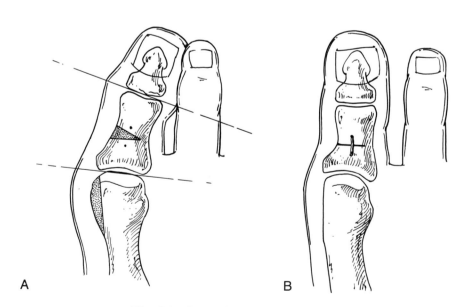

**Fig. 8-7.** (**A & B**) Distal Akin procedure.

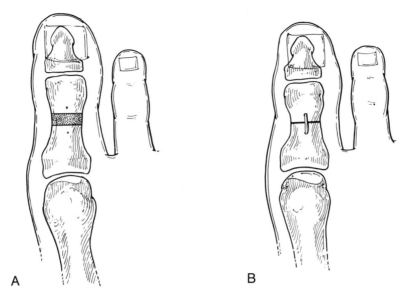

**Fig. 8-8.** (**A & B**) Cylindrical Akin procedure.

dure should be utilized to correct a deformity distal to the first metatarsophalangeal joint and, in particular, an asymmetric proximal phalanx with the medial aspect longer than the lateral. In this light, the most valuable use of the procedure appears to be adjunctive.

## DISTAL AKIN PROCEDURE

When the apex of the deformity is identified to lie in the distal aspect of the proximal phalanx, a distal Akin procedure is appropriate for correction (Fig. 8-7) The criteria and performance of the actual procedure are very similar to those described regarding the proximal Akin procedure, with two important exceptions.

First, a primary indication for this osteotomy is an abnormal HAI value. This value is defined as the angle formed by the longitudinal bisection of the proximal and distal phalanges of the hallux. A value in the 5°–10° range, accompanied by signs and symptoms previously described, would suggest that a distal Akin procedure is indicated.[3–5,13] Second, although the shape of the osteotomy is essentially identical to that of the proximal Akin, placement of this wedge is approximately 5 mm proximal to the interphalangeal joint.

Once again, symmetry of the medial and lateral aspects of the proximal phalanx is a major goal.

## OTHER VARIATIONS OF THE PHALANGEAL OSTEOTOMY

Preoperative evaluation often reveals that an excessively long proximal phalanx is the dominant pathology. To rectify this problem, an osteotomy has been described in which a cylindrical portion of diaphyseal bone of appropriate length is removed (Fig. 8-8). As this is a through-and-through osteotomy with violation of all cortices, adequate fixation is mandatory to avoid nonunion.[3,6,13,14]

Reference has also been made to a derotational-type osteotomy of the proximal phalanx. The primary indication for use of this procedure is in the correction of exaggerated valgus rotation of the hallux, which is identified as a structural component of the phalanx itself, and not simply a positional rotation. Once again, adequate fixation is necessary because all cortices are generally osteotomized.[16]

Finally interphalangeal joint arthrodesis is often considered a variation of the Akin-type procedures. This procedure should be considered for correction of sagittal plane deformities of the hallux, such as hallux malleus. However, in cases of degenerative joint disease involving the interphalangeal joint, appropriate wedging can correct nicely for transverse plane deformities identified at the interphalangeal joint.

## COMPLICATIONS

Although phalangeal osteotomy is relatively uncomplicated to perform, surgical complications do occur. Those occurring most frequently include pain, edema, infection, delayed union, nonunion, overcorrection (hallux varus), undercorrection, and sagittal plane hallucal deformities (e.g., hallux extensus, hallux malleus).[14]

Appropriate preoperative planning, intraoperative execution, (including fixation), and postoperative management will not eliminate postoperative complications but will certainly minimize their frequency. In this light, this procedure should not be utilized as a "cheater"-type procedure, used in an attempt to correct for an extensive, more proximal deformity because buckling at the metatarsophalangeal joint is likely to occur, compromising the result and dooming it to failure.

## CONCLUSION

Phalangeal osteotomy can prove to be an extremely useful adjunct to more intricate and sophisticated procedures for the correction of hallux valgus deformity. However, its application is most useful in correction of deformities that lie distal to the metatarsophalangeal joint.

## REFERENCES

1. Akin OF: The treatment of hallux valgus—a new operative procedure and its results. Med Sentinel 33:678, 1925
2. Colloff B, Weitz E: Proximal phalangeal osteotomy in hallux valgus. Clin Orthop 54:105, 1967
3. Gerbert J, Spector E, Clark J: Osteotomy procedures on the proximal phalanx for correction of a hallux deformity. J Am Podiatry Assoc 64:617, 1974
4. Sorto L, Balding M, Weil L, Smith S: Hallux abductus interphalangeus: etiology, x-ray evaluation on treatment. J Am Podiatry Assoc 66: 384, 1976
5. Segal D: Proximal and distal Akin procedures. J Foot Surg 16:57, 1977
6. McGlammary ED, Kitting R, Butlin W: Hallux valgus repair with correction of coexisting long hallux. J Am Podiatry Assoc 60:86, 1970
7. Goldberg I, Bahar A, Yosipovitch Z: Late results after correction of hallux valgus deformity by basilar phalangeal osteotomy. J Bone Joint Surg 69A:64, 1987
8. Mitchell L, Baxter D: A Chevron-Akin double osteotomy for correction of hallux valgus. Foot Ankle 12:7, 1991
9. Longford J: ASIF Akin osteotomy. J Am Podiatry Assoc 71:390, 1981
10. Murphy J, Mozena J, Walker R: J wire technique for fixation of the Akin osteotomy. J Am Podiatr Med Assoc 79:291, 1989
11. Frey C, Jahss M, Kummer F: The Akin procedure: an analysis of results. Foot Ankle 12:1, 1991
12. Seelenfreund M, Fried A: Correction of hallux valgus deformity by basal phalanx osteotomy of the big toe. J Bone Joint Surg 55A:1411, 1973
13. Borovoy M, Mendelsohn E: Wedge osteotomies for correction of hallux abducto valgus with case histories. J Foot Surg 18:47, 1979
14. Gerbert J (ed): Textbook of Bunion Surgery. Futura Publishing, Mount Kisco, NY, 1981
15. Gohil P, Cavolo D: A simplified preoperative evaluation for Akin osteotomy. J Am Podiatry Assoc 72:44, 1982
16. Schwartz N, Ianuzzi P, Thurber N: Derotational Akin osteotomy. J Foot Surg 25:479, 1986

# 9

# Arthrodesis of the Interphalangeal Joint

## RODNEY TOMCZAK

Arthrodesis of the hallux interphalangeal joint is itself a simple procedure. The difficulty originates over misconceptions involving the interpretations and applications of similar original articles. The major problems appear to center around the flexor hallucis longus, the extensor hallucis longus, and exactly what to do with both, as well as whether fusion of the interphalangeal joint is warranted.

## REVIEW OF THE LITERATURE

In 1938, Forrester-Brown[1] described a procedure in which half the flexor hallucis longus was transferred to a new insertion in the extensor hallucis longus during the late stages of poliomyelitis as well as of other paralytic conditions. The deformity arose because of faulty balance among the muscles, that is, the weakness of the tibialis anterior and compensation for the resulting weak dorsiflexion by the extensor hallucis longus. He also stated that the polio patient used the flexor hallucis longus to compensate for this weak dorsiflexion. When there was subluxation of the interphalangeal joint, he recommended arthrodesis of the joint and transfer of the whole tendon. The flexor hallucis longus was freed from a medial approach and sutured into the extensor hallucis longus on the dorsum of the proximal phalanx. If the metatarsophalangeal could not be plantar-flexed, he recommended a dorsal capsulotomy and extensor tendon lengthening. A dorsal wedge was removed from the interphalangeal joint and the opposing bone surfaces sutured. This procedure was theoretically based on the work of Sir

Harold Stiles,[2] who believed that part of the flexor digitorum sublimis in the hand, if transferred to the extensor tendon at the proximal phalanx, would function as an artificial lumbricales and flex the knuckle and extend the interphalangeal joint.

In 1926, Dickson and Dively[3] reported on 56 cases of fusion of the hallux interphalangeal joint with extensor hallucis longus transfer into the flexor hallucis longus tendon just proximal to the first metatarsal head (Fig. 9-1). The authors thought that procedures that used an extensor hallucis longus transfer to remove the deforming force of the clawed hallux and at the same time dorsiflex the foot were not mechanically correct. They based their theory on the supposition that the paralyzed tendon that was causing the deformity was the flexor hallucis longus. They made no mention of a weak tibialis anterior. It is interesting to review the discussion that followed the presentation of the technique in the same article. Willis Campbell (Memphis, TN) and Henry Meyerding (Rochester, MN) stated that the transference of the extensor hallucis longus through the first metatarsal had not given uniformly satisfactory results. C.L. Lowman (Los Angeles), however, identified the weak tibialis anterior, the strong peroneus longus, and the common extensors used to dorsiflex the foot as the cause of claw foot as opposed to merely claw toe. He mentioned that only when the deformity is first corrected more proximally will correction of the claw toe succeed. The claw toe can then be corrected using the Jones procedure. Arthur Steindler (Iowa City) thought that this procedure, in conjunction with the stripping of the os calcis (Steindler stripping) seemed to be

147

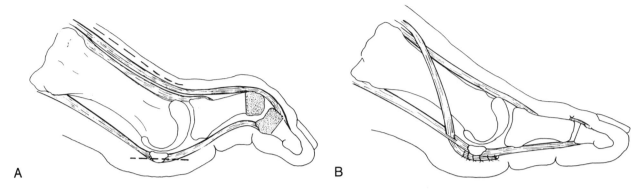

**Fig. 9-1. (A & B)** Dickson-Diveley operation for clawing of great toe. The extensor hallucis longus tendon is transferred to flexor hallucis longus tendon and the interphalangeal joint is arthrodesed after enough bone has been removed to correct deformity. (Adapted from Dickson and Diveley,[3] with permission.)

eminently sound mechanically; the sling constituted by the long flexor of the toes and the extensor of the big toe had the leverage to pull up the sunken head of the first metatarsal.

In 1951, Taylor[4] reported on 68 patients who underwent a procedure developed by G.R. Girdelstone that was then named the Girdelstone procedure. Of these 68 patients, 38 had associated pes cavus, 23 had planovagus deformity, and 7 had no apparent abnormality. Taylor reported that examination of all 68 patients failed to reveal any evidence of paralysis, and no evidence of abnormality of the intrinsic muscles was found at the time of surgery. He further stated that these findings in three different structural foot types make it difficult to account for the deformity, with the exception of ineffective use of the intrinsic muscles.

The technique of the Girdelstone procedure con-

sisted of merely tenotomizing the long and short flexors, transferring them to the lateral side of the extensor expansion through a buttonhole, and suturing them in place (Fig. 9-2). The interphalangeal joints were then arthrodesed. For the hallux, however, Taylor wrote that Girdelstone advocated excision of the interphalangeal joint and transplantation of the extensor hallucis longus into the neck of the first metatarsal so as to form a supporting sling for the head of the first metatarsal.

The Jones procedure[5] itself seems to have its origin in the procedures described by Sherman[6] and Forbes.[7] These procedures advocated the transplantation of the extensor hallucis longus and extensor digitorum longus to the heads of the metatarsals to remove the deforming actions of these tendons on the digits. Jones recommended a Steindler stripping and

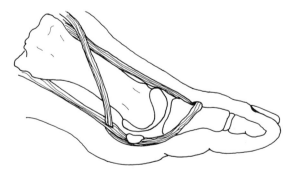

**Fig. 9-2.** Girdlestone-Taylor tendon transfer for clawing of toes. Deformity before surgery. Tendons of long and short toe flexors have been transferred to extensor expansions. The corrected position of each toe is maintained by a suture placed around both the proximal phalanx and the Lambrinudi splint. (From Taylor,[4] with permission.)

transfer of the extensor hallucis longus through the first metatarsal head as surgical treatment for an anterior-flexible claw foot. He did not mention fusion of the interphalangeal joint of the hallux as part of the procedure nor did he mention suturing the attached stub of the extensor hallucis longus tendon to the extensor hallucis brevis tendon.

Ingram, in *Campbell's Operative Orthopaedics,*[8] describes a technique of suturing the remaining portion of the extensor hallucis longus tendon to the soft tissues on the dorsum of the proximal phalanx (Fig. 9-3). He states that the interphalangeal joint may or may not be fused, depending on the age of the patient. Arthro-

desis is preferable, but fusion is difficult to obtain in a child because the epiphysis is largely cartilage. This technique of tenodesis was advocated in almost identical fashion in a 1973 article by McGlamry and Kitting.[9]

Rather than suturing the stub of the extensor hallucis longus to the proximal phalanx, O'Donoghue and Stauffer[10] recommended Kirschner wire (K-wire) fixation to prevent a painful flexion contracture of the joint that may develop secondary to nonunion. Before K-wire fixation, these authors reported that 80 percent of the patients did not progress to bony fusion; with K-wire fixation, however, the rate of bony fusion was 85 percent.

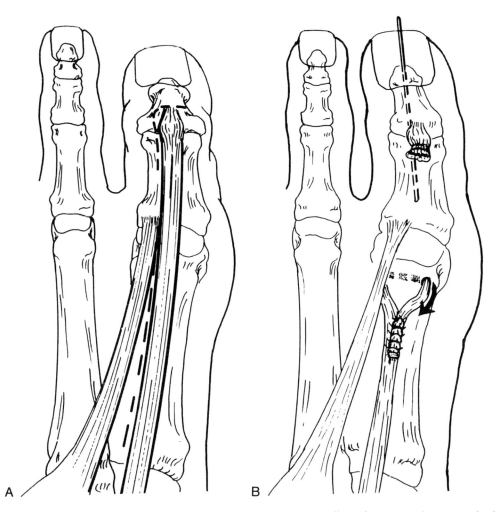

**Fig. 9-3.** Modified Jones operation for clawing of great toe. Extensor hallucis longus tendon is attached to the neck of the first metatarsal; the interphalangeal joint is arthrodesed and fixed by medullary wire and by suturing the distal end of the extensor hallucis longus tendon to soft tissues over the proximal phalanx.

Shives and Johnson[11] from Mayo Clinic reported on the use of a 4.0-mm cancellous bone screw across the denuded interphalangeal joint to achieve rigid internal fixation and compression. This was done through an L-shaped incision parallel with the joint and extending proximally on the medial aspect of the hallux. The extensor hallucis longus tendon was not transected unless it was being transferred. Shives and Johnson implied that extensor hallucis longus transfer did not accompany every interphalangeal joint fusion. A case of hallux hammer toe secondary to an old flexor tendon laceration was treated with joint fusion alone.

Langford and Fenton[12] reported on a similar procedure done through two transverse semielliptical incisions with transection of the extensor hallucis longus tendon. In their procedure they commented that the tendon was approximated at the end of the operation, implying that it was not transferred. In fact, they did not address the subject of extensor hallucis longus tendon transfer in their article.

## CHOICE OF PROCEDURE

Mann[13] states that in cases of congenital hammertoe the articular surface of the hallux interphalangeal joint is abnormal and soft tissue corrections will not suffice. He recommends arthrodesis of the joint without transference of the extensor hallucis longus tendon. In patients who have developed hyperextension of the metatarsophalangeal joint secondary to a combination of weak tibialis anterior and a normal extensor hallucis longus, a transfer of the extensor hallucis longus to the first metatarsal head and arthrodesis of the hallux interphalangeal joint are recommended. It appears that the small amount of growth from the distal phalangeal epiphysis that is arrested with fusion would account for less morbidity to the patient than continued suffering with the deformity.

## ARTHRODESIS OF THE HALLUX INTERPHALANGEAL JOINT USING THE SYNTHES CANNULATED SCREW SYSTEM

The introduction of the Cannulated Screw System (Synthes, Paoli, PA) has simplified the fusion of the hallux interphalangeal joint that was originally de-

scribed by the Association for the Study of Internal Fixation (ASIF) group.[14] The basic principles of the Cannulated Screw System consist of a solid guide wire, a hollow drill bit that is placed over the guide wire to drill the hole through the phalanges, and a hollow screw which is inserted over the guide wire by means of a hollow screw driver.

Two semielliptical incisions are made over the hallux interphalangeal joint and a wedge of skin removed. A second fishmouth incision is made on the distal aspect of the hallux (Fig. 9-4) to allow for skin closure without redundant skin in the shortened toe. The extensor tendon is transected and tagged with suture for retraction. Soft tissues are incised and the interphalangeal joint is exposed. If the long flexor is to be transposed dorsally, it is transected and split longitudinally, and the medial and lateral portions are tagged and moved to the corresponding sides of the incision. Bone is then resected from the head of the proximal phalanx and base of the distal phalanx so that the deformity may be corrected. Thus, the wedge will have its apex plantarly and base dorsally. The joint is then evaluated for adequate alignment by manual reduction.

Utilizing the two incisions, the guide wire is passed in a retrograde fashion to fixate the joint. An intraoperative radiographic technique should now be employed to confirm positioning of the phalanges. The direct measuring device is then slid over the guide wire so that the proper drilling depth can be determined. The following steps are used: the 2.7-mm cannulated drill bit is inserted into the drill guide with stop until the quick coupling end of the bit rests on the drill guide; the drill bit is inserted into the nontapered end of the direct measuring device; the knurled

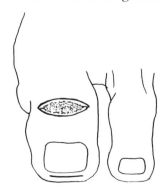

**Fig. 9-4.** Fishmouth incision on distal aspect of the hallux to allow for skin closure. (See text for details.)

nut on the drill guide is loosened; the threaded end of the drill guide is rotated until the drill bit corresponds to the drill depth; and the knurled nut is tightened.

The drill is then placed over the guide wire and the hole drilled. The drill bit will contact the drill guide when the appropriate length has been reached, and the drill should be removed at this point. The cannulated countersink is then placed over the guide wire and the distal aspect of the distal phalanx may be countersunk. The near cortex is tapped by means of the cannulated tap, which is inserted over the guide wire. A small cannulated screw, which is the same length as the depth previously drilled, is then selected and inserted over the guide wire. The guide wire is removed and discarded.

The long extensor tendon is reattached and the long flexor, if it is being transferred dorsally, is juxtaposed to the repaired capsule. Skin is closed in the normal fashion. Non-weight-bearing healing time is suggested if extensive tendon work has been performed.

The screw may be removed with a standard small hexagonal screwdriver if necessary after osseous healing has occurred. Langford and Fenton[12] reported a zero incidence of delayed or nonunions in 29 procedures performed with conventional screw fixation. There is no reason to doubt that similar results should be expected with the Cannulated Screw System.

# REFERENCES

1. Forrester-Brown MF: Tendon transplantation for clawing of the great toe. J Bone Joint Surg 20B:57, 1938

2. Stiles HJ, Forreseter-Brown MF: Treatment of Injuries of the Spinal Peripheral Nerves. Frowde and Hodder & Stoughton, London, 1922

3. Dickson FD, Dively RL: Operation for correction of mild claw foot, the result of infantile paralysis. J Am Med Assoc 87:1275, 1926

4. Taylor RG: The treatment of claw toes by multiple transfers of flexor into extensor tendons. J Bone Jt Surg, 33B:539, 1951

5. Jones R: The soldier's foot and the treatment of common deformities of the foot. Part II, claw foot. Br Med J 1:749, 1916

6. Sherman HM: Operative treatment of pes cavus. Am J Orthop Surg 2:374, 1905

7. Forbes AM: Claw foot and how to relieve it. Surg Gynecol Obstet Jan:81, 1913

8. Ingram AJ: Anterior poliomyelitis. In Edmondson AS, Cremshaw AH (eds): Campbell's Operative Orthopaedics. 6th Ed. CV Mosby, St. Louis, 1980

9. McGlamary ED, Kitting RW: Equinus foot; an analysis of the etiology, pathology and treatment techniques. J Am Podiatry Assoc 63:165, 1973

10. O'Donoghue DH, Stauffer R: An improved operative method for obtaining bony fusion of the great toe. Surg Gynecol Obstet 76:498, 1943

11. Shives TC, Johnson KA: Arthrodesis of the interphalangeal joint of the great toe—an improved technique. Foot Ankle 1:26, 1980

12. Langford JH, Fenton CF: Hallux interphalangeal arthrodesis. J Am Podiatr Assoc 72:155, 1982

13. Mann RA: Surgery of the Foot. CV Mosby, St. Louis, 1986

14. Heim U, Pfeiffer KM: Small Fragment Set Manual: Technique Recommended by the ASIF Group. Springer-Verlag, New York, 1974

# 10
# Sesamoids

MICHAEL GERBER
PATRICK D. ROBERTO

The hallucal sesamoids may seem minute in proportion to all the other bones of the body, but they are a major factor in the function of the first metatarsophalangeal joint. A review of the literature reveals that many have written of the mystique of the sesamoids, particularly the medial sesamoid.[1-5] It was believed that the medial sesamoid was an indestructible seed from which the body would be resurrected on the day of judgment. Helal quotes the writings of Rabbi Ushaia in A.D. 210 from the book *Bereschit Rabbi*[2]:

> This bone (Luz) can never be burned or corrupted in all eternity for its ground substance is of celestial origin and watered with heavenly dew, wherewith God shall make the dead rise as with yeast in a mass of dough.

The name "sesamoid" itself is said to have been coined by Galen, stemming from the flat, oval seeds of the *Sesamum indicum* plant.[1] These seeds were used by the Greek physicians for purging.

The presence of the sesamoids at the third fetal month was detected by Nesbitt in 1736,[1] yet the belief of their existence secondary to trauma of the tendon held on through the late 1800s. Nesbitt's findings were finally confirmed in 1892 by Pfitzner.[1] Through the following years, the question of their origin arose. Some believed their anlage was from that of the tendon, yet others believed it to be from the joint capsule. In any event, the consensus of their constant presence from fetal life was established.

## EMBRYOLOGY AND OSSIFICATION

As mentioned, Nesbitt first published the finding of sesamoid anlage in the third fetal month. Jahss[3] writes that the sesamoids are formed in separate cartilaginous centers and are not from articular budding. Inge and Ferguson[1] noted islands of undifferentiated connective tissue as early as 8 weeks of fetal growth. At 10 weeks this tissue is recognized as precartilaginous, with centers of chondrification at the twelfth week. These authors[1,3] go on to state that by the fifth month these bones reached normal adult shape and only develop further in size. The sesamoids remain as cartilaginous tissue and only begin ossification about 8 to 10 years of life; they ossify earlier in girls than in boys, at 8 to 9 versus 10 to 11 years of age, respectively.

Vranes[6] and Wisbrun, as reported by Inge and Ferguson,[1] report the histologic findings are unique. The trabecular pattern of the sesamoid bones is vertically directed in the dorsal aspect with a horizontally directed pattern in the plantar aspect of the bones. They also noted that the most posterior aspect of the sesamoids appears more dense in relationship to the anterior. Vranes however was not addressing this issue and therefore gave no reasoning for this histologic difference. Wisbrun correlated this histologic difference to a "greater percentage of weight-thrust" being directed through this portion of the sesamoid. The

153

forces placed upon the sesamoids results from their anatomic position, the structural location of tendon attachment, and vector stresses. Indeed, this would follow Wolfe's law of stresses and explain the unique finding.

## ANATOMY

The sesamoids, located inferior to the metatarsal head, articulate via two separate cartilaginous surfaces that are separated by a crista on the metatarsal head. The medial sesamoid is larger than the lateral, both varying in shape and size.

The medial sesamoid ranges in size from 12 to 15 mm by 9 to 11 mm and 7 to 20 mm by 5 to 12 mm, and the lateral sesamoid varies between 9 to 10 mm by 7 to 9 mm and 6 to 16 mm by 4 to 14 mm.[6,7] Their general radiographic appearance on the anteroposterior is ovoid view, and on axial view a concave plantar surface and convex or flat superior surface is noted.[7] The sesamoids can be bi-, tri-, or quadripartite, with the medial sesamoid having a greater incidence of this finding. Partition is covered later in this chapter.

The sesamoids are housed within an intricate network of ligaments, tendons, and capsular structures, all of which function uniformly about the first metatarsophalangeal joint (Fig. 10-1). The sesamoids are enveloped within the flexor hallucis brevis muscle tendon with the exception of the superior aspect, which is covered with hyaline cartilage to articulate with the first metatarsal. The articulating surface on the metatarsal is about 1.2 times greater than that of the corresponding sesamoid.[8] The sesamoids are separated by a crista on the metatarsal head, and the tendon of the flexor hallucis longus muscle passes between them. The abductor hallucis muscle tendon and joint capsule are also attached to the medial sesamoid. The lateral sesamoid has attachments from the adductor hallucis muscle tendon (both the transverse and oblique heads) and also from the joint capsule. The ligamentous structures participating in the network include the intersesamoidal ligament, running between the sesamoids, and the deep transverse intermetatarsal ligament that attaches to the fibular sesamoid. It is also noted that fibers of the plantar aponeurosis attach to both sesamoids.[9]

David et al.[10] also note that the extensor hallucis longus tendon sends expansions to invest into this complex network. These authors in fact refer to the extensor hallucis longus, abductor hallucis, flexor hallucis longus, and adductor hallucis as the sesamoid muscles. Overall, the sesamoids are not merely bones that absorb shock during gait but are an integral part of the function of the first metatarsophalangeal joint. Because of their contribution, any deformity that exists must be addressed if correction of this function is to be attained.

## ARTERIAL SUPPLY

The vascular supply of the sesamoids has recently been noted to be primarily from the first plantar metatarsal artery.[8,11] Pretterklieber and Manivenhaus[8] report three variations. In type A, the sesamoids are supplied by the medial plantar artery and the plantar arch; in type B, they are supplied by the plantar arch alone; type C is solely supplied by the medial plantar artery. The incidence of these types is 52, 24, and 24 percent, respectively. Sobel et al.[11] more recently reported the major vascular supply to the sesamoids as the first plantar metatarsal artery; however, he also notes that the artery branches into a medial and lateral branch. The proximal one-third to two-thirds of each sesamoid was supplied via this route through a further proximal and a plantar branch. A third, distal arterial branch was noted, but was found to be inconsistent, most often only supplying the distal plantar plate. Sobel et al. also noted the absence of vascularity to the lateral capsular and intersesamoidal ligamentous attachments.

Pretterklieber[8] notes that excessive dissection about the lateral border of the fibular sesamoid may disrupt its vascular supply. Sobel et al.[11] reports the arterial supply comes from a proximal location and penetrates through the flexor hallucis brevis muscle tendon before supplying the sesamoids. If the flexor hallucis brevis tendon attachment of the fibular sesamoid is preserved and only an adductor release is performed during hallux abducto valgus surgery, the sesamoid should not become vascularly compromised.

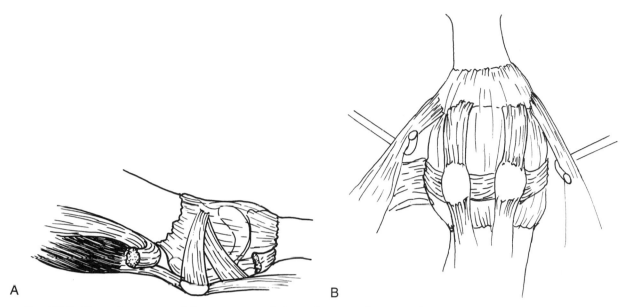

**Fig. 10-1.** Normal anatomy of first metatarsophalangeal joint and sesamoid apparatus **(A)** Lateral view; **(B)** plantar view.

## PATHOMECHANICS

To better understand the pathomechanics of the first metatarsophalangeal joint and sesamoid function therein, one must understand the normal function of this joint. Root et al.[12] described the normal first metatarsophalangeal joint as having two axes of motion: one in the transverse plane, allowing for sagittal plane motion, and another in the sagittal plane, allowing for transverse plane motion albeit small. They further describe the joint as being ginglymus in the transverse plane and ginglymoarthrodial in the sagittal plane. The joint functions as a ginglymus joint in the first 20° to 30° of dorsiflexion, but beyond that range requires the first ray to plantar-flex. The sesamoids at this point articulate more distally with the metatarsal head. Root et al. go on to describe four primary factors necessary for normal function during the propulsive phase of gait, one of which is normal sesamoid function.

As was noted earlier, the flexor hallucis longus tendon passes between and plantar to the sesamoids. This acts as the second pulley system for the flexor hallucis longus tendon, which becomes functional after heel lift and thus as the first ray plantar-flexes. Normal function with the metatarsal is necessary for the flexor hallucis longus tendon to maintain its most mechanical advantage in stabilizing the hallux in the sagittal plane against ground reactive forces. In addition, the sesamoids also absorb shock at forefoot load, distributing the ground reactive forces and thus protecting the metatarsal head.

The sesamoids, with all their soft tissue attachments, will for the most part remain stationary as the first metatarsophalangeal joint begins to function abnormally. This abnormally functioning joint can result in metatarsosesamoid articulation malalignment or may be a direct result of sesamoid dysfunction. Jahss[3] describes disorders of sesamoids as including congenital variations, systemic disorders, heritable disorders, infection, trauma, osteochondritis, and parasesamoid disorders. With reference to congenital variations, congenital absence[3,12,13] and also partition would fall under this category.

Inge and Kewenter in 1936 both reported congenital absence of the tibial sesamoid, and Lapidus in 1939 and Hulay in 1949 subsequently reported single cases. Zinmeister and Edelman[13] in 1985 reported absence of the tibial sesamoid in two cases. Systemic disorders may include collagen vascular diseases and psoriasis. Infections may arise from direct inoculation from trophic ulcerations or may be a result of hematogenous spread. Trauma may result in sesamoiditis or even fractures. Jahss explains parasesamoid disorders as disruption of conjoined tendon and also traumatic neuritis.

Severe hyperextension of the hallux can lead to the sesamoids displacing distally and eventually dorsal to the metatarsal with concomitant rupture of the plantar capsule.[3] When dislocations occur, the sesamoid apparatus will follow the phalanx, which can move either medially or laterally. The lateral position of the fibular sesamoid provides better protection because of the soft tissue of the first intermetatarsal space, which probably accounts for the greater frequency of tibial sesamoid trauma reported in the literature.

In an abnormally functioning foot in which the first ray becomes hypermobile, the first ray rotates in the frontal plane and adducts. This in turn causes all the soft tissue attachments and structures to rotate and thus lose their original balance and mechanical advantages. Because the sesamoids are attached to the tendon and ligaments, they remain relatively stationary. The deep transverse intermetatarsal ligament keeps the sesamoids from moving medially as the metatarsal progressively shifts in that direction. Consequently, the crista on metatarsal head will eventually wear away, thus resulting in a malfunctioning metatarsosesamoid joint. David et al.[10] describe four stages of the loading of the foot in relationship to the functional role of the sesamoids: (1) suspension of the first metatarsal head, (2) fixation of the first metatarsal head, (3) coordination, and (4) the propulsion stage. The first stage corresponds to heel contact to forefoot load in which the first ray plantar-flexes and the sesamoid apparatus suspends the first metatarsal head, acting much like a harness. The second stage consists mainly of fixating the sesamoid apparatus on the ground, making adjustments via isometric contractions of the flexor hallucis brevis, abductor hallucis, and adductor hallucis muscles, and thus acts as the reference point for the later stages. The third stage allows motion of the proximal attachments of the sesamoid muscles with the hallux firmly fixed against the ground, preparing for the fourth stage. The final stage allows for conversion of energy, stored within the flexor hallucis muscle tendon, into kinetic energy allowing for propulsion. David et al. concluded that the function of the sesamoid apparatus is to distribute and coordinate forces placed upon the forefoot for propulsion and balance.

## INFECTION

Infection of either of the sesamoids most often results from ulceration secondary to neuropathy, either diabetic or alcoholic.[3] Acute osteomyelitis from hematologic seeding in the young (9–19 years of age) is rare. Chronic infection secondary to a puncture wound may also occur but again is rare.

Osteomyelitis usually occurs in young males, often with a history of trauma, blunt or penetrating.[14] Early recognition can be difficult, and the differential may include fracture, sesamoiditis, soft tissue abcess, or cellulitis. It should be pointed out that radiographic changes from hyperemic resorption may mimic osteomyelitis and thus careful review of the history and follow-up radiographs may be necessary for differentiation (Fig. 10-2).

Treatment consists of antibiotic therapy, keeping in mind that the infection may recur in subsequent weeks. If it does, then excision of necrotic bone is necessary. The most effective treatment for local ulceration and infection is conservative with local wound care and infection control.

## SESAMOIDITIS

Sesamoiditis may or may not present clinically as a localized redness and swelling about the plantar surface of the sesamoid apparatus. It may present with a callus inferior to either the tibial or fibular sesamoid in cases of a plantar-flexed first ray or may result from a recent onset of athletic activities creating a pathologic process of inflammation of the subsesamoid bursae. In any event, differentiating sesamoiditis from osteochondritis, fracture, or infection is necessary.

Sesamoditis should be differentiated also from neuritis of the medial plantar digital nerve, bursitis, and simple excessive weight-bearing.[15] Radiographic

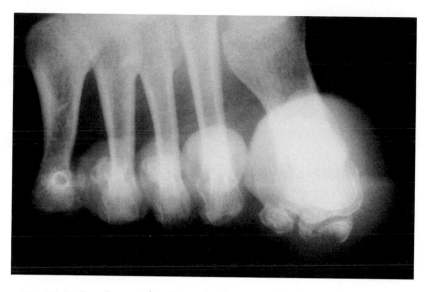

**Fig. 10-2.** Forefoot axial radiograph of osteomyelitis of the tibial sesamoid.

changes are not seen with sesamoiditis, and bone scans may prove equivocal.[16] Thus, diagnosis of sesamoiditis is essentially based on history and clinical presentation of localized pain and tenderness.

Treatment of sesamoiditis is conservative, and may include taping, strapping, or padding to accommodate for a plantar-flexed first ray, or orthoses to decrease the weight-bearing of the first ray and function about the subtalar joint. Local anesthetics or steroids may be injected also. A cast may be utilized to immobilize and decrease weight-bearing of the first metatarsophalangeal joint. If pain persists after all palliative care has been tried, then a sesamoidectomy should be considered.

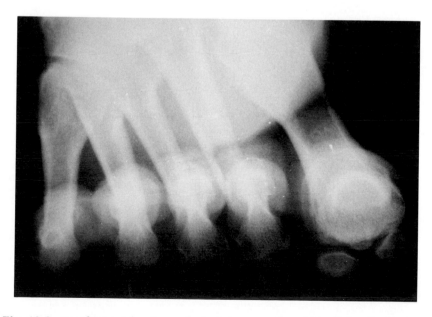

**Fig. 10-3.** Forefoot axial radiograph depicting osteochondritis of the tibial sesamoid.

## OSTEOCHONDRITIS

Some have correlated sesamoiditis with other entities such as osteochondritis.[2] Osteochondritis of the medial sesamoid was first described by Renander in 1924. It may occur either in the medial or lateral sesamoid or rarely, bilaterally. Unlike sesamoiditis, radiographs will ultimately reveal lytic areas, irregularity of the sesamoids, and some areas of sclerosis (Fig. 10-3). It is advised to take multiple views.

## PARTITIONS

The hallucal sesamoids resemble the other sesamoids in that they may present with more than one center of ossification.[1] Ossification of the lateral sesamoid precedes the medial sesamoid.[3] Failure of the multicentric centered sesamoid to fuse will result in a bi-, tri-, or multipartite sesamoid (Fig. 10-4).

The reported incidence of partition varies from 7.8 to 33.5 percent,[3] with partition of the tibial sesamoid occurring with greater frequency,[2,3,6,14] 10 times more often than the lateral sesamoid.[16] Jahss[3] reported 85 percent of partitioned sesamoids are bilateral whereas Inge[1] reported only 25 percent. As described earlier, ossification begins about the eighth year in girls and the tenth year in boys. Multiple centers may exist, and ossification with failure to fuse will result in a partitioned sesamoid. The sesamoids will present with irregular shapes and sizes (Fig. 10-5).

Vranes[6] classified the etiologies of partitioned sesa-

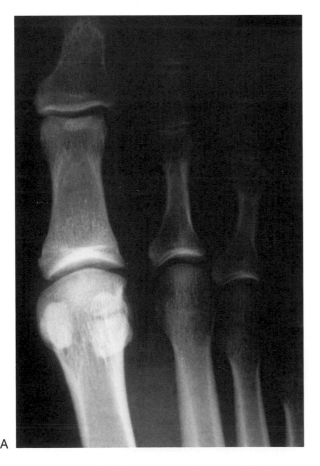
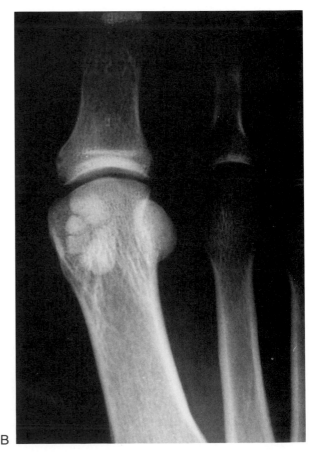

**Fig. 10-4.** **(A)** D-P view of bipartite fibular sesamoid. **(B)** D-P view of multipartite tibial sesamoid.

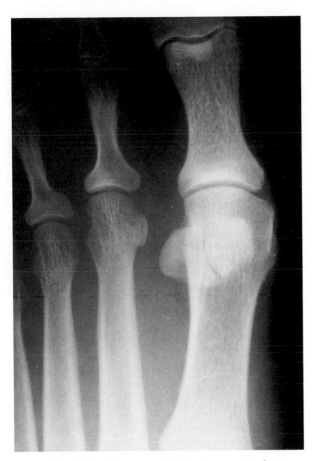

**Fig. 10-5.** Hypertrophic fibular sesamoid.

The frequency of incidence with partition of the tibial sesamoid and weight-bearing load may correlate with the vascular etiology.

With respect to the clinical scenario of a painful first metatarsophalangeal joint, the clinician must ascertain if it may have been direct trauma or indirect trauma. Direct trauma would be a fall from a height landing on the sesamoid apparatus. Indirect trauma may be a hyperextended hallux that thus caused undue stress on the sesamoid apparatus and possibly fracture or ligamentous injury. Therefore, it becomes evident that delineation between a fractured sesamoid and a partitioned sesamoid is necessary. Inge and Ferguson[1] note that incidental finding of a partitioned sesamoid without the complaint of pain is possible. The clinician is thus faced with treating this complaint as a sesamoiditis, fractured sesamoid, or distracted partition.

It should be noted that the radiographic findings differ between a partitioned and fractured sesamoid such that these may help in diagnosing the patient's problem. However, the findings are not always clear-cut and thus may not assist in the diagnostic impression. One should find a smooth edge between pieces in a partitioned sesamoid, whereas a fractured sesamoid will appear jagged[18,19] (Fig. 10-6). It should also be borne in mind that if one were to reassemble a fractured sesamoid, its size should be similar to that of the other sesamoid. In addition, a bipartite sesamoid usually presents with the partition running medial to lateral on anteroposterior view. A higher suspicion of fracture is warranted in cases in which the partition courses obliquely or longitudinally[19] (Fig. 10-7). Oftentimes, however, the patient does not present directly after the trauma and because of this the radiographic criteria mentioned here may not be helpful. The appearance of bilateral partite sesamoids may not help in diagnosing the fractured sesamoid because their incidence bilaterally is less common.[4,6] The only way to ascertain a true fracture from a partition is if previous films have been obtained. To complicate matters further, it would be wise to recall that a partite sesamoid may separate when traumatized and thus become symptomatic and resemble a fracture.[4,14,20] If this proves to be the case, a view can be taken with the hallux in forced dorsiflexion and plantar flexion and the distance between fragments then measured. This will help in delineating between fracture and partition.[19]

moids as phylogeny, congenital, failure of fusion, heredity, constant stress/microtrauma, and biomechanical abnormalities. The results of his study indicate no sex difference, commonality among all age groups, a 19 percent frequency of finding at least one partite sesamoid, and a greater incidence of tibial versus fibular involvement. Others have found similar patterns of frequency with respect to bi-, tri-, and quadripartite sesamoids.[1,17]

It has been mentioned that partitioned sesamoids may be caused by a vascular disturbance.[1,11] This may result from direct trauma or constant microtrauma interrupting the plantar blood supply at the time of ossification. Sobel et al.[11] found that bipartite sesamoids lacked the plantar vessels, thus supporting this finding.

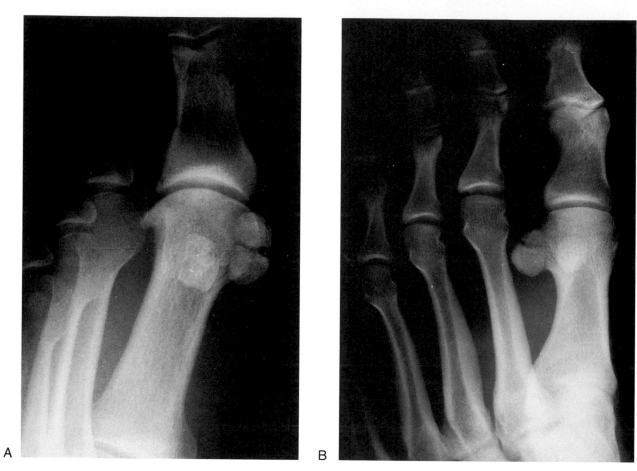

A

B

**Fig. 10-6. (A)** Lateral oblique view shows fractured tibial sesamoid. **(B)** Medical oblique view shows fractured fibular sesamoid.

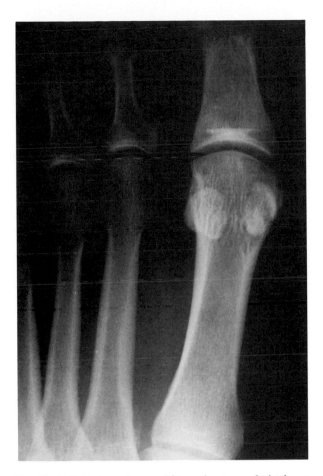

**Fig. 10-7.** D-P view shows oblique fracture of tibial sesamoid.

## SUMMARY

The involvement of the sesamoid apparatus with the function of the first metatarsophalangeal joint is more than distribution of ground reactive forces to protect the metatarsal head, shock absorption, and protection of the flexor hallucis longus tendon; the sesamoids help to maintain the highest mechanical advantage possible with respect to associated muscles and tendons. As with any precision equipment, deviation results in inefficiency and possible wear and degradation. This scenario will eventually cause progressive malalignment and abnormal function, which ultimately lead to hallux abducto valgus deformity and associated sesamoid complications.

## REFERENCES

1. Inge GAL, Ferguson AB: Surgery of the sesamoid bones of the great toe. Arch Surg 27:466, 1933
2. Helal B: The great toe sesamoid bones. Clin Orthop Relat Res 157:82, 1981
3. Jahss MH: The sesamoids of the hallux. Clin Orthop Relat Res 157:88, 1981
4. Scranton PE, Rutkowski R: Anatomic variations in the first ray: Part II, disorders of the sesamoids. Clin Orthop Relat Res 151:256, 1980
5. Aseyo D, Nathan H: Hallux sesamoid bones. Anatomical observations with special reference to osteoarthritis and hallux valgus. Int Orthop 8:67, 1984
6. Vranes R: Hallux sesamoids: a divided issue. J Am Podiatry Assoc 66:687, 1976
7. Nayfa TM, Sorto LA: The incidence of hallux abductus following tibial sesamoidectomy. J Am Podiatry Assoc 72:617, 1982
8. Pretterklieber ML, Wanivenhaus A: The arterial supply of the sesamoid bones of the hallux: the course and source of the nutrient arteries as an anatomical basis of surgical approaches to the great toe. Foot Ankle 13:27, 1992
9. Wooster M, Davies B, Catanzariti A: Effect of sesamoid position on long-term results of hallux abducto valgus surgery. J Foot Surg 29:543, 1990
10. David RD, Delagoutte JP, Renard MM: Anatomical study of the sesamoid bones of the first metatarsal. J Am Podiatr Med Assoc 79:536, 1989
11. Sobel M, Hashimoto J, Arnoczky SP, Bohne WHO: The microvasculature of the sesamoid complex; its clinical significance. Foot Ankle 13:359, 1992
12. Root ML, Orien WP, Weed JH: Normal and abnormal functions of the foot: In Clinical Biomechanics. Vol. II. p. 56, 285. Clinical Biomechanics Corporation, Los Angeles, 1977
13. Zinmeister BJ, Edelman R: Congenital absence of the tibial sesamoid: a report of two cases. J Foot Surg 24:266, 1985
14. Brock JG, Meredith HC: Case report 102. Skcle Radiol 4:236, 1979
15. Jahss MH: Editorial comments on "Pathologic anatomic variations in the sesamoids." Foot Ankle 1:325, 1981
16. Leventen ED: Sesamoid disorders and treatment. Clin Orthop Relat Res 269:236, 1991
17. Stearns LM: Some radiographic, clinical and anatomical considerations of the hallux sesamoids. Curr Podiatry 28:14, 1979
18. Zinman H, Keret D, Reis ND: Fracture of the medial sesamoid bone of the hallux. J Trauma 21:581, 1981
19. Weiss JS, Fracture of the medial sesamoid bone of the

great toe; controversies in therapy. Orthopedics 14:1003, 1991
20. Scranton PE: Pathologic anatomic variations in the sesamoids. Foot Ankle 1:321, 1981

## SUGGESTED READINGS

deBritto SR: The first metatarso-sesamoid joint. Int Orthop 6:61, 1982

Lipsman S, Frankel JP: Criteria for fibular sesamoidectomy in hallux abducto valgus correction. J Foot Surg 16:43, 1977

McCain LR, Nuzzo JJ: The "sesamoidal ligament" and its employ in the suturing of the Keller bunionectomy procedure. J Am Podiatry Assoc 59:479, 1969

McGlamry ED: Hallucal sesamoids. J Am Podiatry Assoc 55:693, 1965

Saxby T, Vandemark RM, Hall RL: Coalition of the hallux sesamoids. A case report. Foot Ankle 13:355, 1992

Shereff MJ, Yang GM, Kummer FJ: Extraosseous and intraosseous arterial supply to the first metatarsal and metatarsophalangeal joint. Foot Ankle 8:81, 1987

Sussman RE, Piccora R: The metatarsal sesamoid articulation and first metatarophalangeal joint function. J Am Podiatr Med Assoc 75:327, 1985

Turner RS: Dynamic post-surgical hallux varus after lateral sesamoidectomy: treatment and prevention. Orthopedics 9:963, 1986

Valinsky MS, Hettinger DF, Schmitt TS: The Valinsky tibial sesamoid planing procedure utilizing Mi-Tech. Foot 1:189, 1992

# 11

# Overview of Distal First Metatarsal Osteotomies

*ALAN J. SNYDER*
*VINCENT J. HETHERINGTON*

Distal first metatarsal osteotomies have played a prominent role in the surgical management of the hallux abducto valgus deformity. This chapter is a brief overview of distal first metatarsal osteotomies. Distal metatarsal osteotomies are usually performed with concurrent remodeling of the medial exostosis or eminance and some form of soft tissue balancing technique.

## REVERDIN OSTEOTOMY AND MODIFICATIONS

In 1881, Reverdin described a closing wedge osteotomy of the first metatarsal head with the apex laterally that also included excision of the medial eminence (Fig. 11-1A). His purpose was to realign the abducted hallux and remove the prominent bump. The procedure effectively reduces an abnormal proximal articular set angle but does not directly address the intermetatarsal angle.[1]

Since the time when Reverdin first described his osteotomy, there have been a number of modifications. Roux, in 1920, described an osteotomy of the first metatarsal in which the capital fragment has a long lateral beak (see Fig. 11-1B). There are three cuts to this osteotomy. The first or distal cut is dorsal to plantar, through and through, made in the metaphyseal region of the first metatarsal head. The second or proximal cut transects the entire first metatarsal, thereby mobilizing the capital fragment. After the capital fragment is mobilized, the third osteotomy is made

perpendicular to the first cut and completes a trapezoidal section of bone, which is resected. The distal capital fragment is then transposed laterally and tilted medially, closing the trapezoidal space.[2,3] Similar in design to the Mitchell osteotomy, the Roux osteotomy addressed both transverse plane deformity of the metatarsal head and the intermetatarsal angle.

Peabody in 1931 reported an operation almost identical in location and purpose to that of Reverdin. Peabody performed this osteotomy more proximately, however, than did Reverdin in the anatomic neck (see Fig. 11-1C). The osteotomy does not quite transverse the entire width of the bone, but leaves the articular or capital fragment attached by a thin segment from the lateral side of the neck and shaft area; at this site, there is undisturbed continuity of capsule and periosteum.[4]

Another modification of the Reverdin is the distal **L** osteotomy, referred to at times as the Reverdin–Green procedure[5] (see Fig. 11-1D). The first cut constructed is transverse, proximal, and parallel to the joint surface. The second dorsal cut is then perpendicular to the shaft of the metatarsal, in the frontal body plane. This creates a wedge that will enable the joint surface to be realigned, properly adjusting the proximal articular set angle. The plantar osteotomy is then made parallel as a shelf protecting the sesamoid articulation surface of the first metatarsal. Transposition of the capital fragment is achieved by completion of the osteotomy laterally.[6]

The Reverdin corrects for abnormality of the proximal articular set angle, but the modifications also address the intermetatarsal angle.

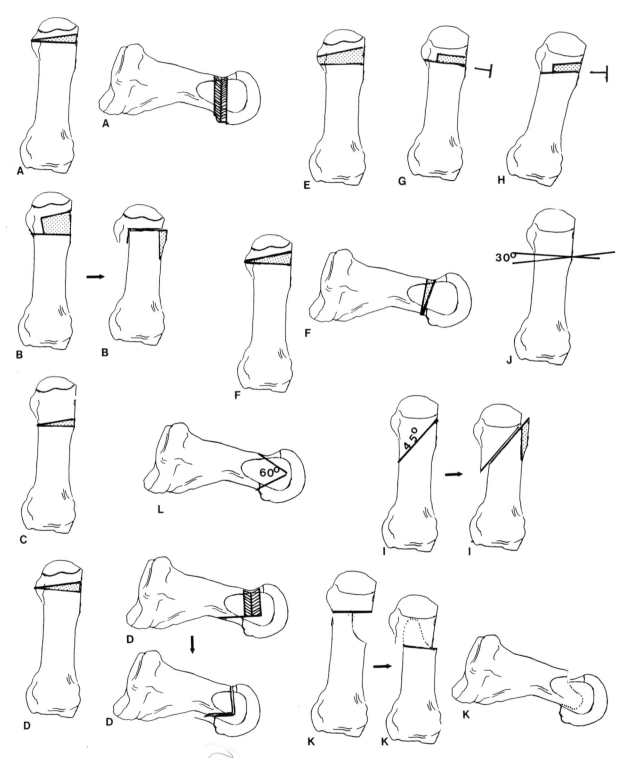

**Fig. 11-1.** **(A)** Reverdin osteotomy. **(B)** Roux osteotomy. **(C)** Peadbody osteotomy. **(D)** Distal L osteotomy. **(E)** Hohmann osteotomy. **(F)** DRATO osteotomy. **(G)** Mitchell osteotomy. **(H)** Miller osteotomy. **(I)** Wilson osteotomy. **(J)** Lindbren and Turan osteotomy. **(K)** Mygind osteotomy. **(L)** Austin osteotomy.

# HOHMANN OSTEOTOMY

Hohmann, in 1923, proposed an operation that would not only correct the valgus deformity of the great toe but also splaying of the forefoot as a whole. The procedure included dissection of the abductor hallucis from the medial head of the flexor brevis, detachment from its insertion into the base of the proximal phalanx, and reflection proximally. The head of the first metatarsal was disconnected from the shaft by a trapezoid or cuneiform osteotomy (see Fig. 11-1E). The trapezoid piece removed was wider on the medial aspect. The capital fragment was then pushed closer to the second metatarsal and the osteotomy closed. The severed end of the abductor hallucis was reattached to a more dorsal point on the medial side of the base of the phalanx.[3,7]

# CAPP OSTETOMY

Suppan in 1974 proposed the cartilaginous articulation preservation principle or CAPP procedure. At all times, the major part of the articulating cartilage is to be preserved. This technique as a general rule corrects the intermetatarsal angle and proximal articular set angle, and allows repositioning of the cartilaginous articulation by rotation of the base of the proximal phalanx to address the valgus component of the hallux. Two cuts approximately $\frac{1}{4}$ in. apart are made through the metatarsal head, and the section of bone is removed. The medial exostosis is also resected, thus leaving the cartilage and subchondral bone of the head of the metatarsal to be positioned freely and correctly within the surrounding capsule. The osteotomy cuts are performed at a right angle to the metatarsal.[8]

# DRATO OSTEOTOMY

The viability of the articular cartilage of the first metatarsophalangeal joint, considered with the congruity or incongruity of the joint surfaces, is important in the assessment of hallux abducto valgus deformity that was stated by Johnson and Smith. They proposed the derotational, angulational, transpositional osteotomy, or DRATO procedure, in 1974 (see Fig. 11-1F). The osteotomy consists of resection of the medial exostosis; a transverse osteotomy is then performed at the neck of the metatarsal perpendicular to its shaft. The capital fragment is either inverted or everted depending on the amount of rotation of the hallux present. A second osteotomy is then performed distal to the first osteotomy, parallel to a line that traverses the metatarsal head, intersecting at the articular margins of that head. The second osteotomy connects with the first at the lateral cortex. The resultant medial wedge is removed to adduct the capital fragment. A third osteotomy may be used to remove a dorsally based wedge to dorsiflex the capital fragment. The metatarsal head is displaced laterally by one-third the width of the bone, and fixated.[9]

# MITCHELL OSTEOTOMY AND MODIFICATIONS

In 1945 and again in 1958, Mitchell described an osteotomy procedure that was used to correct metatarsus primus varus and hallus valgus. The osteotomy is performed by making a incomplete osteotomy perpendicular to the long axis of the first metatarsal. The distal osteotomy is made about $\frac{3}{4}$ in. from the articular surface of the metatarsal head (see Fig. 11-1G). The thickness of the bone formed between the bone cuts depends on the amount of shortening of metatarsal necessary to relax the contracted soft tissue structures. The proximal osteotomy is then completed. The size of the lateral spur depends on the amount of intermetatarsal angle to be corrected with lateral displacement of the capital fragment. The osteotomy is displaced plantarly to accommodate for shortening of the metatarsal and to prevent metatarsalgia. Angulation of the distal bone cut will provide correction for abnormalities of the proximal articular set angle.[3,10,11]

In 1974, Miller described another modification to the Mitchell type of osteotomy (see Fig. 11-1H). He regarded the axis of the foot as more important than the axis of the first metatarsal bone; therefore, the osteotomy was performed perpendicular to the axis of the foot. He obtained lateral displacement in the frontal plane to achieve better correction.[3,12]

# WILSON OSTEOTOMY AND MODIFICATIONS

Wilson in 1963 described an oblique osteotomy for the advantages of simplicity, stability with displacement of the metatarsal head without need for internal fixation, broad osteotomy surfaces that reduce the risks of nonunion, and a large metatarsal head fragment that minimizes the chances of avascular necrosis (see Fig. 11-1I). This technique consists of an oblique osteotomy of the distal third of the first metatarsal, combined with remodeling of the medial exostosis. The line of the osteotomy is on the medial side at the proximal end of the exostosis, extending laterally at an angle of 45°. The osteotomy is cut to displace the distal fragment by angulation of the saw at 45°; the remaining prominent shaft is removed after the osteotomy is in its correct alignment.[13,14]

There have been a number of other modifications to the Wilson osteotomy. One of the first modifications was made by Helal et al.; in 1974, they changed the direction of the osteotomy by tilting it from a dorsal-distal position to plantar-proximal. Because this double oblique osteotomy modification is oblique in two planes, dorsal tilting of the capital fragment is prevented while the area of contact at the osteotomy site is also increased.[15] In 1976, Davis and Litman used Wilson's technique with one exception, that the medial exostosis was not removed, which allowed the first metatarsophalangeal joint to remain undisturbed. Davis and Litman considered that the less interference with the joint, the better.[16]

Allen et al. in 1981 then modified the osteotomy in two ways. First, they used a cancellous screw for rigid internal fixation, and second, they fashioned a medially based wedge that after removal allowed for correction of a laterally deviated cartilage.[17] In another modification, Pittman and Burns in 1984 altered the direction of the osteotomy from a proximal-medial to a distal-lateral direction to address hallux limitus by plantarly displacing the capital fragment.[18]

The Telfer osteotomy for hallux valgus was introduced in 1985. The procedure was developed with modifications to the original simple oblique Wilson osteotomy at the neck of the first metatarsal head that produce a maximum lateral displacement of the distal fragment and retain the ideal position by means of rigid internal fixation. The prominent metatarsal shaft that is created after the osteotomy is transposed is now removed. The author also states that fear of nonunion is now virtually nonexistent, and that greater correction of the hallux valgus is possible by increasing the lateral displacement of the distal fragment because of the internal fixation.[19]

In 1988, Klareskov et al. modified Wilson's osteotomy by plantar-flexing the first metatarsal head as it is shifted laterally. The plantar displacement of the distal fragment allows the first metatarsal to bear more of the weight-bearing forces, thus reducing excessive pressure on the lateral metatarsal heads.[20]

## TRANSVERSE OSTEOTOMY

A transverse osteotomy described by Lindgren and Turan is performed at approximately 30° to a line that transverses the metatarsal head. The osteotomy is displaced laterally and fixated[21] (see Fig. 11-1J).

## PEG-IN-HOLE OSTEOTOMY

Perhaps the most interesting and uncommon modification of dual-plane, lateral and plantar, displacement osteotomy of the distal end of the first metatarsal is that described by Mygind and credited to Thomasen in 1952 and 1953. The peg-in-hole osteotomy is described as primarily indicated in adolescents and young adults with hallux valgus and metatarsus primus. Thomasen's osteotomy modified the oblique osteotomy of the distal end of the first metatarsal. The osteotomy was performed, and a bone spike or peg was made in the proximal portion of the metatarsal with the hole being fashioned in the capital fragment (see Fig. 11-1K). The osteotomy was then laterally displaced so that the osteotomy could interlock, and is then fixated.[3,22]

## AUSTIN OSTEOTOMY

In 1981 Austin published his osteotomy, which is a horizontally directed, V displacement osteotomy of the metatarsal head for the management of hallux valgus and an increase of the intermetatarsal angle[23] (see Fig. 11-1L). In preparation for the osteotomy, the medial exostosis is remodeled, and a drill hole is centered on the medial surface of the metatarsal head. The hole is the apex of the osteotomy cuts. The V osteotomy is horizontally directed, and the cuts are made at a 60° angle that allows the cuts to remain in cancellous bone areas of the head, providing a broad surface for healing. Also, this osteotomy provided excellent stability. The capital fragment is displaced laterally and impacted by hand pressure in the corrected position. The protruding portions of the proximal metatarsal area are now remodeled.

## SUMMARY

Distal metatarsal osteotomies perform four basic functions. They can decrease the intermetatarsal angle; realign structural abnormalities in the transverse plane such as abnormal proximal articular set angles; and shorten or maintain the length of the metatarsal. The Reverdin-type osteotomy is used in correction of an abnormally high proximal articular set angle. This may be also accomplished by biplane osteotomies of the Wilson, Mitchell, or Austin types. Reduction of the intermetatarsal can be accomplished by lateral displacement of those osteotomies. The degree of reduction will be less than that obtained with proximal osteotomies, and therefore lateral displacement osteotomy is used with intermetatarsal angles ranging from 12° to 16°. Distal osteotomies may cause a significant decrease in metatarsal length and therefore should not be used with excessively short metatarsals. Plantar flexion of the capital fragment aids in compensating for metatarsal shortening by retaining the weight-bearing function of the metatarsal. Distal osteotomies may be used to advantage in patients with long first metatarsals.

The osteotomies described by Reverdin, Hohmann, Mitchell, and Austin are described in detail in Chapters 15, 13, 14, and 12, respectively.

## REFERENCES

1. Reverdin J: Antatomie et operation de l'hallux valgus. Int Med Congr 2:408, 1881
2. Roux C: Aux pieds sensibles. Rev Med Suisse Romande, 40:62, 1920
3. Kelikian H: Hallux Valgus, Allied Deformities of the Forefoot and Metatarsalgia. WB Saunders, Philadelphia, 1965
4. Peabody C: The surgical cure of hallux valgus. J Bone Jt Surg 13:273, 1931
5. McGlamry ED, Banks AS, Downey MS: Comprehensive Textbook of Foot Surgery. 2nd Ed. Williams & Wilkins, Baltimore, 1992
6. Zyzda MJ, Hineser W: Distal L osteotomy in treatment of hallux abducto valgus. J Foot Surg 28:445, 1989
7. Hohmann G: Uber hallux und spreizfuss, ihre eatstehung und physidegische behandlung. Arch Orthop Unfall-Chir 21:525, 1923
8. Suppan RJ: The cartilaginous articulation preservation principle and its surgical implementation for hallux abducto valgus. J Am Podiatry Assoc 64:635, 1974
9. Johnson JB, Smith SB: Preliminary report on derotational angulational, transpositional osteotomy: a new approach to hallux abducto valgus surgery. J Am Podiatry Assoc 64:667, 1974
10. Hawkins FB, Mitchell CC, Hedrick DW: Correction of hallux valgus by metatarsal osteotomy. J Bone Joint Surg 27:387, 1945
11. Mitchell CL, Fleming JL, Allen R, Glenning C, Sanford GA: Osteotomy-bunionectomy for hallux valgus. J Bone Joint Surg 40:41, 1958
12. Miller JW: Distal first metatarsal displacement osteotomy. J Bone Joint Surg 56A:923, 1974
13. Wilson JN: Oblique displacement osteotomy for hallux valgus. J Bone Joint Surg 45B:552, 1963
14. Dooley BJ, Berryman DB: Wilson's osteotomy of the first metatarsal for hallux valgus in the adolescent and the young adult. Aust NZ J Surg 43:255, 1973
15. Helal B, Gupta SK, Gojaseni P: Surgery for adolescent hallux valgus. Acta Orthop Scand 45:271, 1974
16. Davis M, Litman T: Simple osteotomy for hallux valgus. Minn Med 12:836, 1976
17. Allen TR, Gross M, Miller J, Lowe LW, Hulton WC: The assessment of adolescent hallux valgus before and after first metatarsal osteotomy. Int Orthop 5:111, 1981
18. Pittman SR, Burns DE: The Wilson bunion procedure modified for improved clinical results. J Foot Surg 23:314, 1984
19. Farguharson-Roberts MA, Osborne AH: The Telfer osteotomy for hallux valgus. J R Navy Med Serv 71:15, 1985
20. Klareskov B, Dalsgaard S, Gebuhr P: Wilson shaft osteotomy for hallux valgus. Acta Orthop Scand 59:307, 1988
21. Lindgren U, Turan I: A new operation for hallux valgus. Clin Orthop Relat Res 175:179, 1983
22. Mygind HB: Operative treatment of hallux valgus. Ugeskr Laeg 115:236, 1953
23. Austin DW, Leventon EO: A new osteotomy for hallux valgus: A horizontally directed "V" displacement osteotomy of the metatarsal head for hallux valgus and primus varus. Clin Orthop Relat Res 157:25, 1981

# 12

# Austin Procedure and Modified Austin Procedures

## VINCENT J. HETHERINGTON

The Austin procedure is primarily a transpositional **V** osteotomy of the head of the first metatarsal for the management of hallux valgus. The procedure was first reported in the podiatric literature and attributed to Dr. Austin by Miller and Croce.[1] The procedure was presented initially by Dr. Dale Austin in his 1981 publication.[2] The procedure as described is a horizontally directed **V** osteotomy performed in the metaphyseal bone of the first metatarsal, with the arms of the **V** at an angle of 60°. Transposition of the head of the metatarsal laterally from one-fourth to one-half the width of the metatarsal shaft addresses the increase in intermetatarsal angle (Fig. 12-1). Redirection by rotation of the metatarsal head is performed to address abnormal transverse plane alignment of the articular surface of the metatarsal head. The osteotomy is fixated by impaction via manual pressure and the protruding portion of the metatarsal shaft is then resected. The osteotomy is combined with soft tissue balancing medially and laterally with tenotomy of the adductor hallucis.

This procedure has also been referred to in the literature as the Austin osteotomy, chevron procedure, or Chevron osteotomy. Subsequent modifications have been described to address components of deformity associated with hallux valgus and first metatarsophalangeal joint deformity. These modifications include a bicorrectional technique for treatment of an associated abnormal proximal articular set angle (PASA) or transverse plane deformity of the head of the first metatarsal,[3] to incorporate shortening or lengthening of the metatarsal, as well as plantar flexion and dorsiflexion of the metatarsal head[4,5] and the correction of metatarsus primus elevatus.[6] The bicor-

rectional technique as described by Gerbert et al.[3] requires the performance of a second bone cut that extends 80 percent through the metatarsal to remove a medial wedge of bone head[3] (Fig. 12-2A).

Duke and Kaplan[4] reported that by angulating the osteotomy from distal-medial to proximal-lateral shortening of the bone will result, and that plantar flexion will accompany an osteotomy that is directed from dorsomedial to plantar-lateral. Combining the techniques described it is possible to effect triplane correction to varying degrees with the osteotomy[5] (Fig. 12-3A and B).

Youngswick[6] performed a second osteotomy paralleling the dorsal arm of the **V** osteotomy to enable plantar flexion for the management of a metatarsus primus elevatus associated with a hallux limitus (see Fig. 12-2B).

Vogler[7] modified the Austin osteotomy to incorporate an extended dorsal arm of the osteotomy, the so-called offset **V** osteoplasty (see Fig. 12-2C). The angle of the **V** reduces from 60° to 40°. The advantages to this modification, according to Vogler, are greater stability of the osteotomy and the ease with which screw fixation in an interfragmentary mode can be applied. Again, modification of the osteotomy allows multiplanar correction. A similar osteotomy has been described by Kalish et al.[8] Modification of the Kalish osteotomy to address an abnormal proximal articular set angle has also been described.[9]

Selection of patients for this procedure includes those complaining of pain associated with a hallux valgus deformity with inability to function comfortably in normal or conventional shoe wear. There should be

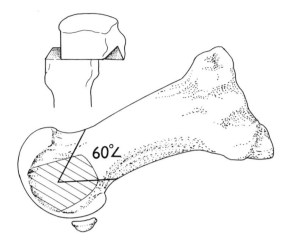

**Fig. 12-1.** Traditional Austin osteotomy.

no pain associated with range of motion with the first metatarsal phalangeal joint. Preoperative examination should reveal a bunion deformity with hallux abductus; a moderate degree of valgus rotation of the great toe is acceptable.

Preoperative radiographic evaluation or criteria include a hallux abductus angle of greater than 16° but less than 40° and a congruous to deviated first metatarsal phalangeal joint, normal or abnormal proximal articular set angle, and an elevation of intermetatarsal angle as great as approximately 16°. The metatarsal width should be assessed because a narrow first metatarsal limits the amount of correction that can be obtained as the potential for transposition is limited. Bone stock in the distal metaphysis of the first metatarsal should be determined radiographically to be healthy and free of cystic changes. A metatarsal index

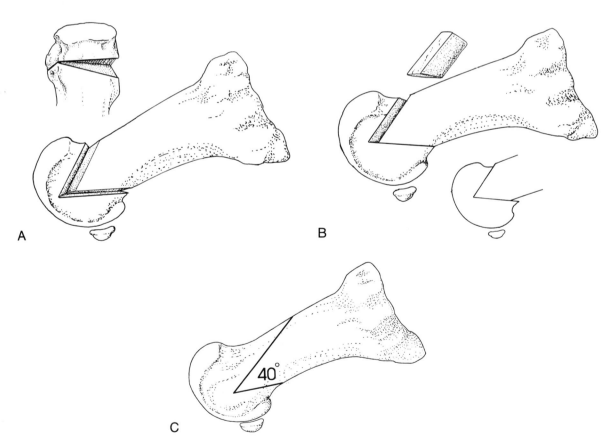

**Fig. 12-2. (A)** Bicorrectional Austin osteotomy (Gerbert). **(B)** Youngswick modification for metatarsus primus elevatus. **(C)** Offset **V** osteotomy of Vogler.

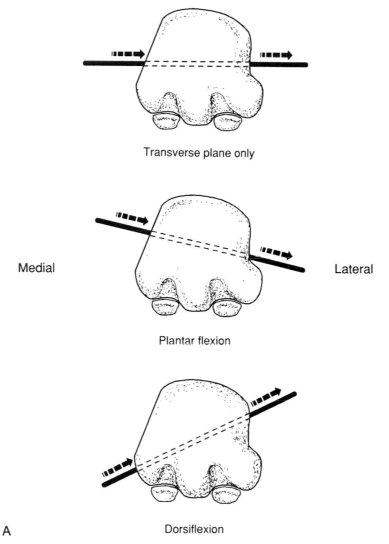

Transverse plane only

Medial

Plantar flexion

Lateral

A    Dorsiflexion

**Fig. 12-3. (A)** Apex orientation to incorporate dorsiflexion or plantar flexion of the capital fragment. (*Figure continues.*)

that is positive, neutral, or negative are all acceptable, provided that they are recognized preoperatively and that the osteotomy is performed in such a matter to address these conditions. A relative guideline to contraindications for the Austin procedure are listed in Table 12-1; each patient should be considered individually. The use of templates may be useful in preoperative assessment of the potential for using the Austin procedure in patients.[10]

The objective of this procedure is to provide patients with postoperative reduction of deformity com-

bined with a pain-free range of motion of the first metatarsal phalangeal joint, reduction of the intermetatarsal angle to less than 10°, and an hallux

**Table 12-1.** Contraindications for Austin Procedure

Limited range of motion in first metatarsophalangeal joint
Radiographic signs of osteoarthritis
Hallux abductus angle greater than 40°
Intermetatarsal angle greater than 16°
Poor quality of bone or cystic metatarsal head changes
Narrow first metatarsal
Geriatric patients

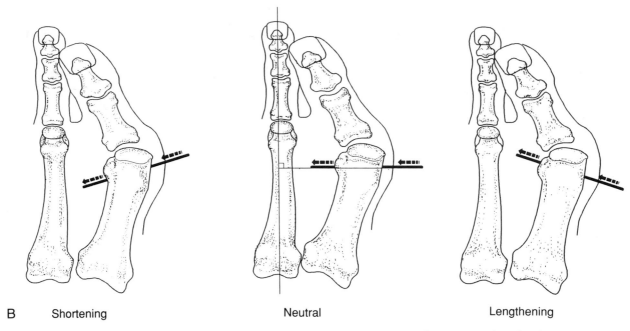

B          Shortening                    Neutral                    Lengthening

Fig. 12-3 *(Continued)*. **(B)** Apex orientation to incorporate shortening or lengthening.

## THE PROCEDURE

The approaches to the first metatarsophalangeal joint for the Austin procedure may be through several initial incisions. These include a dorsomedial linear incision that is placed medial to the extensor hallucis longus tendon, a medial approach, and a plantarmedial approach. The dorsimedial linear incision provides the greatest exposure to the medial aspect of the metatarsal head as well as to the intermetatarsal space. To expose the joint medially, several capsulotomies that can be used include a straight linear incision, one that is **T** or **U** shaped with the flap based distally, as described by Austin,[2] or as the author prefers, an inverted **L**-type capsulotomy. After reflection of the capsule flap and exposure of the metatarsal, remodeling of the exostosis of the metatarsal head is performed using an osteotome and mallet or power equipment.

Minimal resection is required, and aggressive resection of the exostosis is to be avoided; as with all bunion procedures, the exostosis is resected in a dorsomedial attitude.

The attention is next directed to the first intermetatarsal space where the adductor tendon is identified before its insertion in the base of the proximal phalanx and is tenotomized. A linear incision is performed over the fibular sesamoid transecting the fibular sesamoidal ligament, and a vertical capsulotomy of the joint is performed. This lateral **T**-shaped capsulotomy allows reduction of the fibular sesamoid, facilitating effective transposition of the head. This type of approach minimizes the amount of lateral dissection and therefore disruption of the soft tissues. Aggressive dissection should be avoided in the first intermetatarsal space to avoid potential osteonecrosis of the metatarsal head. It is important that anatomic reduction of the sesamoids be performed to ensure favorable long-term results and restore dynamic balance to the first metatarsophalangeal joint.[2]

After the soft tissue procedures have been completed, the osteotomy is performed. The basic osteotomy as described previously is a cut of approximately 60°. The apex of the **V** should rest in the center of the

abductus angle of less than 20°. There should be no resultant metatarsalgia following this osteotomy, which should be associated with a cosmetic result acceptable to the patient and no shoe-fitting problems.

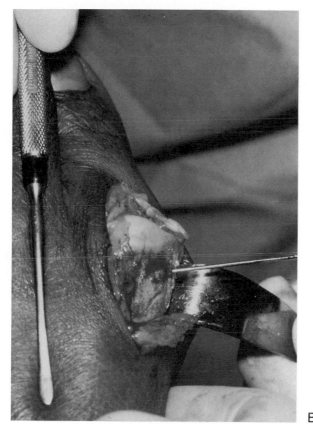
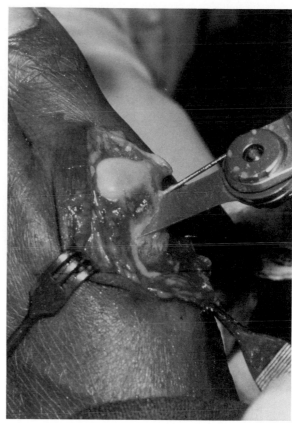

**Fig. 12-4.** **(A)** Apex wire inserted to delineate axis position. **(B)** Wire utilized as guide to direct performance of osteotomy. (*Figure continues.*)

metatarsal head. The center of the osteotomy is marked with a 0.045-in. Kirschner wire[2] (Fig. 12-4) that will then become the apex of the **V** osteotomy. By manipulation of the apex of the osteotomy through the body planes one may obtain, in addition to correction of the intermetatarsal angle, modification to allow lengthening, shortening, plantar flexion or dorsiflexion, or combinations resulting in multidimensional corrections, depending on the position of the apex.[4,5] An apex that approaches the perpendicular relative to the second metatarsal will be neutral, thereby incorporating neither lengthening or shortening (see Fig. 12-3B). If the apex is placed perpendicular to the surface left after resection of the medial eminence (resected primarily dorsomedially), it will incorporate plantar flexion of the metatarsal head (see Fig. 12-3A).

If plantar flexion is not desired, of course, the apex

must be corrected before performance of the osteotomy. To ensure proper alignment of the arms of the **V**, the Kirchner wire (K-wire) is kept in place while cutting the osteotomy, attempting to keep the blade and therefore the plane of the osteotomy maintained in alignment with the apex wire. This simple template, referred to as the apical axis guide,[11] will help ensure performance of the desired osteotomy as well as prevent diversion or conversion of the osteotomy cuts. Before cutting the osteotomy it is useful to score the metatarsal head using the osteotome and mallet in the appropriate 60° angle. The plantar arm should extend proximal to the articular surface for the sesamoids.

Following the osteotomy, the capital fragment is manipulated along the apex for approximately one-quarter to one-half the width of the bone. On completion of the osteotomy and transposition, fixation of the os-

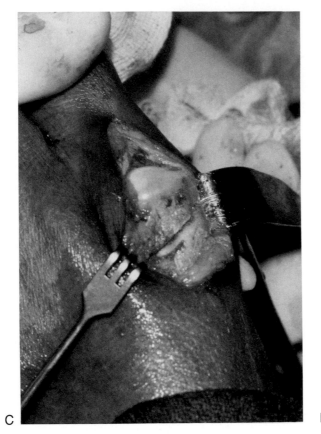
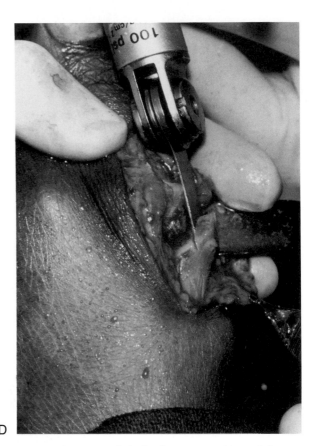

**Fig. 12-4** (*Continued*). **(C)** Completed osteotomy. **(D)** Resection of metatarsal shaft after transposition of the osteotomy.

teotomy may occur by a variety of methods (Fig. 12-5). These methods include impaction of the head of the metatarsal on the shaft of the metatarsal,[2] simple K-wire fixation,[12] buried K-wire technique,[13] monofilament stainless steel fixation,[14] screw fixation[15,16] including the Herbert bone screw,[17,18] staples,[19,20] and absorbable fixation.[21–25] Modification of the osteotomy to accommodate certain types of fixation may be necessary; for example, screw fixation requires elongation of the long dorsal arm. Capsular closure is performed maintaining the toe in correct alignment. Excessive plication of the capsule is not desirable.

Postoperative care may include initially management that is weight-bearing or partially weight-bearing; a cast or postoperative shoes may also be used according to the surgeon's preference. The patient is encouraged to begin range-of-motion exercises in the early postoperative period and gradual return to conventional shoe gear may occur at approximately 4 weeks (Fig. 12-6).

It is important to consider the potential three-dimensional effects of this osteotomy to use these to advantage in correcting the deformity and preventing an undesired result from incorrect osteotomy performance. The key in this procedure lies in the careful evaluation, design, and performance of the osteotomy (Fig. 12-7).

Potential intraoperative problems include an incorrect osteotomy angle that results in an unstable osteotomy or one that extends undesirably and unnecessarily into diaphyseal bone. Incorrect direction of the osteotomy in the transverse plane may cause undesirable shortening, and in the frontal plane may result in undesirable plantar flexion or dorsiflexion (Fig. 12-8).

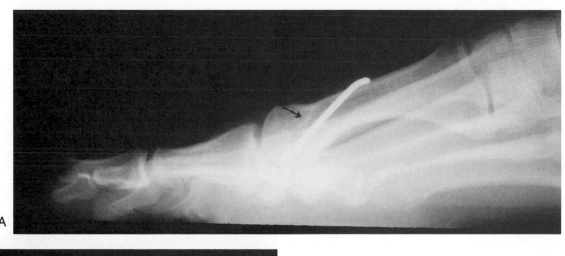

A

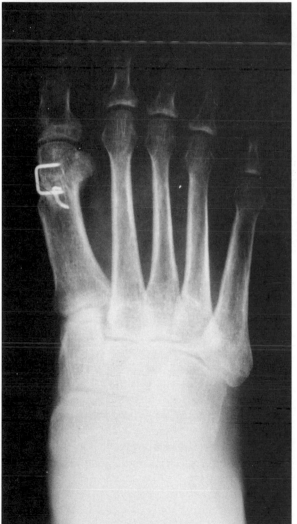

B

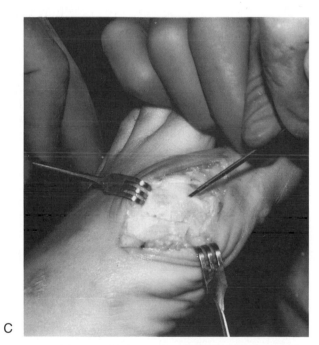

C

**Fig. 12-5.** Examples of internal fixation of the austin osteotomy utilizing **(A)** Kirschner wire fixation; **(B)** bone staples; **(C)** insertion of 1.3-mm Orthosorb pin fixation (Johnson and Johnson, Raynham, MA).

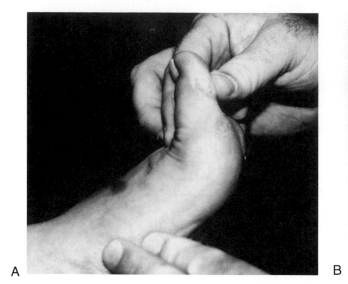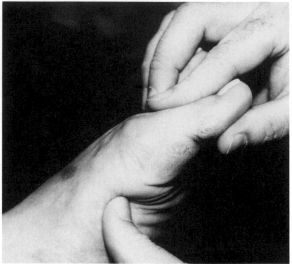

**Fig. 12-6.** Clinical range of motion 4 years after Austin procedure. **(A)** Dorsiflexion; **(B)** plantar flexion.

Care must be taken to not transpose the capital fragment too far laterally, causing instability; conversely, inadequate transposition can result in undercorrection.

The Austin procedure has also been combined with other procedures to address different components of a hallux valgus deformity. Reports on its conjunction with the Akin procedure are favorable when the Akin procedure is used to address structural deformity of the hallux.[26,27] The Austin osteotomy may be performed with simultaneous fibular sesamoidectomy; however, I do not do this on a routine basis, and recommend it be performed only with degenerative changes of the fibular sesamoid and not as a means to extend the correction of the Austin procedure in cases of excessive high intermetatarsal angles.

Lateral dissection with the Austin procedure, advocated by several authors, has been discouraged by others because of potential avascular necrosis of the metatarsal head. The concern regarding avascular necrosis following lateral dissection is still unclear. In those cases utilizing no lateral release, no occurence of osteonecrosis has been reported.[29–32] A 13 percent incidence of osteonecrosis followed transarticular lateral capsular release but did not adversely effect the final clinical result.[34] Others have reported no osteonecrosis to be associated with lateral dissec-

tions.[35–37] Meier and Kensora[38] reported osteonecrosis in 12 of 60 (20 percent) Chevron osteotomies; of 10 patients who underwent an osteotomy plus lateral adductor release, 4 (or 40 percent) developed avascular necrosis. The authors did however conclude that osteonecrosis, even in advanced stages, is not incompatible with satisfactory results. Resch et al.[39] using $^{99m}$Tc bone scans discovered that adductor tenotomy performed through a separate first webspace incision does not increase the risk of osteonecrosis following osteotomy when compared to osteotomy alone.

The advantages of the Austin bunionectomy are that (1) it is a joint-preserving procedure; (2) it is biomechanically sound in that it addresses deformities associated with hallux valgus, although the correction of the intermetatarsal angle is relative as opposed to a direct correction that may be accompanied by a more proximal osteotomy; (3) compensation for structural deformity in three planes is possible; (4) performance of osteotomy in the metaphyseal bone provides good bone healing; and (5) it is accessible to a variety of means of fixation.

Several authors have reported success in the management of hallux valgus using the Austin-type osteotomy.[4,5,11–15,19,21,24,29,37] Variations in technique especially with regards to the performance of any lateral dissection are noted. Various degrees of correction

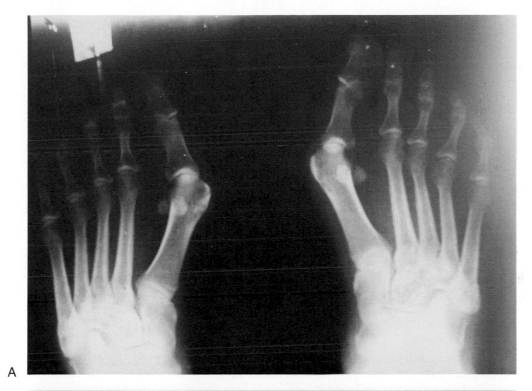

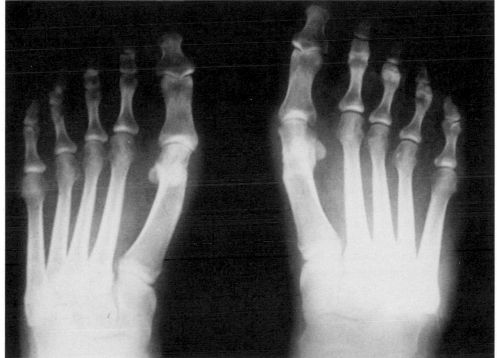

**Fig. 12-7.  (A)** Preoperative radiograph. **(B)** Postoperative radiograph.

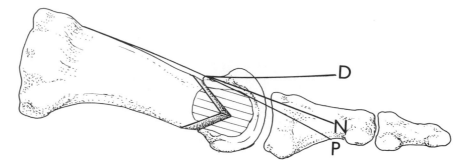

**Fig. 12-8.** Postoperative sagittal plane alignment of the osteotomy. In the author's experience, the neutral (N) and plantarflexed, (P) alignment did not result in metatarsalgia or limitation of first metatarsal phalangeal joint range of motion. The dorsiflexed attitude (D) is associated with metatarsalgia and limited joint motion.

with regards to intermetatarsal and hallux abductus angles are reported and may be attributed in part to individual surgeon's preferences and radiographic measurement techniques. Fixation techniques, postoperative management, and incidences of complications also vary among authors.

In comparisons between the Austin osteotomy and Mitchell osteotomy, Kinnard and Gordon[40] reported the results to be satisfactory both clinically and subjectively and equivalent with regards to outcome, but raised concern about a high, "nearly 40 percent" incidence of metatarsalgia for both groups. They also reported greater correction of the intermetatarsal angle with the Mitchell osteotomy and a tendency to lose correction in the immediate postoperative period for the Austin osteotomy. Meier and Kenzora[38] also reported good to excellent results with both osteotomies in about 90 percent of the cases. Osteonecrosis was reported to occur in 12 of 60 (20 percent) feet operated on by the Austin osteotomy, as opposed to 1 of 12 (8 percent) feet with the Mitchell osteotomy.

When the Austin procedure was compared with Basilar osteotomies, for patients with a intermetatarsal angle of 13° to 16° and a hallux abductus angle of 30°, the V osteotomy provided better subjective findings as well as a lower incidence of metatarsalgia and a better postoperative range of motion of the first metatarsophalangeal joint.[44]

Johnson et al.[42] reported similar postoperative results when comparing a modified McBride bunionectomy with a V osteotomy, noting that greater correction of the intermetatarsal angle and hallux adductus angle resulted with the osteotomy. The

Austin osteotomy applied in a reverse manner has been used for the management of hallux adductus.[43] The Austin osteotomy is also advocated for the management of juvenile hallux valgus.[35,44]

**Table 12-2.** Austin Bunionectomy Complications

| | |
|---|---|
| Insufficient lateral release | Lateral transposition difficult |
| | Rotation versus transposition |
| Angle of osteotomy too large[46] | Instability |
| Angle of osteotomy too small[46] | Osteotomy into diaphyseal bone |
| | Lateral transposition difficult |
| Apex of osteotomy too distal[32,46] | Danger of fracture of distal fragment (intra-articular) |
| Incorrect direction of osteotomy[47] | Deviation resulting in unwanted shortening, plantar flexion, or dorsiflexion |
| Loss of bone substance by saw[36] | Converging and diverging of osteotomy surfaces |
| | Instability |
| | Inadvertent PASA overcorrection[46,48] |
| | Malunion[42] |
| Excessive lateral transposition[46] | Instability, displacement, overcorrection |
| Insufficient impaction[47] | Instability, displacement |
| Excessive or poor soft tissue dissection | Osteonecrosis |
| | Neural injury[33,35,37] |
| Excessive excision of medial eminence[46] | Insufficient bone contact after transposition |
| Incorrect resection of metatarsal shaft[47] | Prominent medial bone |
| Failure to correctly transpose head[36] | Undesired rotation |
| Difficulty with transposition | Incomplete osteotomy; sesamoid blocks transposition |
| Joint pain[37] | Preexisting osteoarthritis |
| Excessive capsular tightening[12,37] | Hallux varus |
| | Joint stiffness |

*Abbreviation:* PASA, proximal articular set angle.

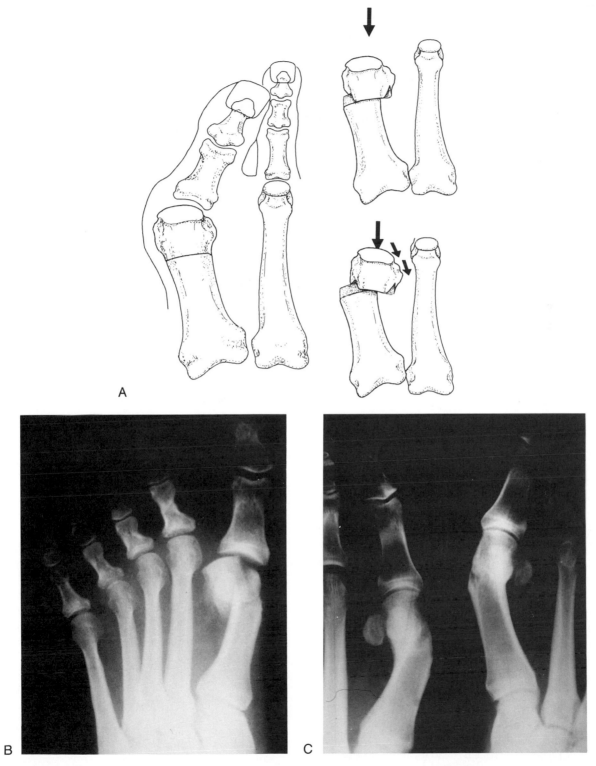

**Fig. 12-9.** Complications following the Austin procedure. **(A)** Dislocation of capital fragment resulting from instability and excessive lateral displacement. **(B)** Radiograph shows dislocation and displacement. **(C)** Radiograph reveals that rotation rather than transposition has occurred. (*Figure continues.*)

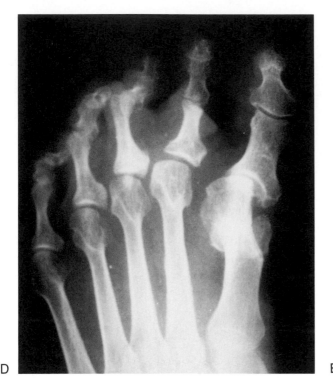 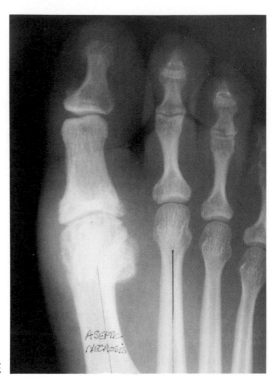

**Fig. 12-9** (*Continued*). **(D)** Hallux varus. **(E)** Osteonecrosis of first metatarsal head.

Like other procedures for the management of hallux valgus, the Austin procedure is not without complications. A review of complications associated with the osteotomy was published by Gerbert.[46] Complications are outlined in Table 12-2 and illustrated in Fig. 12-9. The primary cause of failure to achieve and maintain correction or recurrence of the deformity is the use of this osteotomy in cases that do not fit the preoperative criteria for its use. Hattrup and Johnson[47] reported an increasing rate of dissatisfaction with increasing age of patients, especially patients in their sixties.

The Austin procedure is an effective means of managing mild to moderate hallux valgus deformities using the outlined criteria for both adults and children.[35-37] My experiences have consistently demonstrated high patient satisfaction with the results of the Austin procedure when applied to appropriate patients. Objective clinical evaluation has also demonstrated good clinical results; however, patient subjective evaluations exceeded the clinical ratings. Relative reductions in the intermetatarsal angle have approached 7° to 8°, with a corresponding reduction of the hallux abductus angle of 15° to 17°. The tibial sesamoid position can be reduced in the immediate postoperative period to position 1 but in long-term evaluation a position of 3 was observed.[36,37]

The versatility of the osteotomy allows multiplanar, multidirectional correction with high patient satisfaction and minimal complications. The procedure is effective in reduction of the intermetatarsal and hallux abductus angles. The results of the procedure are reliable and reproducible. Careful attention to detail in the overall performance of the osteotomy will prevent both intraoperative and postoperative complications.

## REFERENCES

1. Miller S, Croce WA: The Austin procedure for surgical correction of hallux abducto valgus deformity. J Am Podiatry Assoc 69:110, 1979
2. Austin DW, Leventen EO: A new osteotomy for hallux valgus. Clin Orthop Relat Res 157:25, 1981
3. Gerbert J, Massad R, Wilson F, Wolf E, Younswick F: Bi-

correctional horizontal V-osteotomy (Austin type) of the first metatarsal head. J Am Podiatry Assoc 69:119, 1979

4. Duke HF, Kaplan EM: A modification of the Austin bunionectomy for shortening and plantarflexion. J Am Podiatry Assoc 74:209, 1984

5. Boc SF, D'Angleantonio A, Grant S: The triplane Austin bunionectomy: a review and retrospective analysis. J Foot Surg 30:375, 1991

6. Youngswick FD: Modification of the Austin bunionectomy for treatment of metatarsus primus elevatus associated with hallux limitus. J Foot Surg 21:114, 1985

7. Vogler HW: Shaft osteotomies in hallux valgus reduction. Clin Podiatr Med Surg 6:47, 1989

8. Kalish SR, Bernback MR, McGlamry DE: Reconstructive Surgery of the Foot and Leg: Modification of the Austin Bunionectomy. Podiatry Institute Publishing Company, Tucker, GA, 1987

9. Hill RS, Marek LJ: Modification of the Kalish osteotomy to correct the proximal articular set angle. J Am Podiatry Assoc 80:424, 1990

10. Gerbert J: Indications and techniques for utilizing preoperative templates in podiatric surgery. J Am Podiatry Assoc 69:139, 1979

11. Boberg J, Ruch JA, Banks AS; Distal metaphyseal osteotomies in hallux abducto valgus surgery. p. 178. In McGlamry ED (ed): Comprehensive Textbook of Foot Surgery, Vol. 1. Williams & Wilkins, Baltimore, 1987

12. Knecht JG, Van Pelt WL: Austin Bunionectomy with Kirschner wire fixation. J Am Podiatry Assoc 71:139, 1981

13. Duke HF: Buried Kirschner wire fixation of the Austin osteotomy bunionectomy: a preliminary report. J Foot Surg 25:197, 1986

14. Turner JM, Todd WF: A permanent internal fixation technique for the Austin osteotomy. J Foot Surg 23:199, 1984

15. Clancy JT, Berlin SJ, Giordan ML, Sherman SA: Modified Austin bunionectomy with single screw fixation: a comparison study. J Foot Surg 28:284, 1989

16. Klein MS, Ognibene FA, Erali RP, Hendrix CL: Self-tapping screw fixation of the Austin osteotomy. J Foot Surg 29:52, 1991

17. Vanore JV: Austin bunionectomy with Herbert bone screw fixation. Promotional Educational Literature, Zimmer Inc, Warsaw, IN, 1986

18. Palladino SJ: Fixation of the Austin procedure with the Herbert screw. J Am Podiatry Assoc 80:526, 1990

19. DeFronzo D-J, Landsman AR, Landsman AS, Stern SF: Austin bunionectomy with 3-mm stabilizer fixation. J Am Med Assoc 81:140, 1991

20. Kaye JM: New staple fixation for an Austin bunionectomy. J Foot Surg 31:43, 1992

21. Brunetti VA, Trepal MJ, Jules KT: Fixation of the Austin osteotomy with bioresorbable pins. J Foot Surg 30:56, 1991

22. Yen RG, Giacopelli JA, Granoff DP, Steinbroner RJ: The biofix, absorbable rod. J Am Med Assoc 81:62, 1991

23. Anderson S, Nielsen PM, Brems E: Chevron osteotomy with biodegradable fixation for hallux valgus. Acta Orthop Scand 62(suppl. 243):2, 1991

24. Hirvensalo E, Bostman O, Tormala P, Vainionpaa S, Rokkanhen P: Chevron osteotomy fixed with absorbable polyglycolide pins. Foot Ankle 11:212, 1991

25. Gerbert J: Effectiveness of absorbable fixation devices in Austin bunionectomies. J Am Med Assoc 82:189, 1992

26. Mitchell LA, Baxter DE: A Chevron–Akin double osteotomy for correction of hallux valgus. Foot Ankle 12:7, 1991

27. Bishop JO, Clifford R, Britt B, Braly WG, Tullos HS: Chevron–Akin procedure for hallux valgus correction. Foot Ankle 7:305, 1987

28. McDonald KC, Durrant MN, Drake R, Paolercio NL: Retrospective analysis of Akin–Austin bunionectomies on patients over fifty years of age. J Foot Surg 27:545, 1988

29. Johnson KA, Cofield RH, Morrey BF: Chevron osteotomy for hallux valgus. Clin Orthop Relat Res 142:44, 1979

30. Lewis RL, Feffer HL: Modified Chevron osteotomy of the first metatarsal. Clin Orthop Relat Res 157:105, 1981

31. Shepherd BD, Giutronich L: Correction of hallux valgus. Med J Aust 1:131, 1982

32. Velkes S, Ganel A, Negris B, Lokiec F: Chevron osteotomy in the treatment of hallux valgus. J Foot Surg 30:276, 1991

33. Williams WW, Barrett DS, Copeland SA: Avascular necrosis following chevron distal metatarsal osteotomy: a significant risk? J Foot Surg 28:414, 1989

34. Horne G, Tanzer T, Ford M: Chevron osteotomy for treatment of hallux valgus. Clin Orthop Relat Res 183:32, 1984

35. Grill F, Hetherington V, Steinbock G, Altenhuber J: Experiences with the Chevron (V) osteotomy on adolescent hallux valgus. Arch Orthop Trauma Surg 106:47, 1986

36. Steinbock G, Hetherington V: Austin bunionectomy: transpositional "V" osteotomy of the first metatarsal for hallux valgus. J Foot Surg 27:211, 1988

37. Hetherington V, Steinbock G, LaPorta D, Gardner C: The Austin bunionectomy: a follow-up study. J Foot Ankle Surgery 32:163, 1993

38. Meier PJ, Kenzora JE: The risks and benefits of distal first metatarsal osteotomies. Foot Ankle 6:7, 1985

39. Resch S, Stenstrom A, Gustafson T: Circulatory disturbance of the first metatarsal head after Chevron osteotomy as shown by bone scintigraphy. Foot Ankle 13:137, 1992

40. Kinnard P, Gordon D: A comparison between Chevron and Mitchell osteotomies for hallux valgus. Foot Ankle 4:241, 1984

41. Tzvi B, Trpal MJ: A retrospective analysis of distal Chevron and basilar osteotomies of the first metatarsal for correction of intermetatarsal angles in the range of 13 to 16 degrees. J Foot Surg 30:450, 1991

42. Johnson JE, Clanton TO, Baxter DE, Gottlieb MS: Comparison of Chevron osteotomy and modified McBride bunionectomy for correction of mild to moderate hallux valgus deformity. Foot Ankle 12:61, 1991

43. Butler M, Keating SE, DeVincentis AF: Reverse Austin osteotomy for correction of acquired static hallux adductus. J Foot Surg 27:162, 1988

44. Zinner TJ, Johnson KA, Klassen RA: Treatment of hallux valgus in adolescents by the Chevron osteotomy. Foot Ankle 9:190, 1989

45. Brahm S, Gerber J: A potential cause of hallux adductus in bi-correctional Austin bunionectomies. J Am Podiatry Assoc 73:155, 1983

46. Gerbert J: Complications of the Austin-type bunionectomy. J Foot Surg 17:1, 1978

47. Hattrup SJ, Johnson KA: Chevron osteotomy: analysis of factors in patient dissatisfaction. Foot Ankle 5:327, 1985

48. Palladino SJ, Kemple T: Proximal articular set angle changes with uni-correctional Austin bunionectomies. J Am Med Assoc 76:636, 1986

## SUGGESTED READINGS

Cleary RF, Borovoy M: A traumatically displaced Austin bunionectomy: a case report. J Am Podiatr Assoc 70:247, 1980

Guerin G: Geometric Austin osteotomy. J Foot Surg 27:528, 1988

Harper MC: Correction of metatarsus primus varus with the Chevron metatarsal osteotomy. Clin Orthop Relat Res 243:180, 1989

Leventen EO: The Chevron procedure. Orthopedics 13:973, 1990

Piccora RN: The Austin bunionectomy: then and now. Clin Pod Med Surg 6:179, 1989

# 13

# Hohmann Osteotomy

*JOHN V. VANORE*

Osteotomy for hallux valgus in the 1990s has evolved from those procedures of simple design with inadequate or no fixation to extremely complex osteotomies designed to allow relatively straightforward internal screw fixation.[1-3] The Hohmann osteotomy is an efficacious time-proven procedure for the correction of hallux valgus that has progressed with our concepts of rigid internal fixation to yield an important procedure in today's surgical armamentarium.[1,4]

Hohmann recognized the potential to address deformity on more than one cardinal body plane.[5-10] Most procedures were attempts to correct only one aspect of the deformity. For example, the Reverdin operation utilized wedge resection within the metatarsal head to reduce the valgus or abduction of the great toe while the Mitchell procedure shifted the metatarsal head laterally to reduce splaying of the first metatarsal.[11,12]

Kelikian called the Hohmann procedure a dual-plane displacement osteotomy,[13] as Hohmann described both lateral and plantar displacement. The addition of a medially based trapezoidal wedge allows for reduction of hallucal abduction as well as for reduction of metatarsus primus varus or elevatus corresponding to lateral or plantar shift of the capital fragment.

Variations of the Hohmann procedure have been used in cases of hallux valgus and hallux valgus rigidus with good success. Although originally described as a trapezoidal osteotomy, this osteotomy has undergone several modifications or versions in the literature. The British literature somewhat confuses a number of these distal osteotomies as being much the same. Turnbull and Grange referred to Peabody or Mitchell modifications of this procedure as well as drawing similarities between the Hohmann and Wilson osteot-

omies.[14-17] Grace et al. described an osteotomy and labeled it a Hohmann; however, it appears to be more akin to a Peabody.[18]

The Hohmann osteotomy to be discussed is also performed as a closing-wedge-type procedure similar to the Peabody[15] or Barker,[17] performed obliquely although not to the same degree as a Wilson,[16,19] but with transposition of the capital fragment much as described by Hohmann[20] (Fig. 13-1). These are somewhat different osteotomies with a certain variation between authors. The orientation of the osteotomies and their potential for correcting various aspects of a hallux valgus deformity does vary as well as their potential complications.[21] The Mitchell osteotomy is associated with a greater amount of shortening than are the Hohmann- or Wilson-type osteotomies.[22,23]

## THE OSTEOTOMY

The Hohmann osteotomy was originally described as an extra-articular osteotomy,[5-10] although today it is usually performed in conjunction with other procedures, for example, capsule tendon balance of the first metatarsophalangeal joint. The osteotomy itself is usually performed as a closing-wedge-type osteotomy in the first metatarsal neck.

The transverse plane orientation of the osteotomy in relationship to the long axis of the second metatarsal determines whether the first metatarsal will shorten or lengthen as a result of the lateral transposition of the capital fragment (Fig. 13-2). The Hohmann osteotomy has been effective particularly in its ability to reduce lateral adaptation of the articular surface of the first metatarsal or the proximal articular set angle

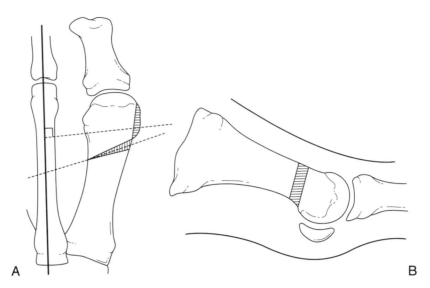

**Fig. 13-1.** (**A & B**) The proposed modified Hohmann osteotomy, generally performed as a closing-wedge or medially based cuneiform osteotomy in the metatarsal neck.

(PASA). If this is elevated, the surgeon may reduce the PASA through a medially based, cuneiform-shaped osteotomy. If the PASA is within normal limits, the osteotomy is performed as an oblique single cut.

After removal of the medial wedge of bone, the lateral hinge is feathered, and the osteotomy is then completed so as to provide optimal bone-to-bone contact. Whether a wedge of bone is removed or simply a solitary osteotomy is performed, the osteotomy is completed through the lateral cortex. This allows for transpositional and rotational movements of the capital fragment (Fig. 13-3). Lateral transposition moves

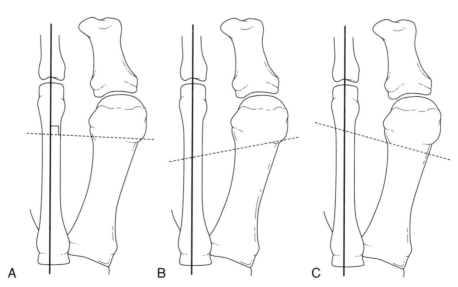

**Fig. 13-2.** Axis of the osteotomy. (**A**) An osteotomy perpendicular to the long axis of the second metatarsal will neither lengthen nor shorten the first metatarsal. An osteotomy therefore may be designed to either shorten (**B**) or lengthen (**C**) the first metatarsal.

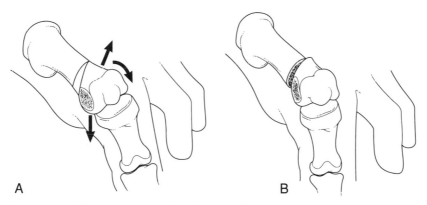

**Fig. 13-3.** Displacements of the osteotomy. (**A**) Reduction of PASA and plantar flexion. (**B**) The capital fragment may be transposed laterally to reduce intermetatarsal angle, rotated to correct axial rotation, or transposed plantarly to improve the sagittal plane alignment of the first metatarsal. In addition to removal of a medial wedge to correct cartilage adaptation, these displacements give the Hohmann osteotomy the potential of significant multiplanar correction of a hallux valgus deformity. The Hohmann may also be utilized as a shortening osteotomy to provide joint decompression through linear reduction of the first metatarsal.

the first metatarsal head closer to the second, thereby achieving a relative reduction of the intermetatarsal angle. The osteotomy is usually performed so that some shortening of the first metatarsal will accompany lateral shift. Shortening of the metatarsal segment will provide decompression of the first metatarsophalangeal joint.

The capital fragment may also be transposed plantarly. This is desirable in cases of mild to moderate metatarsus primus elevatus or to compensate for the shortening that may have occurred. Caution is recommended as both lateral and plantar transposition may significantly reduce bony contact between the metatarsal head and shaft. The capital fragment may also be rotated in the frontal plane before fixation to accomplish reduction of hallucal axial rotation or an oblique range of motion. It is recommended that the toe be placed through a range of motion before preliminary fixation. Adequate and good-quality range of sagittal plane motion is an objective (See Fig. 13-3.)

## OBJECTIVES

The goals of surgery are correction of the hallux valgus deformity and restoration of a functional and pain-free first metatarsophalangeal joint. This procedure is indicated in cases of moderate to severe hallux

valgus where specific osseous abnormalities must be addressed (Table 13-1). The procedure is particularly beneficial in the reduction of the PASA and intermetatarsal angles to as much as 18 degrees. Indications are as follows:

Hallux Valgus
  moderate to severe deformity
  particularly effacious in cases of very high PASA
  the more flexible the foot, the greater the potential for transverse plane correction (intermetatarsal and hallux abductus angles).
Recurrent Hallux Valgus
  excellent procedure in cases of revision surgery; allows for multisegmental correction
Hallux Valgus Rigidus
  in cases of combined deformity, particularly a mild deformity in a rigid foot type; use as a decompression osteotomy

**Table 13-1.** Hohmann Osteotomy for Hallux Valgus

| Segment of Deformity | Corrective Maneuver |
| --- | --- |
| Elevated PASA | Medial wedge |
| Tight joint | Shorten |
| Elevatus or short first metatarsal | Plantar-flex |
| Valgus (axial) rotation | Rotation of capital fragment |

In cases of a rigid foot type or limited range of first metatarsophalangeal joint motion, decompression through shortening aids in the reduction of deformity and improvement of joint function. This enables reduction of joint subluxation as well as realignment of the osseous segments of the deformity. As mentioned earlier, axial rotation of the hallux and mild to moderate sagittal plane deformities of the first metatarsal may be addressed, and the necessity for their correction is an important consideration regarding the choice of procedure. In the case of a long first metatarsal with an index plus, this is an excellent technique to reduce its length.

Our use of the Hohmann osteotomy is similar to the objectives of the derotational, angulational, transpositional osteotomy (DRATO) by Johnson and Smith[24]; that is, multiplanar correction with a single osteotomy. The Hohmann osteotomy for hallux valgus is always performed in conjunction with soft tissue components of capsule/tendon balance, which may include medial capsulotomy and capsulorrhaphy, lateral release, and fibular sesamoidectomy or adductor transfer, in addition to removal of the medial eminence.

## SURGICAL TECHNIQUE

The procedure may be performed from a medial or dorsal longitudinal incision. The dorsomedial approach is preferred, as it allows for greater ease of first intermetatarsal space exposure.

In cases with a very large medial eminence or a large hallux abductus, a significant amount of capsule is removed with the capsulotomy. This may be performed either with a lenticular capsulotomy, which is my preference, or with an inverted **L**, in which a section of capsule is then removed from the vertical arm.

The lenticular capsulotomy allows expedient and adequate exposure to the first metatarsal for performance of the osteotomy and its fixation. Subperiosteal dissection is carried out dorsally and medially with severing of the medial collateral ligaments. A screw will be placed from the dorsal cortex of the first metatarsal, and therefore this area is included in the dissection. Consideration must be given for the potential of avascular necrosis with distal first metatarsal osteotomies, and thus no dissection of the plantar or lateral aspects of the metatarsal is performed at this time. If

osteophytosis or periarticular lipping of either the phalangeal or metatarsal segment is present, then certainly a decision to remodel these areas would necessitate greater exposure and dissection.

The first intermetatarsal space is entered between the first and second metatarsophalangeal joints. The deep transverse metatarsal ligament is severed. A long transverse incision is made into the lateral joint capsule along the upper aspect of the sesamoidal bulge. This is deepened between the sesamoid and joint capsule laterally to dissect it free from the conjoined adductor tendon. Subsequently, the fibular sesamoid may be systematically released through severing its proximal and distal attachments to the lateral head of the flexor hallucis brevis and oblique head of adductor hallucis tendon/aponeurosis. The conjoined tendon is usually left undisturbed from its insertion into the lateral aspect of the proximal phalanx. If an adductor transfer is deemed necessary, it may be dissected free at this time. On occasion, the fibular sesamoid may be completely excised in the presence of severe deformity or degenerative changes. Symptoms associated with the sesamoids should be assessed preoperatively.

The medial eminence of the first metatarsal is resected. Caution should be taken with removal of the bump, erring on the side of less resection. The medial eminence is usually resected slightly oblique in the coronal plane so that the tibial sesamoidal groove is left intact plantarly. The osteotomy is then marked on the bone with an osteotome and mallet before its actual performance to allow assessment of the geometry of the cuts. The osteotomy is made in a cuneiform orientation with the base medially. The most distal cut begins just behind the tibial sesamoid, and the second is proximal enough to correct the lateral adaptation of the articular surface. The lateral apex is oriented somewhat proximal so that some degree of shortening will occur with lateral shift of the capital fragment. As is the use of a medially based wedge, this is a patient-dependent variable and must be assessed individually.

Before the actual performance of the osteotomy, some additional dissection is required. Lateral and plantar subperiosteal dissection is performed at the exact site of the marked osteotomy. Usually only the width of a #15 blade is all the dissection that is necessary, in an effort to preserve the vascular integrity of the first metatarsal head. The osteotomy is then begun perpendicular to the medial resected surface at both the proximal and distal arms of the wedge. Once the osteotomy is begun the cuts may be redirected proximally as outlined or marked on the bone. (This just helps to ensure the desired amount of bone is removed.) The wedge is completed before the lateral cortex so that the hinge may be "feathered" to allow flush apposition of the cut surfaces after cutting through the lateral cortex. As a result of even slight shortening, decompression of the joint and displacement (lateral or plantar) of the capital fragment is accomplished quite readily.

Frontal plane position is determined by placing the toe through a range of motion, thus aligning the toe and its excursion of motion in the sagittal plane. This usually involves varus rotation of the capital fragment.

This osteotomy must be fixated. Indications are as follows:

Correction of moderate to high PASA
Correction of hallucal axial rotation
Good technique for shortening the first metatarsal joint decompression
Revision bunion surgery
Hallux abductus valgus or hallux valgus rigidus (rigid foot type, metatarsus adductus)

The osteosynthesis provides stability to achieve osseous union, but more importantly rigid internal fixation should maintain the optimal position of the osseous fragments in correction until union is achieved. For the Hohmann, this is usually in the form of screw fixation. A cancellous screw from the dorsal surface of the metatarsal shaft directed in a distal and plantar direction is the preferred fixation (Table 13-2). There are numerous variations of the exact direction of the screw, the screw utilized, and the technique, but the principles of interfragmentary compression with a lag technique are followed (Fig. 13-4). Generally a partially threaded screw is chosen that purchases only the cancellous bone of the capital fragment. The lag geometry of the screw draws the capital fragment into or up against the shaft tightly so that there is no movement between the two. In addition to an interfragmentary screw, a second point of fixation is recommended as this is a through-and-through planar osteotomy. This second point of fixation will protect the screw from rotatory and potentially disruptive forces. A 0.062-in.

**Table 13-2.** Hohmann First Metatarsal Osteotomy with 4.0-mm Cancellous Screw

*Preliminary fixation*
  Place a 0.045-in. Kirschner wire from the medioplantar aspect of metatarsal proximal to the osteotomy and drive the wire in a distal and dorsal direction.
*Pilot hole*
  A 2.0-mm twist drill is utilized; the hole is begun 15 mm proximal to the osteotomy and in the center of the metatarsal shaft; the hole is drilled in a plantar-lateral direction.
*Countersink*
  Performed with a 5.5-mm oval side cutting burr; the countersinking must be coaxial; performed in the *same* direction as pilot hole and *only* of the proximal cortex.
  A trough is created in the dorsal cortex that allows oblique insertion of the screw.
*Depth measurement*
  Utilizing a small fragment depth gauge, or preferably use a 0.045-in. K-wire.
  The K-wire is inserted dorsally through the pilot hole entirely through the metatarsal head.
  The base of the proximal phalanx is plantar-flexed, and then abutted against the metatarsal head; this will push the K-wire proximal until it is flush with the articular surface.
  Clamp the wire with a curved stat at the bone edge within the dorsal trough; remove the wire still clamped, and measure it against a ruler.
*Tap*
  The 3.5-mm diameter, 1.75-mm pitch tap is utilized.
*Insertion of the 4.0 mm cancellous screw*
  Usually the exact screw length as measured (or 1 mm less if odd size) is inserted while maintaining retrograde pressure on the capital fragment. The screws most commonly used are 28- and 30-mm; range: 26–38 mm.
*Removal of preliminary fixation*
  The K-wire used for initial fixation is removed.
*Two-point fixation*
  A 0.062-in. K-wire is inserted from proximal lateral to medial plantar to provide rotatory stability and further rigidity of fixation.
*Resection of the medial prominence of first metatarsal*
  The overhanging ledge of metatarsal shaft is resected flush with medial shaft
*Lavage, check of fixation, wound closure*
  Copious wound lavage/irrigation.
  Recheck screw tightness and rigidity of fixation.

Kirschner wire is usually used as the neutralization pin described. The exact technique of osteosynthesis is further described by means of the illustrations of Fig. 13-4. Large deformities often require capsuloplasties or an adductor transfer. Once the osteotomy is fixated, the necessity for additional capsule tendon procedures can be evaluated.

Avoidance of unrestricted weight-bearing is essential to maintaining the integrity and compression of the osteosynthesis. Functional bracing in the form of a

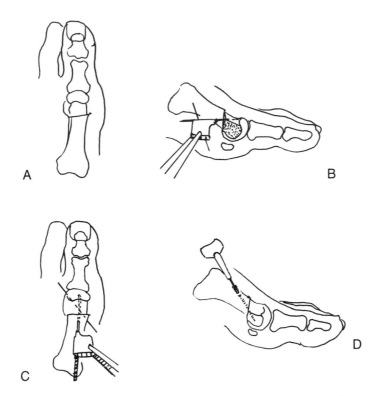

**Fig. 13-4.** Technique of internal fixation. (See also Table 13-2.) (**A**) Performance of the osteotomy. (**B**) Preliminary fixation. (**C**) Pilot hole (equivalent to screw core diameter). (**D**) Countersink. (*Figure continues.*)

below-knee walker is recommended. This is used by the patient for 4 to 6 weeks until the osteotomy is clinically solid and edema has resolved. The Kirschner wire is usually removed at 3 to 4 weeks postoperative when little or no dressing is required. The use of bracing offers the advantage of early range of motion of the joint reconstruction while allowing for easy dressing changes and wound care. A below-knee cast is certainly an alternative but is not conducive to postoperative rehabilitation.

The patient is usually able to put on a pair of gym shoes immediately when coming out of the brace. Initially, it is better to wean the patient from the immobilization device by first allowing use of the gym shoes around the house. Ambulation and activities should be guarded until approximately 6 weeks postoperative. Radiographs are recommended at 2 and 6 weeks, and at 3 months, postoperatively. If any resorption is noted at the 6-week radiograph, an unstable osteosynthesis is

indicated and the patient should be followed closely until osseous union is observed (Fig. 13-5).

## RESULTS

Grace et al.[18] noted loss of position of the Wilson osteotomy in 10 of 31 feet; no internal fixation was utilized. This did not occur with the Hohmann, which was fixated with a Kirschner wire. They acknowledged that neither of the original authors utilized any fixation even though the osteotomies are inherently unstable. Pedobarographic analysis demonstrated increased loading of the lateral metatarsals following either of these osteotomies. Grace et al. also cautioned use of the Hohmann procedure in older patients with preexisting osteoarthritic findings as it was associated with degenerative changes postoperatively.

Winston and Wilson[25] performed a true trapezoidal

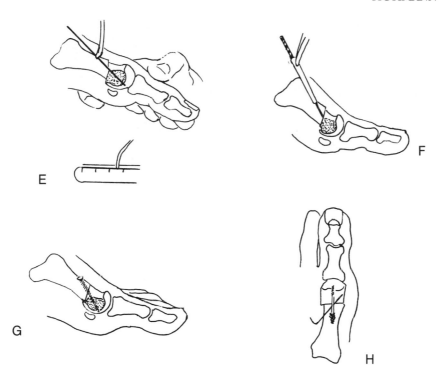

**Fig. 13-4** (*Continued*). (**E**) Depth measurement. (**F**) Tap. (**G**) Insertion of the 4.0-mm cancellous screw. (**H**) Removal of preliminary fixation; two-point fixation; resection of the medial prominence of first metatarsal; lavage, check of fixation, wound closure.

wedge Hohmann but cautioned on the amount of bone removal to minimize shortening. Their paper discussed surgical technique, and they admitted to good results in their 15 cases although no analysis was provided. They discussed divergent postoperative courses allowing immediate weight-bearing in a surgical shoe or a below-knee cast for 5 to 6 weeks with an initial non-weight-bearing period. No comparison of results or further details was given.

Warrick and Edelman[4] described an oblique elongated Hohmann as this would be more amenable to AO fixation and principles. In 11 patients (15 feet), they lagged a 3.5-mm cortical screw from medial proximal to lateral distal. They reported good results and maintenance of osseous position with screw fixation.

Tangen[26] recommended a modified technique of the Hohmann-Thompson osteotomy using a peg-and-hole plantar lateral and wire suture fixation. Tangen reported 97% good to excellent results on 177 patients (109 feet) with an average follow-up of 4 years.

Non-weight-bearing was instituted for the first 2 weeks followed by unrestricted walking in a cast shoe.

A similar type of modified osteotomy that was described by Rowe et al.[27] appeared much like a Roux-modified Mitchell. These authors reported long-term, complete relief of symptoms in all 20 patients (32 feet) postoperatively. The osteotomies were fixated with a Kirschner wire for 6 weeks and ambulation was limited to weight on the heel for the same period of time. Interestingly, with followup, these authors now recommend routine prophylactic osteotomy of the second and third metatarsals to prevent callosities postoperatively.

Excessive shortening may be a problem and a relative contraindication to the procedure would be a short first metatarsal, index minus of more than 4 mm. Our results from more than 150 procedures do show that lateral weight transfer may be an occasional problem, but that capsulitis/metatarsalgia is responsive to orthotic management and that a keratotic lesion is un-

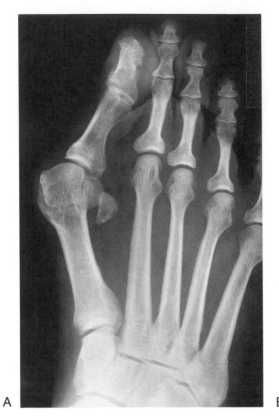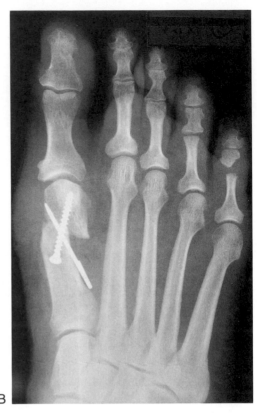

A    B

**Fig. 13-5.** Case of severe hallux valgus. (**A**) A 63-year-old woman with severe hallux valgus deformity. Components of the deformity include an elevated intermetatarsal angle, increased PASA, axial rotation of the hallux, tibial sesamoid position of 7, and a large hallux abductus angle with lateral joint subluxation. (**B**) Postoperative radiograph at 2 weeks illustrating reduction of deformity and restoration of a congruous joint space. Fixation was accomplished with a 3.5-mm fully threaded cancellous screw (1.75-mm pitch) with a 5-mm head and a 0.062-in. Kirschner wire used as a neutralization pin to protect the interfragmentary screw. (*Figure continues.*)

likely unless already present preoperatively or displacement occurs before clinical union. Judicious use of plantar transposition is the best cure for this problem. The modified Hohmann osteotomy has become a versatile procedure that allows correction for some very difficult types of deformities of the first metatarsophalangeal joint.

## DISCUSSION

The Hohmann osteotomy has continued to show its usefulness. This procedure fills a gap between distal osteotomy of the Austin or short Z variety and the closing-base wedge of the first metatarsal. When comparing the Hohmann and chevron-type distal metatarsal osteotomies,[28] the use of the Hohmann procedure has been reserved for the more severe deformity (see Fig. 13-5). Often these deformities require correction at more than one level; for example, joint subluxation, adaptation of the articular surface, or increased intermetatarsal angle.

In the more severe, long-standing hallux valgus deformities, an increase in the intermetatarsal angle is usually accompanied by lateral joint adaptation at the head. The Hohmann osteotomy has been useful in allowing correction of both segments of the deformity with a single osteotomy. Certainly there are limits, but the Hohmann has been effective in intermetatarsal an-

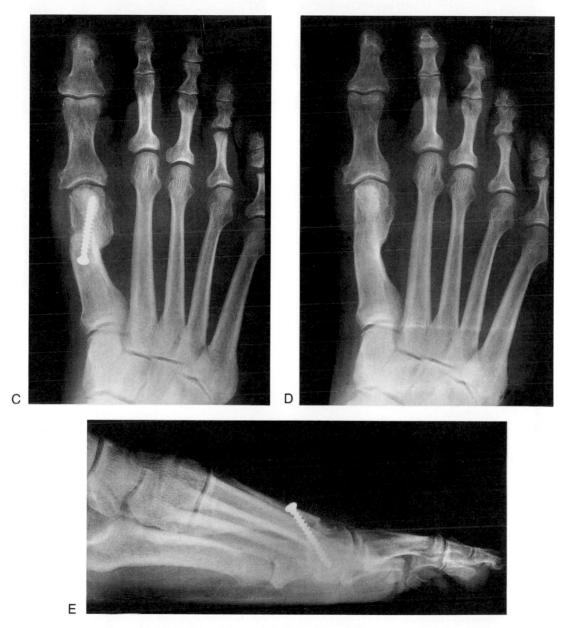

**Fig. 13-5** (*Continued*). Radiographs were taken (**C**) at 6 months and (**D**) 2 years postoperatively. The screw was removed at approximately 1 year postoperatively. Excellent range of motion was maintained throughout. Lateral radiograph (**E**) demonstrates proper placement of the interfragmentary screw. The screw can best prevent dorsal tilting and stabilize the capital fragment against ground reactive forces if the screw crosses the osteotomy in its plantar half and purchases the plantar portion of the metatarsal head.

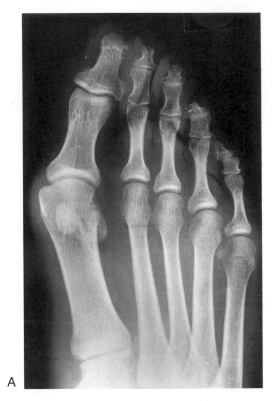
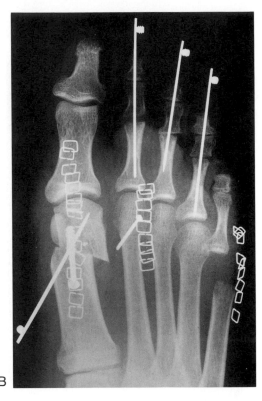

**Fig. 13-6.** Case of hallux valgus rigidus in a 40-year-old man. (**A**) The transverse plane deformity is not that significant but the patient has a limitation of motion and the entire forefoot possesses a certain rigidity. The long first metatarsal was shortened through lateral shift of an oblique osteotomy. Postoperative radiographs (**B**) at 2 weeks. (*Figure continues.*)

gles upwards of 18 to 19 degrees, depending on the flexibility of the forefoot. The Hohmann offers correction of the frontal plane bunion deformity, that of hallucal axial rotation. Not only is the cosmetic appearance of the toe restored but the procedure also provides for a return of sagittal plane motion. This is unique in hallux valgus procedures, and it certainly fills a void when the indications present.

Decompression is usually accomplished by shortening of the osseous segment, thereby widening or increasing the adjacent joint space. Such techniques are useful to provide a restoration of normal joint motion or at least to attempt to maintain a reasonable joint excursion. Joint decompression is a useful adjunct in correcting severe transverse plane abnormalities associated with hallux valgus, recurrent hallux valgus deformities with limited joint motion, or cases of hallux valgus rigidus (Fig. 13-6).

The Hohmann also has been effective in the rigid foot type of deformity. The deformity might not be that severe, but soft tissue releases are inadequate to allow freedom of joint excursion and correction of the deformity. These are feet that are probably best described by the European label of hallux valgus rigidus in which aspects of both pathologies coexist. The Hohmann osteotomy is an excellent technique to provide for joint decompression of the first metatarsophalangeal joint. The Hohmann provides joint relaxation, probably as a result of some shortening, but allows repositioning of the hallucal proximal phalanx on the metatarsal head and joint movement. Actually, it is this finding that lead to the use of the Hohmann in cases of metatarsus adductus where the deformity may not be that impressive but attaining correction and maintaining the great toe in a good position may be difficult.

The form of fixation most often utilized has been a

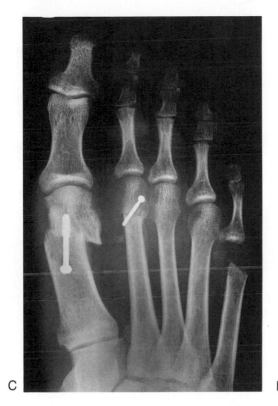
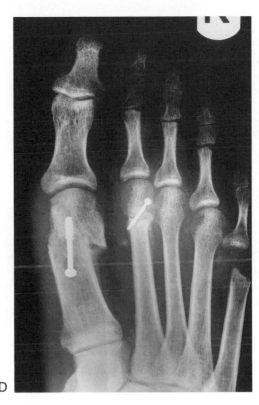

**Fig. 13-6** (*Continued*). Postoperative radiographs at (**C**) 6 weeks and (**D**) 3 months. The postoperative radiographs reveal maintenance of position with gradual filling-in of lateral overhang by displacement of the capital fragment. Only with rigid internal fixation can patients such as this immediately begin range of motion and, as the surgery was intended, to restore or improve the available motion.

4.0-mm, partially threaded, cancellous screw. This screw is placed in a dorsal-proximal to plantar-distal direction. The screw should cross the osteotomy in the plantar half (Fig. 13-7). In this manner, the screw orientation provides an optimal vector of mechanical stability opposing any ground reactive forces that would tend to cause either dorsal displacement of the entire head or simply a dorsal tilt. A medial to lateral orientation of the screw also in the proximal to lateral direction does allow perforation of the lateral cortex for purchase of the screw but at the expense of limiting adequate resection of the medial aspect of the first metatarsal shaft. This medial to lateral screw placement also offers less mechanical stability to ground reactive forces that tend to displace the osteotomy.

A second point of fixation is always recommended, which has usually been an obliquely placed, 0.062-in. Kirschner wire. This may be placed from dorsolateral proximal and to plantar-medial and distal, piercing the medioplantar cortex. An alternative technique pierces the articular surface dorsolateral; the wire is then driven out the medial side of the first metatarsal shaft. The wire may then be retrograded medially until the tip underlies the articular surface. I have also utilized Orthosorb as a secondary point of fixation, but overall my impression is that the Orthosorb provides little if any contribution to the stability of the osteosynthesis.

Regardless how stable the osteosynthesis appears, it is still recommended to limit weight-bearing through the limb and operated foot. Early weight-bearing has resulted in loss of fixation, dorsal tilt of the capital fragment, pathologic fracture of the dorsal cortex, and prolonged morbidity or reoperation from osseous displacement or nonunion. Part of the discontent with this and similar procedures results from the complications of osteotomy displacement and mal-

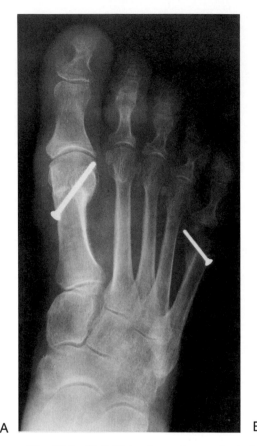

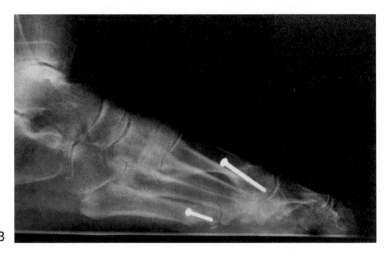

A

B

**Fig. 13-7.** (**A & B**) An alternative method of fixation is placement of the screw in a medial to lateral direction with purchase of the lateral cortex. Commonly a 2.7-mm cortex screw such as this is used. The problem with this technique is the head of the screw may impede resection of the medial shaft of the metatarsal after transposition and fixation of the osteotomy. This is a concern because the patient is usually presenting with an unsightly medial bump. Note the sagittal plane position of the screw; it is unlikely to withstand much loading, and adequate external immobilization is recommended. Results of this case actually are quite acceptable, mainly as a result of the negligible lateral shift of the capital fragment. (Case courtesy of Robert G. O'Keefe, Chicago.)

union. Careful attention to the osteosynthesis and adherence to the prescribed postoperative course minimizes their occurrence.

A definite consideration for the performance of this osteotomy is an adequate bone density to allow some type of fixation. Union is fairly predictable so long as the stability of the fixation is maintained during the postoperative period. Even the postmenopausal female with some degree of osteopenia is capable of undergoing this osteotomy, but control of the postoperative weight-bearing is essential. Experience with the Hohmann-type procedures verifies both the favor-

able comments as well as the difficulties or complications that may ensue. Iatrogenic metatarsus primus elevatus is a complication of nonfixated or poorly fixated first metatarsal osteotomies. Rigid fixation is probably the major contribution to the recent success of this procedure.

This osteotomy is powerful in its ability to correct deformity particularly when combined with joint decompression (shortening), fibular sesamoidectomy, and adductor transfer/medial capsulorrhaphy. Caution is suggested, as hallux varus has occurred with overzealous capsule-tendon balancing techniques. The

Hohmann osteotomy has continued to show its usefulness during the past 12 years. It is particularly valuable for more severe bunions wherein correction at more than one level of deformity is desirable.

## SUMMARY AND CONCLUSIONS

Osteotomy for hallux valgus and hallux valgus rigidus in the 1990s involves sophisticated multicut osteotomies, and usually a secure osteosynthesis to preserve the correction obtained through osteotomy as well as to encourage a successful and timely period of osseous healing.

The Hohmann osteotomy as performed today is really a hybrid of several of the distal first metatarsal osteotomies. The thought processes and techniques of its application reflect the potential usefulness of the procedure. Hohmann recognized the potential to address deformity on more than one cardinal body plane although most procedures were attempts to correct only one aspect of the deformity. Kelikian called the Hohmann procedure a dual-plane displacement osteotomy, as Hohmann described both lateral and plantar displacement; in addition, however, a medially based trapezoidal wedge allowed for reduction of hallucal abduction and the reduction of metatarsus primus varus through lateral shift or elevatus as a result of plantar shift of the capital fragment.

The modified Hohmann osteotomy has become a versatile procedure that has allowed correction for some very difficult types of deformities of the first metatarsophalangeal joint. The host of variations possible has allowed this procedure to correct hallux valgus and hallux valgus rigidus with a good amount of success.

## REFERENCES

1. Vanore JV, Bidny MA: Internal fixation in the correction of hallux valgus. In Scurran B (ed): Manual of Hallux Valgus. Churchill Livingstone, New York (in press)
2. Funk JF, Wells RE: Bunionectomy with distal osteotomy. Clin Orthop 85:71, 1972
3. Zygmunt KH, Gudas CJ, Laros GS: Z Bunionectomy with internal fixation. J Am Podiatr Med Assoc 79:322, 1989
4. Warrick JP, Edelman R: The Hohmann bunionectomy utilizing AO screw fixation: a preliminary report. J Foot Surg 23:268, 1984
5. Hohmann G: Symptomatische oder physiologische Behandlung des hallux valgus. Muench Med Wochenschr 33:1042, 1922
6. Hohmann G: Uber ein Verfahen zur Behandlung des spreizfuss. Zbl Chir 49:1933, 1922
7. Hohmann G: Uber hallux und spreizfuss, ihre entstehung und physiologische Behandlung. Arch Arthop Unfall-Chir 21:525, 1923
8. Hohmann G: Zur hallux valgus-operation. Zentralb Chir 51:230, 1924
9. Hohmann G: Der hallux valgus und die uebrigen Zehenverkruemmungen. Ergeb Chir Orthop 18:308, 1925
10. Hohmann G: Fuss und Bein, p. 145. JF Bergmann, Munich, 1951
11. Jenkin WM, Todd WF: Osteotomies of the first metatarsal head: Reverdin modifications, Hohmann, Hohmann modifications, p. 223. In Gerbert J (ed): Textbook of Bunion Surgery, 2nd Ed. Futura Publishing, Mount Kisco, NY, 1991
12. Mitchell CL, Fleming JL, Allen R, Glenney C, Sanford GA: Osteotomy-bunionectomy for hallux valgus. J Bone Joint Surg 40A:41, 1958
13. Kelikian H: Osteotomy, p. 163. In Hallux Valgus and Allied Deformities of the Foot and Metatarsalgia. WB Saunders, Philadelphia, 1965
14. Turnbull T, Grange W: A comparison of Keller's arthroplasty and distal metatarsal osteotomy in the treatment of adult hallux valgus. J Bone Joint Surg 68B:132, 1986
15. Peabody CW: Surgical cure of hallux valgus. J Bone Joint Surg 13:273, 1931
16. Wilson JN: Oblique displacement osteotomy for hallux valgus. J Bone Joint Surg 45B:552, 1963
17. Barker AE: An operation for hallux valgus. Lancet i:655, 1884
18. Grace D, Hughes J, Klencrman L: A comparison of Wilson and Hohmann osteotomies in the treatment of hallux valgus. J Bone Joint Surg 70B:236, 1988
19. Holstein A, Lewis GB: Experience with Wilson's oblique displacement osteotomy for hallux valgus, p. 223. In Bateman JE, Trott AW (eds): The Foot and Ankle. Brian C Decker, New York, 1980
20. Vanore JV: Capital osteotomies for hallux valgus. First Ray 10:9, 1983 (publication of the Illinois Podiatric Medical Students Association)
21. Ruch JA, Merrill TJ, Banks AS: First ray hallux abducto valgus and related deformities, Part 1, p 133. In McGlamry ED (ed): Comprehensive Textbook of Foot Surgery. Williams & Wilkins, Baltimore, 1987
22. Zlotoff H: Shortening of the first metatarsal following

osteotomy and its clinical significance. J Am Podiatry Assoc 67:412, 1977

23. Jahss MH, Troy AI, Kummer F: Roentgenographic and mathematical analysis of first metatarsal osteotomies for metatarsus primus varus: a comparative study. Foot Ankle 5:280, 1985

24. Johnson JB, Smith SD: Preliminary report on derotational, angulational, transpositional osteotomy: a new approach to hallux valgus surgery. J Am Podiatry Assoc 74:667, 1974

25. Winston L, Wilson RC: A modification of the Hohmann procedure for surgical correction of hallux abducto valgus. J Am Podiatry Assoc 72:11, 1982

26. Tangen O: Hallux valgus, the treatment by distal wedge osteotomy of the 1st metatarsal (Hohmann-Thomasen). Acta Chir Scand 137:151, 1971

27. Rowe PH, Coutinho J, Fearn BD: Fixation of Hohmann's osteotomy for hallux valgus. Acta Orthop Scand 56:419, 1985

28. Pring DJ, Coombes RRH, Closok JK: Chevron or Wilson osteotomy: a comparison and follow-up. J Bone Joint Surg Br 67:071, 1985

# 14

# Mitchell Bunionectomy

*ALLAN M. BOIKE*
*JOHN M. WHITE*

The Mitchell operation for hallux valgus was first described in the literature in 1945 by Hawkins and associates.[1] Mygind, in 1952, described a similar procedure.[2] C. Leslie Mitchell subsequently published an article in 1958 describing this procedure, and from this point on it became known as the Mitchell bunionectomy. Mitchell's original description of this procedure included an osteotomy of the distal portion of the first metatarsal, lateral displacement and angulation of the head of the metatarsal, and exostectomy and capsulorrhaphy.[3]

The following is a description of the operative technique as it appeared in 1958. A dorsal medial incision is made on the foot, curving above the bursa and callus. A Y-shaped incision is made through the medial capsule and periosteum of the first metatarsal. The arms of the Y should meet $\frac{1}{4}$ in. proximal to the metatarsophalangeal joint. If the arms of the Y extend too far proximally, insufficient tissue is left to obtain secure medial capsulorrhaphy.

The neck and shaft of the metatarsal are then stripped subperiosteally. The lateral capsular attachments are not disturbed, because these structures are the only remaining source of blood supply to the metatarsal head. The exostosis is removed flush with the shaft of the metatarsal.

Two holes are drilled, one being $\frac{1}{2}$ in. and the other 1 in. from the articular surface. The distal drill hole is slightly medial so the holes will be in line when the lateral shift of the head is accomplished. Care is taken to place these holes perpendicular to the metatarsal shaft. A #1 chromic catgut suture is placed through the holes by means of a ligature carrier or straight needle.

A double incomplete osteotomy is then done $\frac{3}{4}$ in. from the articular surface between the drill holes and perpendicular to the shaft. The thickness of the bone between the two cuts is dependent on the amount of shortening of the metatarsal that will be necessary to relax the contracted lateral structures. About 2–3 mm ($\frac{1}{8}$ in.) of bone is usually removed. The size of the lateral spur depends on the amount of metatarsus primus varus to be neutralized by the lateral shift of the metatarsal head. In a moderate deformity, one-sixth of the width of the shaft is left to form the lateral spur, while in severe deformity one-third of the shaft remains. The osteotomy is completed proximally with a thin sawblade (Fig. 14-1).

The metatarsal head is shifted laterally until the lateral spur locks over the proximal shaft. Lateral angulation of the head is slight so the articular surface parallels the axis of the second metatarsal. Slight plantar displacement or angulation is desirable. At this stage, the suture is tied, giving surprising stability to the osteotomy site. Medial capsulorrhaphy is carried out with the hallux held in slight overcorrection. Chromic 00 is commonly used for capsular repair.

Splints made of padded tongue depressors are applied with the toe in slight overcorrection and with 5° of plantar flexion, to avoid displacement or angulation at the osteotomy site. Splints are worn for 10 days, and after suture removal a short walking cast is applied to the leg, encompassing the great toe.[3]

With the exception of a few changes in the execution of the Mitchell, the procedure has not changed over the years from the technique just described. In many of the studies performed since 1958, the operation was performed exactly as described by Mitchell.[4,5]

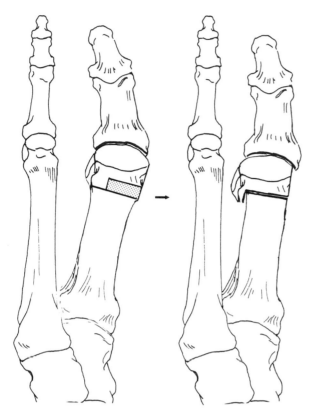

**Fig. 14-1.** Diagrammatic representation of Mitchell osteotomy.

As late as 1987, suture material was still being used for fixation as it is today.[6]

The Mitchell osteotomy has proven itself as originally described; advancement in surgical techniques and fixation methods have given it a stable place in a surgeon's armamentarium for the correction of hallux valgus deformity.

## SURGICAL TECHNIQUE

The dissection of the first metatarsophalangeal joint in light of anatomic dissection for hallux abducto valgus deformity is basically the same for most procedures performed. We recommend a lateral release to mobilize the sesamoid apparatus before the lateral shift of the capital fragment. We have not found avascular necrosis, a complication that was alluded to by Mitchell and Meier. As a matter of fact, avascular necrosis is a rare event with the Mitchell procedure.[4-8] Correction

via medial capsulorrhaphy may be achieved by the surgeon's preferred capsulorrhaphy technique.

Depending on the amount of shortening of the first metatarsal desired by the surgeon, fail-safe holes can be drilled using 2-mm, 3-mm, or 4-mm burrs. This eliminates the guesswork about how much shortening will result (Fig. 14-2).

Fixation with Chromic 00, which was described by Mitchell and others, should be replaced with more rigid forms of internal fixation. Reports in the literature and our experience is that better results are achieved with rigid fixation.[9,10]

The medial eminence, which is usually resected before lateral displacement in most osteotomies on the first metatarsal, should be minimal to nonexistent with this procedure. This will ensure that there is adequate bone-to-bone surface contact to provide enough reduction of the deformity.

Because of the rigidity acquired with internal fixation coupled with accurate capsulorrhaphy, the splint described by Mitchell can be substituted. Ideally, non-weight-bearing is the best suggested method for bone healing. We find that a modification of a surgical shoe to decrease weight-bearing of the first metatarsophalangeal joint complex is adequate for good healing and sagittal plane stability of the osteotomy.

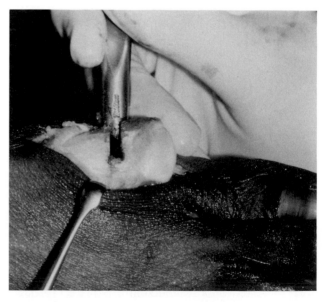

**Fig. 14-2.** Intraoperative view of the osteotomy before completion of the proximal cut. The fail-safe hole is apparent.

## FIXATION

The method of fixation, as described by Mitchell and others utilizing suture material, although reported to have adequate results seems to lend itself to potential complications. The most serious complication is dorsal displacement of the capital fragment after fixation is in place. This may lead to lesser metatarsalgia, lesser metatarsal lesions, and hallux limitus or rigidus.

With the advances in fixation devices available to the surgeon over the years since the Mitchell procedure was first described, better and more sound fixation principles are available that will yield better results. The cross-Kirshner wire (K-wire) technique is one of the more frequently used fixation methods. By having two references of fixation, the likelihood of dorsal displacement of capital fragment is greatly decreased.

For the surgeon with more expertise, the Herbert bone screw provides an excellent type of fixation that ensures stability. This is currently the method of fixation being used by the authors, along with the crossed K-wire technique. Both of these provide rigid internal stability, decreasing the chance of movement of the metatarsal head postoperatively while at the same time allowing early joint range of motion to prevent joint stiffness. Another alternative is insertion of a screw using the A-O guide lines. It is the recommendation of this author and others that all osteotomies be secured with some form of internal fixation because of the instability of the Mitchell procedure when relying on the lateral spicule, soft tissue, and splinting techniques to maintain correction.[9]

## INDICATIONS

The indications for the use of the Mitchell rather than another type of osteotomy or procedure are based mostly on specific radiographic criteria. As is the case for most bunion procedures, pain, aesthetic dissatisfaction, and difficulty in fitting proper shoes are the most probable causes bringing the patient to the foot surgeon. Pain has been indicated as the most dominant presenting factor in which a Mitchell osteotomy was performed.[3,8,11–13]

Radiographically, the selection of the Mitchell procedure has specific guidelines that must be met for a successful outcome. Five basic features must be addressed when considering this procedure: hallux ab-

ductus angle, proximal articular set angle (PASA), intermetatarsal angle (IMA) between the first and second metatarsals, the relative length of the first metatarsal, and the amount of metatarsus primus elevatus. Other factors such as quantity of bone stock, osteoarthritis, width of the metatarsal head, tibial sesamoid position, and metatarsus adductus must also be considered, although the previously mentioned factors will eventually allow one to select or rule out the use of the Mitchell osteotomy.

### Hallux Abductus Angle

The upper limits of the hallux abductus angle (HAA) in which a good result can be obtained have been consistent, being somewhere in the 30° ± 5° range.[6,14] Similarly, angles greater than 40° have been reported to be associated with poor results.[14,15] The average amount of correction of hallux abductus with the Mitchell osteotomy is dependent on the surgeon performing the operation. Averages of correction have been stated in the literature, but they have appeared very sporadically.[5,6,11–13] The most likely cause of failure of success in reduction of the HAA is the inadequate amount of soft tissue rebalancing performed around the first metatarsophalangeal joint. From our experience, all hallux abductus deformities can be brought into the normal range of 10°–15° when the Mitchell is utilized with soft tissue correction techniques such as a modified McBride procedure, provided the intermetatarsal angle (IMA) is not excessive.

### Proximal Articular Set Angle

When performing the Mitchell procedure as described in his original article, it is important that the PASA be within normal range. This matter will be discussed further in the modifications section.

### Intermetatarsal Angle Between the First and Second Metatarsal

Unlike the HAA, there is some controversy as to how high an IMA can be to provide a good result with the Mitchell. It is suggested that the maximum angular relationship be 15°.[5,12,15] Some authors advocate the use of the Mitchell in IMA as high as 20°, but in our experience this is too great an angle to provide enough lateral displacement of the capital fragment to reduce the IMA to within normal range. The width of the metatarsal head is directly proportional to the amount of correction that can be achieved, so it is feasible that some IMAs greater than 15° can be corrected with this procedure. We find a basal osteotomy to be more appropriate with these greater IMAs.

## Length of the First Metatarsal

The length of the first metatarsal is a very important criteria that must be evaluated carefully. It is obvious that the Mitchell bunionectomy is a shortening osteotomy, providing on the average approximately 4.9 mm of shortening.[6] Although Mitchell found no correlation between the amount of shortening and second metatarsalgia, since his report other authors have noted this as being a problem[16]; more than 7 mm of shortening appears to yield poor results.[3,4] Mitchell and associates were reassured by the Harris and Beath[17] study, which concluded that a "short first metatarsal seldom, if ever, is the cause of foot disability." A closer reading of their data, however, shows that only 4 percent had a first metatarsal that was 5 mm or more shorter than the second. It is logical then to conclude that if a first metatarsal is short preoperatively, the amount of shortening acquired postoperatively will result in a difference between the two metatarsals that can be several millimeters beyond the normal range. This in turn correlates with the poor results reported in the literature.[3,4]

## Metatarsus Primus Elevatus

When metatarsus primus elevatus is present, the first metatarsal is not bearing the weight it should during the propulsive phase of gait. This results in a dumping effect onto the second metatarsal. Assessing this is important so that when the lateral displacement is performed, some plantar displacement can be incorporated to allow the first metatarsal to bear weight. Also, to compensate for the inherent shortening of the osteotomy, plantar displacement is required to prevent an iatrogenic metatarsus primus elevatus, which could cause metatarsalgia of the lesser metatarsals.

## CONTRAINDICATIONS

Most contraindications for the Mitchell osteotomy fall into the same category as do contradictions for other joint preservation procedures: degenerative joint disease, inadequate bone stock, and any other general contraindications to surgery must be elevated.

Specific to the Mitchell bunionectomy, these contraindications are mostly radiographic entities. HAAs greater than 40° are considered to produce a poor result, as was mentioned. A PASA greater than the normal limits combined with a Mitchell osteotomy will produce a joint that is not likely to have a normal range of motion or an incongruous joint that can result in degenerative joint or recurrence of the hallux valgus deformity. The IMA between the first and second metatarsal should be 15° or less. The most important contraindication is a short first metatarsal, that is, one that is more than 5 mm shorter than the second metatarsal.[6,17] We prefer that the final outcome be such that the length of the first metatarsal is between that of the second and third metatarsal.

Another contraindication mentioned in the literature is that of age. Some authors recommend not performing the Mitchell procedure after a certain age.[9,15] They mention problems in healing as a complication. Perhaps what should be considered, however, is the physiologic versus the chronologic age of each patient.

## MODIFICATION

When considering a modification of the Mitchell osteotomy, the eponym Roux osteotomy is often mentioned as this modification. This modification takes into account the PASA or deviation of the effective articular cartilage in relationship to the long axis of the first metatarsal. The standard Mitchell osteotomy does not address this problem.

The difference between the two osteotomies is the manner in which the first or distal cut is performed. The Mitchell cut is performed perpendicular to the shaft of the metatarsal, which would make it parallel with the articular cartilage assuming the PASA is within normal limits. With the Roux, this bone cut is not perpendicular to the shaft of the metatarsal but remains parallel to the articular surface. When the remaining

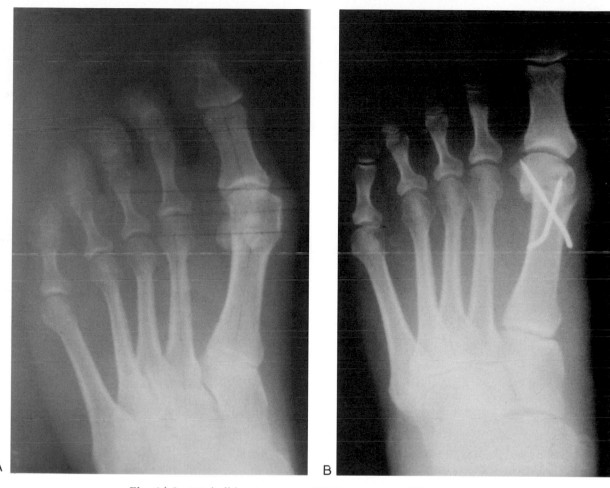

**Fig. 14-3.** Mitchell bunionectomy. (**A**) Preoperative; (**B**) postoperative.

cuts are performed and the wedge of bone is removed, the increased PASA will return to normal range because of the inherent design of the cuts. The remaining stages of the operation are unchanged from the Mitchell: dissection, fixation, and closure.

The indications for the Roux are the same as for the Mitchell except for the additional criterion of a PASA greater than 10°. The contraindications are also the same with the exception of having a normal PASA.

The osteotomy was originally proposed by Roux[18] in 1920 in his original article. According to research, the Roux osteotomy appears to be a modification of Reverdin's original operation rather than a modification of the Mitchell osteotomy.[1,19] Mitchell's original

article was published some 25 years after Roux's publication.

## SUMMARY AND CONCLUSIONS

The Mitchell bunionectomy is one of many distal metaphyseal osteotomies for the correction of the moderate hallux valgus deformity with or without mild hallux limitus. The procedure has proven successful in individuals in whom a long first metatarsal bone is confirmed radiographically. The procedure has clear advantages over the Austin type of osteotomy in situations in which shortening of the first metatarsal is clearly desired. When it is performed properly, a favorable outcome can be expected with minimal complications. Accurate surgical technique with appropriate fixation is most important to ensure a successful outcome. It is our opinion that this procedure, although not commonly indicated, has a place in the armamentarium of foot surgeons (Fig. 14-3).

# REFERENCES

1. Hawkins HB, Mitchell CL, Hedrick DW: Correction of hallux valgus by metatarsal osteotomy. J Bone Joint Surg 27:387, 1946
2. Mygind H: Operations for hallux valgus. J Bone Joint Surg 34B:529, 1952
3. Mitchell CL, Fleming JL, Allen R, Glenney C, Sanford GA: Osteotomy-bunionectomy for hallux valgus. J Bone Joint Surg 40A:41, 1958
4. Carr CR, Boyd BM: Correctional osteotomy for metatarsus primus varus and hallux valgus. J Bone Joint Surg 50A:1353, 1968
5. Glynn MK, Dunlop JB, Fitzpatrick D: The Mitchell distal metatarsal osteotomy for hallux valgus. J Bone Joint Surg 62B:188, 1980
6. Wu KK: Mitchell bunionectomy: an analysis of 430 personal cases plus a review of the literature. Foot Ankle 26:277, 1987
7. Miller JW: Distal first metatarsal displacement osteotomy. J Bone Joint Surg 56A:923, 1974
8. Shapiro G, Heller L: The Mitchell distal metatarsal osteotomy in the treatment of hallux valgus. Clin Orthop 107:225, 1975
9. Broughton NS, Winson IG: Keller's arthroplasty and Mitchell osteotomy: a comparison with first metatarsal osteotomy of the long-term results for hallux valgus deformity in the female. Foot Ankle 10:201, 1990
10. Gibson MM, Corn D, Debevoise NT, Mess CF: Complications of Mitchell bunionplasties with modification of indications and technique (by invitation). Washington, DC.
11. Kinnard P, Gordon D: A comparison between Chevron and Mitchell osteotomies for hallux valgus. Foot Ankle 4:241, 1984
12. Meier PJ, Kenzora JE: The risks and benefits of first metatarsal osteotomies. Foot Ankle 6:7, 1985
13. Vittas D, Jansen EC, Larsen TK: Gait analysis before and after osteotomy for hallux valgus. Foot Ankle 8:134, 1989
14. Mann RA: The great toe. Orthop Clin North Am 20:519, 1989
15. Das De S, Kamblen DL: Distal metatarsal osteotomy for hallux valgus in the middle-aged patient. Clin Orthop 216:239, 1987
16. Merkel KD, Katoh Y, Johnson EW, Chao EY: Mitchell osteotomy for hallux valgus: long-term follow-up and gait analysis. Foot Ankle 3:189, 1983
17. Harris RI, Beath T: The short first metatarsal: its incidence and clinical significance. J Bone Joint Surg 31A:553, 1945
18. Roux C: Aux pieds sensibles. Rev Med Suisse Romande 40:62, 1920
19. Reverdin J: De la deviation en dehors du gros orteil (hallux valgus, vulg. "oignon bunions"), et de son traitement chirurgical. Trans Int Med Congr 2:408, 1881

# 15

# Reverdin Procedure and Its Modifications

*WILLIAM F. TODD*
*RANDALL K. TOM*

The Reverdin osteotomy was first described for use in the hallux abducto valgus deformity by J.L. Reverdin in 1881. It was originally described as a procedure in which, after removal of a medial eminence, a wedge-shaped portion of bone was resected proximal to the articular surface of the head of the first metatarsal. This procedure results in correction of the proximal articular set angle as well as reduction of the prominent bunion deformity.[1] Since Reverdin's original description, several modifications have been made to the original procedure. All the modifications are designed to effect structural correction of the hallux abducto valgus deformity occurring at the first metatarsal head level.

The Reverdin procedure is indicated for a mild to moderate hallux abducto valgus deformity in which the primary pathology is a lateral shift of the articular facet of the first metatarsal head. Physical examination will reveal a stable metatarsocuneiform joint that may shift into metarsus primus varus as the valgus deviation of the hallux occurs. The resulting first metatarsophalangeal joint reveals a hallux valgus deformity with an enlarged medial eminence, an adapted joint, and lateral deviation of the articular cartilage in response to the new angle of function of the hallux. A congruous to slightly deviated freely movable joint with pain-free range of motion should be present on examination[2] (Fig. 15-1). Additional indications include an increased hallux abductus angle with an increased proximal articular set angle (PASA). A valgus rotation or sagittal plane deformity of the first metatarsal head

may also be present. Additional radiographic criteria for performing the Reverdin procedure include adequate bone density and a normal metatarsus primus adductus angle, because no transposition of the capital fragment will occur. A normal to increased metatarsal protrusion distance should be present, as each of the osteotomy cuts will remove a 1-mm portion of bone. This shortening must be taken into account when determining the size of bone wedge to be resected.[3]

The Reverdin procedure is ideally performed on patients less than 60 to 70 years of age *depending on bone structure and quality*. The procedure may be performed on older patients if adequate bone stock is present and their activity level warrants doing the procedure. The age of the patient is also important because the first metatarsal sesamoid articulation of the younger patient adapts more quickly and completely to the new position of the head of the metatarsal and the sesamoid. This may reduce further degeneration of the metatarsal sesamoid articulation if present.[4] Preoperative templates should be made to ascertain the amount of correction desired. This allows for a more accurate evaluation of the results and decreases the chance of error.[5] An alternate method is to create a distal osteotomy parallel to the articular surface of the first metatarsal head and a proximal cut perpendicular to the long axis of the first metatarsal shaft.[6]

A standard approach to the first metarsophalangeal joint is utilized with a dorsolinear skin incision and a linear or inverted L-shaped capsulotomy to expose the joint. The first metatarsal head is freed from the

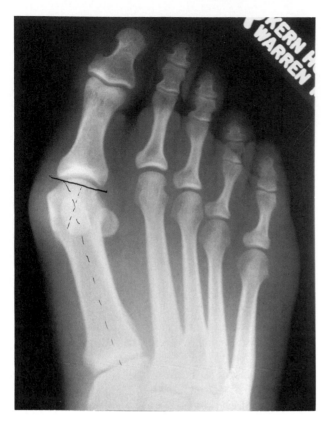

**Fig. 15-1.** Radiograph of bunion deformity with an increased proximal articular set angle and an adapted joint.

surrounding capsular and ligamentous structures and delivered medially through the wound site. The medial eminence is then resected. Release of the conjoined adductor tendon and a lateral capsulotomy are performed along with a tenotomy of the extensor digitorum brevis tendon if contracture is present. A fibular sesamoidectomy may also be performed at this time if significant deviation or degeneration is noted.

A sagittal saw is utilized to make two transverse cuts in the first metatarsal head to allow for removal of a predetermined wedge of bone, leaving the lateral cortex intact. The first osteotomy is created 1 cm proximal to the articular surface of the first metatarsal head. This osteotomy must be parallel to the articular surface to ensure adequate reduction of the PASA. The second osteotomy is performed proximal to the first osteotomy to allow for removal of a predetermined wedge of bone with the base medial and apex lateral. The

lateral cortex is left intact to provide a cortical hinge to stabilize the osteotomy.

The bone wedge is removed and the osteotomy closed, reducing the PASA. The joint is reevaluated to confirm that an adequate wedge has been removed. A significant reduction in the PASA will be noted, with increased joint congruity. This procedure does not require fixation because of the stability provided by the lateral cortex and the retrograde force of the hallux on weight-bearing (Fig. 15-2).

Ambulation is permitted on the first postoperative day in a postoperative shoe as tolerated with crutch assistance. The patient is instructed to avoid prolonged periods of dependency, which can lead to increased edema.

The dressings are changed at weekly intervals with suture removal at 10 to 14 days. The dressings serve to splint the toe in the corrected position to maintain reduction of the hallux abductus deformity. Postoperative radiographs are taken at 2 and 4 weeks to evaluate alignment and healing of the osteotomy site. Physical therapy, consisting of active and passive range-of-motion exercises, is utilized starting at 1 week postoperatively to increase the range of motion and to prevent fibrosis of the joint.

The postoperative shoe is worn for approximately 3 to 4 weeks, at which time the patient is allowed to wear shoes having a wide roomy forefoot. Once the swelling has decreased postoperatively, the patient is casted for orthoses to reduce any abnormal pronatory forces.

The greatest advantage to performing the Reverdin procedure is reduction of the PASA, allowing realignment of the joint. The osteotomy is stable because of its distal placement along with compression from weight-bearing forces. Rapid healing occurs because the osteotomy is placed in metaphyseal bone. Additionally, the procedure may be performed in the presence of uncontrollable pronatory forces and thus allows for increased joint range of motion from shortening of the metatarsal. The shortening results in a decrease in cubic content of the joint that provides increased range of motion. This procedure can also be performed on children before epiphyseal closure because the placement of the osteotomy is distal to the epiphysis.

The disadvantages and complications to performing the Reverdin procedure may include under- or over-

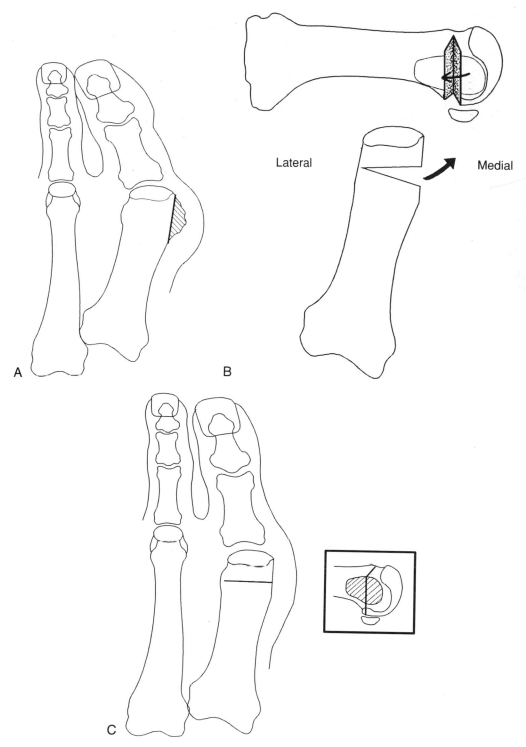

Lateral

Medial

A

B

C

**Fig. 15-2.** Reverdin procedure. (**A**) Portion of the medial eminence to be resected. (**B**) Demonstration of bone wedge removal to allow for PASA correction. (**C**) Completed osteotomy with reduction of the hallux and realignment of the first metatarsophalangeal joint.

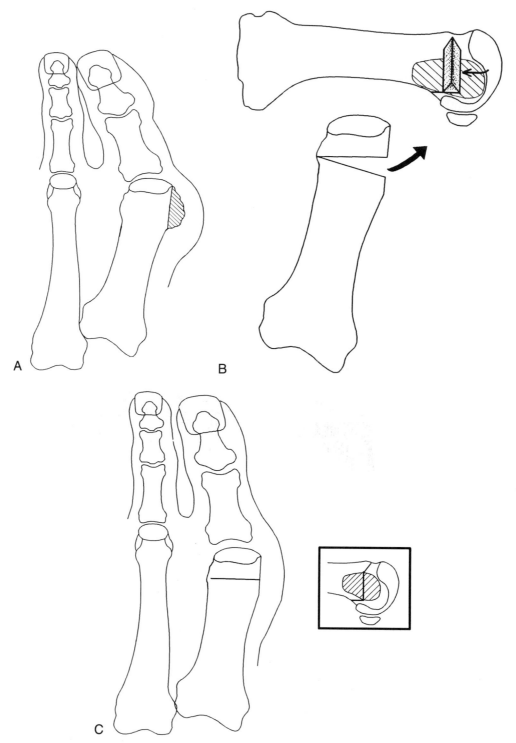

**Fig. 15-3.** Reverdin–Green procedure. (**A**) Portion of the medial eminence to be resected. (**B**) Wedge resection and plantar transverse Green osteotomy. (**C**) First metatarsal after reduction of the osteotomy.

correction caused by inadequate or overaggressive wedge resection, limitus from joint incongruity created by the correction, hallux varus deformity, and disruption of the metatarsal sesamoid articulation resulting in joint limitus and arthritis. As no transposition of the capital fragment occurs, reduction of the intermetatarsal angle or of sagittal plane deformities cannot be addressed. Dislocation of the osteotomy may occur if the lateral cortex is fractured or osteotomized. Nonunion and aseptic necrosis rarely occur, because the osteotomies are created in highly vascular metaphyseal bone while maintaining the lateral cortex and soft tissue structures.

The Reverdin–Green procedure was described by D.R. Green in 1977. The original Reverdin procedure is modified by performing an additional osteotomy designed to prevent disruption of the first metatarsal sesamoid articulation.[4] This osteotomy is created parallel to the plantar weight-bearing surface of the first metatarsal, 1 cm proximal to the articular surface and superior to the plantar aspect of the first metatarsal head. The osteotomy is a through-and-through cut

made from medial to lateral, exiting proximally through the metatarsal neck. The subsequent cuts are made as described for the original Reverdin procedure, extending plantarly to the level of the initial osteotomy (Fig. 15-3).

The indications for the Reverdin–Green procedure are the same as those for the Reverdin procedure. The advantages are as listed for the Reverdin procedure with the additional advantage of preventing the disruption of the metatarsal sesamoid articulation. The disadvantages include the potential for adherence of the flexor plate to the plantar metatarsal neck in the region of the plantar osteotomy, which may result in a limitus deformity. Postoperative care is identical to that listed for the Reverdin procedure.

The Reverdin–Laird procedure, developed by P. Laird in 1977, is a modification of the Reverdin–Green procedure that involves transecting the lateral cortex with the dorsal cuts, allowing lateral transposition of the capital fragment. This procedure allows for reduction of an increased intermetatarsal angle in addition to reduction of the PASA.[4]

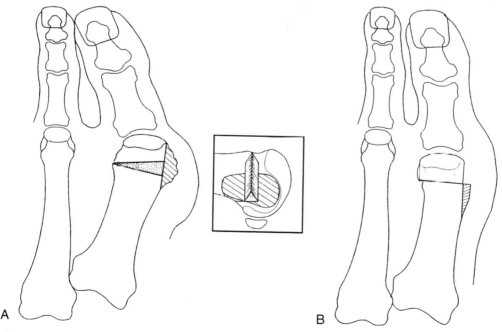

**Fig. 15-4.** Reverdin–Laird procedure. (**A**) Demonstration of eminence resection and wedge removal. The inset shows plantar Green osteotomy. (**B**) Transposed capital fragment before fixation. The remainder of the prominent metatarsal shaft is resected.

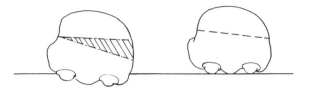

**Fig. 15-5.** Modification for correction of hallux valgus rotation. Wedge removal medially allows for reduction of valgus rotation. (Adapted from Laird et al.,[7] with permission.)

The indications for the Reverdin–Laird procedure include the previously listed indications for the Reverdin procedure. An additional indication is an increased intermetatarsal angle, which may be addressed through transposition of the capital fragment.

The Reverdin–Laird procedure involves exposure and soft tissue releases identical to those performed for the Reverdin procedure. The medial eminence is resected and the plantar osteotomy cut is created from medial to lateral. The dorsal osteotomy cuts are created initially, leaving the lateral cortex intact. This prevents both excessive bone resection and the creation of a U-shaped apex to the osteotomy from excessive resection of the lateral cortex. The wedge of bone is removed, and the lateral cortex is osteotomized. The capital fragment is then transposed laterally to allow for the desired amount of correction of the intermetatarsal (IM) angle. The osteotomy site is approximated, and fixation is achieved based on the surgeon's preference (Fig. 15-4).

The advantages of the Reverdin–Laird procedure include a reduction of the IM angle in addition to preventing disruption of the plantar metatarsal sesamoid articulation. The disadvantages include decreased stability from transposition of the capital fragment and increased difficulty in performing the procedure. Fixation is also required for this procedure as disruption of the lateral cortex is necessary to allow transposition of the capital fragment. Postoperative care is identical to that described for the Reverdin procedure.

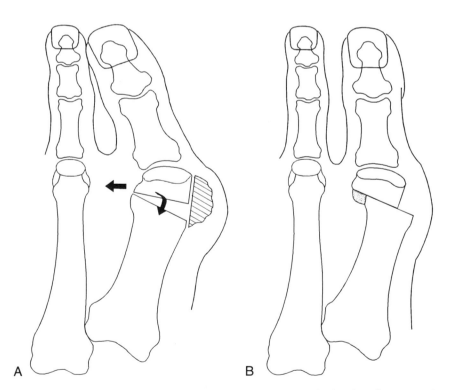

A                                          B

**Fig. 15-6. (A & B)** Modification to reduce shortening of the first metatarsal. The dorsal osteotomies created to remove the bone wedge are angulated to decrease shortening of the first metatarsal on lateral transposition of the capital fragment. (Adapted from Laird et al.,[7] with permission.)

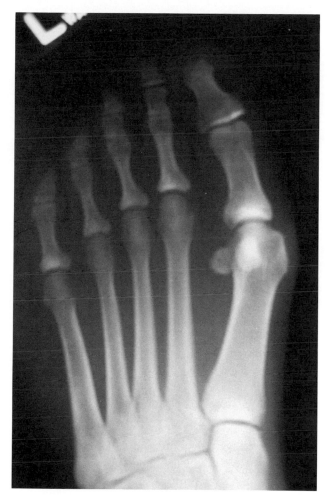

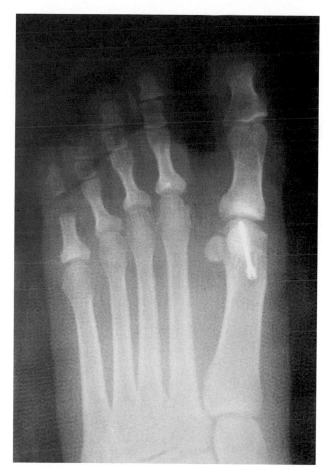

**Fig. 15-7.** Preoperative radiograph demonstrating increased proximal articular set angle before Reverdin–Laird procedure.

**Fig. 15-8.** Postoperative radiograph demonstrating Reverdin–Laird procedure with Herbert screw fixation. The dorsal osteotomy was angulated to decrease shortening of the first metatarsal.

In 1988, Laird introduced two modifications to the Reverdin–Laird procedure. The first involves correction of a valgus rotation of the first metatarsal head; the second procedure is designed to decrease shortening of the first metatarsal when performing the Reverdin–Laird procedure.[7] Both modifications require the same postoperative management as for the previously mentioned procedures.

The modification for correcting hallux valgus rotation involves a modification of the plantar osteotomy cut. A second plantar osteotomy is created dorsal to the first osteotomy cut. The osteotomy is created from dorsomedial to plantar-lateral with the base medial and apex lateral. The wedge of bone is removed and the capital fragment is reapproximated onto the metatarsal shaft. Fixation is used to maintain correction (Fig. 15-5).

The modification to decrease shortening of the first metatarsal is indicated in instances in which a negative metatarsal protrusion distance is present. This procedure involves a modification of the dorsal osteotomy cuts. The dorsal cuts are created from proximal-medial to distal-lateral. This allows distal transposition of the capital fragment when it is shifted laterally (Figs. 15-6 to 15-8). This modification is not recommended

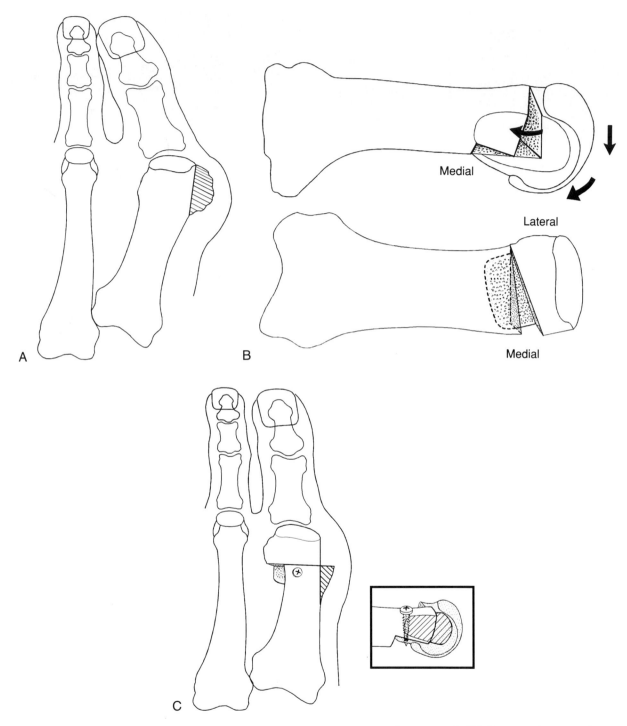

**Fig. 15-9.** Reverdin–Todd. (**A**) Portion of the medial eminence to be resected. (**B**) Bone wedge resections allowing for plantar displacement of the capital fragment and PASA correction. (**C**) Osteotomy after lateral transposition of the capital fragment and screw fixation.

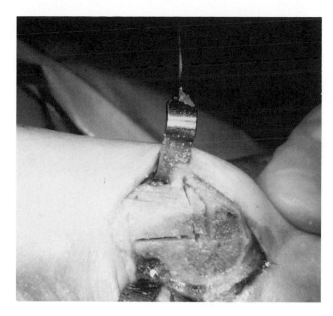

**Fig. 15-10.** Reverdin–Todd osteotomy. The procedure was modified with minimal angulation of the dorsal proximal cut because significant plantarflexion of the capital fragment was not necessary.

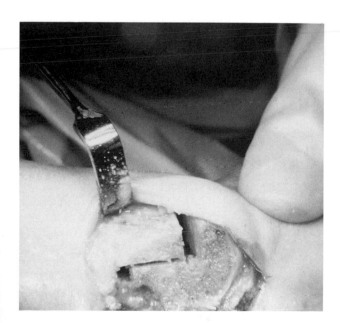

**Fig. 15-11.** Reverdin–Todd osteotomy before transposition of the capital fragment demonstrating dorsal and plantar wedge resections.

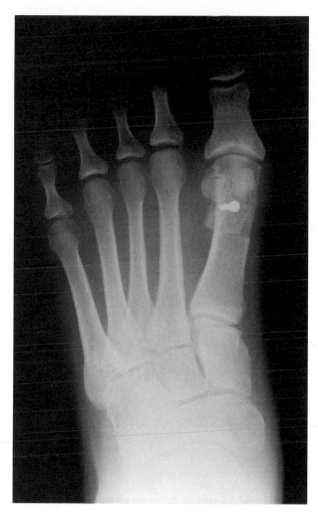

**Fig. 15-12.** Postoperative radiograph shows osteotomy after screw fixation.

for lengthening a metatarsal as the contracture of soft tissue structures would tend to limit lateral displacement of the capital fragment and may result in increased joint limitation. Advantages, disadvantages, and complications are the same as those listed for the Reverdin–Laird procedure.

The Reverdin–Todd procedure was developed by W.F. Todd at the California College of Podiatric Medicine in 1978. It is a modification of the Reverdin–Laird procedure that allows for correction of a sagittal plane deformity.[4] The indications for the Reverdin–Todd procedure include a dorsiflexed metatarsal, adequate bone stock to allow screw fixation, and an increased intermetatarsal angle. Adequate metatarsal width for transposition of the capital fragment is also necessary to allow for reduction of the IM angle and to permit screw fixation.

The Reverdin–Todd procedure involves lengthening the skin incision proximally to expose the distal one-third of the metatarsal shaft. The medial eminence is resected, and appropriate soft tissue releases and fibular sesamoidectomy are performed. The initial plantar osteotomy is made through the medial and lateral cortices, transecting the plantar one-third of the shaft of the metatarsal and extending proximally to the distal one-third of the metatarsal shaft. The dorsal osteotomy is made perpendicular to the plantar cut. The dorsal proximal cut is then made, angulated from dorsal-distal to plantar-proximal an appropriate amount to remove a predetermined wedge of bone to allow for plantar flexion of the capital fragment.

After removal of the bone wedge, the lateral cortex is transected. A second plantar osteotomy is created, dorsal to the first plantar cut, and angulated to the same degree as the amount of plantarflexion created by the proximal dorsal cut. The cut is made through both cortices with the base proximal and the apex located distally. The capital fragment is then transposed the predetermined amount and approximated to the shaft of the metatarsal. The position is maintained utilizing a bone clamp or K-wire, and screw fixation is achieved utilizing standard AO technique and one or two 2.0-mm screws. Additional eminence resection is then performed, and the wound site is closed in the appropriate fashion (Figs. 15-9 to 15-12).

An additional modification to decrease a valgus rotation of the capital fragment can be achieved by angulating the plantar osteotomies to allow resection of a wedge of bone with the base medially and apex laterally. The key steps to performing this procedure involve appropriate preoperative determination of the size of bone wedges to be resected and proper execution and angulation of the osteotomies to prevent errors in angulation or overcorrection. Postoperative care is the same as that described for the Reverdin procedure. Ambulation with crutch assistance is allowed as tolerated by the patient.

The advantages of the Reverdin–Todd procedure are that it allows correction of a sagittal plane deformity, unlike the other modifications. It also allows internal screw fixation. The disadvantages and complications may include an increased difficulty of the procedure due to the angulation of the osteotomies, delayed healing from extension of the osteotomy into diaphyseal bone, weakening of the first metatarsal by a decrease in dorsal to plantar width, and an increased potential for fracture or displacement. Excessive plantar flexion of the capital fragment may be an additional complication.

## SUMMARY

The Reverdin procedure and its most commonly performed modifications have been described. The variety of modifications reveal the versatility of the procedure as well as its many indications. The distal placement of the Reverdin osteotomy makes it a stable procedure that heals rapidly. Additionally, it is technically easier to perform than other procedures indicated for these criteria, such as the bicorrectional Austin osteotomy. The Reverdin procedure and its modifications should be considered in the surgical treatment of hallux abducto valgus deformities with angulational or rotational components to the first metatarsal head.

## REFERENCES

1. Reverdin J: Anatomic et operation de l'hallux valgus. Int Med Congr 2:408, 1881
2. Fielding M: Surgical procedures. p. 31. In: The Surgical Treatment of the Hallux Abducto Valgus and Allied Deformities. Futura Publishing, Co. Mt. Kisko, NY, 1973
3. Todd WF: Osteotomies of the first metatarsal head. Reverdin, Reverdin modifications. Peabody, Mitchell, and Drato. p. 166. In Gerbert J (ed): Textbook of Bunion Surgery. Futura Publishing, Mt. Kisko, NY, 1981
4. Beck E: Modified Reverdin technique for hallux abducto valgus (with increased proximal articular set angle of the first metatarsophalangeal joint). J Am Podiatry Assoc 64:657, 1974

5. Gerbert J: The indications and technique for utilizing pre-operative templates in podiatric surgery. J Am Podiatry Assoc 69:139, 1979

6. Boberg J, Ruch J, Banks A: Distal metaphyseal osteotomies in hallux abducto valgus surgery. p. 173. In McGlamry E (ed): Comprehensive Textbook of Foot Surgery. Vol. 1. Williams & Wilkins, Baltimore, 1987

7. Laird P, Silvers S, Somdahl J: Two Reverdin-Laird osteotomy modifications for correction of hallux abducto valgus. J Am Podiatry Assoc 78:403, 1988

# 16

# Middiaphyseal Osteotomies

GORDON W. PATTON
JAMES E. ZELICHOWSKI

Hallux abducto valgus is a progressive deformity. As the deformity increases, the retrograde force from the abducted hallux results in ever-increasing metatarsus primus varus. The subchondral bone of the first metatarsal head adapts resulting in deviation of the proximal articular set angle (PASA).

When metatarsus primus adductus is combined with hallux abducto valgus deformity, it must be corrected in addition to repair of the first metatarsophangeal joint. More than 130 different surgical approaches have been utilized in the correction of hallux valgus. Further, approximately 75 percent of these procedures are modifications of certain basic operations, thus suggesting at very least there is no perfect procedure available. One must remember the primary goal of surgical treatment of the patient with hallux abducto valgus deformity is to reduce pain, restore the articular congruency to the first metatarsophangeal joint, and restore the alignment of the first ray. With this in mind, let us delve into the possibilities of correction of deformity at the level of the first metatarsal.

Middiaphyseal osteotomies to correct the metatarsus primus varus component associated with hallux abducto valgus deformity have been described by Ludloff, Mau, and Meyer. Each operation is based on its author's concept of the relative importance of the various aspects of the pathologic anatomy.

## THE LUDLOFF OSTEOTOMY

The Ludloff osteotomy was first described in 1918 as a through-in-through, middiaphyseal osteotomy extending from dorsal proximal to plantar distal. The design of the osteotomy allows the distal capital fragment to rotate or slide laterally in the transverse plane for the correction of the metatarsus primus varus component associated with hallux valgus deformity (Fig. 16-1).

Unfortunately, without the use of rigid internal fixation techniques the Ludloff osteotomy was subject to complications resulting from the loading force placed on the first metatarsal during weight-bearing. Today, with the introduction of the Swiss technique of rigid internal fixation, middiaphyseal osteotomies can be successfully executed, resulting in primary bone healing.

## Preoperative Signs and Symptoms

The following are indications suggesting use of the Ludloff osteotomy:

Hallux abducto and/or valgus deformity
Presence of splay foot
Presence of adductus forefoot
Pressure of the hallux against the second digit
Pain with shoe gear

## Preoperative Radiographs

The following views should precede surgery:

Intermetatarsal angle greater than 13° in a rectus foot and greater than 11° in an adductus foot type
Abnormal hallux abductus angle
Normal-to-negative metatarsal protrusion distance
Normal PASA
Normal bone density without osteoporosis

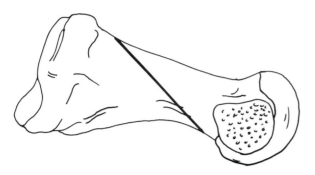

**Fig. 16-1.** Ludloff first metatarsal osteotomy.

## Operative Technique

A 7-cm dorsolinear incision is made, immediately medial and parallel to the extensor hallucis longus tendon over the first metatarsophangeal joint. The incision is deepened, using sharp and blunt dissection with careful attention to maintain hemostasis to the level of the joint capsule. The wound margins are retracted laterally over the first interspace. The extensor hallucis longus tendon is retracted medially, with care to avoid violation of its tendon sheath. The first interspace is entered by sharp and blunt dissection until the appropriate soft tissue structures have been released.

Attention is then directed medially to the first metatarsophangeal joint capsule, where a linear or inverted L capsular incision is performed. Capsular and soft tissue structures are freed with great care to avoid disturbing the dorsal synovial fold of the first metatarsophangeal joint. The medial eminence is removed with an osteotome and mallet or power instrumentation.

The initial skin incision is extended 3 cm proximally to the first metatarsocuneiform joint. A linear periosteal incision is made medial and parallel to the long extensor tendon. Periosteal tissues are reflected gaining exposure to the location of the osteotomy site. A through-in-through osteotomy is performed from medial to lateral, using a power sagittal saw. The osteotomy is angled through the middiaphyseal region of the bone from dorsal proximal to plantar distal. The distal segment can be laterally translated and swiveled. The distal segment may be lengthened by sliding it

forward on the osteotomy axis, permitting distal and plantar migration of the first metatarsal (Fig. 16-2).

A bone clamp is used to gain temporary fixation, and intraoperative radiographs are obtained to ensure proper alignment. If overcorrection is noted on the intraoperative radiograph, then it is a simple matter of releasing the bone clamp and repositioning the distal capital fragment without any further bone resection. The osteotomy is then fixated, most frequently using two 2.0- or 2.7-mm cortical screws.

The medial capsule of the first metatarsophangeal joint is repaired using simple interrupted sutures of 2-0 Dexon. The periosteum is closed with 3-0 Dexon sutures, and the subcutaneous tissues are reapproximated and closed with suture material of the surgeon's choice.

## Postoperative Management

The following steps are recommended after the Ludloff osteotomy:

Below-the-knee, non-weight-bearing cast for 6 weeks.
Initial postoperative radiographs are taken following the surgery and during the postoperative course to evaluate bone healing.
Cast may be bivalved postoperatively and sutures removed 1 week to 10 days postoperative.
Cast is removed at week 6, although final determination for discontinuing casting should be made by clinical and radiographic examination.
Patients are expected to return to normal shoe gear approximately 7 to 8 weeks if there are no complications.

## Advantages and Disadvantages

The Ludloff osteotomy uses the principle of the plane of motion, to rotate or slide the distal segment on the most proximal aspect of the osteotomy. This allows the surgeon to direct the distal segment using a single cut, sliding or rotating the osteotomy along the plane created by the osteotomy and taking advantage of the long axis arm provided by the osteotomy.

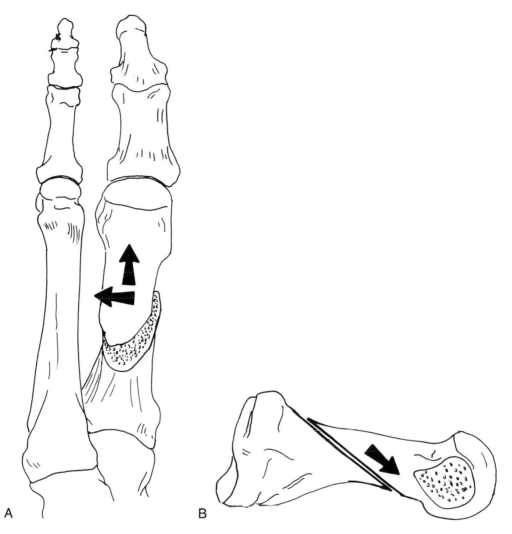

**Fig. 16-2.** (**A**) Dorsal view. Displacement of the distal segment, lateral and lengthened distally. (**B**) Lateral view. Distal translation; lengthen and plantar-flex the first metatarsal.

The concept of the plane of motion is utilized in other metatarsal osteotomies such as the Austin bunionectomy and the scarf or Z osteotomy. The distal segment is moved in a single plane created by the osteotomy. This single cut will allow the surgeon to move the distal segment a number of times until satisfied with the correction, without fear of further wedge resection and fracture of the medial cortical hinge as seen in wedge resection osteotomies (Fig. 16-3).

The Ludloff osteotomy lacks intrinsic stability and requires A-O osteosynthesis with non-weight-bearing (NWB) cast immobilization. Troughing of the metatarsal can result if the distal capital fragment slides laterally beyond the cortical walls of the metatarsal, resulting in frontal plane motion.

## MAU OSTEOTOMY

Mau, in 1926, modified the Ludloff osteotomy by changing the direction of the cut. Angled from dorsal

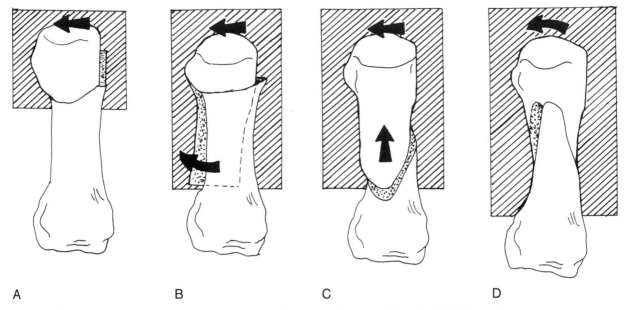

A                    B                    C                    D

**Fig. 16-3.** Plane of motion for four osteotomies: (**A**) Austin; (**B**) Scarf; (**C**) Ludloff; (**D**) Mau. All use transverse cuts to laterally displace or rotate the distal capital fragment for correction of metatarsus primus varus component associated with hallux abducto valgus deformity.

distal to plantar proximal, the osteotomy attempted to prevent dorsiflexion of the distal segment during weight-bearing. Again, without the use of interfragmentary AO screws, the Mau lost its popularity because of the lack of intrinsic stability (Fig. 16-4).

With the introduction of rigid internal fixation techniques, both the Ludloff and Mau osteotomies can now be successfully executed utilizing the concept that the crescentic osteotomy tried to employ. The transverse osteotomies rely on correction by degrees in the transverse plane rather than millimeters of bone by wedge resection. Both the Ludloff and Mau osteotomies take advantage of its long radius arm to provide sufficient lateral displacement of the distal segment, correcting large adductus deformities (Fig. 16-5).

## Preoperative Signs and Symptoms

The following are indications for employing the Mau osteotomy:

Hallux abductus and or valgus deformity
Presence of splay foot
Presence of adductus forefoot

Pressure of the hallux against the second digit
Pain with shoe gear

## Preoperative Radiographs

These views should precede surgery:

Intermetatarsal angle greater than 13° in a rectus foot and greater than 11° in an adductus foot type
Abnormal halux abductus angle
Normal-to-negative metatarsal protrusion distance

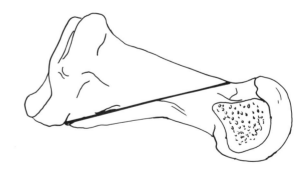

**Fig. 16-4.** Mau first metatarsal osteotomy.

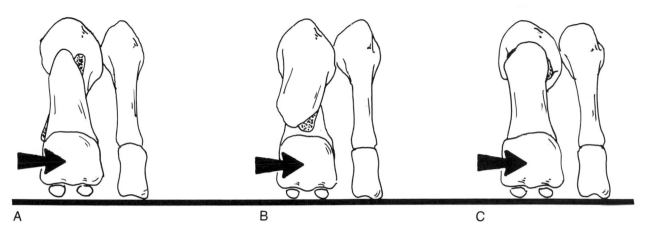

**Fig. 16-5.** Three osteotomies: (**A**) Ludloff; (**B**) Mau; (**C**) crescentic. These move the distal segment in the transverse plane without wedge resection, taking advantage of a long radius arm.

Normal PASA unless corrected by additional procedure

Normal bone density without osteoporosis.

## Operative Procedure

The surgical approach used in the Mau osteotomy is the same as in the Ludloff procedure. However, the osteotomy should be made parallel to the weight-bearing surface from dorsal distal to plantar proximal through the shaft of the first metatarsal. The obliquity of the osteotomy is limited by the pitch of the proximal lateral cortex of the first metatarsal shaft. Care should be maintained to avoid entering the first metatarsocunieform articulation. Once the osteotomy is completed, an axis guide is established at the proximal portion of the osteotomy using a small Kirschner wire. The Kirschner wire is angled perpendicular to the osteotomy, allowing the distal fragment to pivot laterally and thus reducing the intermetatarsal angle. Once the distal segment is moved, the osteotomy is temporarily fixated with a bone clamp. Intraoperative radiographs are obtained to ensure proper alignment. If overcorrection is noted on the intraoperative films, then it is a simple matter of repositioning the distal segment to the correct angle before fixation without any further bone resection. The axis wire is then removed, and the medial cortical overlap is reduced with power equipment (Fig. 16-6).

Attention is then directed to the first metatarsophalangeal joint, and the congruency is accessed. Reduction of a large intermetatarsal angle frequently increases the PASA, requiring a distal subcapital osteotomy. This is accomplished by using a Reverdin-Green osteotomy and fixating with two Orthosorb absorbable pins (Fig. 16-7).

The medial capsule of the first metatarsophangeal joint is repaired using simple interrupted sutures of 2-0 Dexon. The periosteum is closed with 3-0 Dexon sutures, and the subcutaneous tissues are reapproximated and closed with suture of the surgeon's choice.

## Modifications to the Mau Osteotomy

Increasing the length of the osteotomy can reduce a severe metatarsus varus deformity with minimal rotation of the distal capital fragment and adequate bone contact. This however is accomplished by extending the proximal cut of the osteotomy into the plantar portion of the first metatarsocuneiform articulation. At first, entering the joint posed some concerns of possible postoperative pain and degenerative arthritis. It is now apparent, after 2 years followup, that no postoperative pain or degenerative changes have been noted when the osteotomy enters the joint at the plantar one-fifth of the first metatarsal base (Fig. 16-8).

By utilizing this modification, the plantar ligamentous structures and insertion of the peroneus longus tendon at the base of the first metatarsal provides stability to the distal segment. This eliminates the need for an Kirschner wire guide to rotate the capital fragment. The distal segment can be easily rotated using

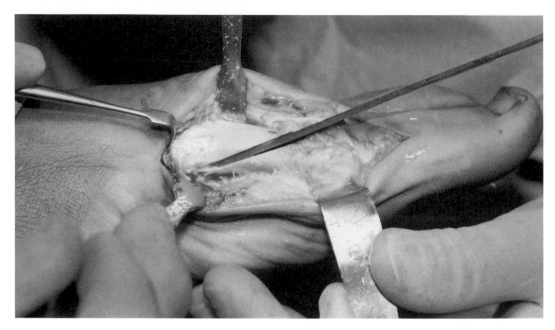

**Fig. 16-6.** Mau osteotomy. Cut is angled from dorsal distal to plantar proximal through the shaft of the first metatarsal. A small osteotome is used to free plantar soft tissues before displacement.

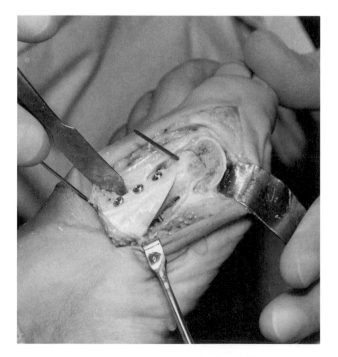

**Fig. 16-7.** Mau osteotomy completed and fixated using three 2.0-mm cortical screws. Distally, a Green-Reverdin subcapital osteotomy is fixated with two Orthosorb absorbable pins.

the plantar structures attached to the base of the first metatarsal as its axis guide (Fig. 16-9).

## Postoperative Management

These conditions should be met after the Mau osteotomy:

Below-the-knee, non-weight-bearing cast for 6 weeks.
Initial postoperative radiographs are taken following the surgery and during the postoperative course to evaluate bone healing.
Cast may be bivalved postoperatively and sutures removed 1 week to 10 days postoperative.
Cast is removed at week 6 although final determination for discontinuing casting should be made by clinical and radiographic examination.
Patients are expected to return to normal shoe gear after approximately 7 to 8 weeks if no complications.

## Advantages and Disadvantages

The Mau, like the Ludloff osteotomy, can effectively reduce the metatarsus varus component associated

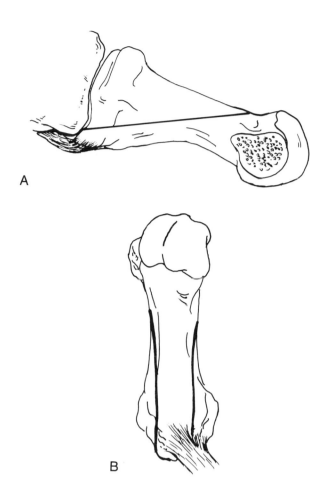

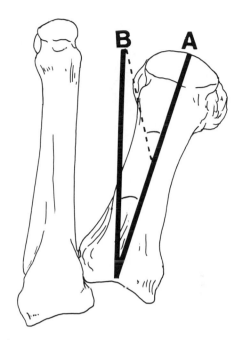

**Fig. 16-9.** Radial arm theory. Doubling the length of the arm reduces the degrees required to move from point A to point B.

**Fig. 16-8.** (**A & B**) Modifications of the Mau osteotomy. The proximal cut is extended into the plantar portion of the base of the first metatarsal. The modification increases the length of the distal fragment, reducing a large intermetatarsal angle with minimal displacement. The plantar intrinsic provides stabilization of the plantar segment during displacement.

with hallux abducto valgus deformity. Both osteotomies are transverse plane osteotomies correcting the deformity in degrees rather than by wedge resection.

However, the Mau osteotomy offers some inherit stability with the aid of internal fixation. Mau modified the angle of the Ludloff osteotomy to prevent dorsal dislocation and elevation of the capital fragment postoperatively. The authors believe that there is a plastic deformation of bone that continues for as much as 6 months in the weight-bearing bones of the feet. Therefore, if the osteotomy is remodeling during this period, the forces of the weight-bearing will affect the

bone until this period of deformation ceases, according to Wolf and Davis Law (Fig. 16-10).

Looking at the forces applied to the first metatarsal during gait, it is clear that elevation will occur at an osteotomy like the transverse wedge if deformation occurs. Studies by Zlotoff, Schuberth, Curda, and Sorto show three main complications following proximal wedge resection osteotomies for the correction of metatarsus varus associated with hallux valgus: hallux varus, first metatarsal elevation, and first metatarsal shortening.

The Mau and Ludloff osteotomies offer an alternative approach to correction of metatarsus primus adductus when criteria are met for a closing abductory base wedge osteotomy. Both osteotomies can not only correct for significant intermetatarsal deviation of the first metatarsal, but do so more effectively by eliminating possibilities of complications inherent to the closing base wedge osteotomy (Fig. 16-11).

## SCARF-MEYER **Z** OSTEOTOMY

A **Z**-type osteotomy of the first metatarsal for the correction of hallux valgus was first described by Meyer

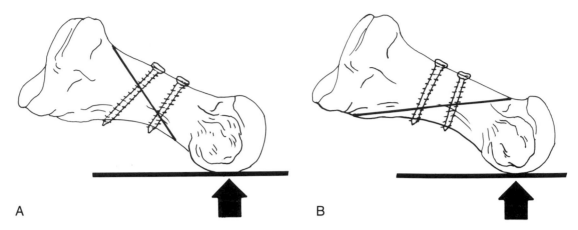

**Fig. 16-10.** (**A & B**) Ground reactive force produces a constant dorsiflexory force during ambulation. Plastic deformation will produce dorsiflexion of the distal segment during remodeling phase. Angulation of the Mau osteotomy closely parallels the weight-bearing surface, preventing elevatus.

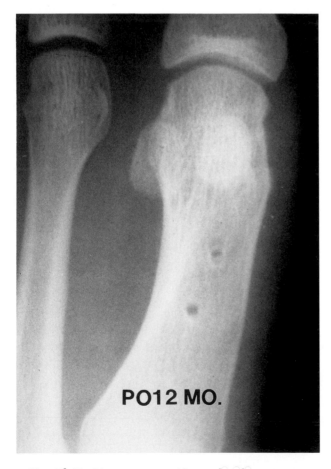

**Fig. 16-11.** Mau osteotomy 12 months after surgery.

in 1926. Gudas, in 1983, popularized the osteotomy to include interfragmentary AO screws. Since this time, the Scarf or **Z** osteotomy has been modified in length and fixation techniques (Fig. 16-12).

The Scarf, described by Gudas, is a horizontally directed **Z**-displacement osteotomy of the head and shaft of the first metatarsal fixated by two cortical screws. Modification of this procedure by shortening the length of the osteotomy was described by Glickman, Pollack, and Gill. By varying the length of the osteotomy, the intermetatarsal angle as well as the PASA can be corrected by taking advantage of the inherited stability of the Scarf cuts. Schwartz and Groves modified the fixation technique by utilizing internally threaded Kirschner wires.

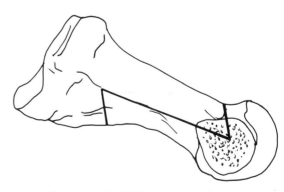

**Fig. 16-12.** Scarf of **Z** first metatarsal osteotomy.

## Preoperative Signs and Symptoms

These are indications for the Scarf or Z osteotomy:

Hallux abductus with medial or dorsomedial bunion deformity
Absence of significant valgus rotation of the hallux
Pain with shoe gear and ambulation

## Preoperative Radiographs

The following conditions should be visualized before osteotomy:

Abnormal hallux abductus angle
Congruous to deviated first metatarsophangeal joint
Mild to moderate increase in the metatarsus primus adductus angle
Absence of cystic changes throughout the metatarsal head
Adequate bone stock without osteoporosis
Normal to moderate increase in PASA

## Operative Technique

A 5- to 6-cm skin incision is made longitudinally, centered over the shaft and head of the first metatarsal halfway between the medial eminence and the extensor hallucis longus tendon. Dissection is carried down to the level of the joint capsule and the periosteum, with care to retract the neurovascular structures. One or two linear semielliptical capsular incisions are made over the medial capsule. The periosteal incision is made by extending the capsular incision proximally, passing over the dorsomedial aspect of the shaft of the first metatarsal. The capsule and periosteum are retracted, and the medial eminence is then removed. A subcutaneous tissue plane is established over the head of the first metatarsal, and the lateral structures are identified and released if contracted.

A transverse Z osteotomy is made horizontally. The central limb is placed at the level of the middle and lower one-third of the metatarsal shaft. The dorsal wing is centered in the metaphyseal region of the head of the first metatarsal, creating a angle of 60°–70°. Proximally, the plantar wing is made at the flare of the base of the first metatarsal at the same angle.

With complete transection of the metatarsal, the bottom segment can be transposed laterally over one-third to one-half of the width of the metatarsal, correcting the metatarsus varus component of hallux valgus. If the PASA needs to be addressed, then the proximal portion of the plantar fragment is displaced slightly farther laterally. Temporary fixation is achieved by the use of a self-centering bone clamp, and permanent internal fixation is then completed using two 2.7- to 3.5-mm cortical screws. The screws are placed perpendicular to the osteotomy but angled slightly of center to obtain maximum bone purchase. The remaining cortex on the dorsal proximal fragment is then removed with a bone saw (Fig. 16-13).

The capsule and periosteum are reapproximated with 2-0 and 3-0 Dexon sutures. The subcutaneous tissue is reapproximated using 4-0 Dexon, and the skin is closed with material of the surgeon's choice.

## Modifications to the Scarf Osteotomy

### Incision

A more medial approach has been utilized to facilitate exposure of the plantar aspect of the first metatarsal, allowing the surgeon to release the lateral sesamoid apparatus through a plantar approach. The skin inci-

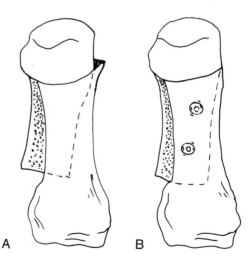

**Fig. 16-13.** Displacement of the Scarf osteotomy consists of two steps. (**A**) Lateral translation of the plantar segment; (**B**) proximal portion of the plantar segment is swiveled into the first interspace for PASA correction.

sion made over the medial to dorsomedial aspect of the first metatarsal but dips down at the level of the first metatarsophalangeal joint.

### Fixation

Permanent, internally threaded 0.062-in. Kirschner wires have been used to replace cortical screws. This method of fixation is relatively simple and very effective. Intrinsic stability in the design of the osteotomy provides that the metatarsal will possess most of the load shearing. Although threaded Kirschner wires do not provide interfragmentary compression such as does a cortical screw in the lag technique, threaded Kirschner wires have proven to maintain compression and the position of the osteotomy provided by the bone clamp.

### Osteotomy Length

The short **Z** bunionectomy has an osteotomy cut of 2.5 to 3.0 cm in length and is utilized for the correction of hallux valgus with or without an increase in the PASA. This technique offers the surgeon good stability and correction, using internal fixation with minimal shortening and less extensive tissue dissection (Fig. 16-14).

## Postoperative Management

The following stages follow the Scarf or **Z** osteotomy:

Parital to full weight-bearing is possible immediately postoperative with a surgical shoe.
Initial postoperative radiographs are taken following the surgery and during the postoperative course to evaluate bone healing.

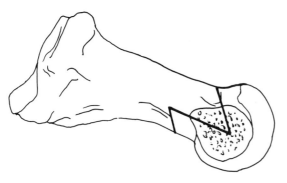

**Fig. 16-14.** Short Scarf or **Z** osteotomy.

Sutures are removed 1 week to 10 days postoperative.
Patient returns to tennis shoes 3 to 4 weeks postoperative.
Patient can return to normal shoe gear 4 to 6 weeks postoperative if no complications occur.

## Advantages and Disadvantages

The Scarf or **Z** osteotomy is another procedure that has found its place in the correction of hallux abducto valgus deformity with the advent of AO fixation techniques. The Scarf osteotomy depends on two maneuvers for correction: the lateral translational shift of the distal segment, and the swing of the plantar wing into the interspace for PASA correction. One should remember that PASA correction is made at the expense of intermetatarsal correction and that intermetatarsal correction is limited by the width of the shaft of the metatarsal. Troughing is seen if lateral displacement exceeds the cortical margins in the diaphyseal region of the bone, resulting in frontal plane rotation of the capital fragment. Fracture through the dorsal cortex at the proximal wing of the osteotomy can result from improper bone cuts or poor bone stock.

Rigid compression of the large bone-to-bone contact along with the inherent stability of the osteotomy provides a good environment for primary bone healing of the Scarf osteotomy. No casting is required, and the patient can ambulate immediately following this procedure, which makes the Scarf osteotomy desirable to both the patient and the surgeon. One should be aware that the Scarf osteotomy is a technically precise procedure and that familiarity with AO/ASIF fixation techniques, which are demanding, is essential.

## SUGGESTED READINGS

Curda GA, Sorto LA: The Mcbride bunionectomy with closing abductory wedge osteotomy. J Am Podiatry Assoc 71:349, 1981

Elkouri E: Review of cancellous and cortical bone healing after fracture or osteotomy. J Am Podiatry Assoc 72:464, 1982

Gerbert J: Textbook of Bunion Surgery. Futura Publishing, Mt. Kisco, New York, 1981

Gill P: Modification of the scarf bunionectomy. J Am Podiatr Med Assoc 78:187, 1988

Glickman S, Zaghari D: Short "Z" bunionectomy. J Foot Surg 25:304, 1986

Ludloff K: Die besetigung des Hallux Valgus durch die schraege planto-dorsale osteotomie des metatarus 1 (Erfahrungen und Erfolge). Arch Klin Chir 110:364, 1918

Mau C, Lauber HT: Die operative behandlung des hallux valgus (Nachuntersuchungen). Dtsch Z Chir 197:363, 1926

Meyer M: Eine neue modifikation der hallux valgus operation. Zentrabl Chir 53:3215, 1926

Neese DJ, Zelichowski JE, Patton GW: Mau osteotomy: an alternative procedure to the closing abductory base wedge osteotomy. J Foot Surg 28:352, 1989

Patton GW, Tursi FJ, Zelichowski JE: The dorsal synovial fold of the first metatarsophangeal joint. J Foot Surg 26:210, 1987

Root ML, Orien W, Weed JH: Normal and abnormal function of the foot. Clinical Biomechanics Corp., Los Angeles, 1977

Sorto LA, Balding MG, Weil LS, Smith SD: Hallux abductus interphalangeus. J Am Podiatry Assoc 66:384, 1976

Schenk R, Willenegger H: Morphological findings in primary fracture healing. Symp Biol Hung 7:75, 1967

Schuberth JM, Reilly CH, Gudas CJ: The closing wedge osteotomy: a critical analysis of first metatarsal elevation. J AM Podiatry Assoc 74:13, 1984

Schwartz N, Groves R: Long-term follow-up of internal threaded kirschner-wire fixation of the scarf bunionectomy. J Foot Surg 26:313, 1987

Zlotoff H: Shortening of the first metatarsal following osteotomy and its clinical significance. J Am Podiatry Assoc 67:412, 1977

Zygmunt KH, Gudas CJ, Laros GS: Z-Bunionectomy with internal screw fixation. J Am Podiatr Med Assoc 79:322, 1989

# 17

# Proximal Osteotomy

*VINCENT J. MANDRACCHIA*
*DENISE M. MANDRACCHIA*
*TRACY A. MERRELL*

## FIRST METATARSAL PROXIMAL OSTEOTOMIES

Many components in various severities come together to form the hallux abducto valgus/metatarsus primus adductus condition commonly known to our patients as a "bunion." In this chapter, we are concerned with what could be called, in layman's terms, a "severe bunion," necessitating osteotomy at the base of the first metatarsal (Fig. 17-1).

There are numerous procedures and even more numerous variations for the correction of a severe metatarsus primus adductus. Those most commonly used today, which we cover in some depth, include the closing base wedge osteotomy, the opening base wedge osteotomy, the crescentic osteotomy, and the Logroscino double osteotomy. We also present some procedures that are less often used and historically interesting.

Our chief concern is presenting broad preoperative, postoperative, and fixation principles applicable to all the base osteotomies. Particulars are covered under specific sections.

## Criteria

Hallux abducto valgus surgical criteria have been identified and recognized by many authors for years. We believe that strict adherence to preoperative criteria helps ensure a satisfactory surgical outcome. Templates can be very useful in determining the size of a wedge or position of an osteotomy, but should be used together with preoperative measurements.[1] A major problem in any osteotomy is shortening of the bone. We believe that any and all osteotomies shorten bone to some degree.

The purpose of this chapter is to describe the surgical correction of a specific first metatarsal deformity. It is imperative that consideration can be given to the biomechanical evaluation of the hallux valgus foot. Inman and other authors have identified excessive pronation of the foot as contributing to the formation of hallux valgus.[2,3] Hypermobility of the first ray has been implicated in the formation of significant hallux valgus deformity. Proper biomechanical evaluation allows the surgeon to functionally accommodate the postsurgical foot with better long-term results.

When considering base wedge osteotomy procedures, the intermetatarsal (IM) angle determination is vital. Hardy and Clapham determined the intermetatarsal measurement in a 1951 study.[4] The intermetatarsal angle is the most significant measurement used in deciding to perform an osteotomy at the base of the first metatarsal.

The Logroscino and Golden procedures correct a high IM angle and an abnormal proximal articular set angle (PASA). However, if the IM angle is easily corrected by a head or midshaft osteotomy, then biplane angling of the osteotomy will help to change the proximal articular set angle as well, thus eliminating the need for the double osteotomy. We believe therefore that proper IM angle determination is crucial.

The intermetatarsal angle is the relationship between lines bisecting the first and second metatarsal

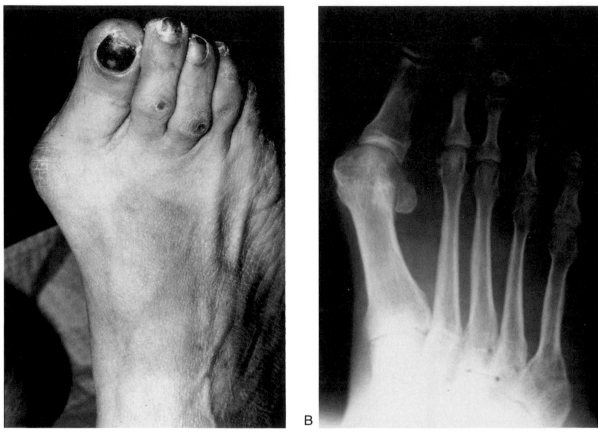

**Fig. 17-1.** (**A**) Clinical appearance of a severe hallux abducto valgus deformity. Note the position of the hallux in relationship to the second toe. (**B**) Anteroposterior radiograph demonstrating severe hallux abducto valgus with high intermetatarsal angle and displacement of the sesamoid apparatus.

shafts (Fig. 17-2A and B). The normal IM is a source of controversy; however, it can be safely said that in a rectus foot as much as 10° is normal, and in an adductus foot, to 8° is normal.[5] We believe that a base osteotomy should be considered in patients who have an intermetatarsal angle of 15° in a rectus foot or more than 12° in an adductus foot. It has been our experience that a head or shaft osteotomy can sufficiently correct an IM angle up to 15° (Fig. 17-2C to E). As always, clinical correlation is important. Visual examination of the foot may at times change the surgeon's mind about a head versus a base osteotomy. If the intermetatarsal angle exceeds 22°, we suggest the use

of the first metatarsal medial cuneiform joint fusion or Lapidus procedure (Fig. 17-3).

The second important measurement criteria is the proximal articular set angle (PASA). The PASA is an angle determined by drawing a line transversely through the effective articular cartilage of the first metatarsal head, then dropping a line perpendicular to that. This perpendicular is then compared to the bisection of the first metatarsal shaft (Fig. 17-4). A normal PASA is considered to be 8° or less. Gudas and Marcinko[6] describe an "effective proximal articular set angle," which they state is usually greater than the radiographic measurement. This effective PASA is de-

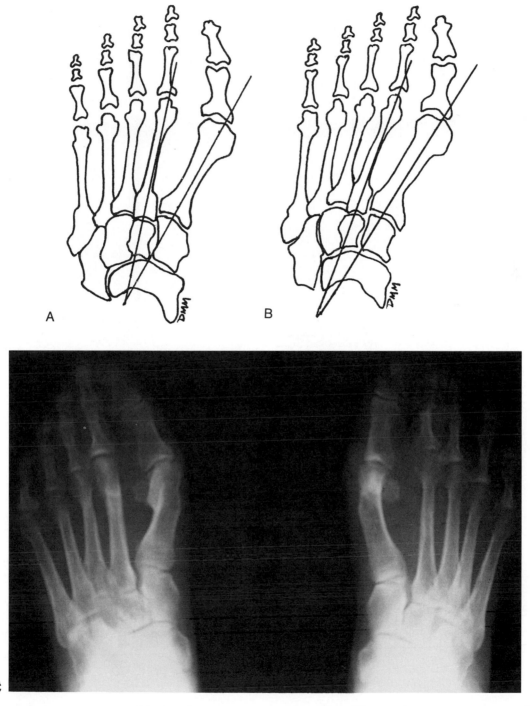

**Fig. 17-2.** (**A**) Intermetatarsal (IM) angle measurement in a rectus foot. (**B**) IM angle measurement in an adductus foot. (**C**) Radiograph demonstrating failed head osteotomy bilaterally. An attempt was made to correct a significantly large IM angle by means of a head osteotomy. Consideration should have been given to a base osteotomy as the IM angle was higher than 15°. (*Figure continues.*)

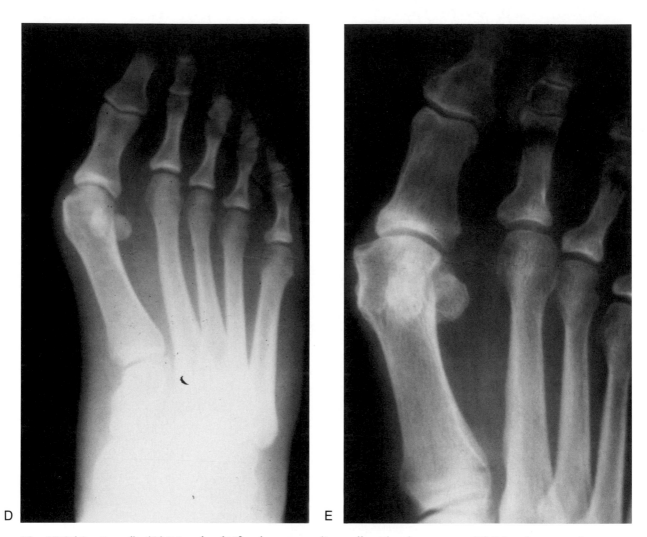

**Fig. 17-2** (*Continued*). (**D**) IM angle of 15° or less responding well to a head osteotomy. (**E**) IM angle greater than 15°, necessitating base osteotomy.

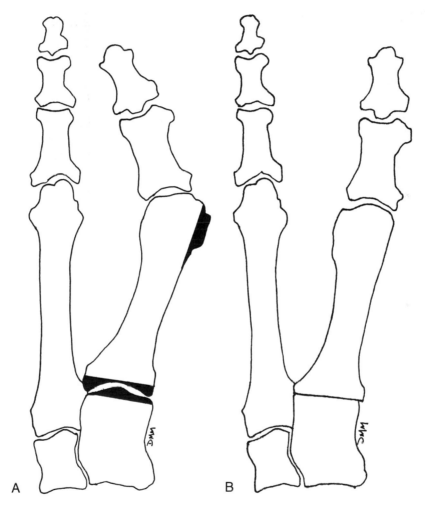

**Fig. 17-3.** (**A**) Diagram of Lapidus procedure demonstrating the bone to be resected, including the hypertrophied medial eminence and cartilagenous surfaces of the base of the first metatarsal and corresponding distal aspect of the medial cuneiform. (**B**) Completed Lapidus procedure.

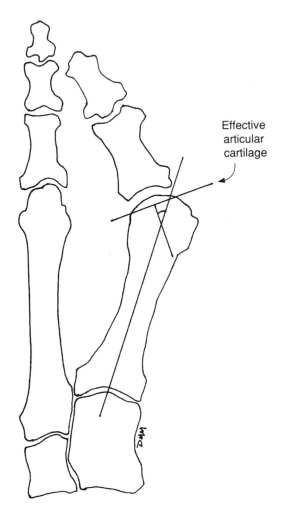

Effective
articular
cartilage

**Fig. 17-4.** Diagram demonstrating the proximal articular set angle measurement. Note the line demonstrating the effective articular cartilage on the head of the first metatarsal.

termined intraoperatively following medial eminence exostectomy.[7] Indeed, we have noted that radiographic measurement of the PASA is difficult at best. Gerbert attempted arthrography of the first metatarsal phalangeal joint (MTPJ) to identify the relationship between a radiographic PASA measurement and a dye-aided view.[8] Differences in the measurements were noted. Further study in this area is both necessary and encouraged. We think that intraoperative measurements of the PASA after visualization of the cartilage

compared to the preoperative radiographic evaluation would be a good study.

The radiographic position of the first metatarsal phalangeal joint should be considered. A congruous joint demonstrates no angulation within the joint. Lines representing the effective articular cartilaginous surfaces of the base of the proximal phalanx and the head of the first metatarsal are parallel (Fig. 17-5A).[10] In a deviated joint, the lines representing the effective articular cartilage of the joint appear to be intersecting outside the joint (Fig. 17-5B)[11]; a subluxed joint shows these lines intersecting within the joint (Fig. 17-5C). Evaluation of congruity of the joint and range of motion are necessary for determining the viability of joint preservation versus joint destructive procedures. Base osteotomies may be performed with either a joint destructive or a joint preservative procedure at the metatarsal head.

The relative metatarsal protrusion is measured on the radiograph preoperatively. A normal protrusion measurement demonstrates the second metatarsal as being longer than the first metatarsal, although a range of plus or minus 2 mm is considered within normal limits (Figs. 17-6 and 17-7).[6] If the first metatarsal is found to be equal in length to the second metatarsal or longer, then a closing base wedge osteotomy can be performed, as a slight shortening of the first metatarsal will take place. This procedure was first described by Loison[10] and Balasescu.[11]

Another method for determining relative metatarsal length is by measuring the metatarsal parabola angle. With the apex at the distal aspect of the second metatarsal, a line is drawn to the distal aspects of the first and fifth metatarsal heads respectively. An angle is formed, the average of which is found to be 142.5° (Fig. 17-8).[12] The normal metatarsal length relationship in order of decreasing length is 2:1:3:4:5.[12]

As in any surgery, the patient's overall physical and emotional condition must be taken into account preoperatively. Of course, circulatory status must be adequate to ensure healing. Bone stock quality is also extremely important. In the case of any base osteotomy where internal fixation is absolutely essential, bone quality becomes crucial. Osteoporotic or cystic bone should be avoided at all costs when considering a base osteotomy (Fig. 17-9).

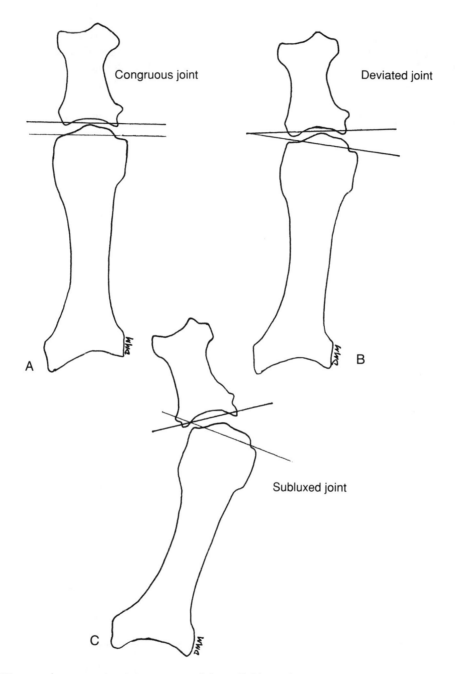

**Fig. 17-5.** Diagram demonstrating joint position. (**A**) Parallel lines demonstrating effective articular cartilage in a congruous joint. (**B**) Intersection of the lines outside the joint show a deviated joint. (**C**) Lines intersecting within the joint demonstrating a subluxed position.

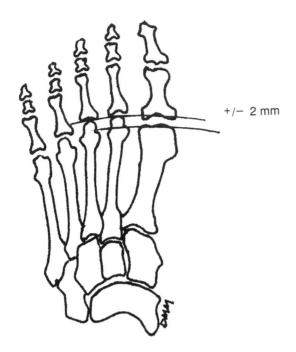

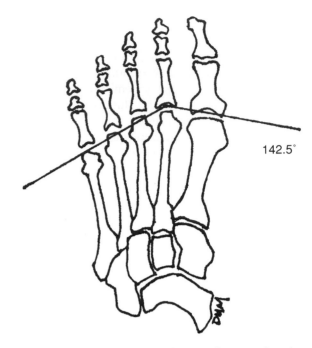

**Fig. 17-6.** Relative metatarsal protrusion. A normal is ±2 mm relative to the first and second metatarsal heads.

**Fig. 17-8.** Metatarsal parabola angle. Note the normal angle of 142.5°.

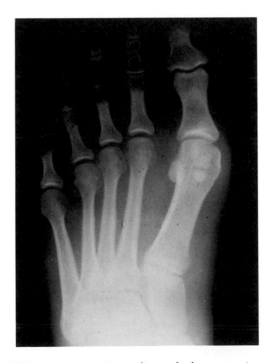

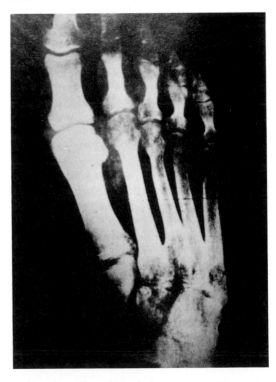

**Fig. 17-7.** Anteroposterior radiograph demonstrating normal metatarsal protrusion.

**Fig. 17-9.** Radiograph demonstrating poor bone stock, contraindicating an osteotomy procedure.

234

## Preoperative Planning

Sharpe,[9] in determining the size of the wedge of bone to be resected for a closing base wedge osteotomy, presented a mathematical formula (Fig. 17-10). Gerbert[1] talks about the use of templates to determine wedge size as is shown in the illustration (Figs. 17-11A to D). It has been suggested that determining the amount of correction desired will aid in choosing the size of the wedge necessary. For example, if an intermetatarsal angle of 18° is noted preoperatively and an angle of 8° is desired postoperatively, then a 10° wedge should be made in the bone.

Others believe that the osteotomy should be made in the traditional fashion, with one cut perpendicular to the shaft of the first metatarsal, and the second cut parallel to the desired articular surface of the head (Fig. 17-12). Another theory involves the "hinge axis concept,"[13] which stresses the importance of keeping the cuts perpendicular to the weight-bearing surface, rather than perpendicular to the surface of the bone (Fig. 17-13). It is believed that dorsiflexion of the capital fragment can be prevented by keeping the cuts perpendicular to the weight-bearing surface. Each method of determination of osteotomy size is presented here.

## Surgical Approach

The surgical approach for the first metatarsal base osteotomy consists of a dorsilinear skin incision approximately 10 to 12 cm long (Fig. 17-14). The incision begins distally at the interphalangeal joint dorsal crease, medial to the extensor hallucis longus (EHL) tendon, and courses proximally until it eventually ends at the metatarsal cuneiform articulation. An 18-gauge needle can be used to demonstrate the location of the metatarsal cuneiform joint and to aid in making the incision (Fig. 17-15). The subcutaneous tissues at the base of the first metatarsal are divided just medial to the extensor hallucis longus tendon. Sharp dissection removes the capsule and periosteal tissues. With careful dissection over the hinge area of the proposed wedge, the capsule and periosteal tissues can be left intact to help strengthen the hinge.[13] Important neurovascular structures to be aware of in this area are the dorsal vein that traverses the base of the first metatarsal, the deep plantar artery between the base of the

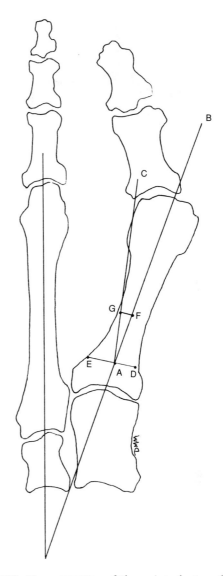

**Fig. 17-10.** Demonstration of Sharpe's technique for determining the size of the wedge of bone to be resected for a closing base wedge osteotomy. (1) The IM angle is drawn. The portion along the first metatarsal shaft is labeled A–B. (2) A line is drawn where the osteotomy is planned. This line is labeled D–E. (3) A line is drawn showing the eventual position of the first metatarsal. This line is labeled A–C. (4) Line D–E is measured. This line is then projected from point A along line A–B to point F, and then from point A along line A–C to point G. (5) Joining points F and G determines the width of the base wedge necessary to obtain the desired correction. (6) If an opening base wedge is to be performed, the width of the graft equals the distance between points F and G.

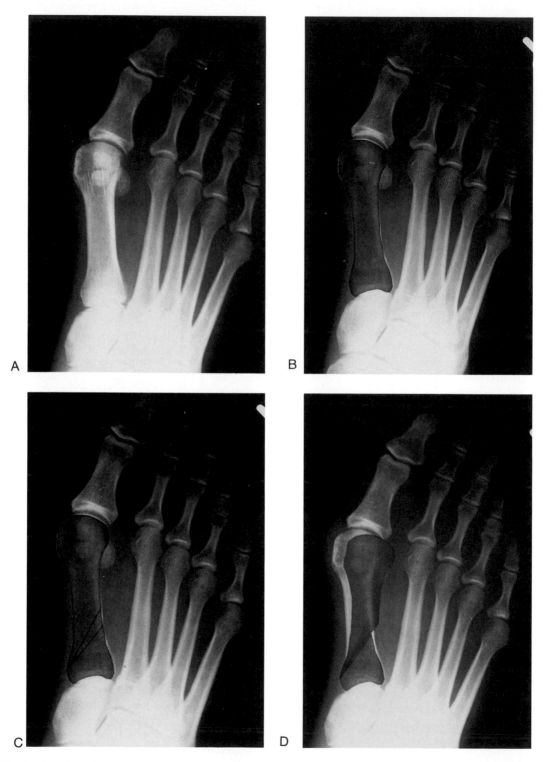

**Fig. 17-11.** (**A–D**) Radiographs demonstrating template cutout technique for determining osteotomy size.

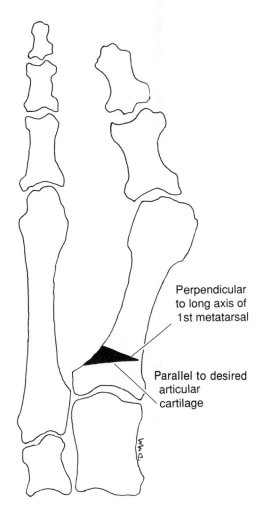

**Fig. 17-12.** Traditional orientation of osteotomy cuts for closing base wedge.

Perpendicular to long axis of 1st metatarsal

Parallel to desired articular cartilage

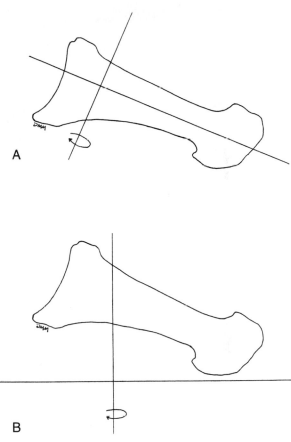

A

B

**Fig. 17-13.** Hinge axis concept. (**A**) The osteotomy is made perpendicular to the shaft of the first metatarsal, which causes a metatarsus primus elevatus postoperatively. (**B**) The osteotomy cut is demonstrated perpendicular to the supporting surface, which helps to prevent metatarsal dorsiflexion postoperatively.

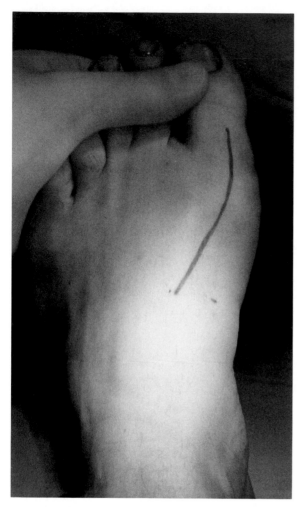

**Fig. 17-14.** Surgical approach for a first metatarsal base osteotomy. Note the dorsilinear skin incision starting just medial to the extensor hallucis longus tendon.

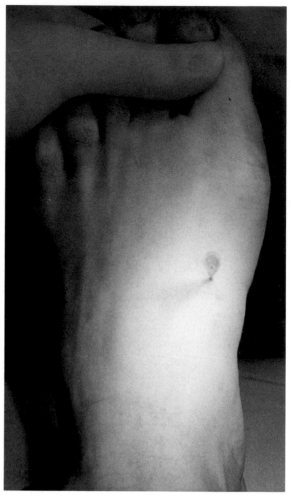

**Fig. 17-15.** Identification of the metatarsocuneiform articulation at the base of the first metatarsal by means of an 18-gauge needle. This aids in determining where the base osteotomy should take place, as an adjunct to making the initial skin incision.

first and second metatarsals, and the medial dorsal cutaneous nerve which crosses within the base of the first metatarsal (Figs. 17-16 to 17-24).

At the level of approximately 1 to 1.5 cm distal to the metatarsal cuneiform joint, the chosen osteotomy is performed. The decision to perform a closing, opening, or crescentic base osteotomy is made by carefully evaluating the relative metatarsal protrusion. On completion of the osteotomy, the surgeon's choice of fixation is utilized and the area is closed in the normal fashion. Cast immobilization of 6 to 8 weeks is necessary, with 4 to 6 weeks being non-weight-bearing. Bony healing will be evidenced on serial x-ray evaluation postoperatively.

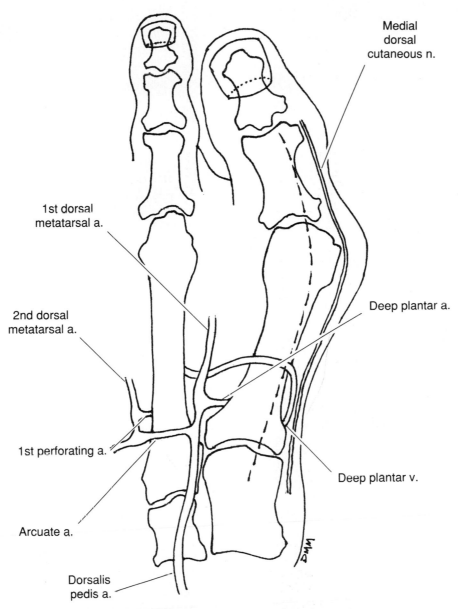

Medial
dorsal
cutaneous n.

1st dorsal
metatarsal a.

2nd dorsal
metatarsal a.

Deep plantar a.

1st perforating a.

Deep plantar v.

Arcuate a.

Dorsalis
pedis a.

**Fig. 17-16.** Diagram demonstrating the superficial and deep structures encountered with the dorsilinear incision over the first metatarsal. Note in particular the dorsal vein traversing the base of the first metatarsal, which many surgeons believe to be a good landmark for placement of base osteotomy.

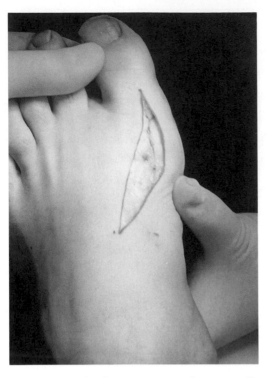

**Fig. 17-17.** Superficial venous network surrounding the first MTPJ.

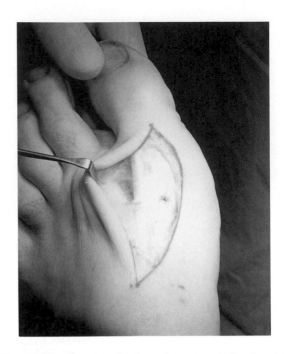

**Fig. 17-19.** Entering the lateral aspect of the first MTPJ. Note the extensor hallucis longus tendon.

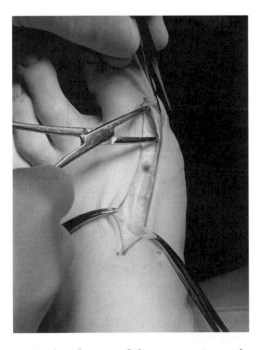

**Fig. 17-18.** Identification of the proper tissue plane between the superficial fascia and the capsule of the first MTPJ by means of blunt dissection. This pocket is found both distally and proximally at the base of the first MPTJ. The joining of these two pockets allows for easy layer dissection.

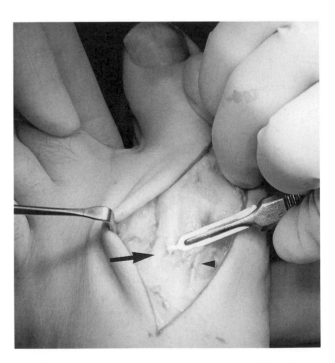

**Fig. 17-20.** Sharp tenotomy of the extensor hallucis brevis tendon (arrow). Note the position and presence of the extensor hallucis capsularis (arrowhead).

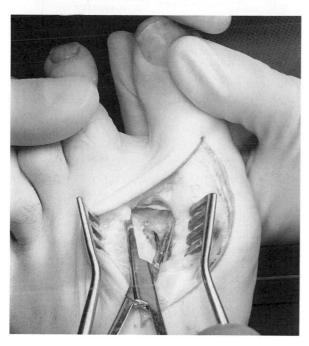

**Fig. 17-21.** The conjoined adductor tendon in the first interspace, prior to tenotomy.

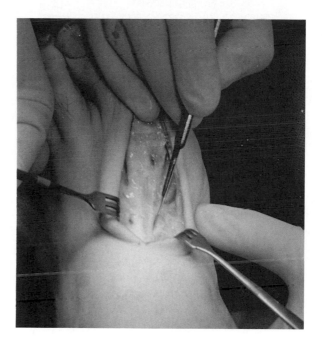

**Fig. 17-23.** The periosteum and capsular tissues being incised by sharp dissection over the base of the first metatarsal.

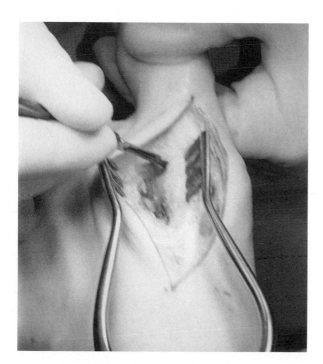

**Fig. 17-22.** Sharp lateral capsulotomy.

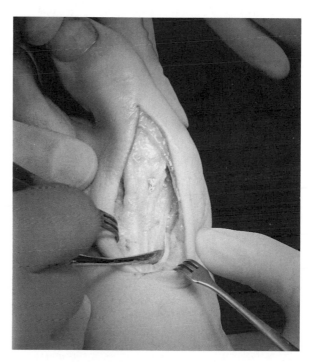

**Fig. 17-24.** Periosteal stripping via Freer elevator in preparation for base osteotomy.

## CLOSING ABDUCTORY BASE WEDGE OSTEOTOMY

### History

The most commonly used base osteotomy is a traditional closing base wedge, first described by Loison in 1901[10] and performed by Balasescu[11] in 1903. The Loison and Balacescu osteotomy was first described as a linear osteotomy at the base of the first metatarsal.

### Surgical Procedure

This osteotomy can be described as a closing abductory base wedge with the apex facing medially and the base directed laterally (Fig. 17-25). Ruch and Banks[13] find it helpful to drive a Kirschner wire (K-wire) perpendicular to the metatarsal shaft where the apex of the wedge should fall (Fig. 17-26). This serves as a guide to ensure preservation of the medial hinge. As pressure is applied to the medial aspect of the first metatarsal head in an attempt to close the intermetatarsal angle, the hinge is "feathered" using the power saw until closure of the osteotomy site is achieved. This is also referred to as reciprocal planing by Patton and Zelichowski.[14] The intermetatarsal angle is corrected, and correction is maintained by rigid internal fixation. The capsule and periosteal tissues are closed over the osteotomy using layer closure (Figure 17-27).

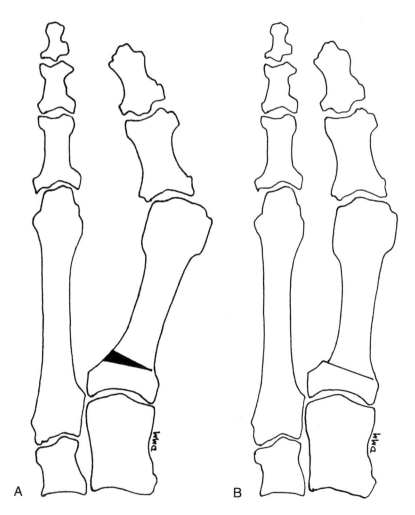

**Fig. 17-25.** (**A**) Diagram demonstrating a closing base wedge abductory osteotomy with section of bone to be removed. (**B**) Completed closing base wedge osteotomy.

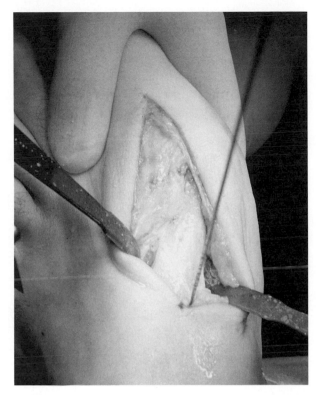

**Fig. 17-26.** Demonstration of the hinge axis concept using hinge axis guide by means of a 0.045 K-wire driven from dorsal to plantar perpendicular to the supporting surface.

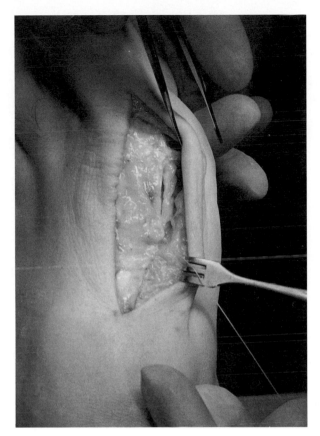

**Fig. 17-27.** Capsule and periosteal closure in a layer fashion using 3-0 vicryl suture.

## OBLIQUE ABDUCTORY BASE WEDGE OSTEOTOMY (JUVARA)

### History

In 1919, Juvara first performed an oblique base wedge osteotomy from proximal medial to distal lateral, angled at approximately 40° to the long axis of the first metatarsal shaft.[15] Originally, the shape of the resected bone was trapezoidal with the medial and lateral cortices transected and the lateral base wider than the medial.[16] Juvara also described a reversed version of his osteotomy in which the wedge ran from proximal lateral to distal medial with a wider base laterally. In the 1970s, the Juvara, which had fallen out of favor because of instability, was revived with the introduction of Arbeitgemeinschaft für Osteosynthesisfragen/American Society of Internal Fixation techniques and the modification of the cut to a true wedge with an intact medial hinge.[14]

### Surgical Procedure

The base wedge should be planned with its medial hinge 1 to 1.5 cm distal to the metatarsal cuneiform articulation. The distal cut is performed at an angle to the long axis of the metatarsal determined by the intermetatarsal correction needed. It must be kept in mind that the proximal cut will be made at approximately 40° to the long axis. The oblique design of the osteotomy not only allows for ease of fixation, but also provides a longer radius arm for rotation of the capital fragment around the hinge axis. This causes greater reduction of the intermetatarsal angle for each degree of rotation.[13] It is suggested that the distal cut be made first so the proximal cut can be made in relatively stable bone, disrupting the hinge as little as possible (Figs. 17-28 to 17-32). The head of the metatarsal is

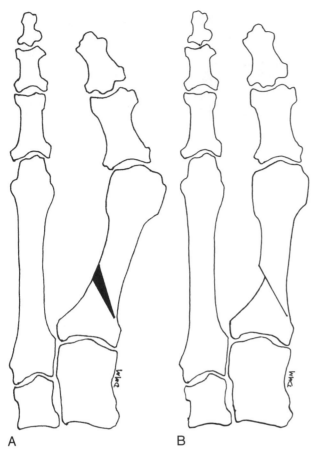

A B

**Fig. 17-28.** (**A**) The Juvara base wedge abductory osteotomy with demonstration of bone to be resected. (**B**) The completed Juvara osteotomy.

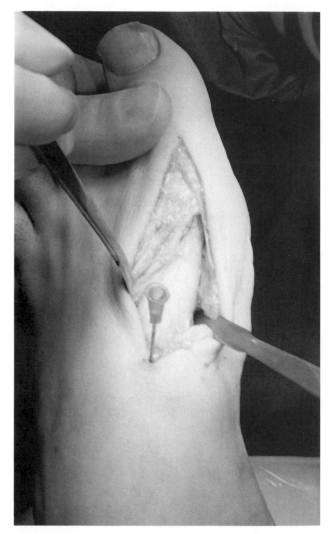

**Fig. 17-29.** Base of the first metatarsal stripped of its periosteal tissue in preparation for osteotomy. Note identification of the first metatarsocuneiform articulation by means of an 18-gauge needle.

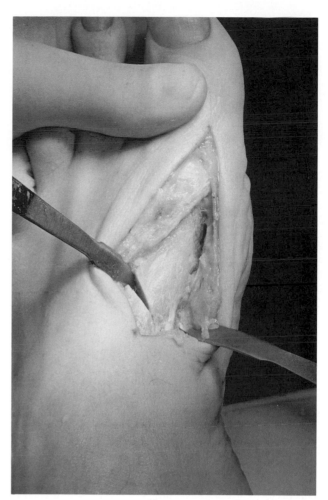

**Fig. 17-31.** The completed Juvara osteotomy before reciprocal planing and feathering of the medial aspect for proper closure.

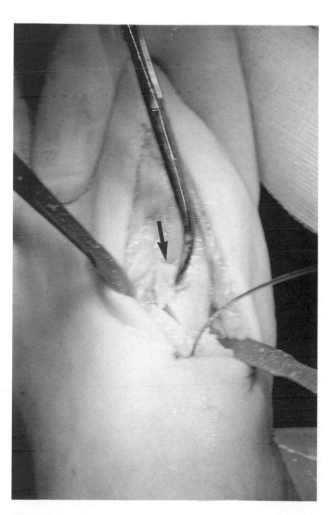

**Fig. 17-30.** The hinge axis guide is in place. The Juvara osteotomy completed, demonstrating the section of bone to be removed (arrow).

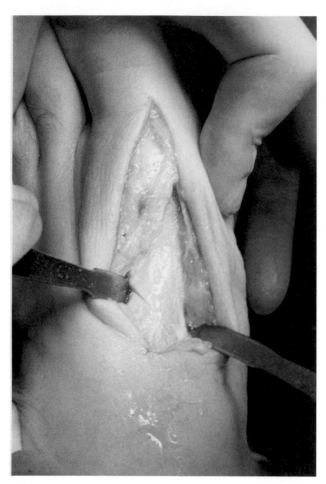

**Fig. 17-32.** The completed Juvara osteotomy with good approximation of the ostetomy site.

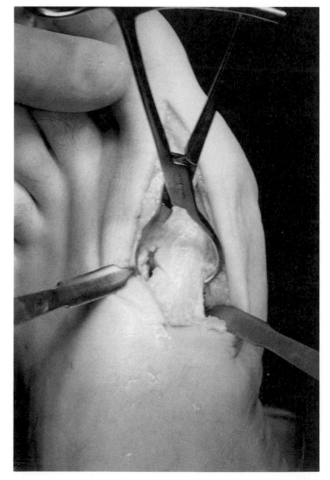

**Fig. 17-33.** Maintenance of closure of the IM angle before internal fixation by means of bone clamp.

moved laterally, and the intermetatarsal angle is closed. A bone clamp is then used to stabilize the osteotomy site while it is fixated (Fig. 17-33). The choice of fixation technique is left to the surgeon; however, we strongly recommend screw fixation. As a rule, one screw is used, but a rule of thumb is that "two screws are better than one." So long as the osteotomy is long enough to allow for the use of two screws without jeopardizing cortical strength, it is preferable to use two screws instead of one. In the case of one screw, if the fixation is lost or fracture of the medial hinge should occur, then rotation and dorsiflexion of the capital fragment may be the result. If,

however, the surgeon is not proficient in AO/ASIF techniques, crossed K-wires are an alternate form of fixation (Fig. 17-34).

## CRESCENTIC/ARCUATE BASE OSTEOTOMY

### History

The development of the arcuate or crescentic saw blade lead to the development of the crescentic base osteotomy. The advantages of this osteotomy include the fact that no wedge of bone is removed; thus, it is suitable for use in short first metatarsals (i.e., those in which the first metatarsal is more than 2 mm shorter than the second metatarsal). The proximal and curved nature of the osteotomy cut helps ensure maximum correction of the intermetatarsal angle with a minimal displacement of the osteotomy (Fig. 17-35). The main drawback of this procedure has been its inherent instability and difficulty in achieving sufficient fixation; thus, it has not been widely used.

### Surgical Procedure

Mercado[17] and Patton and Zelichowski[14] all recommended making a longitudinal score in the metatarsal shaft at the level of the proposed osteotomy. This is referred to as a "register mark," and shows subsequent displacement of the metatarsal shaft (Fig. 17-36). The size of the crescentic blade is chosen according to the width of the first metatarsal shaft. This is essential, because these blades must be kept perpendicular to the shaft and cannot be torqued or they will break. The osteotomy is made so the apex of the arc faces proximally. Mercado[17] suggested that care must be taken so that the plantar cortex remains intact, whereas most other authors recommend transecting the plantar cortex completely.[14] Lateral pressure is then applied to the medial aspect of the first metatarsal head, closing the IM angle. The register mark should only move a couple of millimeters to prevent overcorrection of the IM angle.

Fixation of crescentic osteotomies is notoriously difficult. Keeping the plantar cortex intact, although difficult, helps to stabilize the osteotomy, but excessive motion with resultant malunions or nonunions is common. We recommend crossed K-wires as the fixa-

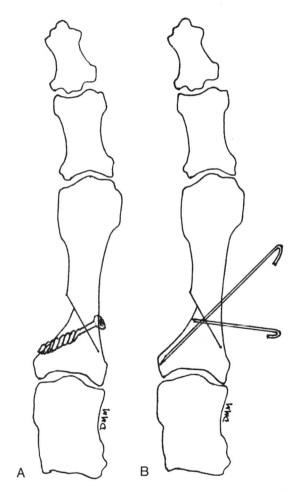

**Fig. 17-34.** Diagram demonstrating internal fixation of the Juvara osteotomy. (**A**) A single Lag screw is used. (**B**) Alternative use of crossed 0.062 K-wires.

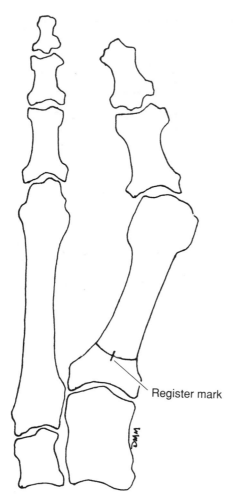

**Fig. 17-35.** Placement of the crescentic base osteotomy. Note the register mark.

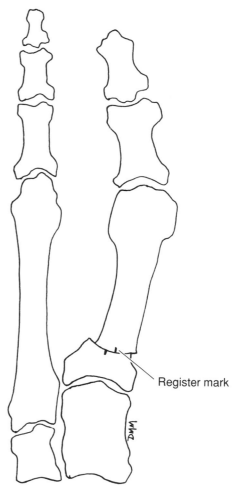

**Fig. 17-36.** Completion of the crescentic osteotomy with lateral displacement of head and medial displacement of register mark.

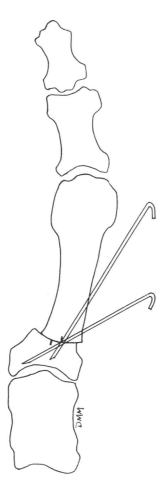

**Fig. 17-37.** The completed crescentic osteotomy stabilized by crossed K-wires.

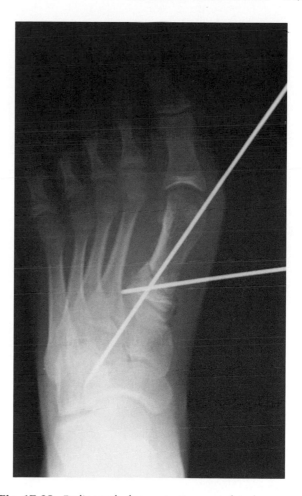

**Fig. 17-38.** Radiograph demonstrating completed crescentic base osteotomy fixated by crossed K-wire technique.

tion method of choice, or the use of a single screw (Figs. 17-37 and 17-38).

# OPENING BASE WEDGE OSTEOTOMY

## History

The original opening base wedge osteotomy was described by Trethowan in 1923.[18] The most common modification was that performed by Stamm in 1957.[16] Trethowan's technique is best described as an opening wedge on the tibial side of the first metatarsal base. The osteotomy is filled with a portion of bone removed from the hypertrophied medial emminence of the first metatarsal head. Stamm described a similar technique[16] in which he used a graft from the base of the proximal phalanx of the hallux (as in the Keller procedure) to insert into the base osteotomy.

## Surgical Procedure

When an opening base wedge is performed, the apex of the cut faces laterally and the base medially. A bone graft is used to hold open the space that is formed on closure of the IM angle (Fig. 17-39). Stable internal fixation is necessary to allow the graft to remain in place. Although this choice remains with the surgeon, we find that a bone staple is the most effective form of fixation (Fig. 17-40). The staple prongs purchase the

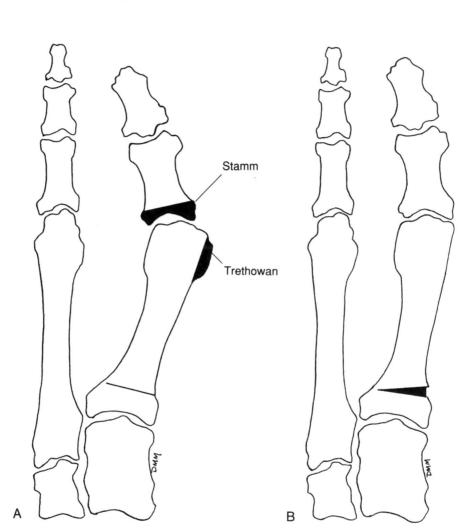

**Fig. 17-39.** (**A**) Opening abductory base wedge osteotomy. This diagram demonstrates proper placement of the osteotomy at 1–1.5 cm distal to the metatarsocuneiform articulation. Note that the bone removed from the hypertrophied medial eminence (Trethowan) or from removal of the base of the proximal phalanx (Stamm) may be used as a bone graft. (**B**) Placement of the bone graft in the opening wedge osteotomy.

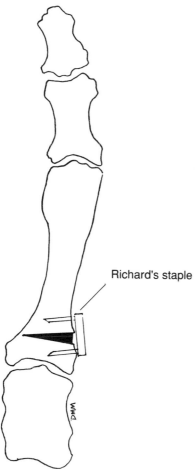

Fig. 17-40. Stabilization of bone graft in an opening wedge osteotomy by means of a Richard's staple.

Richard's staple

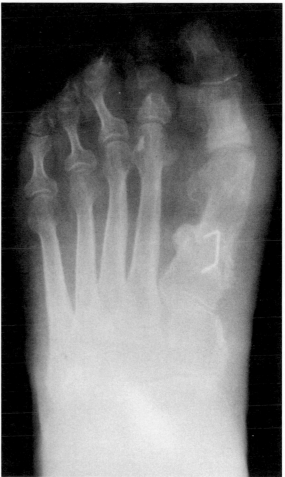

Fig. 17-41. Radiograph demonstrating opening base wedge osteotomy with staple fixation.

medial shaft on either side of the graft, with the body of the staple helping to further stabilize the graft (Fig. 17-41).

## DOUBLE FIRST METATARSAL OSTEOTOMY (LOGROSCINO)

### History

In 1948, in response to a rising number of new surgical procedures for the correction of the hallux valgus deformity, Logroscino recommended a double osteot-omy of the first metatarsal. His initial article described two osteotomies, one at the base and one at the head of the first metatarsal. He used this procedure primarily for the correction of severe inclination of the first metatarsal.[19] Logroscino combined the techniques that had previously been performed by Reverdin (1881), Loison and Balasescu (1902), and Trethowan (1923). The procedure consisted of a distal closing adductory osteotomy as described by Reverdin[20] and a proximal metatarsal osteotomy performed with either a closing abductory wedge osteotomy as described by Loison and Balasescu[10,11] or an opening abductory wedge osteotomy as described by Trethowan.[18]

Reverdin described this technique as a linear resection through the distal portion of the first metatarsal. This procedure is best summed up as removal of a medial closing adductory wedge from the head or the neck of the first metatarsal and resection of the medial eminence. Logroscino identified two types of osteotomies performed at the base of the first metatarsal, the closing abductory wedge osteotomy and the opening abductory wedge osteotomy. The choice of procedure is made by the surgeon on the basis of careful evaluation of the length of the first metatarsal and the metatarsal protrusion measurement. The closing or opening base wedge portions of the procedure were described previously in this chapter.

Joshua Gerbert[21] advocated the use of the Logroscino technique when a bicorrectional Austin would not correct a very high IM angle, or in the case of an abnormally long or short first metatarsal. Kelikian[22] states that he fails to see the advantage of the Logroscino procedure. In his opinion, it creates unnecessary problems in maintenance of position, and prolongs convalescence while increasing surgical trauma. In

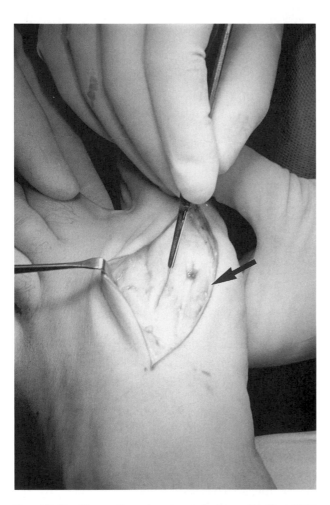

**Fig. 17-42.** Sharp dissection is made into the first MTPJ capsule. Care is taken to avoid the proper digital branch of the medial dorsal cutaneous nerve (arrow).

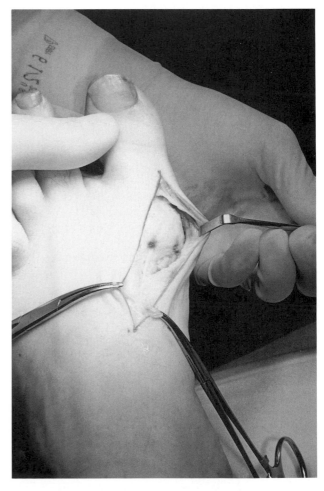

**Fig. 17-43.** Lenticular capsulotomy of first MTPJ with exposure of the hypertrophied medial eminence.

1971, however, Weil and Smith[23] reported excellent results with the Logroscino procedure.

## Surgical Procedure

The incisional approach to the Logroscino double osteotomy is identical to that for other base osteotomies, as discussed earlier. With the Logroscino, however, dissection must be carried out at the level of the first

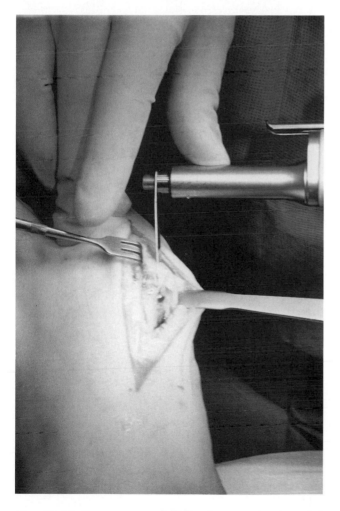

**Fig. 17-44.** Power removal of the hypertrophied medial eminence in line with the sagittal groove.

metatarsal phlangeal joint (MTPJ) as well, to accommodate the distal osteotomy.

The subcutaneous tissues at the level of the MTPJ are divided by sharp and blunt means. The scalpel can be used for both sharp and blunt dissection. Blunt dissection is performed by turning the cutting edge of the blade on an angle toward the capsular tissue. This allows the surgeon to push away the soft tissue with the back end of the scalpel with only a partial exposure of the capsule and soft tissue interface to the cutting edge of the blade. As always, care is taken to avoid neurovascular structures, especially the proper digital branch of the common peroneal nerve (Fig. 17-42). The capsule is entered and reflected from the first metatarsal head dorsally, medially, and plantarly. The choice of capsulotomy (i.e., L-shaped, lenticular, Washington Monument, etc.) rests with the surgeon (Fig. 17-43).

Extensor hallucis brevis tenotomy and lateral capsulotomy are performed in the first interspace (see Figs. 17-16 to 17-24). We do not recommend fibular sesamoidectomy, because a base wedge osteotomy is being performed and the risk of a hallux varus increases with overzealous closure of the IM angle. The medial eminence is resected parallel to the sagittal groove, leaving a slightly wider plantar medial shelf (Fig. 17-44).

We recommend that the base wedge osteotomy be performed first. We strongly believe that closure of the IM angle effectively increases the PASA measurement. Care must of course be taken to ensure that the base osteotomy remains stable while the distal first metatarsal cuts are made. Attention is then redirected to the head of the first metatarsal, where a Reverdin-type procedure, a closing adductory wedge osteotomy, is performed. The apex of this osteotomy faces laterally and the base medially. There are several famous modifications of the original Reverdin, including but not limited to Green's distal L procedure, Laird's, and Todd's; however, in conjunction with the base osteotomy, the simple Reverdin procedure will suffice. On completion of the Reverdin, fixation is once again utilized to maintain the osteotomy position. An opening or closing base wedge osteotomy is then performed to complete the double osteotomy procedure (Fig. 17-45).

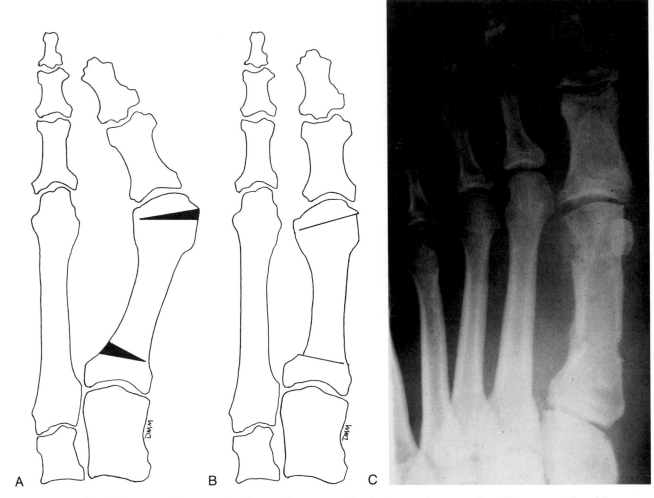

**Fig. 17-45.** (**A**) Diagram demonstrating bone to be resected for the Logroscino procedure. Note correction of the high IM angle as well as abnormal proximal articular set angle. (**B**) The completed Logroscino procedure. (**C**) Radiograph demonstrating the Logroscino double osteotomy.

## GOLDEN BASE OSTEOTOMY WITH DISTAL SOFT TISSUE RELEASE

### History

The Golden osteotomy was designed in 1961 to be used when there was a high IM angle but the PASA did not warrant the marked correction produced by the Logroscino. This procedure is not commonly used in its original form, because of the technical difficulty in making the osteotomy cuts and the inherent instability.[16]

## Surgical Procedure

Golden originally described his base wedge as similar to Roux's, Peabody's, or Mitchell's[16]; that is, a trapezoidal abductory wedge, the base of which faced laterally, the apex medially. A lateral ledge of bone was preserved to provide additional stability. Both the medial and lateral cortices were transected, thus causing stability problems (Fig. 17-46). Distally, Golden performed a resection of the hypertrophied medial eminence and the release of the adductor hallucis tendon laterally. As was discussed earlier, this procedure is

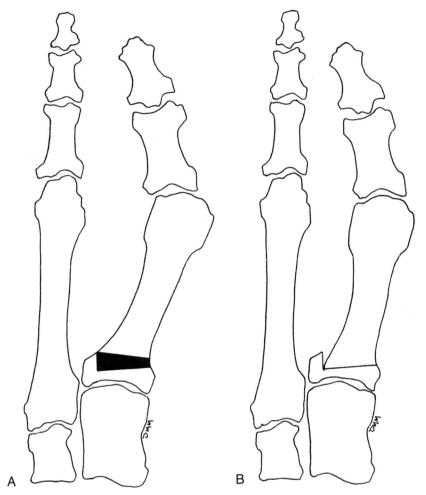

**Fig. 17-46.** (**A**) Bone to be removed in a Golden trapezoidal abductory wedge osteotomy of base of first metatarsal. (**B**) The completed Golden trapezoidal osteotomy.

not very popular because the proximal osteotomy is not stable.

## LUDLOFF AND MAU

### History

In 1918 Ludloff proposed an oblique osteotomy of the first metatarsal shaft from dorsal proximal to plantar distal for the correction of metatarsus primus varus. This procedure was revised by Mau in 1926 to course from dorsal distal to plantar proximal to prevent some of the dorsiflexion of the capital fragment experienced with the Ludloff version.[24,25]

Modern AO/ASIF fixation methods have revived interest in the Mau osteotomy; however, the midshaft location of the osteotomy in diaphyseal bone causes healing concerns.

### Surgical Procedure

The incision used for the Mau is similar to those for base osteotomies, but may be slightly more medially

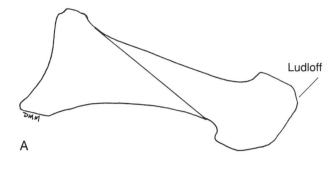

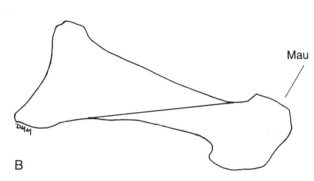

**Fig. 17-47.** The Ludloff and Mau procedures, oblique osteotomies of the first metatarsal shaft. (**A**) Ludloff performed the osteotomy from dorsal proximal to plantar distal. (**B**) Mau made the oblique osteotomy from dorsal distal to plantar proximal.

placed. The main difference, and one of the drawbacks of this procedure, is the denuding of periosteum on the metatarsal shaft medially along almost its entire length. The periosteum must be reflected to provide exposure for the osteotomy. Care should be taken to preserve the periosteal attachments at the plantar proximal and dorsal distal aspects of the metatarsal to help stabilize the resultant osteotomy.

The osteotomy is cut through both cortices from medial to lateral along an oblique line (Fig. 17-47). Once the osteotomy is complete, Patton and Zelichowski[14] recommend using a K-wire as the "axis guide." Driven from dorsal to plantar perpendicular to the metatarsal shaft, the wire acts as a pivot point while

the metatarsal head is shifted laterally to reduce the IM angle (see Fig. 17-26). Once the intermetatarsal angle has been sufficiently reduced, a bone clamp is used to preserve the correction while two screws are inserted to provide rigid internal fixation.

## V-TYPE BASE OSTEOTOMY (KOTZENBERG AND LENOX BAKER)

### History

Both the Kotzenberg (1929) and the Lenox Baker (1953) base osteotomies employed V-shaped cuts. Kotzenberg's V was located in the medial face of the metatarsal and the Lenox Baker was located in the dorsal face of the metatarsal. Neither of these procedures is widely employed today; they are presented mainly for historical purposes.

### Surgical Procedure

In the Kotzenberg procedure, a V-shaped through-and-through osteotomy is made from medial to lateral with its apex proximal and its wings at a 45° angle (Fig. 17-48). The distal fragment is then shifted laterally and impacted on the base. This corrects the IM angle. Fixation is attained using K-wires. This is a fairly stable osteotomy and may well deserve to be more widely utilized. It also has the potential, like the distal Austin, for biplaning to help correct an abnormal PASA.

The Lenox-Baker procedure is approached dorsally and involves a V-shaped through-and-through osteotomy from dorsal to plantar with its apex distal and wings at a 45° angle. A second, more proximal cut is then made on the lateral side at 60° to the long axis of the first metatarsal. The bone wedge that is subsequently removed is used as a graft in the medial cut. As the metatarsal head is shifted laterally, closing the intermetatarsal angle, the medial cut opens, allowing insertion of the graft.[26] The osteotomy and graft must then be fixated. We would recommend the K-wire and bone staple combination. As may be suspected, this osteotomy is technically difficult to perform and control and even more difficult to properly fixate, which explains its infrequent use (Fig. 17-49).

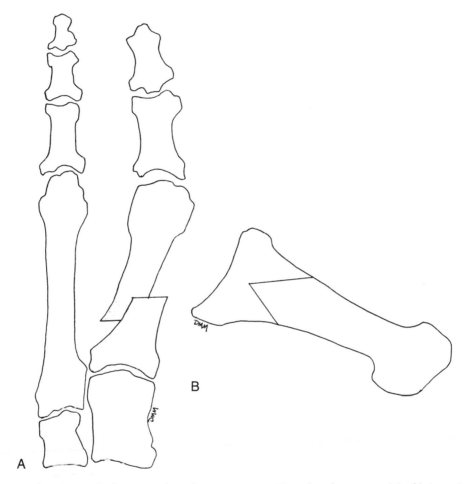

**Fig. 17-48.** (**A & B**) The Kotzenberg base osteotomy. Note the placement of the V-shaped cuts.

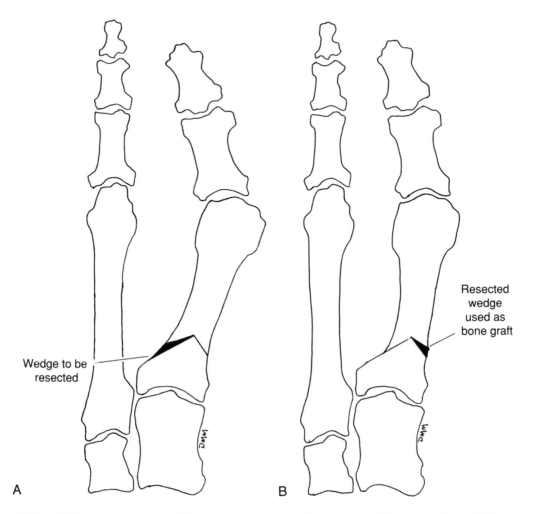

**Fig. 17-49.** (**A**) Proper placement of the base osteotomy cuts in the Lenox-Baker procedure. (**B**) Completion of the Lenox-Baker osteotomy. Note that the wedge removed from the lateral aspect of the first metatarsal (Fig. A) is used as a bone graft in the medial aspect of the osteotomy cut on completion.

## PEG-AND-HOLE BASE OSTEOTOMY (ROCYN JONES)

### History

In 1948, Rocyn Jones suggested a proximal first metatarsal peg-and-hole type procedure for the correction of metatarsus primus varus in adolescents.[16] This procedure is also provided for historical purposes because it is technically difficult to perform and commonly fails. This makes it a poor choice in light of the success achieved with other methods.

### Procedure

This base osteotomy is approached dorsally. An oblique osteotomy is performed from proximal lateral to distal medial at an angle of 40° to 45° from the long axis of the first metatarsal. A second "wedge" is then cut in the distal fragment. The wedge only encompasses the medial two-thirds of the width of the metatarsal, leaving a lateral "peg." The peg is then impacted into the proximal fragment, allowing proper closure of the IM angle.[27]

This osteotomy is obviously difficult to fixate and prone to instability, fracture, and failure. We cannot recommend this procedure, and included it merely for completeness (Fig. 17-50).

## Fixation

In all cases, the choice of fixation for the base and head osteotomies rests with the surgeon. Options include bone staples, K-wires, Steinman pins, monofilament stainless steel wire, screw fixation with or without the use of plates following the AO/ASIF techniques, and casting, among others.

Staples are favored by the authors for their stability and ease of installation, although size must be carefully chosen to prevent fracture of the bone edges and loss of purchase (Fig. 17-51A).

K-wires and Steinmann pins, although easy to install, can have some drawbacks. When using pins, it is preferable to use a crossed K-wire technique to guard against rotation/dorsiflexion of the capital fragment, should fracture of the cortical hinge occur. K-wires or Steinmann pins, in conjunction with staples or screws, provide a good alternative (Fig. 17-51B to D).

Monofilament stainless steel wire can be used in a four-cortex or box technique. A figure of eight or ten-

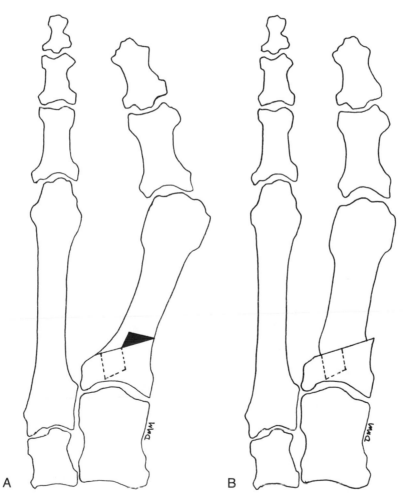

A    B

**Fig. 17-50.** (**A**) The Rocyn-Jones peg-and-hole base osteotomy. (**B**) The completed peg-and-hole base osteotomy.

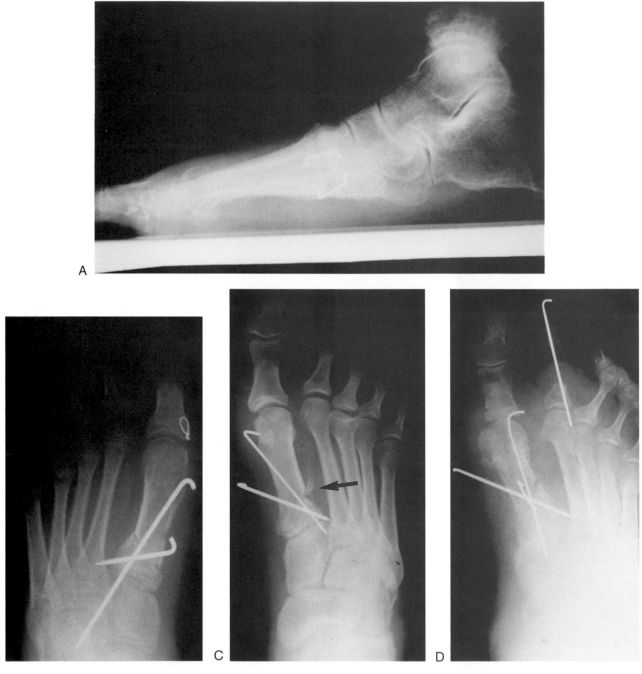

**Fig. 17-51.** (**A**) Radiograph demonstrating staple fixation of a first metatarsal base osteotomy. (**B**) Two 0.062 K-wires in a crossed fashion, securing a first metatarsal base wedge osteotomy. (**C**) Note the crossed K-wires in the closing base abductory osteotomy. Also note the bony fragment in the first interspace, demonstrating a portion of the wedge of bone that was not removed during the osteotomy. Arrow indicates loose bony body after wedge resection. (**D**) Combination of crossed K-wire and staple fixation.

sion technique has been utilized as well (Fig. 17-52). However, if the metal fails or the "knot" slips, fixation is lost. We have used screw or plate fixation with success; however, it is the most technically demanding option and requires previous experience and success with A/O fixation methods (Figs. 17-53 to 17-59).

Casting alone is not recommended as a fixation option, although we do recommend it strongly as an adjunct to internal fixation. Postoperatively, the patient should be placed in a non-weight-bearing short leg cast following a base osteotomy for a total of 6 to 8 weeks of immobilization.

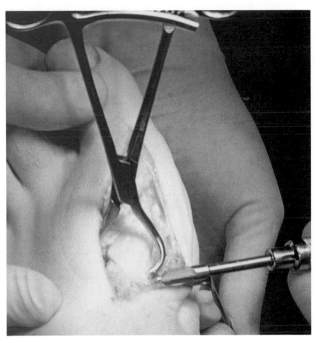

**Fig. 17-53.** The completed Juvara base wedge osteotomy, held in place by a bone clamp. A 2.0-mm drill hole has been placed perpendicular to the osteotomy site; a countersink is now being used to allow for proper positioning of the head of the 4.0 cancellous bone screw.

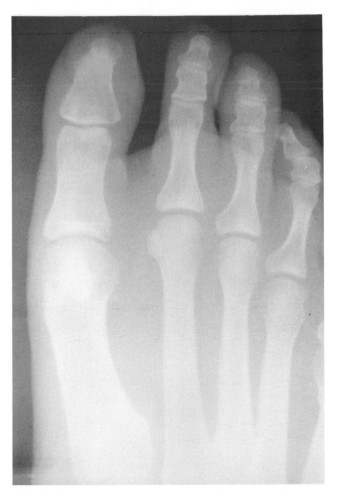

**Fig. 17-52.** Radiograph shows monofilament wire fixation following base osteotomy.

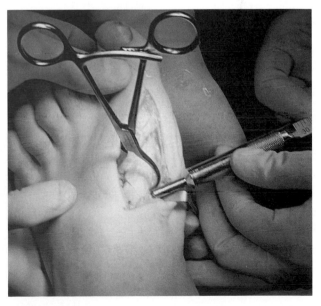

**Fig. 17-54.** A depth gauge used to identify proper length of the cancellous bone screw.

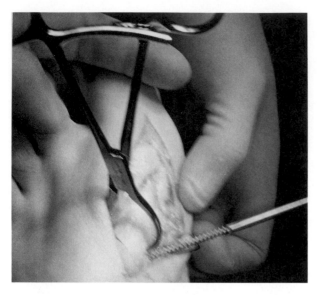

**Fig. 17-55.** A 3.5 tap cutting the proper grooves for placement of the cancellous bone screw.

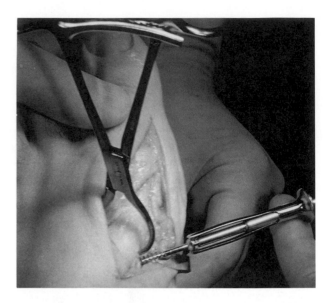

**Fig. 17-56.** A 4.0 cancellous (lag) screw being placed perpendicular to osteotomy site.

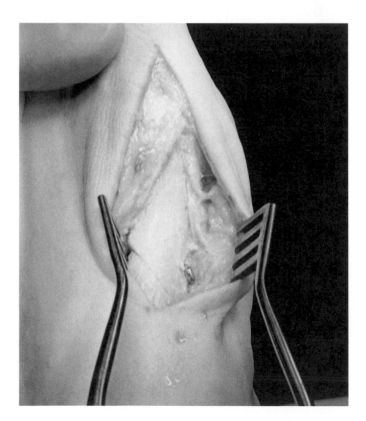

**Fig. 17-57.** Closure of IM angle and proper placement of cancellous bone screw.

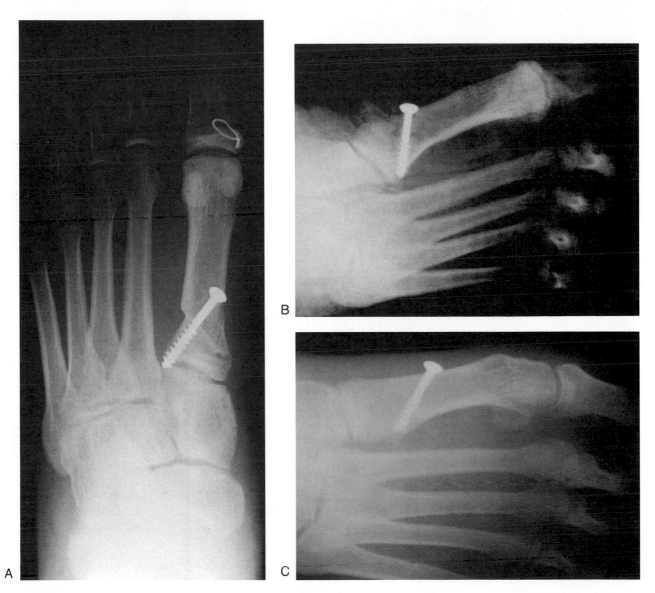

**Fig. 17-58.** (**A–C**). Radiographs demonstrating closure of IM angle following Juvara base osteotomy, using 4.0 cancellous bone screw.

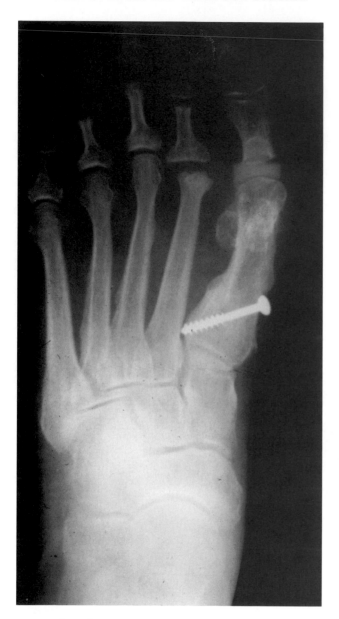

**Fig. 17-59.** Closure of the abductory base osteotomy with screw fixation in conjunction with a hemi-implant, joint-destructive procedure at the first MTPJ.

## Complications

Complications of any of the base procedures include hallux varus caused by overzealous reduction in the IM angle (Fig. 17-60). This, along with shortening of

the first metatarsal, causes a decrease in the abductory force on the hallux by the extensor hallucis longus tendon. Therefore, the lower the postoperative IM angle, the more prone the hallux will be to drift medially. Dorsiflexion of the metatarsal head is usually caused by too much bone being removed dorsally compared to plantarly when preparing the wedge in a base wedge osteotomy. Care must also be taken in placement of the osteotomy; placement too distally in the shaft adversely affects healing, but too proximally could interfere with the metatarsocuneiform articulation.

The major complication in base osteotomies is shortening of the first metatarsal. This can lead to

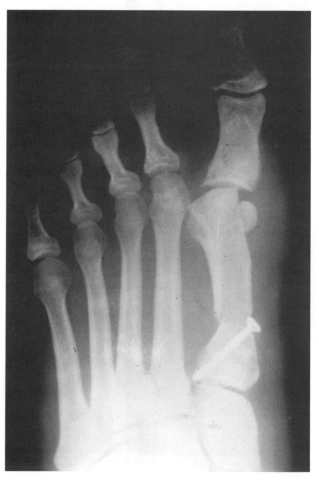

**Fig. 17-60.** Overzealous correction of IM angle. Complete fibular sesamoidectomy resulted in hallux varus deformity.

many subsequent problems such as lesser metatarsalgia, transfer lesions, stress fractures of the lesser metatarsals, and decreased propulsive force in toe-off (called Morton's Foot syndrome). These problems often stem more from elevatus of the capital fragment than from the position or shape of the wedge resected (Fig. 17-61).

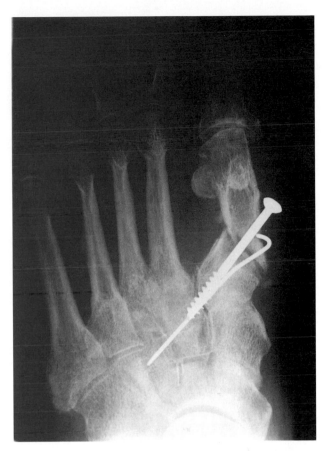

**Fig. 17-62.** Improper fixation of a base osteotomy, resulting in non-union.

As in any surgical procedure involving osteotomies, malunion or nonunion is always a possibility. This is best prevented by rigid internal fixation and external casting for the prescribed period of time (Fig. 17-62).

## SUMMARY

Various base osteotomies have been presented in this chapter, from those used most often to those presented only for the sake of history and completeness. To review our guidelines for selecting procedures, an intermetatarsal angle (IM) greater than 12° in an adductus foot or 15° in a rectus foot calls for a base osteotomy. If the IM angle is greater than 22°, we suggest a Lapidus procedure. When an abnormal PASA is also involved with a high intermetatarsal angle, a head

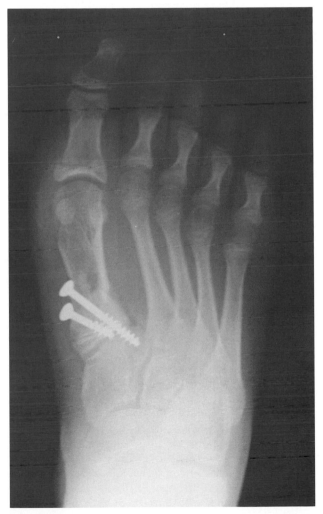

**Fig. 17-61.** Improper placement of cancellous bone screws. Note the proximal screw is placed at the wrong angle to the osteotomy site, necessitating a second screw. Note also the excessive length of the distal screw and its entrance into the metatarsocuneiform joint.

procedure should be used in conjunction with a base osteotomy (Logroscino, Golden). A biplane, base, V-osteotomy may also be considered (Kotzenberg).

Metatarsal protrusion measurements must be taken into consideration before choosing a procedure. If the first metatarsal is within 2 mm of the length of the second metatarsal, a closing base wedge osteotomy (Loison and Balasescu, Juvara) can be employed. If the first metatarsal is shorter than the second by more than 2 mm, an opening base wedge osteotomy (Trethowan, Stamm), crescentic, or V-type base osteotomy is appropriate.

Ease and stability of fixation must also be taken into consideration when choosing a surgical procedure. The final choices and decisions are the responsibilities of the surgeon. Careful preoperative planning, intraoperative technique, and postoperative management should yield satisfying results. Remember, surgery is both a science and an art—do not fear being an artist.

# REFERENCES

1. Gerbert J: The indications and techniques for utilizing pre-operative templates in podiatric surgery. J Am Podiatry Assoc 69(2):139, 1979
2. Inman VT: Hallux valgus: a review of etiologic factors. Orthop Clin North Am 5:5, 1974
3. Root ML, Orien WP, Weed H: Forefoot deformity caused by abnormal sub-talar joint pronation in normal and abnormal function of the foot. p. 349. In Clinical Biomechanics, Vol. 2. Clinical Biomechanics Corp., Los Angeles, 1977
4. Hardy RH, Clapham JCR: Observations on hallux valgus. J Bone J Surg Br 33:376, 1951
5. Haas M: Radiographic and biomechanical considerations of bunion surgery. p. 23. In Gerbert J (ed): Textbook of Bunion Surgery. Futura, Mt. Kisco, NY, 1981
6. Gudas CJ, Marcinko DE: The complex deformity known as hallux abducto valgus. In Marcinko DE (ed): Comprehensive Textbook of Hallux Abducto Valgus Reconstruction. Mosby, St. Louis, 1992
7. Amarnek DL, Mollica A, Jacobs AM, Oloff LM: A statistical analysis of the reliability of the proximal articular set angle. J Foot Surg 25:39, 1986
8. Gerbert J, Spector E, LaPorta G: A preliminary report on arthrography of the first metatarso-phalangeal joint. Arch Podiatr Med Surg 1:75, 1973
9. Sharpe DA: Double first metatarsal osteotomy for a particular type of hallux abducto valgus deformity. Arch Podiatr Med Foot Surg 1:262, 1974
10. Loison M: Note sur le traitement chirurgicale du hallux valgus d'apres l'etude radiographique de la deformation. Bull Mem Soc Chir Paris 27:528, 1901
11. Balasescu J: Un caz de hallux valgus simetric. Rev Chir 7:128, 1903
12. Gamble FO, Yale I: Clinical Foot Roentgenology, 2nd Ed. Krieger, Melbourne, FL, 1975
13. Ruch J, Banks A: Proximal osteotomies of the first metatarsal in the correction of hallux abducto valgus. In McGlamry ED (ed): Comprehensive Textbook of Foot Surgery, Vol. 1. Williams & Wilkins, Baltimore, 1987
14. Patton GW, Zelichowski JE: Proximal osteotomies for correction of hallux abducto valgus with metatarsus primus adductus deformity. In Marcinko DE (ed): Comprehensive Textbook of Hallux Abducto Valgus Reconstruction. CV Mosby, St. Louis, 1992
15. Juvara E: Cure radicale de l'hallux valgus par la resection cuneiforme de la portion moyenne de la diaphyse du metatarsien, suivie de l'osteosynthese des fragments. Lyon Chir 23:429, 1926
16. Kelikian H: Hallux Valgus, Allied Deformities of the Forefoot and Metatarsalgia WB Saunders, Philadelphia, 1965
17. Mercado OA: An Atlas of Foot Surgery, Vol. 1, Forefoot Surgery. Carolando Press, Oak Park, IL, 1979
18. Trethowan J: Hallux valgus. In Choyce AL (ed): System of Surgery. Hoeber, New York, 1923
19. Logroscino D: Il trattamento chirurgico dell'alluce valgus. Chir Organi Mov 32:81, 1948
20. Reverdin J: Anatomie et operation de l'hallux valgus. Int Med Congr 2:408, 1881
21. Gerbert J: Double first metatarsal osteotomy. p. 265. In Gerbert J (ed): Textbook of Bunion Surgery. Futura, Mt. Kisco, NY, 1981
22. Kelikian H: Osteotomy. p. 163. In Kelikian H (ed): Hallux Valgus, Allied Deformities of the Forefoot and Metatarsalgia. WB Saunders, Philadelphia, 1965
23. Weil LS, Smith S: Northlake Surgical Seminar. Chicago, Oct 1971. Symposia Specialists, New York, 1972
24. Ludloff K: Die besetigung des hallux valgus durch die schraege planto-dorsale osteotomie des metatarsus 1 (erfahrungen und erfolge). Arch Klin Chir 110:364, 1918
25. Mau C, Lauber HT: Die operative behandlung des hallux valgus (nachtuntersuchungen). Dtsch Z Chir 197:363, 1926
26. Baker LD: Diseases of the foot. Am Acad Orthop Surgeons 10:327, 1953
27. Jones AR: Hallux valgus in the adolescent. Proc R Soc Med 41:392, 1948

# 18

# Arthrodeses of the First Metatarsophalangeal Joint

*DOMENICK A. CALISE*
*PRAYA MAM*
*VINCENT J. HETHERINGTON*

A versatile procedure in the armamentarium of the foot surgeon is arthrodesis of the first metatarsophalangeal joint. Considering the large number of indications for metatarsophalangeal joint fusion, there are relatively few contraindications. Since Clutton[1] first described fusion of the first metatarsophalangeal joint, there have been numerous modifications and alterations to the procedure. Advances in fixation technique and in biomechanics have allowed for improved methods of fusion and greater ease of performance. This chapter discusses indications and contraindications for fusion of the first metatarsophalangeal joint. Technical considerations such as surgical approach, position of fusion fixation techniques, and postoperative care are also discussed.

## PREOPERATIVE CONSIDERATIONS

The versatility of first metatarsophalangeal joint (MPJ) fusion is evident in the number of indications that exist for this procedure (Table 18-1). The most commonly cited indications for fusion are hallux valgus and hallux rigidus.[2–11] Other indications include rheumatoid arthritis,[12–18] salvage of failed hallux valgus surgery (including failed Keller procedures),[5,8–10,18–21] posttraumatic arthrosis,[8,11] postosteomyelitis, and sep-

**Table 18-1.** Indications

| |
|---|
| Severe hallux valgus |
| Hallux rigidus |
| Rheumatoid arthritis |
| Salvage of failed surgery |
| Failed Keller procedure |
| Postinfection arthrosis |
| Posttraumatic arthrosis |
| Neuromuscular disease |

tic arthrosis[10] (Fig. 18-1). Stroh and Yee presented the use of first MPJ fusion in cases in which both hallucal sesamoids were fractured and there was a failure of conservative care.[22] First MPJ fusion is the procedure of choice in cerebral palsy patients and others with a hallux valgus deformity from neuromuscular disorders.[8,23–25]

There are relatively few contraindications to MPJ fusion (Table 18-2). The most commonly cited contraindication is preexisting arthrosis of the interphalangeal joint of the hallux.[5–7,11] One must take special precautions preoperatively to inform the patient that there will be no motion present at the great toe and that changes in footwear will be necessary. Because osteoporotic bone may cause difficulty with placement of fixation devices, alternative procedures may be of more benefit to the patient.

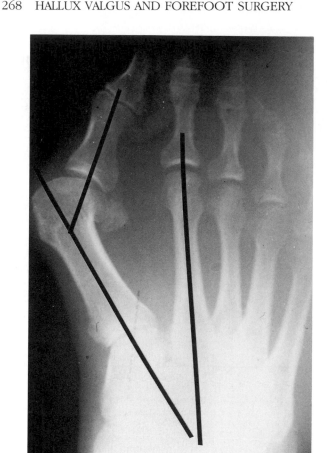
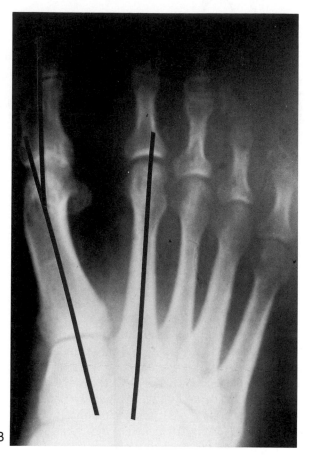

**Fig. 18-1.** Preoperative and postoperative radiographs demonstrating various indications for first MPJ fusion. (**A & B**) Severe hallux valgus. Fig. A: preoperative radiograph; Fig. B: radiograph taken years postoperatively. (*Figure continues.*)

Preoperative evaluation should include a careful radiographic review including anteroposterior (AP), lateral, and oblique views to ensure competence of the hallucal interphalangeal joint. It may be of benefit to construct templates of the planned resection to obtain precise joint resections and optimal alignment. Ginsburg suggests obtaining a lateral radiograph of the foot with the patient wearing a shoe normally used so that the optimal sagittal plane position of the fusion could be determined.[8]

The question of intermetatarsal angle relationships in first MPJ fusion has been raised by Mann and others.[4,10,26–29] The need for ancillary first metatarsal osteotomy has been presented by relatively few authors.[28–31] It has been noted that the stability of the fusion in addition to the effect of the adductor complex will help to decrease the intermetatarsal angle by approximately 4° to 6°.[4,10,26,27] Mann states that the

**Table 18-2.** Contraindications

Interphalangeal joint arthritis
Osteoporotic bone
Active infection
Noncompliance with shoe wear (high heels)

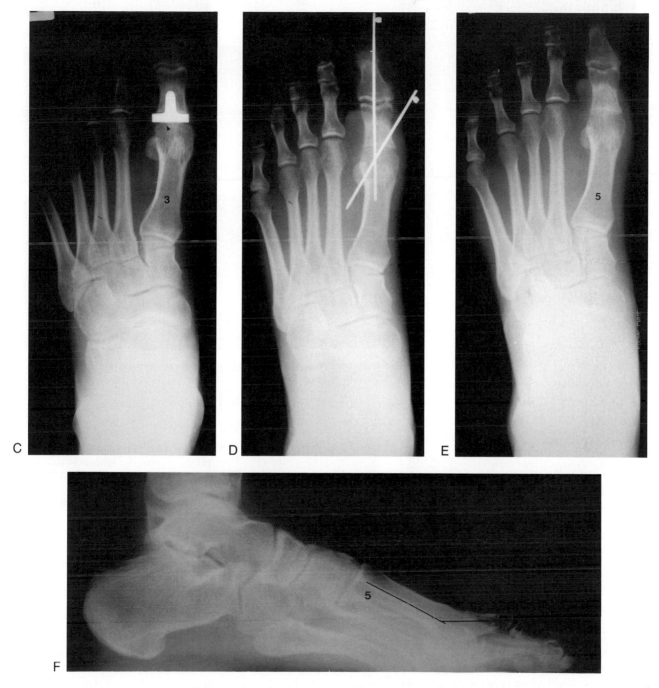

**Fig. 18-1** (*Continued*).  (**C–F**) Salvage of failed implant. Fig. C: preoperative radiograph of a painful first metatarsophalangeal joint postimplant arthroplasty; Fig. D: postoperative radiograph showing K-wire fixation; Figs. E and F: other postoperative views. (*Figure continues.*)

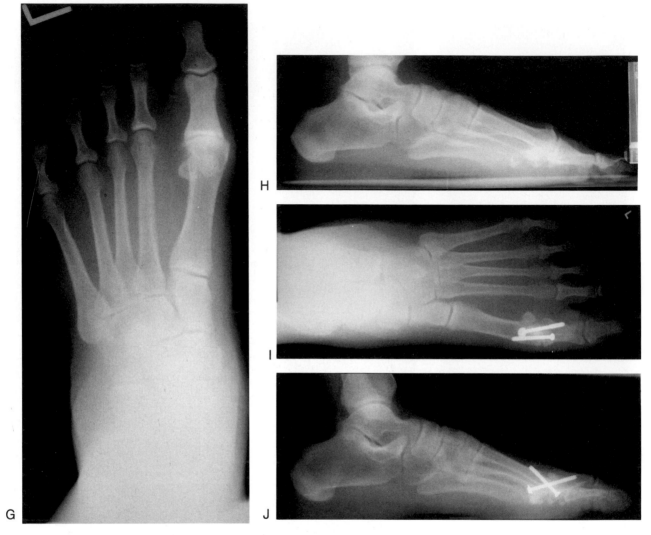

**Fig. 18-1** (*Continued*). (**G–J**) Hallux rigidus. Fig. G: preoperative view; Fig. H: preoperative lateral view (note doasal flag sign); Figs. I and J: postoperative views.

change in the intermetatarsal angle is directly proportional to the preoperative intermetatarsal angle and that concomitant first metatarsal osteotomy is not indicated.[26] Once the hallux is rigidly fused to the metatarsal, the adductor hallucis tendon and lateral soft tissue structures are no longer a deforming force. In fact, the adductor tendon gains mechanical advantage in this situation, and can now function to pull both the meta-

tarsal and the proximal phalanx toward the midline of the foot, which decreases the intermetatarsal angle[4] (Fig. 18-2). Interspace soft tissue dissection is discouraged in this procedure because release of the adductor tendon may lead to increased metatarsal splaying postoperatively. Postoperative splaying of the first metatarsal with a fused MPJ will lead to a hallux varus (Fig. 18-3).

# FUSION POSITION

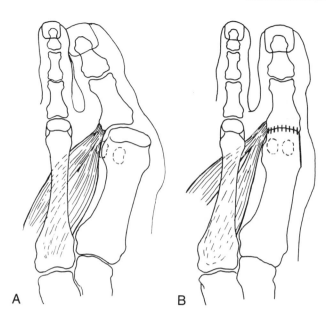

**Fig. 18-2.** Decrease in intermetatarsal angle. (**A & B**) Schematic diagram of role of adductor hallucis in intermetatarsal angle reduction with first MPJ fusion.

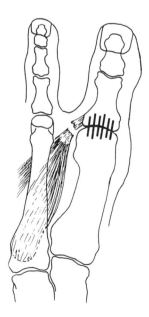

**Fig. 18-3.** Diagram of hallux varus as result of extensive dissection of first intermetatarsal space. Note loss of stabilization with transection of adductor tendon.

The most critical aspect of MPJ fusion is the position of fusion. This key component of the procedure has been a point of great discussion since the inception of MPJ fusion. Although there is today a general consensus of opinion regarding toe position, there have been no randomized, controlled, prospective studies comparing one fusion position to another. Further, there is a paucity of research into the optimal length pattern of the first metatarsal in MPJ fusion. Although Duckworth has supplied research using pedobarographic measurements comparing gait in arthroplasty versus arthrodesis of the first MPJ, there is no statistical comparison of various fusion positions and no mention of metatarsal length patterns.[32–34] These pedobarographic comparisons of first MPJ arthroplasty versus fusion have shown that fusion is more stable than arthroplasty.

Perhaps one of the greatest factors concerning disagreement over fusion position is the question of reference point. Many authors supply varying degrees of valgus and toe dorsiflexion; however, no proper reference point for the particular angle has been given. When discussing the dorsiflexion angle, it is necessary to state whether this measure is taken in relationship to the ground and the hallux or to the metatarsal and the hallux. Further clouding the picture are the questions of metatarsal angulation to the ground and of heel height differences worn by men and women.

For MPJ fusion, we must consider rotation of the hallux in the frontal plane, valgus angulation of the hallux in the transverse plane (more appropriately termed *abduction angle*), and dorsiflexion of the hallux in the sagittal plane (Table 25-3).

Most authors agree that there should be no frontal plane rotation of the hallux.[2–5,9,11,18,30] Rotation of the hallux will result in undue pressure along either nail border, keratosis along a prominent medial or lateral condyle, or increased weight-bearing stress through the interphalangeal joint. Intraoperatively, the surgeon should use the nail plate as a guide to the degree of rotation present at the hallux.

Positioning of the hallux in the transverse plane (valgus angulation) should be such that the hallux appears to sit in natural alignment with the lesser toes. The patient should be made aware preoperatively that the great toe will not be "straight." An excessively rec-

**Table 18-3.** Fusion Position Summary

| Sagittal | 10°–15° | Dorsiflexion |
|---|---|---|
| Transverse | 15°–25° | Abduction |
| Frontal | 0° | Rotation |

tus transverse plane alignment could cause problems with shoe fit and increased stress across the interphalangeal joint. Care should be taken when determining valgus position so as to not cause impingement between the first and second toe, which could lead to painful interdigital corn formation. General consensus regarding valgus angulation of the hallux has yet to be determined; from 5° to 30° of valgus have been proposed as a suitable transverse plane angulation.[2–7,9–11,16,18,20,30] Fitzgerald, in a long-term follow-up study, noted that in cases in which the MPJ was fused in less than 20° of valgus the incidence of postoperative degenerative changes at the interphalangeal joint of the hallux was three times greater than those fused in excess of 20° of valgus.[6] Smith noted that rheumatoid patients could tolerate a greater degree of valgus because of the laterally deviated position of the lesser toes with less possibility of the first and second toes impinging on each other. Smith went on to recommend that rheumatoid patients could be fused in 25° to 30° of valgus.[18] In general, the hallux should be placed in 15° to 25° of valgus and in line with the lesser toes.

The final plane that needs to be addressed is the sagittal plane or dorsiflexion angle. Various authors have proposed values from 0° to 40° of hallux dorsiflexion.[2–5,9,11,18,30,35–37] These values can be somewhat misleading in that a plane of reference is not given. In determining dorsiflexion angles of the hallux in relationship to the horizontal surface of the ground, there may be difficulty in duplicating this angle in a non-weight-bearing foot on the operating room table. The first metatarsal forms a much better point of reference for measurement of the dorsiflexion angle. To properly position the hallux in the sagittal plane, preoperative measurements on weight-bearing radiographs are of the utmost importance. The relationship of the hallux to the first metatarsal and the first metatarsal to the ground can be determined on the lateral view. According to Ginsburg, an extra measure of accuracy can be achieved by obtaining a lateral weight-bearing radiograph while the patient is wearing a shoe with the preferred heel height[8] (Fig. 18-4).

The first metatarsal is usually angulated 15° to the ground (first metatarsal declination angle), which would translate to the hallux being angled 15° to the first metatarsal on stance. Most authors agree that 10° of dorsiflexion of the hallux above the horizontal plane is sufficient for pain-free ambulation.[9,18,30] If the usual first metatarsal declination angle of 15° is added

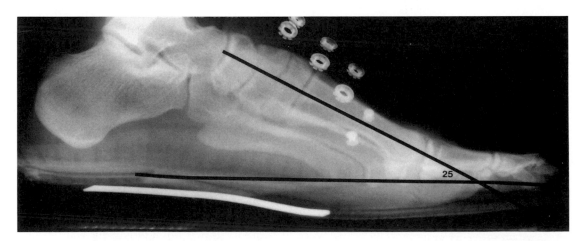

**Fig. 18-4.** Preoperative lateral radiograph with patient wearing a shoe. Note first metatarsal declination angle that will be the frame of reference for determining the sagittal plane position of fusion intraoperatively.

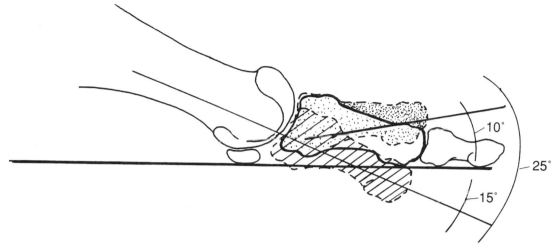

**Fig. 18-5.** Determination of hallux sagittal plane positioning; 10°, hallux dorsiflexion angle; 15°, preoperatively measured first metatarsal declination angle; 25°, angle of fusion between hallux and metatarsal. The hallux dorsiflexion angle should not exceed 15°.

to the recommended 10° of dorsiflexion above the horizontal, a hallux to first metatarsal dorsiflexion angle of 25° results (Fig. 18-5). This angle can easily be measured intraoperatively with a sterile goniometer (Fig. 18-6). A great toe that is fused in less than 10° of dorsiflexion above the horizontal will subject the pa-

tient to pain at the distal tip of the toe and increase stress at the interphalangeal joint of the hallux. Insufficient dorsiflexion will also lead to excess callus formation at the plantar aspect of the hallucal interphalangeal joint. Dorsiflexion angles greater than 15° above the horizontal will cause excessive retrograde pres-

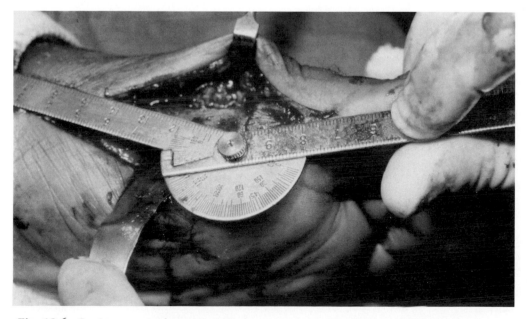

**Fig. 18-6.** Goniometer used intraoperatively to ensure precise position of first MPJ fusion.

sure on the metatarsal head, which will lead to excessive callus formation and pain beneath the first metatarsal[2,6,10] (Fig. 18-7). In summary, the hallux should be fused 10° to 15° above the horizontal; this value should be added to the preoperatively measured metatarsal declination angle to allow for accurate positioning of the hallux on the metatarsal in the sagittal plane.

To ensure exact positioning of the fusion site, Sullivan[38] has proposed the use of the Reese osteotomy guide (Reese, Peoria, AZ). This instrument allows for the precise placement of a sagitally directed chevron fusion site, which will provide for simple placement of a cancellous screw. Another system allowing exact fusion positioning intraoperatively is the truncated cone reamer device (Biomet Inc., Warsaw, IN). This instrument prepares the fusion site into a perfectly matched peg and hole and allows for proper angular adjustments. Although the system facilitates placement, it is

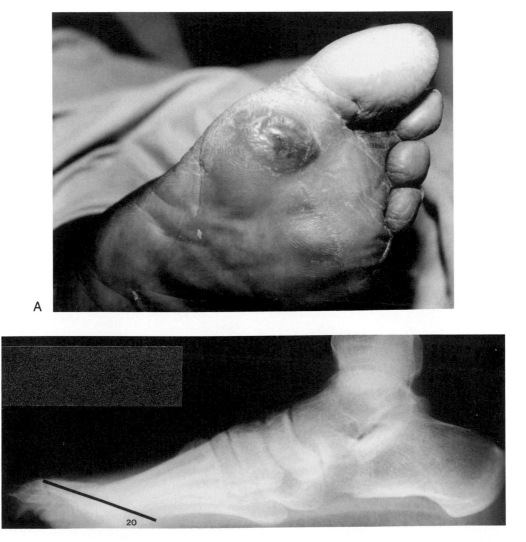

**Fig. 18-7.** Complication of improper sagittal plane positioning of fusion site. (**A**) Sub-first metatarsal tyloma. Note preulcerative appearance of lesion. (**B**) Lateral radiograph of same foot shows excessive dorsiflexion of hallux on first metatarsal.

rather cumbersome in its use, and the instrumentation involved is somewhat complex. Improper use of the truncated cone reamer can lead to severe soft tissue damage.

## FIXATION METHODS

Many different methods of fixation for first MPJ fusion have been proposed.[2,4,7–9,18,30,39–44] McKeever[2] presented the use of screw fixation via a plantarly placed screw running from distal to proximal. Harrison and Harvey[4] proposed the use of a Charnley clamp for fixation. The fixator was left in place for 3 weeks then replaced with a walking cast that completely incorporated the hallux. The cast was left in place for an additional 3 weeks. There have been no other reports to support or refute the use of external fixation devices for first MPJ fusions. Salis-Soglio has discussed the use of the dynamic compression plate applied to the dorsum of the first MPJ for fixation of the fusion site[7]. They made no comment regarding the advantages of this form of fixation.

The use of K-wires and Steinman pins for fixation of MPJ fusion has been supported by many authors.[8,9,18,20,40] The advantages to pin fixation include ease of the procedure, ability to provide stability in porotic bone, and ability to manipulate the fusion site if minor angular changes are necessary. Disadvantages include the possibility of pin tract infection and lack of compression. Wilson has presented the use of the Rush pin as a method of fixating MPJ fusions.[39] The intramedullary Rush nail supplies considerable compressive force across the fusion site, a factor that Wilson states "allows for rapid arthrodesis." Various other methods of fixation have been presented including the use of Herbert screws, wire loop, suture, and combinations of wire and pins.[40–44] The use of cannulated screws is an excellent method of first MPJ fusion which, to our knowledge, has yet to be presented in the literature.

Sykes performed an elaborate biomechanical study using cadaveric specimens to determine the stability of various fixation devices used in first MPJ fusions.[43] He compared cancellous screws used with dome arthrodesis and planar arthrodesis with planar surfaces held by Charnley clamps and various wire constructs. The use of K-wires, Stienman pins, or plate fixation was not investigated. The study concluded that

the best method of fixation was the use of planar surface fusion with a 4.0 cancellous screw; the method of fusion that was second in resistance to load was screw fixation with domed fusion surfaces. The study also noted that the critical component in screw fixation was an intact plantar flange on the proximal phalanx base. Screws were placed from plantar medial distal to dorsal lateral proximal. The head of the screw must impact against the intact plantar flange to obtain sufficient compression across the fusion site.

## SURGICAL PROCEDURE

The surgical approach to the first MPJ is relatively straightforward, consisting of either a dorsomedial or a medial incision. The incision starts at about midshaft on the first metatarsal and extends out to the distal aspect of the proximal phalanx. Dissection is kept to a minimum because there is no need for interspace procedures or sesamoid rotation. The incision is carried down to the level of the first MPJ capsule where a linear capsulotomy is performed in line with the skin incision. The extensor hallucis longus tendon is reflected laterally, and the MPJ is disarticulated. Resection of the medial eminance is performed as needed, taking care to avoid excessive bone removal. At this point one must decide on what type of fusion is to be performed; options include end-to-end flat surface fusion, peg-in-hole fusion, or simple cartilage resection.[2,3,5,7,8,11,30,31,35,36] Each option has its advantages and disadvantages, but the final aim is the same; with any method used, there should be good bone-to-bone contact with no cartilaginous or soft tissue interposition.

End-to-end fusion provides excellent bone apposition for increased stability and greater surface area for fusion. However, if the position of the hallux is not satisfactory, revisional bone cuts will be necessary. Repeated bone cuts may result in excessive shortening of the metatarsal, which may ultimately result in lesser metatarsalgia.

Peg-in-hole and conical fusions provide remarkable stability and allow for angular adjustments but may cause excessive shortening. Peg-in-hole and conical fusions also require greater wound manipulation, are technically more demanding, and may require the use of specialized instrumentation such as power reamers.

Simple cartilage removal allows for minimal loss of bone and provides for a high degree of angular adjustment from the ball-and-socket architecture of the first MPJ. However, this ability to easily adjust position also renders simple cartilage resection highly unstable. Another shortcoming of simple cartilage resection is that the subchondral bone is relatively dense, a factor that may delay union. To overcome this problem, it is necessary to drill multiple holes in the subchondral surface of the metatarsal head and phalangeal base. These holes will increase the surface area for fusion and allow for vascular bridging and bone formation at the site. This is easily accomplished by using a 1.5-mm drill bit.

Another method of increasing surface area for ingrowth is the "fish-scale" technique. Using a small sharp osteotome, multiple small cuts are made in the subchondral surface on both sides of the joint. These cuts should penetrate only through the subchondral bone, and care should be taken not to create fractures that propagate up the shaft of either the metatarsal or proximal phalanx.

When the surfaces of the metatarsal head and base of the proximal phalanx are prepared, the next step in the procedure is the mating of the two surfaces and a check of angular relationships. This step is facilitated by the use of a goiniometer or intraoperative radiographs. Once the position of fusion is deemed accept-

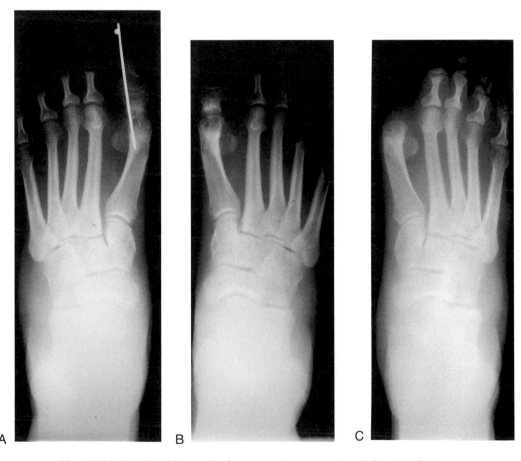

**Fig. 18-8.** (**A–C**) Radiographs demonstrating nonunion of first MPJ fusion.

able, a method of fixation is selected. Recommended fixation techniques include screws, plates, and K-wires. On completion of fixation, intraoperative radiographs are obtained as necessary and closure is performed in the usual fashion. One should keep in mind the words of Fitzgerald: "the precise operative technique is not important provided it maintains the position obtained at operation until the arthrodesis is sound."[6] The patient is then placed in a non-weight-bearing cast for approximately 6 to 8 weeks.

## COMPLICATIONS

Complications associated with first MPJ fusion are relatively few in number. Wound complications involving dehiscence, postoperative infections, and prolonged edema present at a rate similar to any other podiatric procedure and are not a major concern. Improper positioning of the fusion is a serious complication that can be avoided by proper preoperative planning and intraoperative decision making. Fusions that have been improperly positioned present with various signs and symptoms including inability to fit into shoes, interdigital helloma, incurvated or painful nails, lesser metatarsalgia, sub-first metatarsal pain, and tyloma formation. One of the more significant complications associated with malpositioning of the fusion is plantar ulceration at the first metatarsal head. This is particularly true in cases in which a fusion has been performed for a rheumatoid first MPJ. Thin plantar skin with the loss of the plantar fat pad in rheumatoid patients puts these patients at risk for developing plantar ulceration with an error in sagittal plane positioning of the fusion.

Another possible complication of MPJ fusion is that of nonunion (Fig. 18-8). Nonunion rates have been noted to range from 2 to 23 percent with an average of 10 percent.[4,5,9–11,16,18,30,45] In most cases, the non-union develops into a painless pseudoarthrosis and no further intervention is needed. Possible causes for nonunion include hardware failure, improper or no fixation, and steroid or methotrexate use in rheumatoid patients. Patients occasionally will have problems with painful internal fixation devices, most often noted in plantarly placed screws.

A final complication to consider is that of interphalangeal joint arthrosis. This complication can be avoided by ensuring proper transverse and sagittal plane positioning intraoperatively, thereby relieving abduction and dorsiflexion forces on the interphalangeal joint.

## REFERENCES

1. Clutton HH: The treatment of hallux valgus. St. Thomas Rep 22:1, 1984
2. McKeever D: Arthrodesis of the first metatarsophalangeal joint for hallux rigidus and metatarsus primus varus. J Bone Joint Surg 34:129, 1952
3. Marin G: Arthrodesis of the first metatarsophalangeal joint for hallus vallus and hallux rigidus. Guy's Hosp Rep 109:174, 1960
4. Harrison MHM, Harvey FJ: Arthrodesis of the first metatarsophalangeal joint for hallux valgus and rigidus. J Bone J Surg, 45A:471, 1963
5. Marin G: Arthrodesis of the first metatarsophalangeal joint for hallux valgus and hallux rigidus: a new method. Int Surg 50:175, 1968
6. Fitzgerald JAW: A review of long term results of arthrodesis of the first metatarsophalangeal joint. J Bone Joint Surg 51B:488, 1968
7. Salis-Soglio G, Thomas W: Arthrodesis of the metatarsophalangeal joint of the great toe. Arch Orthop Trauma Surg 95:7, 1979
8. Ginsburg AI: Arthrodesis of the first metatarsophalangeal joint. J Am Podiatry Assoc 69:367, 1979
9. Mann RA, Oates JC: Arthrodesis of the first metatarsophalangeal joint. Foot Ankle 1:159, 1980
10. Riggs SA, Johnson EW: McKeever arthrodesis for the painful hallus. Foot Ankle 3:248, 1983
11. Johansson JE, Barrington TW: Cone arthrodesis of the first metatarsophalangeal joint. Foot Ankle 4:244, 1984
12. Leavitt DC: Surgical treatment of arthritic feet. Northwest Med 55:1086, 1956
13. Du Vreis HL: Surgery of the foot. 2nd Ed. CV Mosby, St. Louis, 1965
14. Morrison P: Complications of forefoot operations in rheumatoid arthritis. Proc R Soc Med 67:110, 1974
15. Watson MS: A long term follow-up of forefoot arthroplasty. J Bone Joint Surg 56(B):527, 1974
16. Mann RA, Thompson FM: Arthrodesis of the first metatarsophalangeal joint for hallux valgus in rheumatoid arthritis. J Bone Joint Surg 66A:687, 1984
17. Geppert MJ, Sobel M, Bohne WO: Foot fellows review: the rheumatoid foot; part I, forefoot. Foot Ankle 13:550, 1992

18. Smith RW, Joanis TL, Maxwell PD: Great toe metatarsophalangeal joint arthrodesis: a user friendly technique. Foot Ankle 13:367, 1992

19. Henry APJ, Waugh W: The use of footprints in assessing the results of operations for hallux valgus. A comparison of Keller's operation and arthrodesis. J Bone J Surg 57(B):478, 1975

20. Coughlin MJ, Mann RA: Arthrodesis of the first metatarsophalangeal joint as a salvage for the failed Keller procedure. J Bone Joint Surg 69(A):68, 1987

21. Thompson FM: Complications of hallux valgus surgery and salvage. Orthopedics 13:1059, 1990

22. Stroh KI, Altman MI, Yee DY: First metatarsophalangeal joint arthrodesis: treatment for sesamoid fractures. J Am Podiatr Med Assoc 80:595, 1990

23. Thompson FR, McElvenny RT: Arthrodesis of the first metatarsophalangeal joint. J Bone Joint Surg 23:555, 1940

24. Renshaw T, Sirkin R, Drennan J: The management of hallux valgus in cerebral palsy. Dev Med Child Neurol 21:202, 1979

25. Richardson GE: The foot in adolescents and adults: hallux valgus in cerebral palsy. p. 879. In Crenshaw AH (ed): Campbell's Operative Orthopedics. 7th Ed. CV Mosby, St. Louis, 1987

26. Mann RA, Katcherian DA: Relationship of metatarsophalangeal joint fusion on the intermetatarsal angle. Foot Ankle 10:8, 1989

27. Humbert JL, Bourbonniere C, Laurin CA: Metatarsophalangeal fusion for hallux valgus: indications and effects on the first metatarsal ray. Can Med Assoc J 120:937, 1979

28. Kampner SL: Total joint prosthetic arthroplasty of the great toe—a 12-year experience. Foot Ankle 4:249, 1984

29. Raymakers R, Waugh W: The treatment of metatarsalgia with hallux valgus. J Bone Joint Surg 53(B):684, 1971

30. Coughlin MJ: Arthodesis of the first metatarsophalangeal joint with mini fragment plate fixation. Orthopedics 13:1037, 1990

31. Gould N: Surgery of the forepart of the foot in rheumatoid arthritis. Foot Ankle 3:173, 1982

32. Duckworth T, Betts RP, Franks CI: Foot pressure studies: normal and pathological gait analysis. p. 484. In Jahss MH (ed): Disorders of the Foot and Ankle. 2nd Ed. WB Saunders, Philadelphia, 1991

33. Duckworth T, Betts RP, Franks CI, Burke J: The measurement of pressures under the foot. Foot Ankle 3:130, 1982

34. Betts RP, Stockley I, Getty CJM: Foot pressure studies in the assessment of forefoot arthroplasty in the rheumatoid foot. Foot Ankle 8:315, 1988

35. Kellekian H: Hallux valgus, allied deformities of the forefoot and metatarsalgia. pp. 236–241. WB Saunders, Philadelphia, 1965

36. Zadik FR: Arthrodesis of the great toe. Br Med J 2:1573, 1960

37. Lipscomb PR: Arthrodesis of the first metatarsophalangeal joint for severe bunions and hallux rigidus. Clin Orthop Relat Res 142:48, 1979

38. Sullivan BT: Use of the Reese osteotomy guide system for fusion of the first metatarsophalangeal joint. J Bone Joint Surg 30:43, 1991

39. Wilson CL: A method of fusion of the metatarsophalangeal joint of the great toe. J Bone Joint Surg 40(A):384, 1958

40. Wilson JN: Cone arthrodesis of the first metatarsophalangeal joint. J Bone Joint Surg 49(B):98, 1967

41. Chana GS, Andrew TA, Cotterill CP: A simple method of arthrodesis of the first metatarsophalangeal joint. J Bone Joint Surg 66(B):703, 1984

42. Phillips JE, Hooper G: A simple technique for arthrodesis of the first metatarsophalangeal joint. J Bone Joint Surg 62(B):774, 1986

43. Sykes A, Hughes AW: A biomechanical study using cadaveric toes to test the stability of fixation techniques employed in arthrodesis of the first metatarsophalangeal joint. Foot Ankle 7:18, 1986

44. Wu KK: Arthrodesis of the metatarsophalangeal joint of the great toe with Herbert screws: a clinical analysis of 27 cases. J Foot Ankle Surg 32:47, 1993

45. Moynihan FJ: Arthrodesis of the metatarsophalangeal joint of the great toe. J Bone Joint Surg 49B:544, 1967

# 19

# Arthrodesis of the First Metatarsocuneiform Joint

## CHARLES GUDAS

Abduction of the first metatarsal to correct metatarsus primus varus and hallux valgus was first described by Albrecht in 1911.[1] Lapidus in 1934 advocated fusion of the first and second metatarsals with the first cuneiform.[2] Overall uses of the procedure since its initiation have been dedicated to hallux valgus with a relatively high intermetatarsal angle. Clark, Veith, Sangeorzan, and Hansen have utilized the Lapidus procedure for correction in postadolescent hallux valgus.[3,4] Bacardi and Saffo have advocated the utilization of the procedure for severe metatarsus primus varus.[5,6] The procedure has gained popularity in the past 10 years, perhaps because The Association for the Study of Internal Fixation (ASIF) fixation techniques, with more precise placement of the distal first metatarsal and high fusion rates, have been used. Objectives of the procedure include reduction of the high intermetatarsal angle and stabilization of obliquity/hypermobility at the first metatarsocuneiform joint. Previous complications of the procedure included less than optimal position of the first metatarsal head, secondary to elevation, or nonunion, which may produce moderate to severe forefoot instability.[1,2,5–7]

Patient selection varies with age; however, most procedures have been targeted to the adolescent-to-50-year-old population. In most instances, the patient complains of shoe-fitting difficulties as well as appearance problems, pain, ambulatory difficulties, and impingement syndromes to the lateral forefoot, including formation of metatarsalgia, hammer toes, and Morton's neuroma. Specific indications for the procedure include juvenile hallux valgus with obliquity or hypermobility at the first metatarsocuneiform joint,

paralytic hallux valgus (either spastic or flaccid in nature), osteoarthritis, traumatic degenerative joint disease secondary to an old Lisfranc injury, severe adult hallux valgus with intermetatarsal angles exceeding 18° (Fig. 19-1), and as an ancillary procedure for the correction of flatfoot of an idiopathic nature or secondary to a posterior tibial tendon rupture, generalized ligamentous laxity, or medial column instability.

The procedure is usually combined with a distal first metatarsal procedure, including exostectomy, sesamoid release, distal or midshaft first metatarsal osteotomy, implant and proximal phalangeal techniques, prosthetic implant, proximal phalangeal techniques, including the modified Keller bunionectomy or Regnauld procedure.

Arthrodesis is used less frequently than proximal metatarsal osteotomies or distal osteotomies, which may be secondary to the complications encountered in performing the technique. Excess bone removal or elevation of the distal fragment will cause severe forefoot dysfunction, a result that is less than optimal. Patient selection is of paramount importance in the procedure. The long-term effects of fusion of the first metatarsocuneiform joint in the adolescent population are not specifically known at this time. The incidence of nonunion approaches 10 percent and is also a factor in increasing the complication rate with this procedure.[5]

Specific preoperative criteria can be highlighted in three areas: (1) hallux valgus; (2) osteoarthritis of degenerative joint disease of the metatarsocuneiform articulation; and (3) as an adjunct procedure to increase

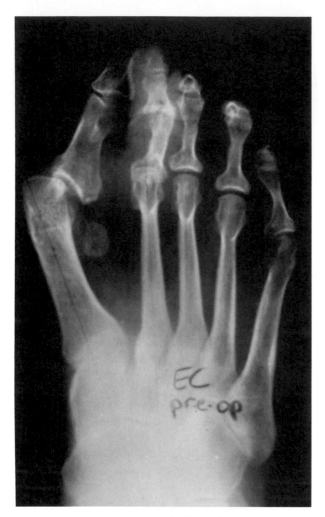

**Fig. 19-1.** Severe hallux valgus.

medial column stability secondary to paralytic dysfunction or tendon rupture.

Hallux valgus-specific criteria include an intermetatarsal angle exceeding 18° and hypermobility or obliquity of the first metatarsocuneiform joint. The distal first metatarsophalangeal joint should have a hallux abductus angle exceeding 25°, with moderate to severe hallux valgus present. There is no contraindication in performing this procedure on an arthritic joint; however, ancillary procedures such as a Keller bunionectomy or Silastic prosthesis may be utilized in cases in which arthritis is present. Care must also be

taken to assess the articular surface because in severe cases of hallux valgus, the functional articular surface is 20–30 percent of the total joint area. Repositioning in instances such as these may cause increased evidence of osteoarthritis and future disability.

Fusion of the first metatarsocuneiform joint is indicated in cases of degenerative joint disease or osteoarthritis (Fig. 19-2), which is often secondary to Lisfranc's fracture/dislocation or overt injury to this area.

Distal medial column stabilization procedures are indicated by the use of this technique when there has

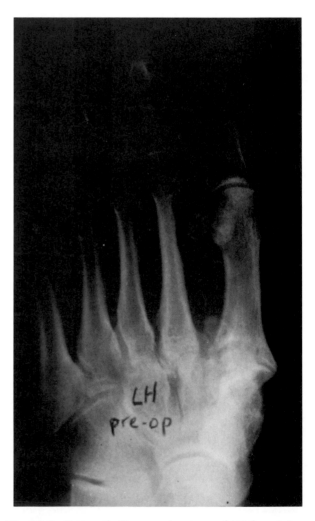

**Fig. 19-2.** Osteoarthritis secondary to an old Lisfranc injury.

been a disturbance to the medial column, secondary to a tendon injury such as a partial or complete rupture of the posterior tibial tendon or an overt or subtle Lisfranc's derangement. Paralytic deformities that affect muscle tendon units surrounding this joint system are also indications for this procedure. Stabilization in the presence of spastic or flaccid paralysis of the external or intrinsic muscle groups is indicated for direct control of the unstable area.

Whether one fuses the joint for osteoarthritis or for correction of severe hallux valgus, two factors are of primary importance. The first is fusion. Throughout literature reviews, nonunion of the joint has been as high as 10 percent. Although most authors state that they have very little problem with nonunions in this area, the long-term effect can be disastrous. The second is exact placement of the metatarsal so that proper metatarsal declination is achieved. It is a common tendency to elevate the first metatarsal, thus imparting undue stress on the lateral metatarsals. The overall principles of the procedure have changed, especially with the introduction of small ASIF screws and plates. Crossed Kirschner wires (K-wires) were formerly the procedure of choice, with long-term non-weight-bearing for fusion. In the mid-1970s, screws became the procedure of choice, as advocated by Clark, Hansen, Veith, and others in the latter part of the 1970s and early 1980s.[3,4] During the past 7 years, we have used a small plate combined with screw fixation to achieve more exact reduction (Fig. 19-3). The use of a soft template allows the proper declination to be imparted to the fusion site, and from this template, the plate can be prebent to achieve this process. The plate can also be utilized with or without a bone graft. Other technical considerations include protection of the medial nerve, which courses along the incision sites in many cases. Care also must be taken not to remove excess bone to avoid shortening with subsequent lateral forefoot dysfunction. When more than 2 mm of bone removal is anticipated, the utilization of a small bone graft from the medial cuneiform is extremely helpful.

## THE PROCEDURE

The first metatarsophalangeal joint is generally exposed, and distal procedures are performed initially. If an osteotomy is performed or an implant is to be inserted, the cuts are made without fixation until the fusion site is stabilized proximally.

Before the proximal incision is made, the outline of the joint is marked with a skin-marking pencil. This allows the incision to be placed correctly and provides maximum exposure to the bean-shaped joint. The incision is made approximately 1 to 1.5 in. long dorsomedially, with great care being taken to protect the medial nerve. Care must also be exercised to preserve the attachment of the tibialis anterior, as well as the

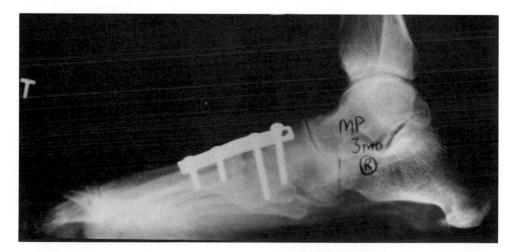

**Fig. 19-3.** Plate fixation of first metatarsocuneiform fusion.

distal attachments of the posterior tibial tendon. A sharp incision should be made to the joint and a very sharp periosteal elevator utilized to elevate both the ligaments and the capsule from the articulation for later repositioning over the fusion site.

The area and amount of bone removed depend on the desired result. Generally, however, as little bone as possible is removed. Enough bone should be removed plantarly to allow some plantar flexion of the first metatarsal. A laminar spreader may be helpful in visualizing the plantar surface of this somewhat irregular bean-shaped joint. If failed reconstructive bunion surgery or severe intermetatarsal angle correction is necessary, 3–5 mm of bone graft may be necessary to avoid shortening. The bone can be obtained from the posterior iliac crest or as a small wedge from the first cuneiform. The graft should be wedged safe with the base directed dorsally. The metatarsal should be plantar-flexed in approximately 15°–20° of plantar flexion. When there is significant diastasis between the first and second metatarsals, the medial aspect of the second metatarsal metaphysis should be incorporated into the fusion.

Once the bone cuts have been made and the graft inserted (if necessary), a simple technique allows preliminary manipulation of the fusion site before final fixation is applied. We utilize this in not only first metatarsocuneiform, but also great toe joint fusions. The techniques involve driving a 0.45 or 0.62 K-wire through the fusion site and graft, if inserted. The distal metatarsal is then plantar-flexed and abducted the desired amount until correct positioning is achieved. Once this position is achieved, we use a small plate and one or two screws for fixation. We previously utilized a 2.7 or 3.5 semi-tubular plate to achieve rigid stability, but now use the titanium limited contact dynamic compression plate for this joint (Fig. 19-4). The plates are thinner, lighter in weight, and rigid, and can be prebent more easily. In most instances, two holes are utilized for the cuneiform and two holes for the first metatarsal. As previously mentioned, the plate should be prebent to approximately 15°–20° of plantar flexion, as well as the desired amount of abduction, to achieve correction. Sangeorzan, Veith, and Hansen advocate the use of 3.5–4.0 cortical screws for stabilization of the fusion site.[3,4] One screw is used to stabilize the first metatarsocuneiform joint and the second to stabilize the first metatarsal against the medial as-

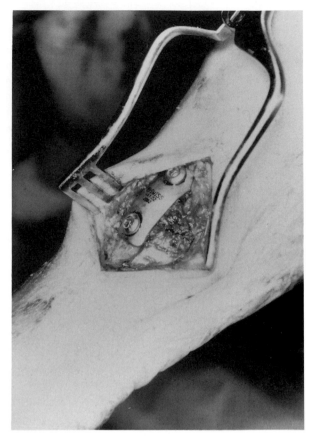

**Fig. 19-4.** Titanium limited contact dynamic compression plate fixation with bone graft.

pect of the second metatarsal. We have also used this technique, but found that limited metaphyseal curvature on the bone may make insertion of these screws somewhat difficult. Other types of fixation that can be utilized are crossed K-wires and staples.

It is important to realize the dimensional analysis of this procedure. In cases of hallux valgus, the average intermetatarsal angle exceeds normal by 10°–12°. When the osteotomy is completed, the intermetatarsal angle should be reduced to less than this; this angle should be carefully measured at the operative site to avoid overcorrection. It is also extremely important to achieve 15°–20° degrees of plantar declination of the distal first metatarsal. As mentioned before, this is best achieved by the use of a combination of plate and screw fixation techniques to achieve good alignment. Great care also must be taken to measure the length of the first metatarsal pre- and postoperatively, to assess the amount of shortening that is likely to occur. Excess shortening of the first metatarsal can create an adverse biomechanical situation on the lateral forefoot, resulting in disability and pain. The key points of the procedure include protecting the medial nerve from transection or irritation, obtaining adequate position of the distal first metatarsal in plantar flexion and abduction if necessary, good compression across the osteotomy site (our preference is plates and screws), utilization of a bone graft when necessary to prevent shortening, and careful tissue handling to avoid necrosis and infection.

Potential intraoperative difficulties include damage to the neurovascular bundle, elevation of the first metatarsal, excess bone removal, and excessive soft tissue damage. Additional complications can occur distally where severe hallux valgus may render the first metatarsophalangeal joint (MPJ) cartilage less than optimum. Therefore, the patient should understand that ancillary procedures may have to be performed, including fusion or limited-resection Keller bunionectomy, or first metatarsal osteotomy to achieve first MPJ mobilization. Care must be taken not to overcorrect the hallux so that a varus occurs.[7] The procedure is extremely technically demanding and should be attempted only by a surgeon familiar with the area, and who has had some previous training in this technique. The criteria for excellent results, similar to those established by Bonney and McNab,[8] include a normal intermetatarsal angle of approximately 8°, a normal hallux abductus angle of approximately 15°, elimination of pain at the joint site or first metatarsophalangeal joint, elimination of first-ray hypermobility, functional and cosmetic patient satisfaction, ability to wear normal shoe gear, and absence of stiffness of the first metatarsophalangeal joint.

Specific complications of this procedure include medial neuralgia, which has been mentioned in many studies because of the close proximity of the nerve medially. Great care must be taken to protect the nerve to avoid this complication. Nonunion has been mentioned in as many as 10 percent of cases by Clark,[3] and in 6 of 54 feet by Saffo et al.[6] Mauldin et al. reported 50 percent formation of plantar osteophytes at the fusion site (Fig. 19-5). Transfer lesions have been found in as many as 14 percent of the patients[6] secondary to elevation or shortening of the first metatarsal. In 54 procedures, Saffo et al. found the average shortening of the first metatarsal to be approximately 6 mm.[6] Other studies indicate elevation of the first metatarsal may occur in as often as 20 percent of the procedures. Other complications include hallux varus, noted in 15.7 percent of Mauldin's study (Fig. 19-6).[7] Additional findings/complications include formation of plantar osteophytes between the first metatarsocuneiform plantar fusion site.

Other complications include fractured screws or plates. We have seen a 5 percent screw fracture rate in

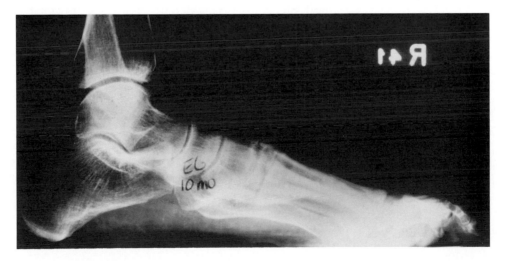

**Fig. 19-5.** Potential nonunion of the first metatarsocuneiform joint.

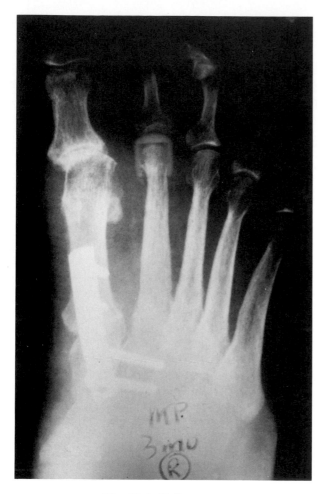

**Fig. 19.6.** Hallux varus.

oblique screws across the first metatarsocuneiform joint. A small percentage of plates will fracture. All plates and screws should be removed 6 to 12 months after surgery.

## Specific Biomechanical Considerations

Fusion of the first metatarsocuneiform joint is believed to help prevent medial column collapse and hypermobility at the first metatarsal cuneiform joint. The proper performance of this technique will lead to increased stability during the midstance and toe-off phase of gait. If shortening or elevation occur, however, medial column rigidity is decreased, with subsequent increase in lateral forefoot pressure and the possibility of metatarsalgia or the formation of hammer toes or claw toes. Elevation of the first metatarsal may cause an iatrogenic primus elevatus leading to hallux limitus or rigidus.

## Postoperative Care

Most authors prefer non-weight-bearing or limited weight-bearing for 6–8 weeks. It has been our experience to note that a total non-weight-bearing regimen should be enforced for the first 6 weeks after surgery, followed by an additional 2 weeks if necessary. After that time, the patient may start gradual touchdown during the next 2–3 weeks. After 3 months, intensive physical therapy may be initiated with walking, exercises, and gradual fitting into a normal shoe. It is not uncommon for mild to moderate edema to be present from 12 to 18 months with this procedure.

## REFERENCES

1. Albrecht GH: The pathology and treatment of hallux valgus. Russ Vrach 10:14, 1911
2. Lapidus PW: The operative correction of the metatarsus primus varus in hallux valgus. Surg Gynecol Obstet 58:183, 1934
3. Sangeorzan BJ, Hansen ST Jr: Modified Lapidus procedure for hallux valgus. Foot Ankle 9:262, 1989
4. Clark HR, Veith RG, Hansen ST Jr: Adolescent bunions treated by the modified Lapidus procedure. Bull Hosp Joint Dis Ortho Inst 47:109, 1987
5. Bacardi BE, Boysen TJ: Considerations for the Lapidus operation. J Foot Surg 25:133, 1986
6. Saffo G, Wooster MF, Stevens M, et al: First metatarsocuneiform joint arthrodesis: a five-year retrospective analysis. J Foot Surg 28:459, 1989
7. Mauldin DM, Sanders M, Whitmer WW: Correction of hallux valgus with metatarsocuneiform stabilization. Foot Ankle 11:59, 1990
8. Bonney G, McNab I: Hallux valgus and hallux rigidus: a critical survey of operative results. J Bone Joint Surg 34:366, 1952

# 20
# Cuneiform Osteotomy

*FRANCIS LYNCH*

While the use of the cuneiform osteotomy for surgical repair of hallux abducto valgus has never gained significant notoriety, there has been a recent heightened interest in this procedure as a potentially valuable tool in the correction of both the adult and juvenile forms of the deformity. As such, this chapter presents specific guidelines for the efficacious application of the cuneiform osteotomy in the repair of select cases of hallux abducto valgus.

## HISTORICAL REVIEW

The deformity of hallux abducto valgus is not a new concept. In fact, the deformity has drawn the attention of clinicians and surgeons for more than a century. Interestingly, however, there is little reported use of the cuneiform osteotomy in the surgical repair of hallux abducto valgus. More commonly, surgical intervention at this level has been reserved for the repair of flexible flatfoot[1] and metatarsus adductus.[2–4]

The first reported use of the cuneiform osteotomy in the repair of hallux abducto valgus was in 1908 by Riedl.[5,6] He recommended a closing wedge osteotomy of the medial cuneiform to address an "atavistic" deformity. This procedure would clearly be technically demanding and is rarely, if ever, performed today.

In 1910, Young[7] initially reported on the use of the opening wedge cuneiform osteotomy for the correction of hallux abducto valgus. Some 42 years later, Bonney and MacNab[8] applied a similar technique to realign the metatarsocuneiform joint without disturbing the proximal metatarsal epiphysis.

In 1935, Cotton[1] described an opening wedge osteotomy of the medial cuneiform with insertion of allogenic femoral graft as a sagittal plane structural correction of the depressed medial column of the arch in pes planus. He reported favorably on the stabilization of the medial column to the supporting surface with the use of this procedure.

In 1958, Joplin[9] modified his sling procedure for the correction of "splay foot," originally described in 1950, to routinely include an opening wedge osteotomy of the first cuneiform. A year later, Fowler et al.[2] advocated the use of the opening wedge cuneiform osteotomy for the correction of residual forefoot adduction in the treatment of talipes equinovarus.

Graver,[10] in 1978, reported on the use of the cuneiform osteotomy in the correction of metatarsus primus adductus. Using an autograft constructed of a triangular piece of bone fashioned from the resected medial eminence of the first metatarsal head and inserted into the cuneiform osteotomy, he claimed excellent reduction of the metatarsus primus adductus component of the bunion, with a significantly reduced healing time and a decreased incidence of long-term complications such as metatarsalgia.

In 1986, Bicardi and Frankel[11] reported on the use of the biplane cuneiform osteotomy for the surgical repair of juvenile metatarsus primus varus. They advocated the use of an appropriately sized wedge of homologous or autogenous bone graft that was wider medially and dorsally and fixated with a bone staple; they thought that this procedure addressed the apex of the deformity, which was the obliquity of the metatarsocuneiform articulation, accounting for the increase in metatarsus primus varus in conjunction with the lack of sagittal plane stability of the first ray. They further advocated the concomitant use of the Hohmann osteotomy bunionectomy to alter the proximal articular set angle (PASA) by realigning the adapted articular cartilage of the first metatarsal head, and also recommended that the capital fragment be transposed laterally for additional intermetatarsal angle correction, and plantarly, to overcome the elevation of the first metatarsal that is often seen with a hypermobile first ray.

Bicardi and Frankel believed that this procedure preserved the length of the first metatarsal, and by increasing the height of the distal-medial arch and the forward inclination of the metatarsocuneiform joint in the sagittal plane, enhanced the durability of correction against recurrence from continued pronatory stress in the flatfoot.

Using pre- and postoperative electrodynagraphy (EDG), Bicardi and Frankel noted significant alterations in the weight-bearing of the forefoot postoperatively. Interestingly, the first metatarsal bore weight relatively earlier in the stance phase of gait and also loaded to a greater extent than preoperatively. They were also impressed with the overall reduction and alignment of the first metatarsophalangeal joint (MPJ). As such, the authors concluded that this particular technique was superior for intermetatarsal angle reduction and realignment of the first metatarsocuneiform joint.

# INDICATIONS

The following represent indications for the use of the cuneiform osteotomy in the repair of hallux abducto valgus:

1. Structural increase in the first intermetatarsal angle or metatarsus primus adductus as a result of atavism or increased obliquity of the distal articular facet of the medial cuneiform
2. Absence of deformity of the first metatarsal proper—no hyperadduction of the long axis of the first metatarsal relative to its base
3. Medial column adductus with or without concomitant metatarsus primus adductus
4. Hypermobility of the first ray with resultant elevatus and instability
5. Patient displaying appropriate degree of maturity of the medial cuneiform (age 6 and older) (Fig. 20-1)

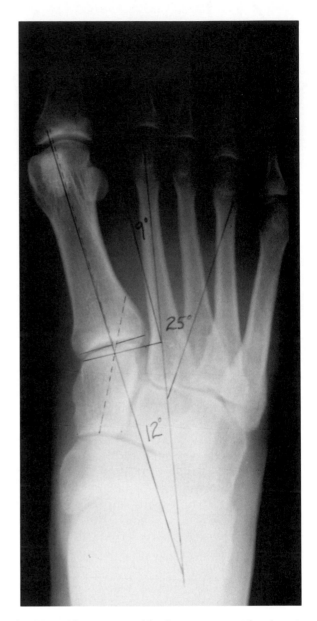

**Fig. 20-1.** This 25-year-old white woman with advancing hallux valgus displays classic radiographic findings that suggest the efficacious applicability of cuneiform osteotomy. Note the increased intermetatarsal angle as a result of structural deformity in the distal articular facet of the cuneiform with absence of deformity within the first metatarsal proper. There is also accompanying medial column adductus of 25°.

## EFFECTS

The following are considered primary effects of the cuneiform osteotomy when applied to the correction of hallux abducto valgus (Fig. 20-2):

1. Reduction in the obliquity of the distal articular facet of the medial cuneiform
2. Reduction of metatarsus primus adductus
3. Reduction of medial column adductus (juvenile patient)

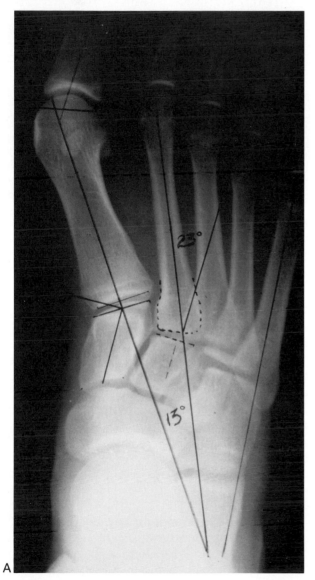
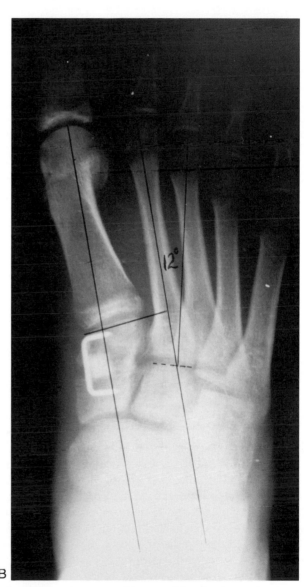

**Fig. 20-2.** **(A)** Preoperative and **(B)** postoperative radiographs reveal reduction in obliquity of the distal articular facet of the medial cuneiform, metatarsus primus adductus, and medial column adductus as a result of performance of the biplane cuneiform osteotomy. Accentuation of the PASA and lengthening of the first ray have been accommodated by bicorrectional first metatarsal head osteotomy.

4. Plantar flexion of the first ray
5. Lengthening of the first ray
6. Accentuation of PASA deformity of the first MPJ

## SURGICAL TECHNIQUES AND APPLICATIONS

The cuneiform osteotomy is reserved for the older child and adult. In children much less than the age of 6 years the ossification of the first cuneiform has not proceeded to an extent that would allow appropriate dissection and osteotomy at this level.[3]

It is imperative that the surgical procedure be carried out in a certain manner for optimal benefit. The sequence of steps in the performance of the procedure are as follows:

1. Complete release of the first MPJ.
2. Biplane cuneiform osteotomy with grafting and fixation.
3. Transpositional, PASA-realigning, and first metatarsal-shortening osteotomy as necessary.
4. Adductor tendon transfer, capsulorrhaphy, and concomitant rebalancing of the first MPJ as deemed appropriate.
5. Performance of ancillary surgical procedures deemed necessary for the overall elimination of associated pedal pathology. This may include lengthening of the achilles tendon, gastrocnemius recession, surgical repair of flexible flatfoot, or additional adjunctive repair of metatarsus adductus.

The surgeon should first direct his attention to the first MPJ. The short extensor tendon is tenotomized and the long extensor tendon is lengthened in a sliding or open **Z** fashion if this structure is taut or displaced laterally to the long axis of the first MPJ. The adductor tendon is freed from the lateral aspect of the base of the phalanx and fibular sesamoid. In cases in which there is a significant lateral deviation of the sesamoids relative to the first metatarsal head and repositioning is deemed appropriate,[12] or when preoperative evaluation suggests additional positional abnormality of the first metatarsocuneiform joint,[13] the adductor tendon is tagged for later transfer (Fig. 20-3). A lateral capsulotomy is performed and a medial inverted **J**-shaped capsulotomy is carried out.

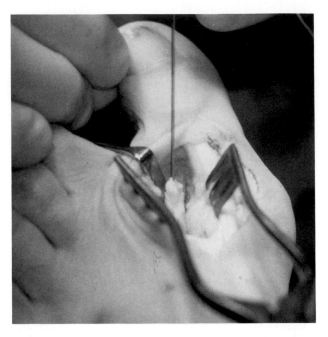

**Fig. 20-3.** Adductor tendon transfer is an important adjunctive maneuver in the overall repair of hallux abducto valgus, serving to reposition the sesamoid apparatus beneath the first metatarsal head and to reduce positional increase in the first intermetatarsal angle.

At this point the first MPJ is considered appropriately released, and further surgical intervention at this level is delayed until the effects of the cuneiform osteotomy can be appreciated. Incision planning for the cuneiform osteotomy is of paramount importance. The two landmarks that are most helpful in this process are the tibialis anterior and extensor hallucis longus tendons. Mapping their course, the surgeon can then plan an incision overlying the substance of the medial cuneiform approximately two-thirds of the way from the tibialis anterior to the extensor hallucis longus tendon.

Few anatomic structures are encountered in dissection from the subcutaneous tissue through to the periosteum overlying the cuneiform. A longitudinal periosteal incision is made, and subperiosteal dissection is carried out exposing the dorsal and medial aspects of the medial cuneiform.

The osteotomy is then created within the substance of the medial cuneiform. Two variations of this osteotomy have been used to date and warrant some degree of explanation.

When the primary transverse plane deformity is metatarsus primus adductus and there is minimal medial column adductus, or in instances in which a moderate amount of medial column adductus exists with or without additional metatarsus primus adductus in the juvenile foot displaying relative lack of maturity of the lesser metatarsocuneiform articulations, the osteotomy is created approximately 1.0–1.5 cm proximal and parallel to the distal articular facet of the first cuneiform (Fig. 20-4).

In instances in which the predominant deformity is medial column adductus with minimal metatarsus primus adductus, and the foot shows maturity at the lesser metatarsocuneiform articulations, the osteotomy must be varied somewhat. In this case, the osteotomy is begun at the midpoint of the medial cuneiform and directed proximal and lateral toward the cuboid. This variation allows the surgeon to continue the cut through the second or third cuneiform bones to allow for optimal abduction of the medial column with avoidance of the second metatarsal base. Although the osteotomy performed in this manner will have less

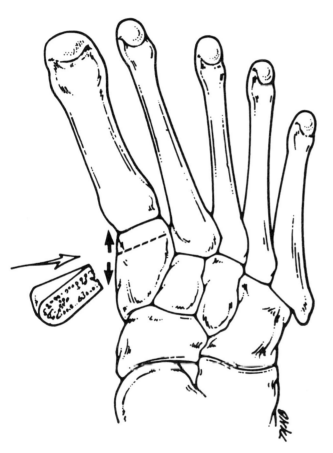

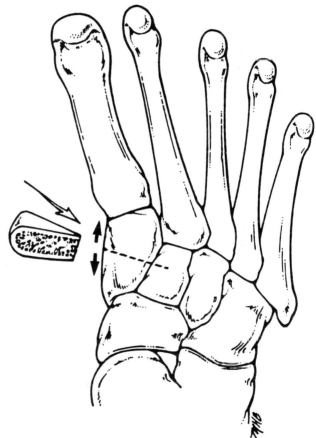

**Fig. 20-4.** Placement of the cuneiform osteotomy just proximal and parallel to the distal articular facet of the medial cuneiform will result in maximal reduction of cuneiform obliquity and intermetatarsal angle. Further, a "domino effect" is observed in the juvenile foot, resulting in significant reduction of medial column adductus. (Courtesy of J.V. Ganley, D.P.M., Norristown, PA.)

**Fig. 20-5.** Placement of the cuneiform osteotomy, beginning at the midpoint of the medial cuneiform and extending through the second or third cuneiforms, is indicated in the mature foot with minimal metatarsus primus adductus, but significant medial column adductus. (Courtesy of J.V. Ganley, D.P.M.)

direct effect on the first intermetatarsal angle proper, it has better ability overall to abduct the entire medial column when this surgical maneuver is deemed of primary importance (Fig. 20-5).

With the osteotomy held open the desired amount, an allogenic corticocancellous graft of appropriate proportions is created and inserted. This graft should be wider dorsally and medially to allow for plantar flexion of the medial column in conjunction with the transverse plane correction. The graft is then secured with Kirschner wire (K-wire) or power staple fixation and remodeled as necessary.

Once the cuneiform osteotomy and grafting have been carried out, a sponge is placed over the surgical site and attention is directed back to the first MPJ. The degree of correction of the intermetatarsal angle and medial column adductus can now be appreciated, and the necessity for any further lateral transposition of the first metatarsal head, shortening of the first metatarsal to prevent jamming of the first MPJ, and degree of correction of the PASA for overall better alignment and function of the first MPJ can be evaluated. To this extent, most cases will require a PASA realigning,

transpositional, and shortening first metatarsal head osteotomy that will complete the structural correction (Fig. 20-6).

If it is deemed appropriate to perform adductor tendon transfer to decrease positional deformity of the first metatarsocuneiform joint or to help in the realignment of the sesamoid apparatus, it should be carried out at this time.

When the procedure has been appropriately performed, examination of the foot before final closure and application of the postoperative dressing will reveal the following (Fig. 20-7):

1. The concavity of the medial aspect of the foot has disappeared.
2. The alignment of the first MPJ is optimal.
3. The first ray is in a rectus to slightly plantar-flexed position relative to the lesser metatarsals.
4. The range of motion of the first MPJ is full and is noted not to jam or track back into the abducted position with dorsiflexion.

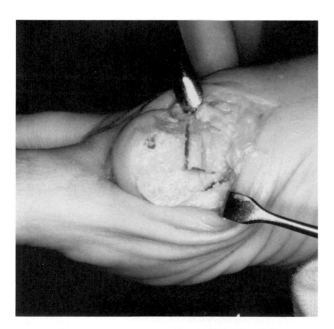

**Fig. 20-6.** Concomitant first metatarsal head osteotomy for realignment of the PASA and decompression of the first MPJ is usually required in conjunction with cuneiform osteotomy for overall optimal alignment of the first MPJ.

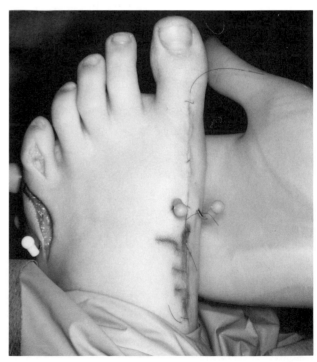

**Fig. 20-7.** Postoperative photograph showing overall improvement in contour of the entire forefoot and alignment of the first MPJ after performance of the cuneiform and first metatarsal head osteotomies.

## ANCILLARY SURGICAL PROCEDURES

On occasion, it is necessary to perform adjunctive surgical procedures to eliminate additional structural pathology. As such, the correction of equinus, flatfoot, and significant residual lateral column adductus may be required.[12]

If preoperative assessment reveals significant contracture of the gastrocnemius or triceps surae complex, then appropriate Achilles tendon lengthening or gastrocnemius recession should be carried out in conjunction with repair of the primary deformity.

In individuals with significant flexible flatfoot whose control postoperatively is tenuous, surgical repair of the flatfoot must be considered. A significant, uncontrollable flatfoot should undergo realignment and stabilization of the rearfoot to eliminate a primary deforming force from continuing its destructive input at the level of the first MPJ postoperatively.

Significant pan metatarsus adductus, while a rare finding, does on occasion exist and may require additional surgical technique. In addition to the cuneiform osteotomy, this particular foot may require closing wedge osteotomy of the cuboid for overall alignment of the foot and better long-term function[14] (Fig. 20-8).

Finally, the repair of lesser digital deformities and rebalancing of lesser MPJs, or metatarsal osteotomies, should be carried out to correct the secondary deformities as the result of advancing hallux valgus as deemed necessary.

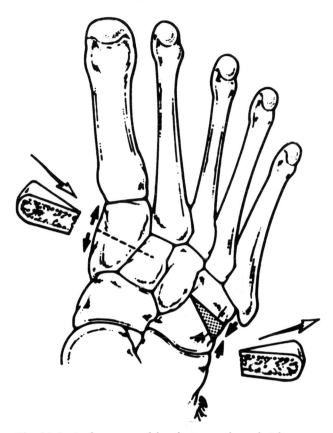

**Fig. 20-8.** Performance of the closing wedge cuboid osteotomy in conjunction with cuneiform osteotomy is indicated in patients with significant lateral column adductus. (Courtesy of J.V. Ganley, D.P.M.)

## POSTOPERATIVE CARE

At the time of surgical repair, a compression dressing and posterior splint are applied holding the corrected components in their appropriate position. This splint should allow the first ray to be held in the slightly plantar-flexed position with optimal alignment of the first MPJ in the transverse plane. Further, the ankle should be kept at a right angle to the leg to prevent contracture of the flexor hallucis longus in the early stages of recovery, which could cause restriction of dorsiflexion of the first MPJ in the long run.

The importance of early mobilization and range of motion of the first MPJ cannot be overstated. The immediate use of continuous passive motion (CPM) to encourage appropriate range of motion of the first MPJ postoperatively should be entertained.[15]

The sutures are removed in 14 days, and the splint is converted to a below-knee cast until 6 weeks from the date of surgery have elapsed. During this entire period, weight-bearing is not permitted and range-of-motion exercises are strongly encouraged.

When the patient begins weight-bearing postoperatively, it should be in a rigid orthotic that affords significant midfoot and rearfoot control with maximal intrinsic forefoot posting, to encourage the first ray to maintain its plantargrade position in the sagittal plane and to remove the deforming forces from the MPJ that may exist postoperatively as a result of continued anteromedial imbalance.

## POTENTIAL COMPLICATIONS OF CUNEIFORM OSTEOTOMY

The following are the most common potential complications that may arise as a result of the cuneiform osteotomy:

1. The procedure may be made difficult by the presence of the tibialis anterior tendon, which traverses the operative field. This, however, is rarely a significant problem and the tendon sheath may be opened and tendon reflected with later repair without significant alteration of the overall surgical outcome.

2. The procedure requires bone grafting, which potentially introduces a separate set of complications. Realistically, however, there has been little problem with the use of allogenic bone graft. It rapidly incorporates into the osseous system of the host with minimal complications. To date there has been only one delayed union that went on to eventual healing with the use of electrical bone stimulation and immobilization. There have been no rejections.

3. That part of the osteotomy bridged by the graft may heal more slowly. This, again, has not been noted, and in fact with the use of allogenic bone graft and power staple fixation, this area seems to be afforded tremendous stability with rapid incorporation and healing.

4. Soft medullary bone is more inclined to collapse with loss of correction. This event is conceivable but has not been observed to happen in this author's experience. The use of the power staple fixation and properties of allogenic graft incorporation prevent this deleterious event from occurring.

5. While graft extrusion may occur, it has not been noted to date by the author. Appropriate fashioning, placement, and fixation will eliminate this potential complication.

6. The surgeon may accidentally osteotomize the second metatarsal base. This can be avoided by leaving the lateral cortex of the medial cuneiform intact and "green-sticking" it when the osteotomy is opened.

7. The patient may experience insertional tendonitis of the anterior tibial tendon. While this has oc-

curred on several occasions, it has been only transitory. Appropriate graft remodeling and fixation placement in conjunction with atraumatic soft tissue dissection will reduce the possibility of this problem.

8. Osteotomy, or staple entrance, into the first metatarsocuneiform joint is possible, but this unfortunate occurrence may be eliminated by complete visualization of this joint before osteotomy or fixation.

9. Irritation of the skin overlying the cuneiform as a result of prominent internal fixation can be eliminated by the use of K-wire or reduced with appropriate staple placement. When staple irritation occurs, the staple can be removed with minimal disability.

10. Misalignment or jamming of the first MPJ may be eliminated with appropriate adjunctive first metatarsal osteotomy, which aligns the PASA and compensates for the lengthening that occurs as a result of the cuneiform osteotomy.

## SUMMARY

The goal of hallux abducto valgus surgery is to create a well-aligned, pain-free joint while removing as many contributory etiologic factors causing misalignment of the first MPJ as possible. Retrospective analysis of both juvenile and adult hallux abducto valgus shows an intimate relationship of misalignment of the first MPJ with metatarsus primus adductus as a result of structural deformity of the distal articular facet of the medial cuneiform, medial column adductus, anterior medial instability of the first ray with elevatus, and varying degrees of flexible flatfoot. The cuneiform osteotomy is ideal for addressing the apex of the deformity, reestablishing a more transverse attitude to the distal articular facet of the medial cuneiform, and thus reducing the intermetatarsal angle and medial column adductus. Further, the first ray is stabilized in the sagittal plane and the anterior medial instability is improved. At the same time, postoperative complications are kept to a minimum and consistent and reliable realignment of the forefoot and MPJ deformity are attained.

We do not present the opening wedge cuneiform osteotomy with adjunctive first MPJ rebalancing and metatarsal osteotomy as a panacea applicable to all foot types. However, in the appropriately applied clinical setting, a consistently reliable result can be attained, and modern podiatric surgeons must consider this procedure as a valuable addition to their surgical armamentarium.

# REFERENCES

1. Cotton F: J Foot statistics and surgery. Trans N Engl Surg Soc 18:181, 1935
2. Fowler B, Brooks AL, Parrish TF: The cavovarus foot. J Bone Joint Surg 41A:757, 1959
3. Hofmann AA, Constine RM, McBride GG, Coleman SS: Osteotomy of the first cuneiform as treatment of residual adduction of the fore part of the foot in club foot. J Bone Joint Surg 66A:985, 1984
4. Lincoln CR, Wood KE, Bugg EI: Metatarsus varus corrected by open wedge osteotomy of the first cuneiform bone. Orthop Clin North Am 7:795, 1976
5. Helal B: Surgery for adolescent hallux valgus. Clin Orthop 157:50, 1981
6. Kelikian H: Hallux Valgus, Allied Deformities of the Forefoot and Metatarsalgia. WB Saunders, Philadelphia, 1965
7. Young JD: A new operation for adolescent hallux valgus. Univ Pa Med Bull 23:459, 1910
8. Bonney G, McNab I: Hallux valgus and hallux rigidus: a critical survey of operative results. J Bone Joint Surg 34B:366, 1952
9. Joplin RJ: Some common foot disorders amenable to surgery. Am Acad Orthop Surg 15:144, 1958
10. Graver HH: Cuneiform osteotomy in correction of metatarsus primus adductus. J Am Podiatry Assoc 68:111, 1978
11. Bicardi BE, Frankel JP: Biplane cuneiform osteotomy for juvenile metatarsus primus varus. J Foot Surg 25:472, 1986
12. Mahan KT, Yu GV: Juvenile and adolescent hallux valgus. p. 61. In McGlamry ED, McGlamry R (eds): Doctors Hospital Podiatry Institute Surgical Seminar Syllabus. Doctors Hospital Podiatric Education and Research Institute, Atlanta, 1985
13. Pressman MM, Stano GW, Krantz MK, Novicki DC: Correction of hallux valgus with positionally increased intermetatarsal angle. J Am Podiatr Med Assoc 76:611, 1986
14. Grumbine N: Cuboid osteotomy. Seminar lecture, Baha Project, Los Angeles, 1986
15. Kaczander B: The podiatric application of continuous passive motion: a preliminary report. J Am Podiatr Med Assoc 81:631, 1991

# 21

# Joint-Destructive Procedures

## GUNTHER STEINBÖCK

The term *joint-destructive procedure* might suggest that a functioning joint is destroyed by the procedure. It is emphasized here, however, that this type of procedure must be reserved for joints with a hallux valgus deformity accompanied by severe, painful osteoarthritis with erosion of cartilage and limitation of motion, various types of arthritis, and severe infections or damage of other origin of this joint.

To relieve pain and restore reasonable function of the first metatarsophalangeal joint in these cases, there are three possible procedures: resection of articulating parts of bones, resection, and using an implant or arthrodesis. All resection arthroplasties have in common that if the entire metatarsal head is not removed, the medial outgrowth (exostosis) of the metatarsal head is resected. Several combinations have been utilized (Table 21-1).

In 1836, Fricke[1] performed "excision of the bones which form the metatarsodigital joint of the great toe" with great success. As the sesamoids belong to the joint, this implicates that they also were extirpated. In 1853, Hilton[2] removed the "articular extremities" of the metatarsal and first phalanx "including the two sesamoid bones."

Heubach[3] reported in 1897 on results of total joint resection including the sesamoids performed by his chief, Rose, of Berlin, in the years 1884–1897. Heubach himself used the removed joints for a detailed description of the pathomorphology of hallux valgus and for staging hallux valgus into three groups relating to the position of the sesamoids.

Clayton,[4] for his forefoot correction in severe rheumatoid arthritis, employed resection of the metatarsal head and the phalangeal base leaving the sesamoids in situ. Kramer (1826) and Roux (1829) were known by Heyfelder[5] to have removed the head of the first metatarsal. Hueter[6] did this procedure for an infected first metatarsophalangeal joint, but later (1877) also applied it to hallux valgus without infection.

Mayo in 1908 modified the operation by removing two-thirds of the metatarsal head, "the section also removing two thirds of the anterior portion of the bony hypertrophy on the inner side." Riedel[7] in 1886 was the first to publish four successfully operated cases of hallux valgus that he had treated by resection of the base of the phalanx and the exostosis of the head of the first metatarsal. He had seen deplorable results with decapitation of the first metatarsal, and intended his publication to serve as a warning to other surgeons treating hallux valgus. In 1887 Davies-Colley[8] described the same surgical technique for the treatment of hallux rigidus ("hallux flexus").

Keller,[9,10] being also impressed by poor results of the metatarsal head resections, in 1904 and 1912 reported his technique of treating hallux valgus, which is essentially the same as that described by Riedl. Brandes,[11] apparently inspired by Billroth, unfortunately recommended resection of two-thirds of the phalanx, causing several generations of surgeons in German-speaking countries to create short and floppy great toes that were often followed by transfer metatarsalgia.

Although Kelikian[12] in 1965 again tried to put straight the fact that Riedel[7] was the first, in 1886, to publish base resection combined with exostectomy for the treatment of hallux valgus, it remained the convention to call this operation after Keller in English-speaking and after Brandes in German-speaking countries.

**Table 21-1.** Resection Arthroplasties for Hallux Valgus

| Resected Part of Joints | Authors |
| --- | --- |
| Metatarsal head | Fricke 1836 |
| Base of phalanx | Hilton 1853 |
| Sesamoids | Rose 1884 (Heubach 1897) |
| Metatarsal head | Clayton 1960 |
| Base of phalanx | |
| Metatarsal head | Kramer 1826 |
| | Roux 1829 |
| | Hueter 1871 |
| Metatarsal head, partial | Mayo 1908 |
| Medial prominence of | Riedel 1866 |
| Metatarsal head, | Keller 1904 |
| Base of phalanx | Brandes 1927 |

## THE KELLER TYPE OF ARTHROPLASTY

### General Discussion of Procedure

The Keller procedure can be defined by Riedel's description[7]: removal of the exostosis from the metatarsal head and of the base of the first phalanx. The numerous variations in respect to details of the operation are discussed and we refer to what has for us proved to lead to acceptable results with this procedure.

Keller[9] recommended a medial skin incision, which has the advantage that the important digital nerves and vessels are avoided and that the scar is scarcely visible.[13] We have observed no problems with pressure caused by shoes.

If a bursa is present, it is not resected; the incision is deepened through it.

The capsule is incised longitudinally at its medial aspect. If reconstruction of the capsuloligamentous apparatus is planned, the sesamoids are mobilized.[13,14] The lateral capsule is also cut in a longitudinal direction[14] to facilitate the cerclage fibreux, which serves to reduce the intermetatarsal angle. Care must be taken to preserve the posteromedial insertion of the capsule just behind the exostosis rather plantarly.[15] At this portion of the capsule the nutrient artery of the metatarsal head penetrates the capsule. If this vessel is cut, the metatarsal head is at risk for osteonecrosis.[15]

Although several authors have contended that the intermetatarsal angle is reduced by removal of the base of the phalanx,[16–18] it was noticed that an intermetatarsal angle less than 10° usually was not achieved.

Bonney and MacNab,[19] in analyzing a series of operations to correct hallux valgus, concluded that the most important of two main causes of poor ("indifferent") results was failure to correct "metatarsus primus varus," which in this case apparently means the intermetatarsal angle. In my experience[18] the average reduction of the intermetatarsal angle was from 14° to 11.8° in the simple procedure, while in the group with cerclage fibreux the average intermetatarsal angle was altered from 16.6° to 9.3° at follow-up in an average of 8.5 years. Although as Jahss indicates,[20] the value of this procedure was doubted by Kelikian, Jahss[20] emphasizes that the cerclage holds with his experience of 10 years of follow-up.

With a mobile first ray, intermetatarsal angles up to 25° can be treated with this method. We therefore made it an indispensable step in the procedure. If there is doubt of reductibility, radiographs are done with an elastic bandage around the forefoot to see whether the forefoot narrows sufficiently. If the deformity is rigid, which is very rare, an osteotomy of the Trethowan type is performed.[21]

The disarticulation of the base of the phalanx should be achieved by sharp dissection with a knife. If a sharp elevator is used to free the phalanx laterally, a piece of bone may break off that must be removed. However, Bonney and MacNab[19] in their study on operative results after Keller procedures found fragments of bone left behind to have little influence on the results, "provided this untidiness is not carried too far."

Contrary to Keller and followers we do not resect the phalanx subperiosteally but remove the base with the periosteum adhering to it; this prevents neosteogenesis, which may be expected from a tissue with osteogenetic potency.

Because some controversy is apparent from the literature regarding the size of the resected part of the phalanx, several opinions may be of interest. Riedl[7] did not give any details as to the amount of resection of the base of the phalanx, nor did Keller.[8,9] In his second publication in 1912, Keller[10] advised that enough of the "phalangeal head" is removed to enable the distal portion to be placed in an overcorrected position medially without impinging on the first metatarsal. Brandes[11] strictly insisted on resection of two-thirds of the phalanx. Gilmore and Bush[22] removed one-third to one-half of the proximal phalanx. Cleveland and Winant[23] postulated removal of at least one-half of the phalanx to prevent the postoperative development of hallux rigidus.

Kelikian recommended resection of at least half the phalanx. He attributed proliferative new bone formation to resection through the cancellous base. Bonney and MacNab[19] in their critical survey of operative results concluded that the optimal length of the resected piece was one-third to one-half of the proximal phalanx.

Wrighton[24] considered the most common technical error to be resection of more than one-third of the phalanx, producing a short, rotated, and floppy toe and a relative projection of the second toe that leads to a hammer deformity. Giannestras[25] recommended removing 1 cm, or not more than 1.5 cm, to avoid an obvious overshortening of the hallux. He also emphasized that the cut should be perpendicular to the long axis of the phalanx. The incidence of the development of a floppy toe appeared to rise significantly when more than one-third of the phalanx was removed. Lelièvre[13] postulated that as "metatarsus varus has been reduced" (by cerclage fibreux) the hallux should be as long as the second toe, calculating that in the following weeks there will be, by shaping of the base of the stump of the phalanx, a reduction in length of 2–3 mm. Thus, an ideal proportion will be gained. He also demands a "joint play" of 10 mm at distraction and thinks that in most cases these conditions are realized by resecting the base at the metadiaphyseal border. Mann[26] resects the proximal part of the phalanx at the metaphyseal flare, which compares well with Lelièvre's prescription. As much as one-half of the phalanx may be removed.

The amount of resection done by Imhoff et al.[27] depends on the valgus angle. At less than 40°, they resect one-third; at angles greater than 40° they resect one-half as recommended by Reiter.[28]

In our experience resection at the metaphyseal flare[13,26] is usually sufficient; this represents approximately one-third of the total length of the phalanx. The plane of resection is perpendicular to the long axis of the bone, as is recommended by most authors.

An oscillating saw is used. Bone-cutting forceps carry the risk of crushing the bone, and the phalanx is at risk for damage, especially in the elderly osteopenic patient.

Replantation of the base of the phalanx was advocated by Regnauld.[29] To make the operation as reconstructive as possible, we began using Regnauld's replantation of the base of the proximal phalanx to provide for cartilaginous joint surfaces. At an early follow-up of 22 operations, we found one replant dislocated; another was partly resorbed, and in one case the replanted base was broken. Because at that time we had found this step of the operation technically difficult, we have discontinued doing it.

The exostosis of the metatarsal head is removed flush with the medial contour of the shaft,[12] which is in agreement with most writers. Keller[10] in his second publication in 1912 recommended making the cut obliquely upward and outward along the length of the metatarsal, extending from the inner sesamoid below to a line above that is well past the middle of the bone. All other outgrowth of bone around the metatarsal head is also removed.

In contrast to other authors,[12] the sesamoids are preserved even if severe osteoarthrosis is present. Osteophytes are removed from the medial sesamoid if they protrude too far medially. Pain stemming from a metatarsosesamoidal osteoarthrosis is extremely rare. Removal of the sesamoid can add to the biomechanical disadvantages of the procedure.

We have occasionally added interposition of a distally pedunculated capsuloperiosteal flap, doubled with a resorbable suture and sewn over the resection surface of the phalanx using the lateral periosteum or a drill hole in the bone to anchor it. We have not obtained sufficient results to determine whether this improves mobility. Lelièvre[13] has abandoned interposition of a capsular flap. He described early development of a fibrous cartilage that gradually develops into chondroid metaplasia. We also saw this macroscopically when correcting recurrent hallux valgus after Keller-type operations.

In considering tenopexy, at an early follow-up of Keller procedures to which fibrous cerclage was added, metatarsalgia had developed at the second and sometimes third metatarsal in 5 of 21 feet.[14] Transfer metatarsalgia is attributed to weakened ground pressure of the great toe. According to Ellis,[30] in normal function of the foot the posture of the great toe is flat and straight on the ground. He explained that the proximal phalanx is pressed to the ground by the short flexors as a presupposition for the long flexor to act as a pressor on the distal phalanx. If the proximal

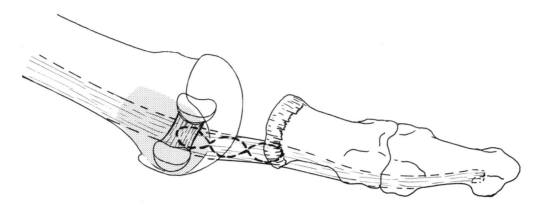

**Fig. 21-1.** Tenopexy according to Viladot. A Bunnel-type suture connects the long flexor tendon with the intersesamoid ligament.

phalanx is not stable, the long flexor causes knuckling at the interphalangeal joint.

When the base of the phalanx is removed in a Keller-type procedure, the insertion of the short flexors is severed and the proximal phalanx is left unstable. To compensate for this, several techniques have been developed that aim at reuniting the plantar plate with the stump of the phalanx either directly or via the long flexor tendon. Regnauld[29] places a resorbable suture from between the sesamoids and across the tendon sheath of the long flexor through the capsuloperiosteal tissue of the phalanx. He also describes Viladot's technique of suturing the intersesamoid ligament to the tendon of the flexor hallucis longus muscle (Fig. 21-1) and Buruturan's method of connecting the intersesamoid ligament to the base of the phalanx by using a drill hole. Regnauld[15] advises against including the long flexor tendon in the suture because of the risk of creating a permanent flexion at the interphalangeal joint, thus producing a mallet toe. Lelièvre[13] does not believe that such procedures reduce the frequency of metatarsalgia.

We use Vilatot's technique; in our experience, the sesamoids retract proximally but cock-up deformities seem to be prevented. Lengthening of the extensor longus tendon is usually not necessary, a reason why we continue to add tenopexies in Keller procedures.

The repair of the capsuloligamentous apparatus is done by reconstructing the medial metatarsosesamoidal ligament. This is accomplished with resorbable material of size 1, usually Vicryl (see Fig. 21-1).

Any type of postoperative immobilization of the toe is deemed unnecessary if rehabilitation begins on the day of the operation, or preferably on the preceding day, by instructing the patients about their contribution to the success of the procedure. Although it is recommended by some authors, [12,22,25,31–33] Sherman et al.[33] did not recognize any advantage in Kirschner wire (K-wire) distraction and suspected that degenerative changes in the interphalangeal joint and a subjectively worse result might be the outcome. Use of an external staple creates two portals for possible infection instead of just one for the K-wire.[34]

Bonney and Macnab[19] found when comparing results with and without immobilization in a plaster that incorporated the great toe for 2 weeks that there was no difference in the objective functional results. Although the authors are of the opinion that mobility of the new joint does not depend on what is termed early mobilization, on the other hand the results suggest that immobilization is not necessary.

With respect to metatarsalgia, there was no significant difference in the results of Rogers and Joplin,[35] who "followed Keller's technique" without fixation and those of Bryan[35] who used K-wires and external staples. In 1976 we discontinued distraction with a suture through the pulp of the toe and did not see any disadvantage as to the functional results.

We never resect any skin even if a surplus of skin results after removal of the bunion. The baggy appearance of this skin disappears within 6 weeks postoperatively. Postoperative treatment is continued for 6 weeks using elastic adhesive tape. Movement of the toe is encouraged on the day of operation, and ambulation with sandals or larger tennis shoes as soon as the patient tolerates it.

## OBJECTIVE OF THE PROCEDURE

The goal of this procedure is to eliminate pain caused by the exostosis, and by osteoarthritis, and to restore function of the whole foot as completely as possible. This can be achieved by taking into account all pathologic anatomic alterations accompanying the deformity. The procedure thus must include removal of the exostosis, correction of malposition of the first metatarsal in a transverse and sagittal plane, reposition of the metatarsal head onto the sesamoidal apparatus by lateral release, medial reconstruction of the capsulo-ligamentous structures, and restoration of muscular balance as much as possible.[36]

## PATIENT SELECTION AND INDICATION

The opinion that a joint with good mobility must be treated by a joint-preserving procedure regardless of the patient's age is gaining support.[37] As in all planned surgery, circulatory problems must be evaluated; if necessary, advice of an angiologist should be sought.

The indication for a Keller-type procedure will usually be established with a painful osteoarthritic joint, dorsiflexion less than 30°, and a hallux valgus angle of more than 40°.[12] Candidates for a simple Keller procedure will be patients with nonhealing ulceration at the site of the exostosis, ulcerations and joint destructions initiated by sensory neuropathics, and septic arthritis with destruction of joint surfaces.

In the rheumatoid foot, treatment of the lesser metatarsophalangeal joints, mutilated and dislocated as they are, will usually be metatarsal head resection. To achieve good functional alignment some part of the metatarsal head will also have to be removed,[13] or an arthrodesis of the first metatarsophalangeal joint can provide for even better stabilization of the foot.

## PREOPERATIVE MEASURES

An ankle block is set with 1% Xylocaine after ruling out all contraindications. A tourniquet is put on just above the ankle joint and inflated to a pressure of twice the patient's systolic pressure of the arm. In patients with diabetes or with even slight circulatory problems, a tourniquet is not used.

## THE OPERATION

A medial longitudinal skin incision is made from the crease of flexion of the interphalangeal joint to just proximal to the exostosis. The joint is exposed subcutaneously by blunt dissection using scissors. The capsule is incised longitudinally 5 mm plantar to the insertion of the medial metatarsoscsamoid ligament at the epicondyle of the metatarsal head.

With a knife, using a hook inserted into the proximal joint surface of the phalanx, the base is shelled out separating the abductor hallucis, the adductor hallucis, the flexor brevis, and the extensor brevis tendon from its insertion into the base. The periosteum is left intact. The base is grasped with a small reposition forceps, and while rinsing thoroughly with saline the base of the phalanx is removed with an oscillating saw perpendicular to the longitudinal axis of the bone and just proximal to the site where the reposition forceps gripped, at the proximal metaphyseal flare of the phalanx.

Exostectomy is performed flush with the medial contour of the metatarsal shaft. An osteotome or an oscillating saw is used to remove the exostosis. To prevent intrusion into the shaft, an indentation is made perpendicular to the axis with a smaller osteotome just proximal to the exostosis. The osteotomy may incline 10° to the sagittal plane from dorsolateral to plantar-medial. If present, osteophytes are removed from the dorsal and lateral circumference also.

Adhesions of the sesamoid apparatus to the metatarsal head are separated by a blunt periosteal elevator.[12] The lateral metatarsosesamoidal ligament and capsule is dissected using a Smillie meniscotome. The deep transverse metatarsal ligament is left intact.

Tenopexy of the flexor hallucis longus tendon to the intersesamoid ligament is now added. The tendon sheath is opened longitudinally with a knife from the intersesamoid ligament to the resection plane of the phalanx. With a Bunnel-type suture starting just at the resection plane of the phalanx, the flexor hallucis tendon is fixed to the intersesamoid ligament (see Fig. 21-1). The capsule is sutured with resorbable material. Medial reefing is possible by resection or plication.

With the toe in neutral position and under longitudinal traction of the toe, a U-type mattress suture (Regnauld, personal communication) is set with a resorbable 1-0 thread, usually Vicryl. The needle penetrates the capsule dorsally at the border to the periosteum from outside in, is directed through the plantar lip of the capsule just dorsal to the medial sesamoid at its proximal end, then back through the capsule from outside in at the distal end of the sesamoid and from

inside out through the dorsal origin of the capsule paralleling the thread that is already inserted (Fig. 21-2A). The forefoot is now compressed transversely and the suture is tied under tension, thus repositioning the metatarsal head on the sesamoid apparatus (Fig. 21-2B). The surplus rims of the capsule are now resected and by side-to-side sutures with the same material the capsuloligamentous apparatus, especially the medial metatarsosesamoid ligament, is reconstructed (Fig. 21-

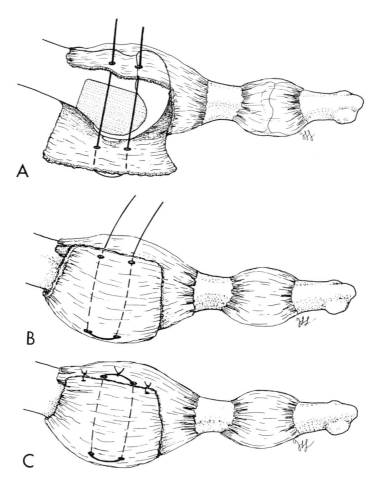

**Fig. 21-2.** (**A**) Reconstruction of the capsuloligamentous apparatus. After resection of the base of the phalanx and the exostosis, freeing the sesamoid bones from the metatarsal head and a lateral capsulotomy a U-type suture connects the dorsal rim of the capsule with the plantar part, passing through it close to the medial sesamoid bone. (**B**) By pulling at the threads of the suture, the sesamoids are replaced on the metatarsal head. (**C**) With the U-type suture tied, the surplus of capsuloligamentous tissue is resected and the suture completed by simple knots.

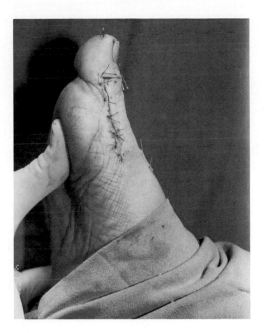

**Fig. 21-3.** Push-up test at the end of the operation. The head of the first metatarsal is supported from below with the ankle joint in a neutral position. If there is extension in the metatarsophalangeal joint, usually with buckling at the interphalangeal joint, the long extensor tendon will have to be lengthened.

2C). The most distal suture connects the periosteum of the phalanx with the capsule and the tendon of the abductor hallucis muscle.

In the case of a rigid first metatarsal fixed in abduction, an opening wedge osteotomy at the base of the first metatarsal is made as described by Trethowan[20,38] A push-up test is performed at the end of the operation (Fig. 21-3). After having performed the operation in the manner described here, there is usually no dorsiflexion in the metatarsophalangeal joint. If there is, the extensor hallucis longus tendon must be lengthened.

## KEY POINTS OF THE PROCEDURE

To reestablish function of the forefoot, the first ray must be stabilized. It has been shown that after head resections of the lesser metatarsals the results were fair if the first ray was stable but poor when it was unstable.[39]

This stabilization is achieved by reducing the intermetatarsal angle by reconstructing the medial metatarsal ligament and by strengthening the ground pressure of the first toe, which can be accomplished by trying to maintain the function of the short flexors. Care must also be taken of the lesser toes in respect to the expected excess length of the second and sometimes also the third toe, hammer toes, and dislocations at lesser metatarsophalangeal joints. The whole foot must always be addressed.[13]

## POTENTIAL INTRAOPERATIVE DIFFICULTIES

Although the Keller operation is considered to be a simple procedure for the treatment of hallux valgus, there are some steps that can cause difficulties for the less experienced. The flexor hallucis longus tendon follows the plantar contour of the first phalanx, which is concave in a plantar direction. If the structures cannot be clearly visualized and the knife does not follow the osseus contour closely, the flexor tendon is at risk to be dissected. This would have to be repaired immediately.

In rather stiff joints, the ablation of the lateral collateral ligament and the adductor tendon can be difficult. A smaller scalpel and patience are often helpful. Care must also be taken to preserve the digital nerves because lesions can create painful neuromas. If the capsular reconstruction is inadequate, the intermetatarsal angle will not be reduced to normal and recurrence of the deformity must be expected.

If the tenopexy of the flexor hallucis longus is situated too far proximally, the flexor longus tendon will aid in pulling the sesamoids proximally and waste much of its power to this purpose.

## CRITERIA FOR ACCEPTABLE RESULTS

A pain-free joint that appears straight with a minimum passive dorsiflexion of 30°, an eliminated exostosis, and the absence of metatarsalgia will usually satisfy the patient. The intermetatarsal angle is expected to be smaller than 10° and the hallux valgus angle less than 20°. The metatarsal head should be relocated on the sesamoid apparatus, and the sesamoids should not retract proximally.

## COMPLICATIONS

Early postoperative complications are rare. If infection occurs, it can usually be cured by antibiotics in an early stage. If empyema develops in the nearthrosis, the wound should be opened and debrided and a drainage applied. A complication that often develops insidiously is hallux varus (Fig. 21-4). If the intermetatarsal angle is reduced to less than 5° or even becomes negative, the patient must be considered at risk to develop hallux varus. The technique of application of

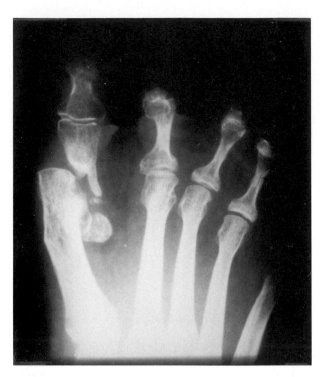

**Fig. 21-5.** Four years after a Keller operation without cerclage fibreux. Intermetatarsal angle is 21°; the phalanx is dislocated into the intermetatarsal space; the metatarsal head protrudes medially.

the dressings must be modified; the elastic adhesive bandage should be looser and a sling pulling the toe medially must be avoided.

Sequelae following too little or too much resection are more frequent. In the first case, either hallux rigidus, or, especially if the metatarsal angle is not addressed, an early recurrence will develop with the phalanx subluxing into the intermetatarsal space (Fig. 21-5). If too much is resected a thick, short, and weak toe will result (Fig. 21-6), sometimes followed by march fractures of one or more metatarsals (Fig. 21-7).

## SPECIFIC PREOPERATIVE CRITERIA

The Keller procedure, consisting of resection of the base of the phalanx and the exostosis, should be restricted to cases in which the most simple intervention is desirable to reduce the risk of complications, espe-

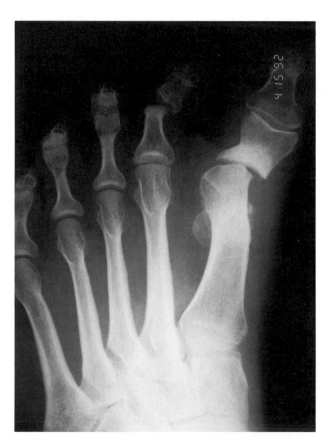

**Fig. 21-4.** Severe hallux varus of 20° after Keller's operation in a 49-year-old woman, 4 years after surgery.

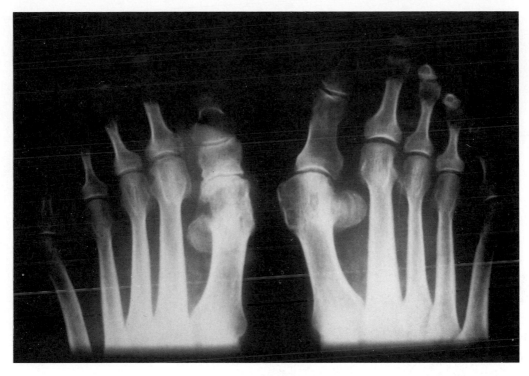

**Fig. 21-6.** Left foot. Excessive resection of base of phalanx in an index minus foot.

cially in patients with circulatory problems, and to such emergency situations as septic arthritis and non-healing ulcers over the joint caused by chronically ulcerating bursitis or by various types of neuropathies, often accompanied by osteoarticular alterations. In an otherwise healthy foot, the expanded procedure addressing the specific situation created by removal of the base of the phalanx should be executed.

## SPECIFIC BIOMECHANICAL CONSIDERATIONS

In a simple Keller procedure the most serious disadvantage that becomes biomechanically relevant is the loss of insertion of the short flexors to the base of the phalanx. These muscles provide for ground pressure of the first ray, enabling the long flexor to develop full power at push-off of the great toe.

If the short flexors are absent, the toe will buckle at the interphalangeal joint, leading to a mallet deformity (Fig. 21-8). The long extensor overpowering the flex-

ion forces will lead to hyperextension in the neoarthros and to recurrence of lateral deviation of the toe because the abductor hallucis tendon is also detached from the base of the phalanx. The aforementioned complementary procedures should therefore be added.

If the intermetatarsal angle is not reduced to less than 10° the bowstring mechanism, especially of the long extensor, will lead to recurrence. Bonney and Macnab[19] found in their series that a main cause of indifferent results is "the failure to maintain correction of the metatarsus primus varus."

## POSTOPERATIVE CARE

Postoperative care begins on the day before the operation by instructing the patient about his rehabilitation program. At the end of the operation, a compression dressing with crêpe-rubber is applied with an adhesive type of gauze bandage. While still in the operating room, the patient is asked to move his toes. Even after

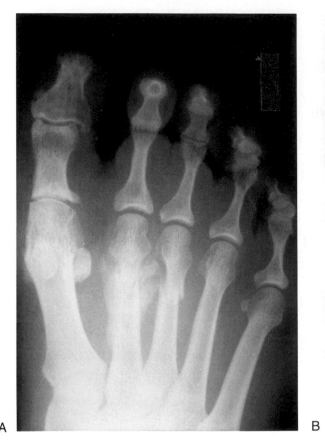
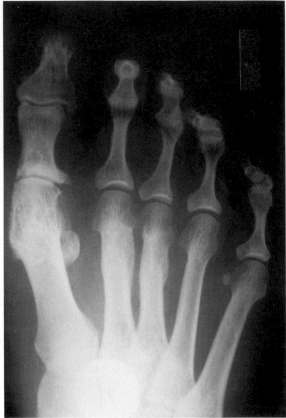

A                                                                B

**Fig. 21-7.** (**A**) March fractures after Keller's operation in a 54-year-old woman. Pain arising in the forefoot 4 months after surgery ceased after 8 weeks. Pain recurred in the forefoot 6 months later. Radiograph showed large callus at second metatarsal and new fracture of third. (**B**) Two years after fracture of third metatarsal, march fractures have healed and the calluses are smoothed out.

the effect of the local anaesthetic has faded, small movements of the toes are possible without causing too much pain. Pain is reduced by analgesics.

As soon after surgery as the patients are able, they are asked to dorsiflex and plantar-flex their ankle joints as if pressing on a pedal and to bend and stretch hip and knee joints in a bycycling type of movement to promote circulation in the foot and the leg as a prophylaxis to the sequelae of venous stasis and for improvement of metabolism at the site of operation. They will have to try active movement of dorsi- and plantar flexion in the metatarsophalangeal joint, eventually supported by their hands.

Swelling is also avoided by administration of certain drugs, such as Reparil, starting on the day before operation. Dressings are changed on the second post-

operative day if soaked through on the day following the operation. The second dressing is fixed by an adhesive bandage that compresses the forefoot moderately. Patients are encouraged to get out of bed on the day following the operation and use a wheeled chair to reach the lavatory. On the fourth day they usually walk using special shoes with a soft upper part and a wooden rocker-bottom sole, using crutches.

Low-dose heparin anticoagulation is started 2 hours before the operation and is maintained until the patient leaves the hospital, usually on the tenth day after operation, or at least until he has gained full mobilization. After a week the crutches are usually no longer needed. The sutures are removed on the tenth day after operation. The adhesive bandage is worn for 6 weeks and is changed weekly because it stretches out.

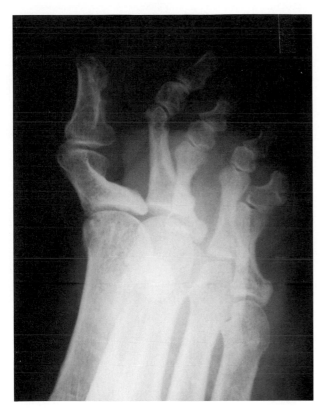

**Fig. 21-8.** Buckling of the interphalangeal joint 12 years after Keller's operation.

After 6 weeks, in addition to exercises to promote mobility actively and passively using the hands, resisted movement in the direction of flexion is started. This rehabilitation program should be continued for at least 3 months. It would be desirable for the patient to continue an exercise program for the feet throughout life. Postoperative care is at least as important as a meticulously performed operation to make the best out of an otherwise regrettable condition.[13] If the deformity can be attributed to pronatory forces during the propulsion phase of gait, orthoses are prescribed to prevent recurrence of hallux valgus and to prevent or treat metatarsalgia.

# REFERENCES

1. Fricke JLG: Exostosis of the ball of the foot. Dr. Fricke's report on the Hamburg Hospital of the first quarter of 1836. Dublin J Med Sci 11:498, 1837

2. Hilton J: Resection of the metatarsophalangeal joint of the great toe. Med Times Gax 7:141, 1853

3. Heubach F: Über hallux valgus und seine operative behanbdlung nach Edm. Rose. Dtsch Z Chir 46:210, 1897

4. Clayton ML: Surgery of the forefoot in rheumatoid arthritis. Clin Orthop 16:136, 1960

5. Heyfelder O: Operationslehre und Statistick der Resektionen. W. Braumüller, Wien, 1861

6. Hueter C: Klinik der Gelenkkrankheiten mit Einschluß der Orthopädie. FCW Vogel, Leipzig, 1877

7. Riedel: Zur operativen Behandlung des hallux valgus. Z Chir 44:754, 1886

8. Davies-Colley N: Contraction of the metatarsophalangeal joint of the great toe (hallux flexus). Br Med J 1:728, 1887

9. Keller WL: The surgical treatment of bunions and hallux valgus. Medical record. (NY Med J Phila Med J 80:741, 1904

10. Keller WL: Further observations on the surgical treatment of hallux valgus and bunions. NY Med J 95:696, 1912

11. Brandes M: Zur operativen therapie des hallux valgus. Zbl Chir 56:2434, 1929

12. Kelikian H: Hallux Valgus, Allied Deformities of the Forefoot and Metatarsalgia. WB Saunders, Philadelphia, 1965

13. Lelievre J, Lelievre JF: Pathologie du Pied. Masson, Paris, 1981

14. Steinböck G, Moser M: Die cerclage fibreux als zusätzliche maßnahme bei der operation des hallux valgus. Orthop Praxis 10:840, 1981

15. Regnauld B: Le Pied. Springer-Verlag, Berlin, 1986

16. McMurray TP: Treatment of hallux valgus and rigidus. Br Med J 2:218, 1936

17. Stockinger G, Ramach W: Erfahrungen mit der modifizierten operation nach Brances-Keller bei hallux valgus. In Murri A (ed): Der Fuß. Med Lit Verlagsges, Uelzen, 1981

18. Vitek M, Steinböck G: Value of cerclage fibreux for the Keller-Brandes procedure. Arch Orthop Trauma Surg 108:104, 1989

19. Bonney G, MacNab I: Hallux valgus and hallus rigidus. J Bone Joint Surg 34B:366, 1952

20. Jahss MH: Disorders of the Foot. Vol. 1. WB Saunders, Philadelphia, 1982

21. Trethowan J: Hallux valgus. In Choyce CC (ed): A System of Surgery. PB Hoeber, New York, 1923

22. Gilmore GH, Bush LF: Hallux valgus. Surg Gynecol Obstet 104:524, 1957

23. Cleveland M. Winant EM: An end result of the Keller operation. J Bone Joint Surg 32A:163, 1950

24. Wrighton JD: A ten-year review of Keller operation. Clin Orthop 89:207, 1972

25. Giannestras NJ: Foot Disorders. Lea & Febiger, Philadelphia, 1976
26. Mann R: Surgery of the Foot. CV Mosby, St. Louis, 1986
27. Imhoff A, Baumgartner R, Blauth W, Büsch HG, Lamprecht E: Fehlschläge mach hallux-valgus-operationen und ihre behandlung. p. 105. In Blauth W (ed): Hallux Valgus. Springer-Verlag, Berlin, 1986
28. Reiter R: Spätresultate nach 1464 hallux valgus operationen. Z Orthop 94:178, 1961
29. Regnauld B: Techniques Chirurgicales du Pied. Masson et Cie, Paris, 1974
30. Ellis TS: Deformities of the great toe. B Med J 1:157, 1887
31. Fitzgerald W: Hallux valgus. J Bone Joint Surg 32:139, 1950
32. Vallier GT, Petersen SA, La Grone MO: The Keller resection arthroplasty: A 13-year experience. Foot Ankle 11:187, 1991
33. Sherman KP, Douglas DL, Benson MKD'A: Keller's arthroplasty: is distraction useful? J Bone Joint Surg 66B:765, 1984
34. Bryan TF: Keller's arthroplasty modified. J Bone Joint Surg 44B:356, 1962
35. Rogers WA, Joplin RJ: Hallux valgus, weak foot and the Keller operation. Surg Clin N Am 27:1295, 1947
36. Steinböck G: Differential indication for the treatment of hallux valgus. In Mann G (ed): Sport Injuries: Proceedings of the Fourth Jerusalem Symposium, Freund Publishing, London, 1988
37. Zollinger H, Imhoff A: Die operative behandlung des hallux valgus. p. 95. In Blauth W. (ed): Hallux Valgus. Springer-Verlag, Berlin, 1986
38. Gore DR, Knavel J, Schaefer WW: Keller bunionecktomie with opening wedge osteotomy of the first metatarsal. p. 147. In Bateman JE, Trott A (eds): The Foot and the Ankle. Brian C Decker, New York, 1980
39. Pinsger M, Forbelsky M, Steinböck G: Metatarsalköpfchen-resektionen in kongreßband 2. In Internationaler Kongreß für Fußchirurgie der Österreichischen Gesellschaft für Orthopädie, Oberlech, 1991

# 22

# Hallux Varus

*ALLAN M. BOIKE*
*GLORIA CHRISTIN*

Hallux varus resulting from both iatrogenic and idiopathic causes has been reported throughout the podiatric and orthopedic literature. Although hallux varus acquired as a complication of bunion surgery occurs much more frequently, those unique cases of congenital deformity may occasionally present to a practitioner's office.

Hallux varus has been reported as a simple transverse plane deformity, and in those cases is referred to as hallux adductus. The classic hallux varus deformity, however, is triplanar, involving supination of the first metatarsophalangeal joint, hyperextension of the first metatarsophalangeal joint, and hyperflexion of the hallux interphalangeal joint (Fig. 22-1). The hallux is deviated or subluxed medially with a nonpurchasing digit in varus rotation with a possible negative angle between the first and second metatarsals.[1,2]

Congenital hallux varus is classified as one of two types. In the primary type, the varus is the only deformity to be noted. The secondary type is associated with congenital metatarsus adductus, equinovarus, or clubfoot, neuromuscular disorders such as are seen with polio, and other teratogenic anomalies.[3–7]

Abnormal insertion of the abductor hallucis muscle is thought to be a cause of the primary type. In only a few percent of individuals does the abductor ride purely on the medial aspect of the foot. Its usual insertion is the plantar medial base of the proximal phalanx along with the flexor hallucis brevis. Altering its insertion would change its directional pull and likewise its function across the metatarsophalangeal joint, leading more to adduction than to stabilization or flexion.[4]

Cases of the second type of congenital hallus varus have been reported in association with supernumerary phalangeal or metatarsal bones. These have involved duplication of the distal phalanx, both proximal and distal phalanges, and occurred in combination with syndactyly. A triangular to trapezoidal malformation of the proximal phalanx, as well as a congenital absence of the fibular sesamoid, has been described.[3,7–11] It should be recognized that true hallux varus is a deformity of the first metatarsophalangeal joint. Medial deviation of the hallux seen with metatarsus adductus and clubfoot is secondary to a deformity whose apex is found more proximally.[12]

Although acquired hallux varus is most often seen following bunion surgery, two other etiologies should not be overlooked. Joint subluxation following a chronic inflammatory process, as seen with rheumatoid arthritis or other systemic disorders, is known to occur. With weakening of the joint capsular structures, the hallux may drift in a medial direction.[2,13,14] Trauma as a source of deformity has also been reported. Sport injuries that disrupt the lateral joint structures can lead to metatarsophalangeal joint instability, resulting in medial deviation of the hallux.[2,13,15]

Numerous procedures or combinations of procedures have been found to predispose the surgical outcome to a varus deformity. Postoperative hallux varus has occurred following most bunion procedures, including but not limited to the Mayo, Stone, Silver, and Peabody bunionectomies and metatarsal shaft osteotomies, but it is most commonly associated with the McBride technique.[2,5,11,12,16–22] Historically, excision of the fibular sesamoid was thought to be the primary etiology; however, a sesamoidectomy done as an isolated procedure will not produce the varus.[1,16,23] It is

307

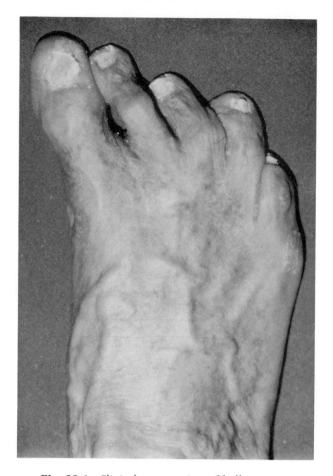

**Fig. 22-1.** Clinical presentation of hallux varus.

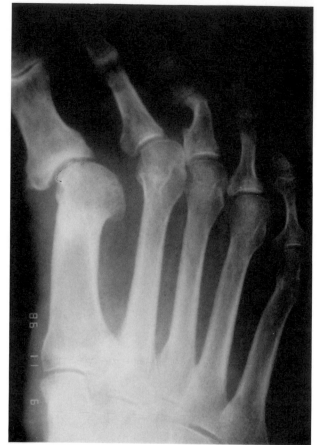

**Fig. 22-2.** Hallux varus following fibular sesamoidectomy.

the combination of surgical errors described below that give rise to this complication.

*Excision of the Fibular Sesamoid.*    Excision of this sesamoid removes the fulcrum about which the lateral head of the flexor hallucis brevis acts, thereby reducing its effectiveness in contraction. This allows the medial head to gain a mechanical advantage and, with time, can cause the hallux to deviate medially (Fig. 22-2).

*Staking of the Metatarsal Head.*    When the first metatarsophalangeal joint is in normal alignment, the medial proximal base of the proximal phalanx travels in the sagittal groove. When this groove is removed by overly zealous osseous resection, its stabilizing effect is lost

and the hallux may drift medially. Plantarly, the groove forms the medial border of the tibial sesamoidal groove. Resection of this border allows medial displacement of the tibial sesamoid and with it the medial head of the flexor hallucis brevis gains a mechanical advantage over the lateral head of the flexor hallucis brevis. Contraction of this muscle then contributes to or increases the deformity (Fig. 22-3).

*Overcorrection and Undercorrection of Osseous Deformities.*    A negative angle between the first and second metatarsals tends to create a varus deformity. As the intermetatarsal angle decreases, the medial vector pull of the soft tissues increases. Once this angle becomes negative, the vector force that helps to correct a hallux valgus deformity now moves in favor of a varus or

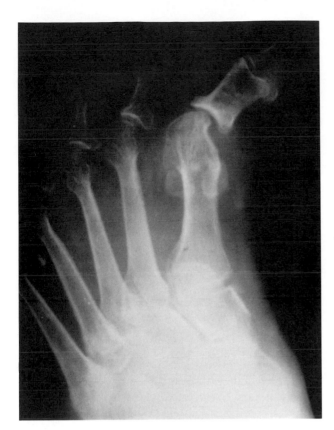

**Fig. 22-3.** Hallux varus resulting from excessive resection of the medial eminence and resulting in a dynamic imbalance.

adducted position. If additional procedures weaken the lateral stabilizing structure, varus deformity may result. When the metatarsal is moved toward a rectus position during hallux valgus surgery, osseous deformity of the metatarsal head and proximal phalanx must be addressed. Failure to recognize an abnormal proximal articular set angle or distal articular set angle or deviation (i.e., overcorrection) in bone shape may result in a varus postoperatively.

*Transection of Adductor Hallucis and Lateral Head of the Flexor Hallucis Brevis Tendons.*    Sacrifice of both these tendons appears to be the significant factor in causing imbalance of the intrinsic musculature around the first metatarsophalangeal joint. Once the balance is disrupted, medial structures will dominate. Incidence of

varus formation is significantly reduced when these procedures are performed individually.

*Overaggressive Medial Capsulorrhaphy.*    This error again alters the balance along the first metatarsophalangeal joint, favoring medial deviation.

*Aggressive or Excessive Postoperative Bandaging.*    When the digit is bandaged in an overcorrected position for a prolonged period of time, adaptive changes and wound scarring occur that then maintain the deformity.

*Medial Tibial Sesamoid Subluxation Following Adductor Transfer.*    Transfer of the adductor hallucis tendon to

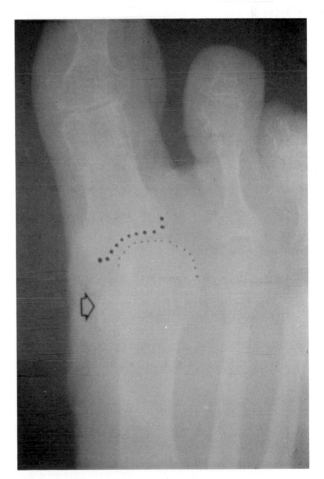

**Fig. 22-4.** Tibial sesamoid subluxation following adductor hallucis tendon transfer.

the medial joint capsule or tibial sesamoideal ligament is done to maintain the corrected sesamoid position following derotation of the apparatus from the first interspace. If the tendon is not of sufficient length or is inserted too far distally, an increase in transverse tension across the joint results. This encourages medial dislocation of the tibial sesamoid, destabilizing the intrinsic musculature and contributing to the deformity (Fig. 22-4).

# CORRECTION OF HALLUX VARUS

When evaluating a varus deformity for correction, it is important to use the same criteria as are employed in hallux valgus surgery. First, inherent genetic factors should be reviewed. The shape of the first metatarsal should be determined. More transverse plane motion is available with a round metatarsal head, whereas less motion can occur if it is more square in shape. A long metatarsal creates an abnormal parabola that affects the biomechanics of gait. Muscle compensation may occur with time, which can contribute to a varus deformity. Any other osseous malformations present that may contribute to the deformity should be identified.

The patient's history and physical examination should include an evaluation for ligamentous laxity. Subclinical Ehlers-Danlos will have an effect on a joint's overall ability to maintain a corrected position. Questions concerning neuromuscular disorders are also important because these disorders can obviously affect gait and may initiate osseous or musculature adaptation over time.

Radiographic parameters should be examined. All angles important to a hallux valgus correction are again used here. Values of the proximal articular set angle, distal articular set angle, and hallux abductus interphalangeus angle should be noted. The degree of splay between the first and second metatarsals should be determined and also whether the deformity involves simply the transverse plane or is multiplanar. Any elevatus should be noted, and the patient's gait should be observed.

Next, it should be determined whether the varus deformity is static or dynamic. Static deformity results from overcorrection following an osteotomy. It is frequently present immediately postoperatively and is usually corrected by an osteotomy aimed at reversing the deformity. Dynamic deformity results from a disruption in the normal balance of muscle, tendon, and capsule around the first metatarsophalangeal joint.[16,20,24] Treatment, then, is determined by the duration, flexibility of the deformity, joint integrity, and any muscle and soft tissue imbalance. Conservative therapy such as bandaging and splinting in a valgus attitude may be helpful only if the complication is recognized quickly. If the deformity has been in existence for some time, a stepwise surgical repair is indicated, using any combination of soft tissue and osseous procedures.

When addressing a varus correction, the soft tissues around the first metatarsophalangeal joint should first be evaluated to determine their influence in creating and maintaining the deformity. The medial capsule should be opened in such a manner as to allow for lengthening and closure, as seen with the V-to-Y or U-flap techniques. A contracted extensor hallucis longus tendon should be lengthened by Z-plasty, and a medially inserted abductor hallucis should be released, lengthened, or transferred laterally. Transecting the deep transverse intermetatarsal ligaments or freeing up its remaining scar will allow for better assessment of first metatarsal flexibility. The lateral joint capsule should be tightened on closure with excision of any redundant tissue. In some cases, total degloving of the first metatarsal head may be necessary to release longstanding adhesions.

Soft tissue corrections alone usually are not sufficient for complete repair. The shape, condition, and position of the first metatarsal must be evaluated. Metatarsals that have been staked or joints which have significant cartilage erosion may be corrected by Keller, implant arthroplasty, or joint fusion procedures. A technique of choice will be determined by the patient's age, activity level, and bone quality. When an implant arthroplasty is being considered, joint stability must be thoroughly evaluated. Implants, by design, are meant only to act as joint spacers and therefore they will not stand up to abnormal biomechanical forces over time.

If the tibial sesamoid is dislocated medially, transferring the adductor hallucis tendon laterally to derotate the apparatus may be attempted. If it cannot be relocated back under the first metatarsal head, the tibial sesamoid should be removed and the interphalangeal joint arthrodesed. The extensor hallucis longus tendon may also be split or transferred in toto to attempt joint realignment. The tendon can be routed deep to the deep transverse intermetatarsal ligament and anchored into the lateral base of the proximal phalanx.

Osseous correction of a negative intermetatarsal angle may be achieved by a reverse distal metaphyscal or reverse base wedge osteotomy, depending on the degree of deformity. A reverse Reverdin-type procedure may be used to correct an abnormal proximal articular set angle, and other osseous deformities of the proximal phalanx may be addressed by Akin or reverse Akin osteotomies.[16,25]

As has been discussed, a sequential approach in the treatment of hallux varus is essential. The reduction must be based on the clinical and radiographic evaluation of the patient. Without appropriate evaluation, procedures may be undertaken that either will not reduce the deformity or will result in recurrence.

# REFERENCES

1. Banks AS, Ruch JA, Kalish SR: Surgical repair of hallux varus. J Am Podiatr Mcd Assoc 78:339, 1988
2. Campbell's Operative Orthopedics. Vol. 2, 7th Ed. CV Mosby, St. Louis, 1986
3. Neil MJ, Conacher C: Bilateral delta phalanx of the proximal phalanges of the great toes. A report on an affected family. J Bone Joint Surg Br 66:77–80 1984
4. Thomson SA: Hallux varus and metatarsus varus. A five year study. Clin Orthop 16:109, 1960
5. Haas SL: An operation for correction of hallux varus. J Bone Joint Surg Am 20:705, 1938
6. Bilotti MA, Caprioli R, Testa J, Cournoyer R Jr, Esposito FJ: Reverse Austin osteotomy for correction of hallux varus. J Foot Surg 26:51, 1987
7. Jahss MH, Nelson J: Duplication of the hallux. Foot Ankle 5:26, 1984
8. Horwitz MT: Unusual hallux varus deformity and its surgical correction. (Case report.) J Bone Joint Surg Am 19A, 1937
9. JAHSS MH: Spontaneous hallux varus: relation to poliomyelitis and congenital absence of the fibular sesmoid. Foot Ankle 3:224, 1983
10. Mills JA, Menelaus MB: Hallux varus. J Bone Joint Surg Br 71:437, 1989
11. Greenfogel SI, Glubo S, Werner J, Sherman M, Lenet M: Hallux varus—surgical correction and review of literature. J Foot Surg 23:46, 1984
12. Joseph B, Jacob T, Chacko V: Hallux varus—study of thirty cases. J Foot Surg 23:392, 1984
13. Hunter WN, Wasiak GA: Traumatic hallux varus correction via split extensor tenodesis. J Foot Surg 23:321, 1984
14. Joseph B, Chacko V, Abraham T, Jacob M: Pathomechanics of congenital and acquired hallux varus: a clinical and anatomical study. Foot Ankle 8:137, 1987
15. Mullis DL, Miller WE: A disabling sports injury of the great toe. Foot Ankle 1:22, 1980
16. Hawkins FB: Acquired hallux varus: cause, prevention and correction. Clin Orthop 76:169, 1971
17. Janis LR, Donick II: The etiology of hallux varus: a review. J Am Podiatry Assoc 65:233, 1975
18. Feinstein MH, Brown HN: Hallux adductus as a surgical complication. J Foot Surg 19:207, 1980
19. Midkiff LC: Surgical hallux varus reduction. J Am Podiatry Assoc 64:160, 1974
20. Miller JW: Acquired hallux varus: a preventable and correctable disorder. J Bone Joint Surg Am 57:183, 1975
21. Johnson KA, Spiegl PV: Extensor hallucis longus transfer for hallux varus deformity. J Bone Joint Surg Am 66:681, 1984
22. Turner RS: Dynamic post-surgical hallux varus after lateral sesmoidectomy: treatment and prevention. Clin Orthop 9:963, 1986
23. Langford JH, Maxwell JR: A treatment for post-surgical hallux varus. J Am Med Assoc 72:142, 1982
24. Zinsmeister BJ, Griffin JM, Rdelman R: A biomechanical approach to hallux varus. J Am Podiatr Med Assoc 75:613, 1985
25. Wood WA: Acquired hallux varus: a new corrective procedure. J Foot Surg 20:194, 1981

# SUGGESTED READINGS

Bateman JE: Pitfalls in forefoot surgery. Orthop Clin North Am 7:751, 1976
Harkless LB, Wallace GF: Clinics in Podiatric Medicine and Surgery; Complications of Foot Surgery. Vol. 8, No. 2. WB Saunders, 1991

Joplin RJ: Sling procedure for correction of splay-foot, metatarsus primus varus, and hallux valgus. J Bone Joint Surg Am 32:779, 1950

Joplin RJ: Follow-up notes on article previously published in the Journal Sling procedure for correction of splay-foot, metatarsus primus varus, and hallux valgus. J Bone Joint Surg Am 46:690, 1984

Kimizuka M, Miyanaga Y: The treatment of acquired hallux varus after the McBridge procedure. J Foot Surg 19:135, 1980

Mann RA: Complications in surgery of the foot. Orthop Clin North Am 7:851, 1986

McGlamry ED, McGlamry R: Reconstructive Surgery of the Foot and Leg. Update '88. Prodiatry Institute, 1988

# 23

# Hallux Limitus and Hallux Rigidus

*VINCENT J. MUSCARELLA*
*VINCENT G. HETHERINGTON*

## DEFINITION

Hallux limitus can be defined as limitation of motion of proximal phalanx at the first metatarsophalangeal joint (MPJ) in the sagittal plane. The normal range of dorsiflexion for this joint is approximately 55°–65°. In hallux limitus, the range of motion is reduced to 25°–30°. With decreased dorsiflexion, symptoms may result in adolescent and early adult life with pain and inability to perform in daily and athletic activities.

With continued loss of dorsiflexion and continued jamming of the joint, degenerative changes occur within the first MPJ with severe restriction of motion, increase in pain, and immobility, which leads to the condition hallux rigidus. In symptomatic hallux rigidus, pain is noted with any attempt at dorsiflexion. The amount of dorsiflexion may be reduced to as little as 0 to 10 degrees with pain on both active and passive motion.

Hallux limitus, and its subsequent counterpart, hallux rigidus, are the most common terms used in the literature as well as the clinical setting. Other terms include hallux equinus,[1] which is described as a deficiency in sagittal plane motion wherein the proximal phalanx is in an attitude of plantar flexion with inability to dorsiflex. In older orthopedic literature, the term dorsal bunion[2] is used similarly to describe the same condition.

## ETIOLOGY

Ever since 1887 when Davies-Colley[3] first used the term hallux limitus, there have been various theories on the formation of this entity. Nilsonne,[4] in 1930, described hallux rigidus as arising from a severely elongated first metatarsal with subsequent jamming of the base of the proximal phalanx. This is caused by the inability of the base of the proximal phalanx to dorsiflex adequately on the head of the first metatarsal. Lambrinudi[5] evaluated the first metatarsal in relation to the remaining lesser metatarsals and found it to be elevated. This condition, termed metatarsus primus elevatus, decreases the available dorsiflexion present at the first MPJ with subsequent jamming. Kessel and Bonney[6] agreed with Lambrinudi in that hyperextension was noted at the first metatarsal in hallux rigidus formation. They also found that in a small percentage of cases osteochondritis dissecans initiated the formation of degenerative changes at the first MPJ with subsequent lack of dorsiflexion.

The belief that osteochondritis dissecans at the head of the first metatarsal was the common cause in the formation of hallux rigidus was further substantiated by Goodfellow in 1966. Goodfellow[7] found that an acute traumatic episode may damage the integrity of the first metatarsal head. This results in osteochondritis dissecans and leads to decreased range of motion as well as the subsequent changes found around the joint margins in degenerative joint disease (Fig. 23-1). McMaster[8] in 1978 further identified the location of the lesion as being subchondral in origin. This lesion was most often found beneath the dorsal tip of the proximal phalanx.

Root et al.[9] described hallux rigidus as being caused by a multitude of factors including hypermobility, immobilization, elongated first metatarsal, metatarsus primus elevatus, osteoarthritis, acute trauma, osteochondritis dissecans, gout, and rheumatoid arthritis. Neuromuscular disorders causing hypermobility or hyperactivity of the tibialis anterior muscle or weakness of the peroneous longus muscle may lead to hallus rigidus by causing instability of the first ray.

Hallux limitus/rigidus can result from biomechanical and dynamic imbalances in foot function.[10,11] The peroneous longus muscle as it courses laterally around the cuboid and inserts on the base of the first metatarsal acts as a stabilizing force during gait to help maintain plantar flexion of the first ray during the midstance phase of gait. This allows relative dorsiflexion of the hallux on the first metatarsal head in the propulsive phase of gait (Fig. 23-2A).

When excessive pronation occurs through the subtalar joint, the peroneous longus tendon loses its fulcrum effect around the cuboid and therefore cannot stabilize the first ray. Hypermobility results in the first ray with subsequent dorsiflexion of the segment and is considered a function elevatus because it occurs during the gait cycle. In contrast, a structural elevatus, if found, is osseous in etiology and may be iatrogenic or congenital in origin. This hypermobility allows for jamming of the base of the proximal phalanx onto the dorsal aspect of the head of the first metatarsal (Fig. 23-2B). With repetitive trauma in this area, osteochondral defects occur. The body attempts to heal this lesion with the formation of new bone in the area (Fig. 23-2C). This new bone formation is seen initially as a dorsal lipping at the first metatarsal head that progresses to involve the dorsal aspect of the base of the proximal phalanx (Fig. 23-3A to C). Through repetitive jamming of the joint and possibly osteochondral fracture, a small circular osteochondral island of bone may be found between the base of the proximal phalanx and head of the first metatarsal, causing further impingement and limitation of dorsiflexion of the hallux (Fig. 23-4A and B).

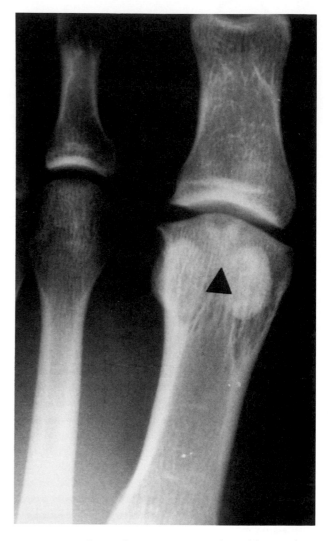

**Fig. 23-1.** Radiographic presentation of an old osteochondral fracture of the first metatarsal head in a patient with a painful hallux limitus associated with restriction of motion, crepitation, and locking. Intraoperatively, a large cartilage tear involving both the metatarsal head and base was identified.

Despite the lack of dorsiflexion of the MPJ in hallux limitus/rigidus, both passive and active plantar flexion is preserved except in advanced cases. Hallux rigidus and limitus may also occur as a complication following surgical procedures of the first MPJ. The restriction of motion may result from fibrosis of the joint or inadvertent elevation of the first metatarsal by distal or proximal osteotomy.

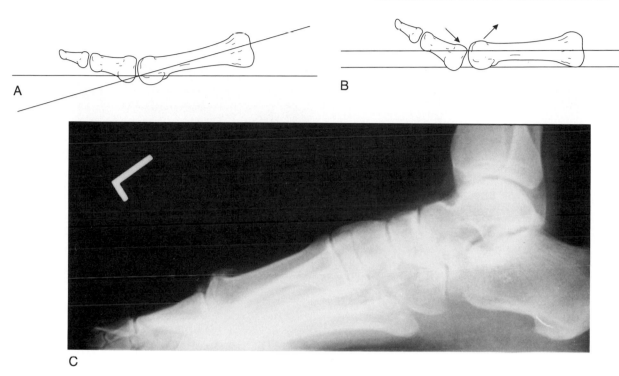

**Fig. 23-2.** (**A**) Normal plantar flexion of the first metatarsal, allowing dorsiflexion of the proximal phalanx. (**B**) Hypermobility resulting in dorsiflexion of the first metatarsal, causing impingement and excessive compression of the joint at the available end range of motion, and ultimately decreased motion and development of arthritic changes. (**C**) Radiographic presentation of hallux rigidus associated with metatarsus primus elevatus. The elevation of the first metatarsal is evident by the divergence of the first and second metatarsal shafts.

## CLINICAL SYMPTOMS

The hallux limitus patient usually presents with a chief complaint of pain at the first MPJ. Pain is most often present with activity. Symptoms include edema and effusion of the first MPJ with palpable pain. There may be associated erythema around the joint, although this usually occurs after extensive or rigorous activity that causes an acute crisis.

The hallux rigidus patient is most commonly seen in early adulthood extending to middle age. Limitation of dorsiflexion is observed, both weight-bearing and non-weight-bearing (Fig. 23-5). A hypertrophy of bone that is present around the joint is evidenced clinically by palpation and by inspection. Pain is present with palpation, and edema and erythema are usually found on examination. Additional clinical symptoms include painful keratosis beneath the interphalangeal joint of

the hallux as a result of the joint compensating for the loss of dorsiflexion of the first MPJ, resulting in an extension deformity of the hallux. A painful plantar lesion, metatarsus primus elevatus, may also result beneath the second metatarsal head as a result of the hypermobility of the first ray.

Biomechanical examination of the patient with early hallux limitus usually yields a pronated foot type with demonstrated increased subtalar joint motion and compensation through the midtarsal joint, as evidenced by eversion of the calcaneus in the stance position. The midtarsal joint is usually maximally pronated, and collapse of the medial arch may be present.

Although pronation is considered a contributing factor in the formation of both hallux limitus and hallux valgus, genetics also plays an important but not fully understood part in the etiology of these conditions.

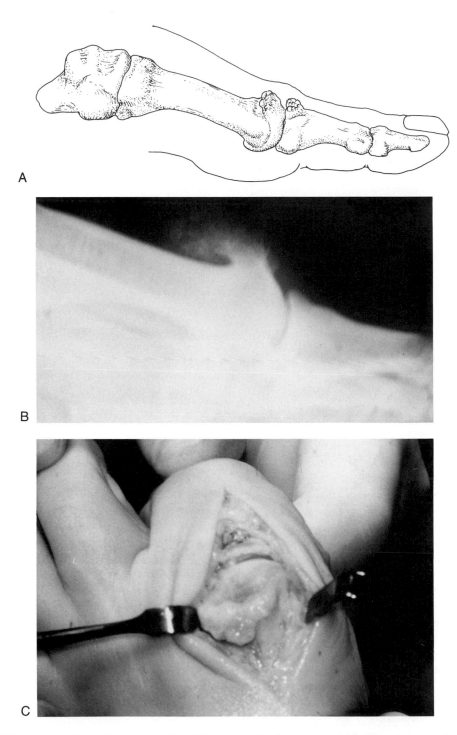

**Fig. 23-3.** (**A**) New bone formation seen as dorsal lipping on the first metatarsal head and proximal phalanx. (**B**) Radiographic presentation. (**C**) Intraoperative presentation.

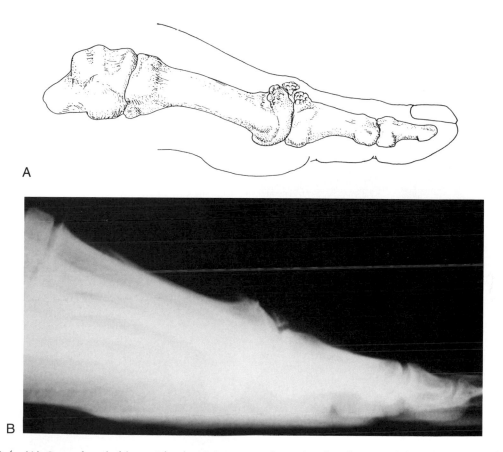

**Fig. 23-4.** (**A**) Osteochondral bone island or joint mouse formed within the joint. (**B**) Radiographic example.

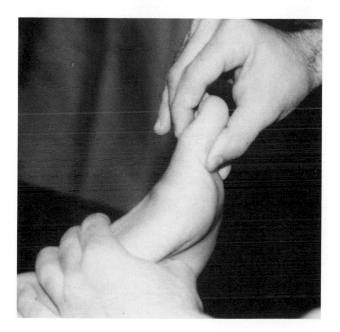

**Fig. 23-5.** Limitation of dorsiflexion of the first metatarso-phalangeal joint in a patient with hallux limitus.

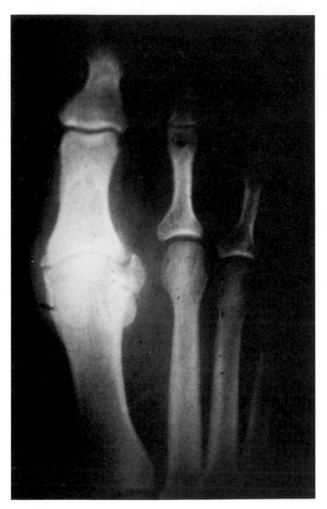

**Fig. 23-6.** Dorsoplantar radiograph demonstrating decrease in joint space and hypertrophy at first metatarsophalangeal joint.

# RADIOGRAPHIC INTERPRETATION FOR EVALUATION

The early stage of hallux limitus may present radiographically with very little sign of a dorsal exostosis at the first metatarsal head. Hypermobility of the first ray may be evidenced by dorsiflexion of the first ray segment as compared to the lesser metatarsals. The foot appears pronated, and on the lateral view, a decrease in the calcaneal inclination angle and increase in the talar declination angle are evident. Joint margins may appear to be equal with little narrowing noted.

The hallux rigidus patient, radiographically, is late stage with severe dorsal flagging and an exostosis noted at the dorsal aspect of the first metatarsal; there is often a concurrent dorsal exostosis at the base of the proximal phalanx. Narrowing of the joint margins on the dorsoplantar view and the presence of an osteochondral circular island are distinguishing features (Fig. 23-6).

The shape of the first metatarsal head may be a significant factor in determining whether a hallux limi-

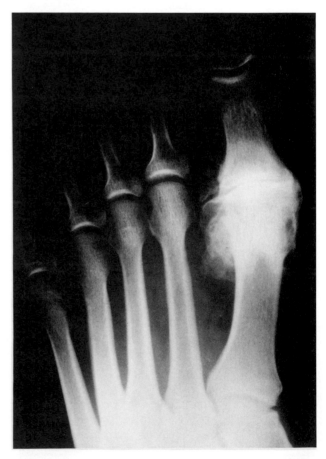

**Fig. 23-7.** Dorsoplanar radiograph demonstrating late-stage hallux rigidus with almost complete absence of joint space at the first metatarsophalangeal joint.

**Table 23-1.** Stages in Progressive Management of Joint Deformity

| Investigator | Stage I | Stage II | Stage III | Stage IV |
|---|---|---|---|---|
| Rzonca et al.[1] | | | | |
| Clinical | DF = 25°–45° <br> Reducible contractures <br> Preschool to teens | DF+ = 5°–20° <br> Minimally reducible contractures <br> Teenaged to geriatric years | No ROM <br> Variable age | None |
| Radiographic | No osseous pathology | Osseous pathology consistent with severity | Joint fusion | None |
| Drago et al.[21] | | | | |
| Clinical | Pain at end ROM <br> Minimal adaptive change | Limited ROM <br> Structural adaptation | Painful ROM <br> Crepitation | <10° ROM |
| Radiographic | Metatarsal primus elevatus | Small dorsal exostosis | Nonuniform joint space | Loss of joint space |
| | Plantar subluxation proximal phalanx | Flattening of metatarsal head | Osteophytic production | Loose bodies |
| | Pronation of rearfoot | Possible osteochondral defect | Large dorsal exostosis <br> Marked flat metatarsal head | Inflammatory arthritis |
| Bonney and McNab[10] | | | | |
| Clinical only | DF = 35° <br> PF = 15° | Limitation of either df or pf | Limitation of df and pf | Loss of ROM |
| Hattrup and Johnson[17] | | | | |
| Radiographic only | Mild osteophytes | Narrow joint space <br> Moderate osteophytes <br> Subchondral sclerosis | Loss of joint space <br> Marked osteophytes <br> Possible subchondral cyst | None |
| Regnauld[12] | | | | |
| Clinical | DF = 40° <br> Pain at end | Decrease in ROM <br> Painful ROM | Little ROM <br> Crepitation | None |
| Radiographic | Slight decrease of joint space <br> Periarticular osteophytes <br> Decreased metatarsal head convexity <br> No sesamoid disease | Narrow joint space <br> Incomplete osteophytes <br> Flattening/broadening of joint surface <br> Osteochondral defect <br> Elevatus of first ray | Loss of joint space <br> Marked osteophytes <br> Incomplete sesamoid involvement <br> Osteochondral defect <br> Loose bodies <br> Hypertrophy of joint | None |

*Abbreviations:* DF, dorsiflexion; PF, plantar flexion; ROM, range of motion.

tus/rigidus condition occurs as opposed to the hallux valgus deformity also seen in pronated foot deformities. Three shapes of first metatarsals are described. A completely rounded metatarsal head may yield to the abductory drift of the hallux and form what we commonly know as hallux abducto valgus deformity. The square metatarsal head is more stable and does not allow the abductory drift, but increases the amount of joint jamming and forms hallux limitus/rigidus. The square metatarsal head with a center ridge appears to be the most stable, which allows no transverse plane motion of the hallux, and with improper pronatory biomechanics appears to subsequently lead to the formation of hallux limitus/rigidus (Fig. 23-7).

## STAGING OF HALLUX LIMITUS/RIGIDUS

Some authors have attempted to stage hallux limitus/rigidus by clinical versus radiographic findings. Table 23-1 summarizes clinical and radiographic staging by various authors; they differ mainly in their interpretation of the amount and quality of the range of motion at the first MPJ.

Radiographic staging demonstrates similarities in the loss of joint space and disruption of the osteochondral defect. The differences include the disruption of the metatarsal head (i.e., flattening), osteophytic formation, and presence or absence of metatarsus primus elevatus.

# CONSERVATIVE TREATMENT

Conservative treatment of the acute flare-up of the hallux limitus consists in reduction of the acute inflammatory phase. Oral nonsteroidal anti-inflammatories in combination with joint steroid injections and physical therapy are usually successful in mild to moderate cases. Also, rest helps alleviate the acute episode. Orthotic control may be beneficial in helping to prevent pronatory forces and stabilize the first ray. Concurrent first MPJ range-of-motion exercises, if successful in increasing the amount of dorsiflexion, may prevent future acute episodes. Patients who do not respond to conservative treatment, especially the hallux rigidus patient in whom there is complete absence of joint motion, inevitably require surgical intervention.

# SURGERY FOR CORRECTION OF HALLUX LIMITUS/RIGIDUS

When conservative treatment has proven inadequate and symptoms are persistent, surgical intervention is indicated. Surgical procedures are tailored to certain factors, such as the patient's age, the amount of deformity, the degree of loss of motion at the first MPJ, and the amount of degenerative changes present both radiographically and intraoperatively.

When planning surgical intervention for the management of hallux limitus, two basic factors must be addressed: deformity of the joint and deformity of the first ray. If one uses Regnauld's[12] classification of hallux limitus, the severity of the symptoms and deformity progress from first degree to third degree (stage I to stage III in Table 23-1). The procedures for management of the joint deformity can be grouped in a progressive fashion, as outlined in Table 23-2, from joint preserving to joint destructive procedures. Additional consideration may be given to management of the osteochondral lesion, a long first metatarsal, and metatarsus primus elevatus. Hallux limitus secondary to a traumatic osteochondral lesion with no elevatus may be managed by arthroplasty of the first MPJ and subchondral drilling or abrasion of the defect.

Procedures such as the Bonney-Kessel phalangeal osteotomy and Waterman osteotomy are joint preservation procedures that attempt to displace the available range of motion in a more dorsal direction. Phalangeal osteotomy with resection for shortening of the hallux may be useful in those cases of hallux rigidus associated with a long hallux. The Waterman procedure redirects the articular cartilage dorsally and provides decompression of the joint. One theory is that in long-standing hallux limitus contracture of the soft tissue of the first MPJ results from the continuing inadequacy of the hallux, hallux flexus, and elevation of the first metatarsal. Decompression as a result of shortening of the first metatarsal by osteotomy also accommodates for the contracture, thereby removing a cause of joint motion limitation. Shortening of an excessively long first metatarsal can be managed by distal osteotomy. Bicorrectional osteotomies can result in shortening (decompression) and plantar flexion. Proximal osteotomies provide a direct approach to the management of metatarsus primus elevatus. Many of the osteotomies used in the management of hallux valgus have been adapted for hallux limitus. The Reverdin-Green osteotomy (distal L) osteotomy and Austin osteotomy, by resection of additional bone from the vertical or dorsal arm of the osteotomies, can provide for plantar flexion. The Z osteotomy performed in the sagittal plane can also be used for metatarsal shortening and plantar flexion.

DuVries[13] in 1965 described the use of a cheilectomy-type procedure that was directed toward the patient with hallux limitus evidenced by the following criteria: (a) decreased range of motion at the first MPJ and dorsiflexion of no more than 20°–30°; (b) pain with range of motion; (c) narrowing of joint space as well as the beginnings of extra-articular bony changes as evidenced on radiography (dorsal flagging); and (d) early to middle-aged adult in whom arthrodesis, joint destructive procedures, or replacement procedures are contraindicated.[16–18]

**Table 23-2.** Staging of Procedures in the Management of Hallux Limitus

| First degree | | Cheilectomy |
|---|---|---|
| | Limitus | Regnauld osteocartilagenous graft |
| | | Bonney-Kessel |
| Second degree | | Waterman or decompression osteotomy |
| | | Implant arthroplasty |
| | Rigidus | Resection arthroplasty |
| Third degree | | Arthrodesis |

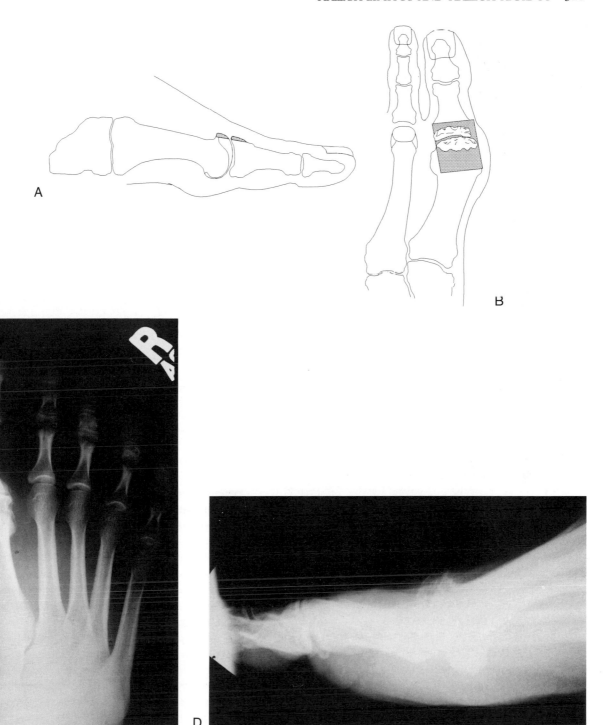

**Fig. 23-8.** (**A & B**) Diagrammatic presentation of cheilectomy surgical procedure. (**C & D**) Preoperative radiographs demonstrating dorsal exostosis of hallus limitus anteroposterior and lateral view. (*Figure continues.*)

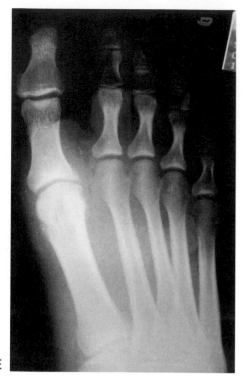

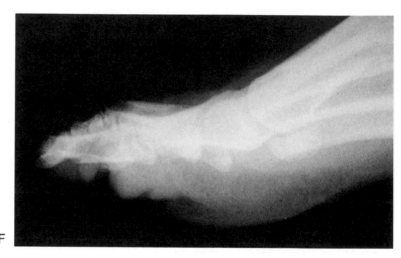

**Fig. 23-8** (*Continued*). (**E & F**) Postoperative cheilectomy anteroposterior and lateral views.

The cheilectomy procedure is sometimes termed a "clean-up arthroplasty." Remodeling of the first metatarsal head is accomplished by removal medially, laterally, and dorsally of all extra-articular bony exostoses that impede the ability of the base of the proximal phalanx to dorsiflex (Fig. 23-8A). Oftentimes a small osteocartilaginous joint mouse is present and is also excised. Dorsally, the base of the proximal phalanx is remodeled, and subchondral bone drilling may be used for any osteochondral defects found in the first metatarsal head (Fig. 23-8B and C).

Early range of motion (usually within 7 to 10 days) following the procedure is extremely important in decreasing the amount of adhesions and fibrosis, which will create a stiff postoperative joint. Early return to motion and activity is an advantage of this procedure.[19] A more aggressive surgical procedure may be indicated in the future, because progressive degenerative joint disease may continue following this procedure. Pontell and Gudas[20] found in their 1988 study good to excellent results at 5-year follow-up occurred with

cheilectomy of the first MPJ. The range of ages of their patients was from 39 to 71 years of age.

Kessel and Bonney[6] described in 1958 a dorsiflexory wedge osteotomy at the base of the proximal phalanx for the adolescent and early stages of hallux limitus. In these early stages of hallux limitus, minimal degenerative changes are present at the articular cartilage but pain is present as the result of jamming of the joint from the lack of dorsiflexion at the first MPJ. There should not be an associated metatarsus primus elevatus or evidence of any bony exostosis or degenerative changes around the joint margins on radiography. With limitation of motion at the first MPJ in the dorsiflexory plane of motion, the osteotomy directed at the base of the proximal phalanx aligns the hallux slightly more dorsiflexed in a resting position and achieves a "relative" increase in dorsiflexion during gait (Fig. 23-9). In this form of hallux limitus, and particularly in this age group, Kessel and Bonney reported good to excellent results utilizing their technique. A disadvantage of the procedure is that because

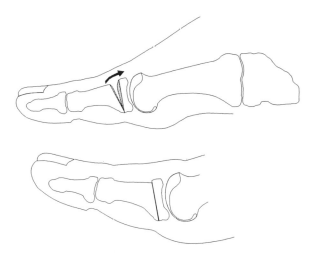

**Fig. 23-9.** Bonney-Kessel procedure.

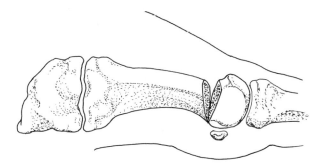

**Fig. 23-10.** Waterman procedure.

an osteotomy is performed, proper bone healing, approximately 4 to 6 weeks, must take place before aggressive therapy is initiated at the first MPJ. This in itself may result in some joint stiffness after removal of the immobilization.

Another procedure indicated in the younger age group was described by Waterman (1927).[19] The healthy articular cartilage of the first metatarsal bone in this condition is directed slightly plantarly. A tile-up osteotomy performed in the metaphyseal portion of the first metatarsal will direct the articular cartilage in a more dorsiflexed, position allowing for increased range of motion (Fig. 23-10). This procedure is successful when articular cartilage damage and bony degenerative changes are absent. It is contraindicated in a severe metatarsus primus elevatus deformity in that this procedure will exacerbate the elevatus and cause increased joint jamming and progression of the disorder.

A closing plantar-flexory wedge osteotomy described by Lapidus (1940)[20] is directed at the first metatarsal cuneiform joint (Fig. 23-11). Creating increased plantar flexion of the first MPJ allows an increase in the ability of the proximal phalanx to dorsiflex on the head of the first metatarsal during the propulsive phase of gait.

An attempt to combine the advantages of a Waterman-type osteotomy at the metatarsal head and plantarflexory osteotomy at the first metatarsal base was

described by Cavolo et al.[19] in 1979. A crescentic type of osteotomy is performed at the first metatarsal base with a concurrent Waterman-type osteotomy at the metatarsal head.

Further modification of this concept by Drago et al.[21] was termed the "sagittal Logroscino." Their technique combined a Waterman-type osteotomy at the metatarsal head with an opening plantarflexory wedge osteotomy at the base of the first metatarsal bone. The procedures described provide structural correction that allow for proper functioning of the first MPJ. They are indicated in the younger, adolescent, or early adult patient in whom again no articular damage is evident as well as no periarticular joint and bone changes.

## JOINT DESTRUCTIVE PROCEDURES

Joint destructive procedures are indicated in hallux rigidus where little or no dorsiflexion is present at the

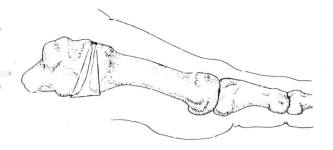

**Fig. 23-11.** Lapidus procedure.

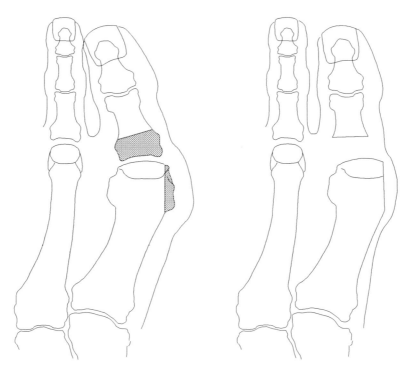

**Fig. 23-12.** Keller procedure.

first MPJ. These joints exhibit severe arthritic changes both radiographically and clinically.

Radiographically there is loss of joint space with squaring of the first metatarsal head and bony proliferation at the joint margins dorsally, medially, and laterally. Clinically the patient usually has such an enlargement around the first MPJ that shoe gear is extremely painful and ambulation is sometimes unbearable. With these late arthritic changes noted, there is complete absence of articular cartilage, and osteochondral defects are present. The aim of these procedures is to either arthrodese or fuse the joint, remove a portion of the joint, or replace the joint.

Arthrodesis of the first MPJ, described by McKeever[22] in 1952, may be an acceptable procedure for certain patients, especially for female patients because of the restriction of shoe gear afforded by the procedure. Its attempt to completely eliminate motion at the first MPJ does alleviate the pain, but compensatory motion at the first ray may occur more proximally and cause, over time, degenerative changes at the first metatarsal cuneiform joint or distally at the interphalangeal joint of the hallux to begin.

The joint arthroplasty described by Keller[23] in 1904 results in resection of the joint by removal of approximately one-third of the base of the proximal phalanx, resulting in an increase in the motion of the hallux relative to the lack of bony substance within the joint (Fig. 23-12). Although this is a common procedure in hallux valgus surgery, especially for the late-middle-aged to geriatric patients, complications are associated with it. These usually include loss of purchase power of the hallux and shortening of the hallux, as well as a dorsal drift of the hallux with the possibility of shoe pressure-induced lesions dorsally on the hallux. Lesser metatarsalgia is often encountered. In the middle-aged patient with severe degenerative changes and a contraindication to joint replacement arthroplasty, the Keller procedure is acceptable (see Fig. 23-12).

## JOINT REPLACEMENT: IMPLANT ARTHROPLASTY

In an attempt to surgically correct severe arthritic first MPJs, Swanson et al.[24] in 1979 described an implant arthroplasty utilizing a silicone-type prosthesis inserted into the proximal phalanx after removal of the base of this bone. This procedure is only indicated in patients more than 50 to 55 years of age because the life of the implant is limited and possible implant complications are associated with it.

Pontell and Gudas[18] found that the use of the hinge silastic implant was a safe and efficacious procedure in patients 60 years or older with severe hallux rigidus. Their follow-up study at 5 years revealed good range of motion and return to an active lifestyle without complications.

Implant arthroplasty, joint destructive procedure, and arthrodesis of the first MPJ are discussed in greater detail in separate chapters.

# REFERENCES

1. Rzonca E, Levitz S, Lue B: Hallux equinus. J Am Podiatry Assoc 74, 1984
2. McKay D: Dorsal bunions in children. J Bone Joint Surg 65A; 1983
3. Davies-Colley N: On contraction of the metatarsophalangeal joint of the great toe (hallax flexus). Trans Clin Soc Lond 20:165, 1887
4. Nilsonne H: Hallux rigidus and its treatment. Acta Orthrop Scand 1:295, 1980
5. Lambrinudi C: Metatarsus primus elevatus. Proc R Soc Med 31:1273, 1938
6. Kessel L, Bonney G: Hallux rigidus in the adolescent. J Bone Joint Surg 40B, 1958
7. Goodfellow J: Etiology of hallux rigidus. Proc R Soc Med 59, 1966
8. McMaster M: The pathogenesis of hallux rigidus. J Bone Joint Surg 60B, 1978
9. Root M, Orien W, Weed J: Normal and Abnormal Function of the Foot, Vol. 3, p. 358. Clinical Biomechanics Corp., Los Angeles, 1977
10. Bonney G, MacNab I: Hallux valgus and hallux rigidus. J Bone Joint Surg 34B, 1952
11. Meyer J, et al: Metatarsus primus elevatus and the etiology of hallux rigidus. J Foot Surg 26, 1987
12. Regnauld B: The Foot (Techniques Chirugicales du Pied). p. 335. Springer-Verlag, New York, 1986
13. Mann R (ed): DuVries' Surgery of the Foot, 4th Ed., p. 263. CV Mosby, St Louis, 1978
14. Mann R, Clanton T: Hallux rigidus: treatment by cheilectomy. J Bone Joint Surg 70A, 1988
15. Feldman R, et al: Cheilectomy and hallux rigidus. J Foot Surg 22, 1983
16. Gould N: Hallux rigidus: cheilectomy or implant? Foot Ankle 1, 1981
17. Hattrup SJ, Johnson KA: Subjective results of hallux rigidus following treatment with chilectomy. Clin Orthop 226:182, 1988
18. Pontell D, Gudas C: Retrospective analysis of surgical treatment of hallux rigidus/limitus. J Foot Surg 27, 1988
19. Cavolo D, Cavallaro D, Arrington L: The Waterman osteotomy for hallux limitus. J Am Podiatry Assoc 1, 1979
20. Lapidus P: Dorsal bunion: its mechanics and operative correction. J Bone Joint Surg 22:627, 1940
21. Drago J, Oloff L, Jacobs A: A comprehensive review of hallux limitus. J Foot Surg 23, 1984
22. McKeever D: Arthrodesis of the first metatarsophalangeal joint of the great toe. J Bone Joint Surg 49B:544, 1967
23. Keller W: The surgical treatment of bunions and hallux valgus. NY Med J 80:741, 1904
24. Swanson A, Lunsden R, Swanson G: Silicone implant arthroplasty of the gret toe. Clin Orthop 142:30, 1979

# 24

# First Metatarsophalangeal Implants

*LAWRENCE M. OLOFF*
*MICHAEL A. FEIST*

Surgical correction of hallux limitus or degenerative articular disease of the first metatarsophalangeal joint (MPJ), whether as singular conditions or in the face of concomitant hallux abductor valgus, is a dilemma with which foot surgeons have struggled with for almost a century. The ideal procedure would provide adequate pain-free motion of the first MPJ without shortening the hallux or unweighting the first metatarsal in gait, and would withstand the rigors of weight, activity, and time. The advent of the implant arthroplasty procedure utilizing silicone-based joint implants was the hopeful solution to this complex problem. After years of clinical experience, however, it has unfortunately become apparent that the silicone implant is not the panacea that many had hoped it would be. Although patient satisfaction has generally been good, complications such as materials and structural failure, foreign body reaction, and short implant life span have forced many surgeons to reconsider its use. However, for a very select patient population implant arthroplasty may still be an acceptable alternative.

Before the development of the silicone implants, the only surgical alternatives available for the "unsalvageable" joint were arthroplasty and arthrodesis. Both these joint destructive procedures had their own individual inherent complications and problems. The development of the silicone implants was an effort to avoid these complications and to try to provide the patient with a functional and cosmetic alternative. The implant arthroplasty is by definition a joint destructive procedure. However, when utilizing the total joint implant, the patient is provided with a spacer to retain hallux length and functional motion for the first MPJ.

This chapter specifically addresses the implant arthroplasty as it is applied to the first MPJ. The bulk of the discussion relates to the total joint implant, although the hemi-implant is also discussed. Implant materials and designs are explained, as are the specifics of the most commonly used implants. Indications, criteria, objectives, and technical aspects of the procedure and postoperative care are also discussed, along with complications inherent to the implant arthroplasty.

## BIOMECHANICAL ASPECTS

The first MPJ is an extremely complex joint, both in its function and with regards to the multiple structures that affect it. The normal function of the first MPJ requires plantar flexion of the first metatarsal to allow dorsiflexion of the hallux. The sesamoids must also be able to glide freely to promote first metatarsal plantar flexion or dorsiflexion. First metatarsal plantar flexion is also required for the appropriate transfer of weight-bearing forces to the first metatarsal.[1] Simultaneously, the hallux must be stabilized by the flexor brevis and longus tendons and collateral ligaments. Transverse plane stabilization is provided by medial and lateral collateral ligaments, which limit sagittal plane motion.

When functioning properly, these structures provide the joint with approximately 90° to 120° of motion, good propulsion, transverse stability, and acceptance of 50 percent of body weight. The axis remains proximal to the joint, centered in the first metatarsal head, and migrates dorsally during dorsiflexion. The

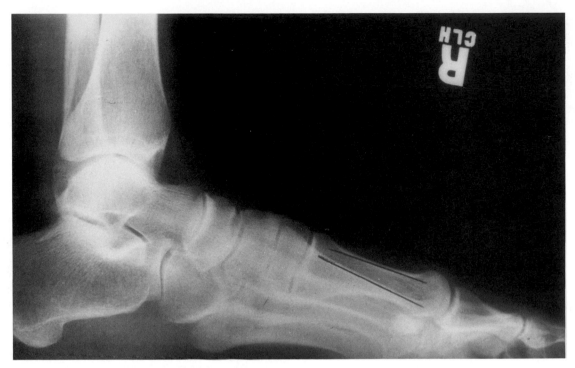

**Fig. 24-1.** Radiographic example of metatarsus primus elevatus.

fact that the axis is mobile is a key to understanding why current one-piece implant designs are unable to provide motion analogous to the original joint. The foregoing are but a few of the complexities that have frustrated attempts to reproduce normal function of the joint using modern implant designs and materials.

Pathologic function of the first MPJ, or hallux limitus and rigidus, has primarily been attributed to pathomechanics in which abnormal pronatory forces act unabated in a rectus foot type. Pes planus and a long first metatarsal will result in similar pathologic function. Structural abnormalities such as metatarsus primus elevatus (Fig. 24-1) and hallux abducto valgus (also a theoretical product of pronation) are also frequently implicated.[2] Eccentric load of the joint eventually compromises the status of the joint and precipitates the development of premature arthritis. Regardless of cause, loss of plantar-flexory ability of the first metatarsal results in dorsal joint impingement and failure of normal dorsal phalanx gliding; tight or contracted plantar intrinsic structures ultimately occur. The excessive forces produced by the host are an effort to "buttress" the areas experiencing abnormal compression forces. Thus, the characteristic findings of dorsal phalanx osteophytes, dorsal metatarsal head osteophytes or so-called dorsal bunion, and squaring of the first metatarsal head are produced (Fig. 24-2). These structural adaptations contribute further to joint limitation and produce excessive cartilage wear and resultant osteoarthritis.

## HISTORICAL PERSPECTIVE

Attempts to reproduce joint function began with Swanson's hemi-implant design.[3] This procedure had hopes of improving on the weaknesses inherent in the time-honored Keller arthroplasty procedure by replacing the resected phalangeal base with a similarly shaped silicone elastomer implant. However, like the Keller procedure, resection of the base of the proximal phalanx to receive the implant resulted in destabilization of the phalanx (caused by resection of the flexor brevis/sesamoid attachment and collateral ligament), thus reducing the hallux purchase and stabilization that assist in first metatarsal plantar flexion. In addi-

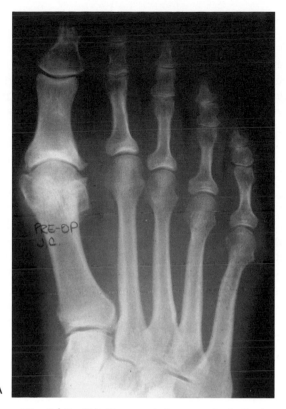

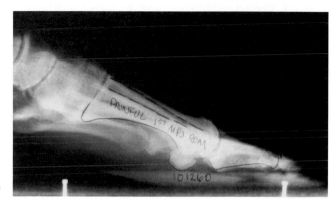

A    B

**Fig. 24-2. (A)** Characteristic osteophytic lipping of the first metatarsal and proximal phalanx seen with hallux limitus. **(B)** Characteristic dorsal osteophytes seen with hallux limitus.

tion, excessive implant wear and eventual implant failure occurred as a result of the implant functioning opposed to irregular and abraded cartilage on the first metatarsal head. This is not unexpected as the presence of arthritis on one side of the joint would be unusual with the possible exception of the early stages following an intra-articular fracture. These factors led to dissatisfaction with hemi-implant use.[4–7]

Designers later attempted to reproduce function by replacing both the proximal phalanx and first metatarsal head with two separate components (e.g., Richards implant.[6] Unfortunately, patients frequently experienced poor transverse plane stability and hallux purchase, loosening of the first metatarsal component, and bony overgrowth of both components.[7] Once again, lack of hallux stability may have contributed to poor joint function, and weight-bearing on the implant (proximal portion) may have contributed to implant loosening and osteophytic production.

The advent of the double-stemmed hinge-type implant provided the transverse plane stability that had previously been lacking in other designs. However, by fixing the axis of motion to the implant, designers inadvertently extended the lever arm for dorsiflexion of the first metatarsal and this produced poor mechanical advantage to the hallux and excess stress at the stem–hinge interface. Continued demands for dorsiflexion at the hinge during dorsiflexion causes flexion and distraction of the stems from their respective stem holes.[1] Thus, a portion of the hinged implant motion is a result of stem pistoning and stem flexion. Efforts to fixate the stems to the proximal phalanx and first metatarsal by use of Dacron mesh resulted in excessive stem–implant interface stress and early implant fracture and failure.[8] Failure of the first metatarsal to plantar-flex also results in excessive transfer of body weight to the second and often third metatarsal. Thus, metatarsalgia and second and third submetatarsal tylomas may result or continue similar to those occurring following Keller arthroplasties. On occasion, second metatarsal stress fractures can even result. In a study specifically addressing second metatarsalgia by Beverly et al.[9] a 33 percent incidence of postimplant second metatarsalgia was found. They also found a 65 percent increase of peak load to the second metatarsal in gait, with a 43 percent decrease in load to the hallux.

It is our opinion and that of other authors writing on this subject[1,4] that the normal function of the first MPJ is not and cannot be reproduced by any of the implant designs currently available. Current designs function only as a flexible spacer that maintains the cosmetic length of the hallux and transverse phalanx stability. We also think that the outlook for a truly functional implant design in the future is promising but that a nonconstrained design is necessary.

## IMPLANT MATERIALS AND DESIGNS

One of the greatest challenges in the development of joint implants has been finding materials that could meet the extensive demands imposed on them by the human body. Ideal characteristics of implantable biomaterials include durability, resistance to deformity and tearing, nontoxicity, and biologic nonreactivity.[3,10] The ideal biomaterial should closely replicate the physical properties of the tissues that it is meant to replace. Initial endeavors involved the use of glass, ivory, metal alloys, and high molecular weight polyethylene, which were promising, given their biologically nonreactive qualities, but their extreme rigidity led to multiple complications.[11] Later, medical-grade silicon elastomer, often praised for its biocompatability, and an elastic modulus similar to cartilage (Table 24-1) was used by Swanson for first MPJ implantation.

### Table 24-1. Comparison of Elastic Modulus (N/m²)

| | |
|---|---|
| Silastic HP[a] | 2.1 × 10⁶ |
| Artic cart | 2.3 × 10⁶ |
| Cancellous bone | 1800 × 10⁶ |
| Cortical bone | 17,700 × 10⁶ |
| Titanium | 120,000 × 10⁶ |

[a] Dow Corning.

Although the material provided the flexibility necessary for a hinged implant, its relative softness provided poor resistance to tear propagation and abrasion. Later, Dow Corning Wright developed its Silastic HP (high performance silicone elastomer), which had a higher durometer reading and elastic modulus. This increased durability reduced related complications, and Silastic is the current acceptable grade of first MPJ implantable silicon.

Silicon elastomers are the most acceptable biomaterials to date available for implantation. Early studies suggested that silicon was extremely nonreactive and that elastomers were simply encapsulated in fibrous tissue. This phenomenon does in fact seem to occur with intact blocks of elastomer. However, clinical experiences with rigid elastomers have shown that microshards are produced from abrasion and wear, and these by-products of implant wear do in fact produce host reactions. Giant cell foreign body reactions, silicon dendritic synovitis, and lymphadenopathy (ranging from 0.01 to as high as 13 percent) have all been reported in the literature.[12–17] Although accentuated immune reactions such as those seen in rheumatoid arthritis have been implicated in the multiple cases of foreign body reactions[5] they cannot account for all the immune-related complications that are reported in the literature.

Mounting concern about the use of silicon biomaterials has led to several studies that have implicated silicon in the alteration of human fibroblast cell metabolism,[18] direct type I and IV immunogenicity,[19] and T-cell activation.[20] Nevertheless, silicon elastomers are still the most acceptable biomaterials available for first MPJ implants and when utilized properly have an "acceptable" level of complications.

### Implant Designs

The hemi-implant, although originally a very popular design (it was introduced in 1967), is rarely used today because of limited indications. The original design (Dow Corning Wright Swanson Great Toe Hemiimplant) has a phalanx base portion that is perpendicular to the square tapered stem. Dow Corning later produced a second design (Weil modification) with a 15° wedged base portion (base of wedge lateral), which is indicated for abnormally angled proximal ar-

**Table 24-2. Implants Most Commonly Used**

| Type | Material | Intrinsic ROM | Sagittal Angulation | Transverse Angulation | Makeup |
|---|---|---|---|---|---|
| * Hemi (Swanson) | Silastic/Siliflex | NLBD | NA | 0° | DC Sutter |
| Angled hemi (Weil) | Silastic/Siliflex | NLBD | NA | 10° | DC Sutter |
| Lawrence | Siliflex | 85° | 15° | 0° | Sutter |
| La Porta | Siliflex | 60° | 15° | 10° | Sutter |
| + Swanson | Silastic | 45° | 0° | 0° | DC |

*Abbreviations and symbols:* *, Now available made of titanium; +, also available with Gromet; NLBD, not limited by design; DC, Dow Corning Wright; Sutter, Sutter Biomedical, Inc.; NA, not available.

ticular set angles such as are often seen with more severe cases of hallux abducto valgus (Table 24-2).

Dow Corning Wright and Sutter Biomedical, Inc. both produce hemi-implants. The Dow Corning model is constructed of Silastic HP in five sizes (0 through 4),[10] with short-stemmed models designated as OS through 4S. The Weil modification hemi-implant (also Silastic HP) is available in sizes 1 through 3. Sutter Biomedical, Inc. produces hemi-implants utilizing Silifex (a medical-grade silicone elastomer) and similar size options are available. Dow Corning Wright has also begun distributing titanium hemi-implants (five sizes). Because research and long-term follow-up studies are not available, we cannot recommend them.

At present, the primary indication for the hemi-implant is arthritis of the base of the proximal phalanx, without concomitant arthritis of the first metatarsal head or limited range of motion. In addition, the phalanx should be stable and without deforming soft tissue or bony structural stresses. Proximal and distal osseous segments must be properly aligned to prevent excessive stresses to the implant and contiguous bone.

Years of experience have shown that, although patient acceptance is generally good, the implant life span can be relatively short and that a significant number of complications have arisen. Problems with implant wear and fragmentation, bony overgrowth, metatarsal cartilage wear, subchondral cysts, and poor phalanx stability have all been reported.[4,6,13,21] Because indications for its use are rather limited and it has a propensity for complications, the hemi-implant is rarely used in podiatry today.

The Swanson double-stem implant (total implant) was first introduced in 1974 and was the first silicone-based double-stem implant.[7] As currently produced, the implant is composed of Silastic HP 100 and has long rectangular stems (proximal stem longer than distal stem) and a U-shaped hinge. Eight sizes are available with the standard stem (0 through 7) and six with small stems (OS through 5S). A titanium grommet set is now also available for each size Swanson total implant. These are thin titanium shields that are press-fitted into the stem hole openings and were developed to reduce abrasion and shear forces at the stem–hinge interface; no long-term follow-up studies are available regarding the success of this innovation. The implant has no transverse or sagittal plane angulation. Although most reports in the literature suggest that the open portion of the hinge should be dorsal when placed, several authors have suggested that inverting the hinge will provide greater dorsiflexion to the hallux.[22]

Along with the indications previously mentioned for total implants, we believe that the Swanson implant is the preferred implant for the correction of hallux varus because of its long stems and inherent rigid and stable hinge. As with other implant usage, deforming soft tissues must be removed concurrently.

Alternative total implant designs have appeared over the years. Produced by Sutter Biomedical Inc., the LaPorta and Lawrence total implants were released in 1982 and were the first centrally hinged implants to enjoy wide use in podiatry. They are both constructed of Silastic, a medical-grade silicone elastomer, and offer design modifications whose intent has been improved function. The LaPorta total implant has cylindrical base portions connected by a central horizontal flexible hinge with 60° of intrinsic motion. The stems are rectangular and tapered with the proximal stem angled 15° in the sagittal plane, which duplicates the

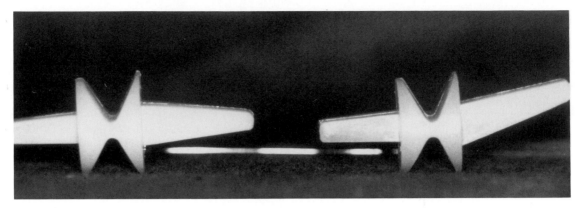

**Fig. 24-3.** LaPorta neutral (left) and standard (right with 15° sagittal plane angulation) total implants.

first metatarsal declination angle. A neutral model is also available with 0° sagittal plane angulation and is indicated for the abnormally low metatarsal declination angle seen with the pes planus foot (Fig. 24-3). A 15° transverse plane angulation is also provided that duplicates the normal anatomic hallux abductus angle (Fig. 24-4). The implant is supplied in four sizes (20, 30, 40, 50) in right left, and reversible neutral configurations. Studies have shown that approximately 40° to 50° of MPJ range of motion can be expected postoperatively,[23,24] and similar results can be expected with the Lawrence implant.[25]

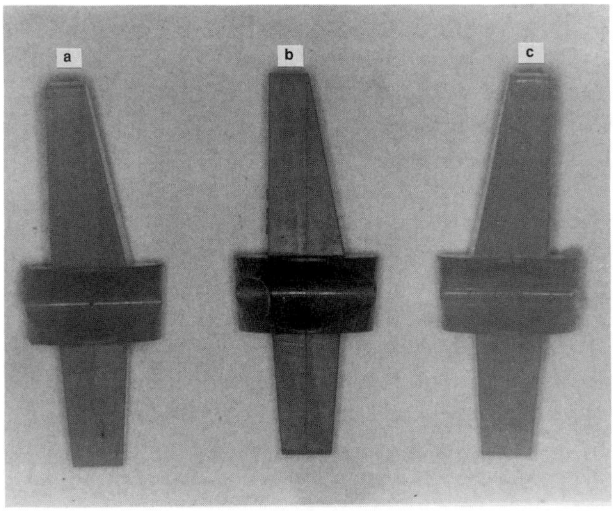

The Lawrence implant is unique in its attempt to preserve the anatomic insertion of the sesamoid apparatus. It does this by angling the proximal phalanx osteotomy from dorsal distal to plantar proximal by 30° from the perpendicular (Fig. 24-5). A guide is available to accurately angle the osteotomy. The implant, like the LaPorta, has tapered square stems with a 15° sagittal plane angulation. The bases are cylindrical with a central horizontal flexible hinge boasting 85° of intrinsic motion. Unlike the LaPorta, the Lawrence has no transverse plane angulation. The implant comes in five sizes (10, 20, 30, 40, 50) and can be used on either foot. Although more technically difficult to place properly, the implant leaves the plantar intrinsics intact and has shown to maintain hallux purchase.[25]

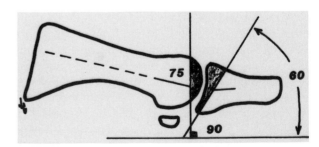

**Fig. 24-4.** LaPorta total implants (*a*, left; *b*, sizer; *c*, right) with 15° transverse plane angulation.

**Fig. 24-5.** Proper osteotomy orientations for the Lawrence total implant.

**Table 24-3.  Indications for Implant Arthroplasty[a]**

Structural hallux limitus/rigidus
Hallux abducto valgus with degenerative arthritis
Painful osteoarthritis
Inflammatory arthridities
Posttraumatic arthritis
Hallux varus with degenerative arthritis
Unstable hallux (flail toe)

[a] The indications listed assume that the joint is not amenable to primary correction (i.e., unsalvageable).

# INDICATIONS AND CRITERIA FOR IMPLANT USE

Dysfunctions of the first MPJ, such as hallux limitus/rigidus, severe degenerative joint processes, or destabilization of the hallux are the primary indications for implant arthroplasty procedures (Tables 24-3 and 24-4).[26] These conditions may present alone or, more commonly, in conjunction with other pathologies of the first MPJ.

Hallux limitus (and hallux rigidus), for the purpose of this discussion, will referr to structural hallux limitus as opposed to functional hallux limitus. Functional hallux limitus is not an indication for implant arthro-

**Table 24-4.  Cause of First Metatarsophalangeal Joint Dysfunction**

Hallux limitus/rigidus
   Functional
      Funtional met primus elevatus (MPE)
      Pes planus
   Structural
      Structural MPE
      Sesmoid abnormalitites
      Osteophytes
      Previous MPJ surgery
      Long first metatarsal
Arthridities
   Inflammatory
      RA
      SLE
      Psoriatic
      Gout
   Degenerative
      Osteochondritis
      Posttraumatic
      Neurotrophic
Stabilizing influence
   Hallux varus
   Flail toe following Keller
   Hallux extensus
   Subluxed hallux with severe hallux abducto valgus

plasty, because the articular cartilage is still intact and joint preservation procedures are thus preferred. Great attention should therefore be placed on discerning functional from structural limitations. Structural hallux limitus and hallux rigidus can be caused by several pathologic conditions (see Table 24-4). Most commonly, osteophytes at the base of the hallux and on the dorsum of the first metatarsal head limit motion by bony abutment during dorsiflexion. Concomitant osteoarthritis is frequently seen in these areas of excessive stress. Structural metatarsus primus elevatus (or a long first metatarsal) can also limit first MPJ motion, as discussed in the biomechanics section. Adhesions of the sesamoid apparatus to the plantar aspect of the first metatarsal head, often caused by chondral erosions, can also limit motion. Iatrogenic hallux limitus following procedures addressing the first MPJ is not uncommon and is frequently the result of fibrous adhesions, tissue contractures, and malunion of osteotomies.

The multitude of procedures available to address hallux limitus/rigidus (Table 24-5) can be divided into two categories: salvage procedures and joint destructive procedures. Determination of joint salvageability is based on the severity of the symptoms experienced by the patient, the physical and radiographic findings, and the actual intraoperative findings. In general, severely painful joints with significant chondral wear and osteophytes are candidates for implantation. However, the etiology of the limitus should be identified and correctable if implant use is to be considered. Ultimately, the surgeon is the one to decide when implantation is warranted.

Osteoarthritis and rheumatoid arthritis are the most common arthritic conditions for which the implant arthroplasty may be indicated (Fig. 24-6). Gout and other inflammatory arthritides on rare occasions may also warrant implantation, but to a far lesser degree than osteoarthritis or rheumatoid arthritis.

The primary objective when considering implantation for arthritic conditions or hallux limitus is the return of function and the relief of chronic pain (Table 24-6). Relief of pain is the objective most easily obtained. However, when considering implant arthroplasty for the correction of hallux varus, severe subluxation secondary to hallux abducto valgus (HAV), or flail hallux (following Keller arthroplasty), the objective becomes stabilization of the hallux. Correction of

**Table 24-5. Alternatives to Implant Arthroplasty for Treatment of Hallux Limitis/Rigidus**

| Type | Advantages | Disadvantages |
| --- | --- | --- |
| Salvage procedures | | |
| Osteotomy procedures | Salvage procedure | Recurrence |
| | | Technically difficult |
| Enclavement (Renault) | Salvage procedure | Recurrence |
| | | Avascular necrosis |
| | | NWB postoperatively |
| Cheilectomy | Salvage procedure | May recur |
| | Technical ease | |
| Joint destructive procedures | | |
| Arthroplasty (Keller) | Less complications | Shortens phalanx |
| | Technical ease | Second Metatarsalgia |
| Arthrodesis | Technical ease | No motion |
| | | Potential for nonunion/malunions |
| | | Transfer weight/motion |

*Abbreviation:* NWB, non-weight-bearing.

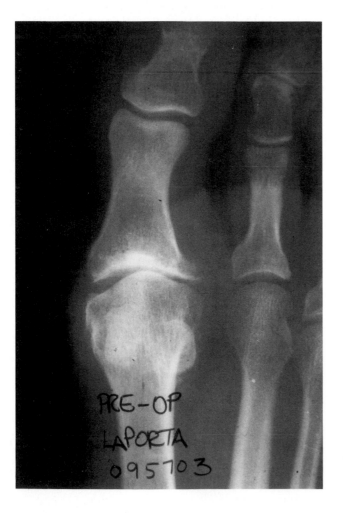

hallux varus using the total implant should only be considered if degenerative articular processes have developed or if soft tissue corrections would result in a severely unstable hallux. All efforts should be made to salvage the first MPJ if at all possible. Soft tissue corrections must be able to fully balance musculotendinous and capsular influences before implant insertion. Improvement of the flail hallux can be achieved using the total implant as a stabilizing force and as a spacer. However, the surgeon should proceed cautiously, because lengthening of neurovascular structures by implant placement might cause a vascular compromise and ultimately threaten the viability of the hallux.

Use of the implant to stabilize the hallux following correction of a subluxed hallux (usually secondary to HAV) should only be considered if articular surfaces have been irreparably damaged. As with hallux varus, all efforts should be made to salvage the joint when possible. If implantation is necessary, then the surgeon must be able to neutralize all deforming soft tissue and structural influences. In particular, an abnormally high intermetatarsal angle (usually seen with severe HAV) must be corrected if an implant is to be used. If the patient is not a candidate for the appropriate base procedure, the implant should not be used.

**Fig. 24-6.** Preoperative radiograph. Note subchondral sclerosis and osteophytes indicative of osteoarthritis.

### Table 24-6. Functional Objectives

Functional/pain-free motion
Stability
Cosmetic length
Durability

### Table 24-8. Ideal Patient

Not overly obese or large
Sedentary life-style
Older
Realistic expectation
Intact immune system
Apropulsive gait

Because the hemi-implant replaces only the base of the proximal phalanx and provides no inherent stability, the authors believe that it is only indicated for posttraumatic arthritides affecting only the base of the hallux. Use for degenerative arthritis is rarely indicated because these processes usually involve wear to both chondral surfaces. Use in the treatment of hallux limitus is not usually indicated, given that surgical remodeling of the first metatarsal head is frequently required, resulting in rough osseous surfaces would rapidly abrade a hemi-implant and likely provide poor motion. Use of the angled (Weil) hemi-implant to correct severe HAV with a subluxed hallux is not advisable if the angled portion is to be used to "buttress" the hallux into the correct position. If the joint is arthritic, then a total implant would be advisable. If the joint is not arthritic, the appropriate osteotomies and soft tissue procedures should be performed to properly correct the HAV deformity.

Once it has been determined that an implant is indicated, then the surgeon must determine if the patient meets the criteria required for implant use (Table 24-7). Evaluation of the bone stock and musculotendinous balance is of particular importance. Soft bone stock or cystic subchondral spaces lack the mechanical support necessary to stabilize the implant, an area of particular importance with the rheumatoid or sedentary elderly patient. When a musculotendinous imbalance is present it must be correctable; if it is left

uncorrected, the abnormal forces could lead to permanent plastic deformation, poor implant function, or even early implant demise.

In addition to the physical criteria required for implant use, the surgeon must also consider the patient population for which implants are acceptable (Table 24-8). The total implants currently available, although durable and reliable, will not withstand the demands of overly obese, large, very active, or athletic patients nor should an implant be expected to last more than 10 to 15 years. Therefore, when considering implantation, the ideal patient should be moderate in weight and size, have an apropulsive gait, and have a relatively sedate life-style. Patient expectations should be realistic with regards to function and expected life span for the implant. The prospect of additional surgery in the future to replace or remove a failed implant should also be clearly explained to the patient, as well as the possibility of requiring orthotic devices to promote proper foot function.

Special consideration should be given to the use of implants in rheumatoid patients because of the increased incidence of complications.[27] Findings of dendritic synovitis, infection, giant cell reactions, and poor bone stock secondary to chronic steroid use have all been reported. Therefore, patients should be very well informed as to possible complications before considering implantation.

### Table 24-7. Criteria for First Metatarsophalangeal Joint Implant Use

Adequate bone stock
Adequate soft tissue strength
Adequate neurovascular status
Adequate skin coverage
No allergy to implant material
Intermetatarsal angle <12–14 (or correctable deformity)
Correctable musculotendinous capsular imbalance
No active infection for 6 months
Adequate immune function

## TECHNICAL CONSIDERATIONS OF IMPLANT SURGERY

The skin incision should be made medial to the extensor hallucis longus tendon, extending from the first metatarsal neck to the interphalangeal joint (IPJ) of the hallux. This exposure will allow for adequate resection of the proximal phalanx base and remodeling of all portions of the first metatarsal head. At this point, correction of any HAV, metatarsal primus adductus, or metatarsal primus elevatus should be completed. Once HAV correction is completed, and hallux should be able to sit in the corrected position without undue deforming stress from lateral capsular structures, tendons, or skin. Excessive abductory force from soft tissue structures will subject the implant to transverse plane stress, which could inhibit pistoning (and thus limit motion) and lead to permanent deformation or fracture of the implant.

While the hallux is held in the corrected position, the base of the proximal phalanx is then resected so that the osteotomy will provide appropriate transverse and sagittal plane orientation for the given implant. If using the Lawrence total implant, the osteotomy angulation guide should be used to properly orient the osteotomy in the sagittal plane. In general, the amount of base being resected should be slightly greater then the base portion of the implant. The excess resection distance allows for pistoning of the implant and slacking of soft tissue structures. The base is then dissected free, taking care to preserve the plantar intrinsic structures and flexor longus tendon. Bone quality of the proximal phalanx can now be assessed, and if necessitated by excessively soft or cystic medullary bone the procedure can be converted to a Keller procedure. A portion of the distal first metatarsal head is next resected. The osteotomy should be distal to the sesamoid articulation, but it should be proximal enough to provide a flat stable surface for the implant to rest upon. Bone quality should again be evaluated to ensure adequate stock for implant placement (see Figs. 24-5 and 24-7).

The sesamoids should now be investigated to ensure that they articulate properly with the first metatarsal head and are not overly arthritic or adherent to the metatarsal head. If the sesamoids are overly

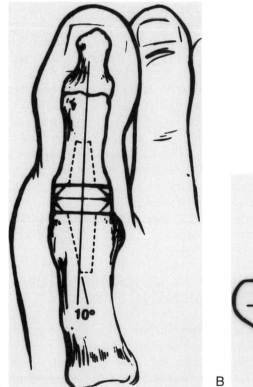

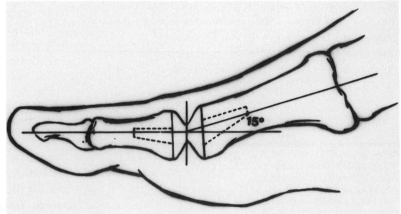

**Fig. 24-7. (A & B)** Proper placement of LaPorta total implant. Osteotomies are perpendicular to weight-bearing surface.

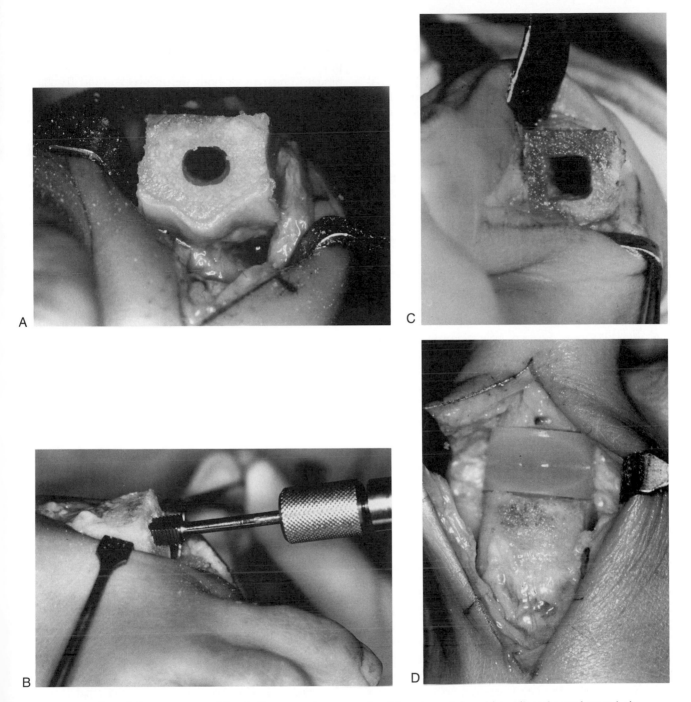

**Fig. 24-8.** **(A)** Fist metatarsal head after osteophyte resection (dorsal, medial, and lateral) and initial stem hole. **(B)** Medullar reaming with manual broach squares corners of stem hole. **(C)** Stem hole after medullar reaming with broach. **(D)** Proper placement of LaPorta implant and appropriate remodeling of surrounding bone. (Note that no bone extends past the edge of implant.)

arthritic, the surgeon may elect to resect them, but he should be conscious of the potential ramifications on short flexor function and ultimately joint stability.

Stem holes can now be fashioned in the proximal phalanx and first metatarsal using a side-cutting burr (four corners). Once the hole is the appropriate depth and diameter, a square broach (manual or power) can be used to square the corners of the hole; this will provide a more exacting stem hole that will assist with rotational stability of the implant.[28] The broach is intended to enlarge and square previously drilled holes and should not be used to deepen a shallow stem hole (Fig. 24-8).

Great care should be taken in the orientation of the proximal phalanx stem hole. The shaft should be parallel to the dorsal cortex of the phalanx and biased to the dorsal aspect of the osteotomy site. The natural plantar concavity of the phalanx and first metatarsal neck place the plantar cortex at risk of being violated if the surgeon orients the stem hole too plantarly. Violation of the plantar cortex may cause inadequate distal stem stability, increased stem abrasion and wear (secondary to pistoning abrasion), fracture of the plantar proximal phalanx cortex, and irritation of surrounding soft tissues. Careful attention must also be given to the coronal plane orientation of both stem holes. Medial and lateral walls should be perpendicular to weight-bearing surfaces to place the hinge horizontal and to prevent torsional forces between the hallux and the first metatarsal.

The surgical site should then be copiously lavaged with a physiologic solution to remove debris created by surgery. Antibiotics may be added to the solution at the discretion of the surgeon, based on host risk factors and any previous breaks in sterile field. As with any joint replacement procedure, prophylactic antibiotics seem best advised. Topical antibiotics remain at the discretion of the operating surgeon.

Acetate implant template sheets can be used preoperatively to estimate which implant size is likely to be required.[10] This is also an excellent illustration for informed consent. Implant sizers can now be used to determine the appropriate size for the arthroplasty site. More accurate sizing lessens the chance for implant size-related complications.

Once placed, the implant should flex and extend freely, and stems should glide freely within the stem holes and should not bind within the hole. The bases of the implant should bridge both cortexes, and no bone should be lipping the implant edge. If the implant is too small, it may telescope into cancellous bone. Hallux position should also be evaluated at this time to ensure that both the transverse and frontal plane orientations are appropriate. Larger sized implants are less likely to be compromised by bone overgrowth. However, larger sized implants require greater bone resection, and if adequate bone resection is not achieved, the motion may be compromised. If stem holes are too tight or if excess bone overlaps the implant base, these conditions should now be modified. Continue to try implant sizers until appropriate motion, position, and bone modeling are achieved. The surgical site should again be copiously lavaged and cleansed of debris.

The appropriate sized implant can now be opened and rinsed in sterile solution (antibiotics are optional) to eliminate any static charge that the implant may carry. The implant should be handled only with atraumatic, toothless forceps to avoid any damage to the implant. All contact with gloves, paper, or linen should be carefully avoided so that no foreign material is carried into the implant site; foreign material such as glove powder, paper fiber, or lint could cause a foreign body reaction. Foreign body reactions often attributed to the implant are in reality reactions to some material that has inadvertently made its way onto the implant during the handling process. Contact with skin edges should also be avoided as this is a potential source of bacterial contamination. If grommets are to be used, they should now be press-fitted into their respective stem holes. Placement of a double-stem implant is easiest if the proximal stem is placed first and the distal stem is then plantar-flexed into the hallux stem hole.

Once placed, the implant should again be tested for proper function. The foot should be loaded in the position of function and again tested for motion. If the implant is functioning properly, the capsule can be closed. Again, function should be evaluated to ensure that capsular closure has not impeded function. Skin closure can then be accomplished and the surgical site dressed. Emphasis should be placed on bandaging of the phalanx in the proper transverse position with compressive dressings to reduce postoperative edema. Postoperative radiographs should be taken on the day of surgery to ensure correct implant placement (Fig. 24-9).

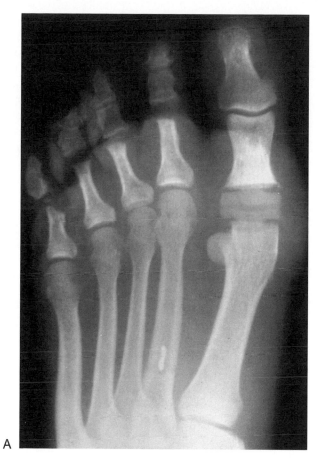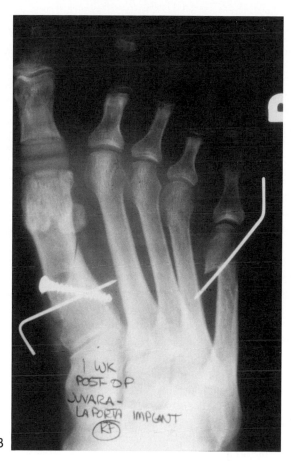

A    B

**Fig. 24-9. (A)** Radiograph of properly placed Swanson implant. **(B)** Radiograph at first postoperative visit. Note that base procedure was required to fully correct metatarsal primus varus and hallux abducto valgus.

## TECHNICAL ASPECTS OF FIRST METATARSOPHALANGEAL JOINT IMPLANT ARTHROPLASTY

The surgical objectives of the implant arthroplasty should be consistently implemented to reduce avoidable complications. These objectives (Tables 24-9 and

**Table 24-9. Technical Objectives of Procedure**

1. Appropriate skin and capsular incisions
2. Complete correction of deforming soft tissue structures
3. Adequate resection of bone with proper orientation
4. Complete correction of structural abnormalities (i.e., IM angle)
5. Proper orientation of stem holes
6. Atraumatic sterile handling of implant
7. Evaluation of function before and during closure

24-10) cannot prevent all potential complications, but they will help avoid correctable problems that consistently lead to implant failures and complications.

### Intraoperative Complications

Complications may arise intraoperatively that would require modification of the procedure or even contraindicate the use of an implant.

The finding of cystic or excessively soft medullary bone is a contraindication to any implant use. Inadequate cancellous strength will lead to failure of the stem holes and result in poor implant stability, failure to maintain proper phalanx position, and potential implant dislocation. The use of bone grafts to pack cystic areas has been suggested. However, we believe this is not advisable because the immobilization required for

**Table 24-10.  Key Points of Procedure**

Proper skin incision placement
Careful capsular reflection from first metatarsal head and proximal phalanx base
Complete release of deforming forces
Adequate resection of articular surfaces with careful attention to orientation of cuts
Remodeling first metatarsal head as required
Fashion stem holes; careful attention for orientation
Evaluate implant function and size with sizor; flush copiously
Place implant atraumatically; correct as necessary
Evaluate, modify, and close capsule
Close skin

proper graft incorporation would seriously compromise rehabilitation of the surgical site.

During resection of the phalanx base, the inadvertent laceration of the flexor longus or flexor brevis tendon may occur. Should this happen, it is imperative that the tendon be sutured to its distal end to prevent total loss of hallux purchase and an eventual hallux extensus. A nonabsorbable suture should be used.

Improper orientation of the stem holes or osteotomies may be corrected by reorientation of the inappropriate osteotomy(ies) of stem hole(s). However, if this would result in overresection of bone or overly large stem holes (and thus an unstable implant site), the surgeon may wish to abandon the attempt at implantation. In some cases, switching to a larger implant may correct the instability. However, this option also carries potential complications and has limitations.

If the proximal phalanx is too short to accommodate a given implant stem length, then the surgeon may alter the implant by cutting the stem to the appropriate length. This is the only alteration that may be made on the implant by a surgeon, and even this may cause increased silicon fragmentation and microfractures. Excessive shortening of the stem should be avoided in that it could produce poor implant stability and potential implant dislocation.

If lapses in sterile technique occur, the authors recommend that the surgical site be lavaged with antibiotic solutions, and the patient should be given prophylactic antibiotics if not given previously. In the case of suspected contamination, antibiotics should be continued for 24 to 48 hours after surgery. This is in contrast to the perioperatively administered one dose of antibiotics recommended for prophylaxis. If the surgical site is grossly contaminated, the surgeon may wish to delay implantation for a minimum of 6 months, or until such time that further documentation as to the sterility of the implantation site can be assessed and assured.

Finally, if the implant fails to function properly once placed, then the surgeon must determine the cause. Failure to resect adequate bone or an implant that is too large often causes difficult or inadequate motion.

Failure of the implant to piston, which can limit joint motion, has several causes. Stem holes that are too small will bind the stems once pressed into the cancellous bone and prevent pistoning. Overzealous medial capsulorraphy and closure during the course of HAV correction also can limit pistoning and should be avoided. As mentioned earlier, adequate soft tissue releases and structural correction must be completed before implantation. Otherwise, excessive stresses placed on the implant will limit function and lead to increased complications and decreased implant life span. The presence of structural metatarsus primus elevatus can also limit implant/toe dorsiflexion.

Once capsular closure is completed, it is imperative that the foot be loaded in a position where the foot is likely to function, in that functional metatarsus primus elevatus may also occur and impeded function.

Recognition of complications intraoperatively and immediate correction of these problems will provide the patient with a more functional foot and the surgeon with a more consistent and reliable result.

## Postoperative Management

In general, postoperative management of an implant arthroplasty site should consist of weight-bearing for 3 to 6 weeks in a postoperative shoe, with the first dressing change at 3 to 7 days and suture removal at 14 days. Both passive and active motion should be started as early as possible. Return to normal shoe gear can begin as soon as patient tolerance will allow.

Immediately following surgery, there are three general areas of concern. First, range of motion should be instituted as early as possible to retain the motion increase achieved at the time of surgery. The patient should be instructed preoperatively in passive range-of-motion therapy and can then begin at home as soon as pain tolerance allows. Eventually, continuous passive motion (CPM) devices will assist with this process. If patient compliance is in doubt, the surgeon may wish to begin a formal physical therapy regimen soon after surgery. The patient should return to flexible weight-bearing shoe gear to promote joint mobilization as early as possible. The vital role of postoperative physical therapy is appreciated with most implant arthroplasty techniques. It is especially important in those patients whose medical conditions predispose them to excessive fibrosis postoperatively, such as in the psoriatic arthritis patient.

Second, aggressive management of potential edema should include compressive dressings (e.g., Coban, Tubigrip), emphasis on postoperative limb elevation, and avoidance of prolonged dependent periods; the use of cryotherapy and nonsteroidal anti-inflammatory medications may even be indicated. Failure to control immediate postoperative edema may lead to prolonged edema, increased fibrosis, and slower joint rehabilitation. A high index of suspicion for early complications, including hematoma, infection, and dislocation, should be maintained.

During the immediate postoperative period, if there are clinical signs and symptoms indicative of a hematoma (Table 24-11), immediate action should be taken. The presence of a hematoma greatly increases the chance of infection and wound complications. In the early postoperative period, the hematoma can be extravasated through the closed wound with gentle manual pressure. A syringe with a large-bore needle can also be used to aspirate focal hematomas, following strict adherence to sterile technique and with consideration for antibiotic prophylaxis. If the blood has clotted, however, extravasation and aspiration are of limited value. If the hematoma is discovered after clotting has occurred, then conservative measures such as heat compression and physical therapy may be used to accelerate the body's normal enzymatic and regenerative processes. If the hematoma is severe or slow to resolve, the surgeon may wish to reenter the surgical site and perform an aggressive sterile wound evacuation.

The best way to handle hematomas obviously is to prevent their occurrence. This can be accomplished by use of meticulous hemostasis intraoperatively, release of pneumatic cuffs before wound closure, and even the use of wound drainage systems. The use of gravity or capillary action drains is not recommended because retrograde flow could contaminate the surgical site. Use of closed pressurized systems has been advocated by several authors,[29,30] although we would caution the surgeon to use careful sterile management of such drains, as they provide potential bacterial portals directly to the implant site.

Infection is probably the most dreaded complication of implant surgery, and as such deserves a high index of suspicion, especially during the early postoperative period. Follow-up visits should always include oral temperature and examination of the surgical site for drainage or pus, elevated skin temperature, cellulitis, lymphangitis, or lymphadenopathy. If in doubt, the surgeon should obtain a complete blood count (CBC), sedimentation rate, and radiographs. Diagnosis and management of postoperative infections are discussed in the complications section below.

If dislocation occurs, it will likely happen in the early postoperative period. Whether caused by trauma, improper implant size, or the failure of soft tissue or bone to adequately contain the implant, dislocation is always a potential complication. When suspected, dislocation can usually be diagnosed with both physical examination and radiographs. The physical examination will usually show poor or no implant motion, deformity, and possibly pain; the radiograph will likely show displaced implant stems or malposition of the hallux. To correct dislocation, the surgeon may try closed manual reduction under anesthesia. However, this is unlikely to be successful. Open surgical relocation or replacement or removal of implant is usually required after dislocation and should be performed as soon as possible after diagnosis of the dislocation.

## Implant Compications

As any other surgery, the implant arthroplasty procedure is subject to potential complications. The implant procedure may be subject to a greater variety of complications because it involves introduction of a foreign body and intrinsic complex demands.

In an effort to logically organize these complications, classification systems have been devised. Vanore

**Table 24-11. Hematoma Signs and Symptoms**

Edema
Tense or fluctuant surgical site
Ecchymosis (plus or minus)
Disproportionate pain

et al.[31] have devised the most widely used system, which separates the complications into four basic areas: problems with the implant itself, alignment problems, tissue problems (soft tissue and bone), and functional problems.

Intrinsic implant failures are those resulting from failure of the implant structure because of environmental stresses. Although silicone is designed to resist permanent deformation and fracture, long-term stresses can surpass the capability of the material. Deformation of the stem or articular surfaces of hemi-implants can result from long-term compressive or torsional forces.

Fatigue fractures of implants are also caused by long-term stresses. Hemi-implants tend to fracture at the base portion or at the stem–base interface, and total implants tend to fracture at the stem–base interface or at a central hinge. Implant fractures such as these have sometimes been difficult to determine from plain radiographs. However, recent studies of fractured MPJ implants have shown that magnetic resonance imaging (MRI) can be very valuable in evaluating implant conditions.[32] The most common intrinsic failure of implants is that of microfragmentation. Even with the advent of the tougher silicone elastomers, it has become apparent that microfragmentation is unavoidable.[33] Given that almost all implants experience some stem pistoning with the stem and base in contact with bone, abrasion of silicone into microfragments can be expected. While in the "solid block" state, silicone is a very nonreactive material that is uneventfully encapsulated[21,33,34] by fibroblasts and collagen. However, microfragments of silicone (10–100 mm) do produce multinucleated giant cell and inflammatory reactions. The effects of these silicone microshards are discussed in the section on tissues. Extrinsic implant failures or structural failures from intraoperative physical insults are almost always iatrogenic. Whether accidental or intentional, any alteration to the implant can lead to microtears that propagate and result in gross fracture or failure.

Alignment problems with implants can be caused by muscle imbalances or improper surgical orientation. Muscle imbalance usually manifests itself in the sagittal plane in the form of hallux extensus. When the extensor hallucis longus overpowers the flexor tendon(s), an extensus results. Evaluation of extensor contractions should be accomplished at the time of implantation and corrected as necessary. However, because intrinsic flexor ability can be disrupted in the process of implantation, hallux extensus may not present until postoperative ambulation has begun. In these cases, a second surgery to balance the tendon or arthrodese the hallux IPJ may be required. Extensus deformities can also result from improper osteotomy orientations. Plantar contractures or plantar-flexed orientation of the hallux are relatively rare and usually result from iatrogenic malpositioning of the proximal implant stem.

Transverse plane malorientation is a problem primarily associated with hemi-implants and is usually caused by imbalance of tendinous or capsular structures. Recurrent hallux abductus is typically caused by inadequate correction of metatarsus primus varus or tight lateral capsular structures. Hallux adductus (varus) is usually caused by overzealous medial capsulorrhaphy. Transverse malorientation is infrequently seen with the total implants, and when it occurs usually results from improper stem hole or osteotomy orientation.

Frontal plane deformities are not a frequent problem, especially when a total implant is used and the stem holes are squared and properly oriented with a manual or power broach. However, oversized stem holes can allow stems to rotate, even in square holes. Therefore, careful attention must be given to proper implant and stem hole sizes intraoperatively.

Tissue problems, both soft tissue and osseous, can be divided into three subjects: infection, host reactions to silicone, and sequelae of the stress of implantation or implant function. Although the incidence of implant infection is similar to that of other lower extremity surgeries (0.38–2 percent),[6,30,35,36] its occurrence can seriously affect the final surgical outcome. Because the body has a drastically reduced tolerance to infection when a foreign body is present (reduced from $10^5$ to $10^2$ bacteria/mm$^3$), the presence of infection may necessitate implant removal.[22]

Infection presentation and its diagnostic picture are best divided into two timeframes, early infection and delayed infection.[36] Early infection, which presents in the first postoperative month, must be differentiated from hematoma and wound dehiscence, which may exhibit similar signs and symptoms. However, the presence of cellulitis, lymphangitis, increased pain, elevated sedimentation rate, and white blood cells

(WBCs) with left shift are all suggestive of infection. Radiographs and radionucleotide studies are generally of little value in this immediate postoperative stage, although some authors have reported increased ability to differentiate infection from surgical sites that are not infected by more specific bone scanning techniques. This is discussed at greater length below. Wound dehiscence, if it occurs, must be differentiated from infection, and deep wound and tissue cultures are a must. Careful investigation of dehiscence sites must be undertaken to determine if sinus tracts or portals to the implant exist. Any exposure of an implant to air in a dehisced or infected wound would mandate removal. If soft tissue infection exists, but is not suspected of extending to the deeper planes, it may be treated with appropriate antibiotics, local wound care, and debridement. Antibiotics should address *Staphylococcus aureus* and *S. epidermidis,* and if prophylactic antibiotics were given, it must be assumed that the offending organisms are resistant to the original antibiotic.

Delayed infections, which can present at any time after the first postoperative month, can be diagnostically challenging. Recent potential causes for bacteremia, such as occurs with certain dental procedures, need to be ascertained. Infection must be differentiated from allergic reactions (i.e., dendritic synovitis or bone inflammation), osseous fracture, osseous proliferation and impingement, and implant malfunction or failure.

Soft tissue infections generally present with new pain, edema, erythema, and possibly lymphangitis. The laboratory tests mentioned earlier may be helpful in differentiating infection from synovitis and implant malfunction. Any presenting sinus tracts or ulcers must be carefully evaluated and differentiated from other pathologies that can produce draining tracts such as rheumatoid nodules or tophaceous gout. Cultures from sinus tracts are notoriously inaccurate in representing actual pathogens, and therefore they should be treated as dubious laboratory information. The use of the radionucleotide indium-111, which has been recommended by multiple studies, has the advantage of being both very sensitive and specific for infection.[37,38] Gallium, which binds nonspecifically to plasma proteins and WBCs,[39,40] can produce a positive scan with many inflammatory situations and thus is falling into disfavor for diagnosis of infections.

If soft tissue infection is suspected, then attempts to obtain cultures should be undertaken. Tissue cultures are likely to provide the most accurate picture of the pathogens involved. If these are not obtainable, aspirations from the site or even blood cultures may be attempted. However, these have very poor yields of pathogens. As for any soft tissue infection, appropriate antibiotic and local wound care should be begun immediately, and surgical debridement and implant removal may be required.

Diagnosis of osteomyelitis, acute or chronic, following prosthetic implants is a difficult task. Because evidence of frank osteolysis or cortical erosions can be difficult to discern around nonfixated implants, plain radiographs are often of little help. Until recently, accurate evaluation of bone around an implant usually required a bone biopsy. Increased experience with radionucleotides and MRI have provided the surgeon with relatively accurate noninvasive diagnostic information. Accuracy of diagnostic ability when combining indium-III with technetium-99 has been reported as 93 percent (versus 70–75 percent for technetium/gallium, 58 percent for aspiration, and 48 percent for plain radiographs),[37,38] with 100% sensitivity for indium alone (25 percent for gallium).[40] These studies were conducted on large fixated orthopedic prostheses, however. It is foreseeable that similar results could be expected for first MPJ prostheses. Use of MRI to diagnose osteomyelitis is becoming more popular and, with increased experience and research, should be a valuable diagnostic tool. If osteomyelitis is diagnosed, then implant removal and appropriate debridement are mandated.

Use of prophylactic antibiotics with implants is an area of considerable controversy. Research specifically addressing first MPJ implants has shown that infection rates necessitating implant removal are reduced with intravenous prophylactic antibiotic use. However, it is arguable that the low rate of infection seen for this procedure would not justify indiscriminate antibiotic use for all patients. It is advisable to use prophylactic antibiotics in patients at high risk for infection, and these would include patients with rheumatoid arthritis, diabetes,[27,36] chronic steroid use, obesity, or advanced age. The authors recommend a 2-g dose of first-generation cephalosporin (e.g., Cephazolin) given intravenously 10 minutes to 1 hour before tourniquet inflation and every 6 to 8 hours thereafter for

24 to 48 hours. For low-risk patients, we believe that surgeons should rely on community standards and their own judgment as to when to use prophylactic antibiotics.

Tissue reaction to silicone microfragments has been attracting more attention as experience with implants has grown. Reactions to silicone can manifest as dendritic synovitis, intraosseous inflammation,[31] cystic bone reactions,[13] and even regional lymphadenopathy with silicone present in the nodes.[12,15–17,41] Although Swanson[15] reported silicone lymphadenopathy as only 0.01 percent, a recent study specifically addressing this problem regardless of symptoms found a 23 percent incidence. Malignant lymphoma has also been found in conjunction with silicone lymphadenopathy, more frequently with rheumatoid arthritis. However, this is a very rare occurrence and neither statistical significance nor causation has been proven.[17,42]

Evidence of intraosseous giant cell and inflammatory reactions to silicone shards has been found (incidence was 57 percent in one study[13]). Radiographic erosive arthritis secondary to silicone-related synovial hypertrophy has also been reported.[14] All these conditions may remain asymptomatic, but symptoms of pain and swelling may necessitate removal of the implant in a few patients.

Bone is the tissue most likely to exhibit complications secondary to the stresses of surgery or implant function. Avascular necrosis, primarily of the proximal phalanx, has been reported[31] and attributed to overzealous medullary reaming and excessive periosteal dissection. Osteophyte production around implants is a very common problem and one that frequently limits motion, produces pain, and may require implant revision. Osteophyte production is likely a response of bone to abnormal forces, but it has also been attributed to osseous generation by remaining periosteum. Incidence of osteophyte production has been reported to be as high as 100 percent by several authors.[6,23] Finally, bone can fail to tolerate or support an implant mechanically.[6] Grooving of the first metatarsal head by hemi-implants is not uncommon[13,31] and can even be seen radiographically. If the implant does not bridge the cortices of the supporting bone, it is also possible for the implant to "telescope" into the softer medullary bone. Osteolysis at the bone implant interface has also been reported (average of 3.4 mm over 7 years),[34] which resulted in shortening of the hallux.

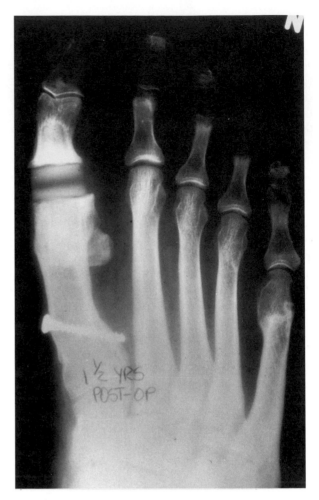

**Fig. 24-10.** Radiograph of LaPorta implant at 1.5 years postoperative. Note sclerotic bone around implant sesamoid retraction.

Fracture of bone around implants is relatively rare, but it may occur if cortexes are burred through or if extreme forces are present at the joint. Sclerosis of bone surrounding the implant and sesamoid retraction are common radiographic findings, but are not considered complications because these are expected findings (Fig. 24-10).

Although many implant complications are not avoidable, many others are. For this reason careful adherence to criteria, indications, and technical recommendations should be practiced.

## NEW TECHNOLOGY

Recent efforts to improve implant life span and function have resulted in several new products. Titanium grommets to protect Swanson total implants at the implant bone interface, released in 1987, were developed to reduce implant abrasion and osteophytic lipping. They are press fitted into the stem hole opening and should cover the osteotomy site. Current reports on their performance is only anecdotal.[43]

Dow Corning has also released a titanium hemi-implant with the hope that implant life span will be improved. This is not a new idea, however, as Swanson's first hemi-implants were also constructed of metal alloys and were abandoned because of numerous complications. The authors think that the titanium hemi-implant has a poor prognosis, given its extreme durometer difference from cartilage, and they cannot recommend its use without thorough long-term follow-up studies.

Several dual-component implants have also been reported,[43–45] but long-term studies of their performance have yet to be published. Historically, implants with these designs have had multiple complications (bony overgrowth, implant loosening, and poor transverse plane stability) and were eventually abandoned. A dual component, or so-called nonconstrained device, if sound in biomaterial and design, is likely to function better than implants presently employed in cases in which the supporting periarticular soft tissues are healthy. With improved function, there is less implant stress and greater chance for implant longevity.

## ACKNOWLEDGMENT

We would like to thank the C.C.P.M. Surgery Department for generously supplying all the photographs for this chapter.

## REFERENCES

1. Orien WP: Biomechanics of implanted joints of the foot. Clin Podiatry 1:29, 1984
2. Gerbert J: Hallux limitus/rigidus. p. 453. In Gerbert J (ed): Textbook Surgery. 2nd Ed. Futura Publishing, Mount Kisco, NY, 1991
3. Frisch EE: Biomaterials in foot surgery. Clin Podiatry 1:11, 1984
4. Sollitto RT: Implant arthroplasty: still a consideration. Clin Podiatr Med Surg 6:149, 1989
5. Glod D, Frykberg RG: Foreign body reaction in a dacron-meshed hemi-implant. J Foot Surg 29:250, 1990
6. Weil LS, Pollak RA, Goller WL: Total 1st joint replacement in hallux valgus and hallux rigidus. Clin Podiatry 1:103, 1984
7. Vanore JV, O'Keefe R, Pikscher I: 1st MPJ joint implant arthroplasty. p. 756. In McGlamry ED (ed): Comprehensive Textbook of Foot Surgery. 2nd Ed. Vol. 3. Williams & Wilkins, Baltimore, 1987
8. Kempner S: Total joint prosthetic arthroplasty of the great toe; a 12 year experience. Foot Ankle 4:249, 1986
9. Beverly MC, Horan FT, Hutton WC: Load cell analysis following silastic arthoplasty of the hallux. Int Orthop 9:101, 1985
10. Burns A: Implant procedures. p. 269. In Gerbert J (ed): Textbook of Bunion Surgery. 2nd Ed. Futura Publishing, Mount Kisco, NY, 1991
11. Kaplan EG, Kaplan GS, Kaplan DM, Kaplan RK: History of implants. Clin Podiatry 1:3, 1984
12. Lazar MA, Morteo DG, De Benycar MA, et al: Lymphadenopathy secondary to silicone hand prosthesis. Clin Exp Rheumatol 8:17, 1990
13. Verhaar J, Vermeulen A, Bulstra S, Walenkamp G: Bone reaction to silicone MPJ hemiprosthesis. Clin Orthop Relat Res 245:228, 1989
14. Schneider HJ, Weiss MA, Stern PJ: Silicon induced erosive arthritis: radiologic features in seven cases. AJR 148:923, 1987
15. Shiel WC, Jason M: Granulomatous inguinal lymphadenopathy after bilateral metatarsophalangeal silicone implantation. Foot Ankle 6:216, 1986
16. Lim WT, Landru K, Weinberger B: Silicone lymphadenitis secondary to implant degeneration. J Foot Surg 22:243, 1983
17. Benjamin E, Ahmed A, Rashid AT, Wright DH: Silicone lymphadenopathy: a report of two cases, one with concomittant malignant lymphoma. Diagn Histopathol 5:133, 1982
18. McCauley RL, Riley DB, Juliano RA, et al: In vitro alterations in human fibroblast behavior secondary to silicone polymers. J Surg Res 49:103, 1990
19. Kossovsky N, Heggers JP, Robson MC: Experimental demonstration of the immunogenicity of silicone-protein complexes. J Biomed Mater Res 21:1125, 1987
20. McCarthy DJ, Kershisnik W, O'Donnel E: The histopathology of silicone elastomer implant failure in podiatry. J Am Podiatr Med Assoc 76:247, 1986
21. McCarthy DJ, Chapman HL: Ultrastructure of collapsed MPJ silicone elastomer implant. J Foot Surg 27:418, 1988

22. Burns A: Implant complications. p. 525. In Gerbert J (ed): Textbook of Bunion Surgery. 2nd Ed. Futura Publishing, Mount Kisco, NY, 1991

23. Dobbs B, Student Research Group: Laporta great toe implant: long term study of its efficacy. J Am Podiatr Med Assoc 80:370, 1990

24. Farnworth C, Haggard S, Nahmians M, Dobbs B: The laporta great toe implant: a preliminary study of its efficacy. J Am Podiatr Med Assoc 76:625, 1986

25. Jarvis BD, Moats DB, Burns A, Gerbert J: Lawrence design first metatarsalphalangeal prosthesis. J Am Podiatr Med Assoc 76:617, 1986

26. Fenton CF, Gilman RD, Yu GV: Criteria for joint replacement surgery in the foot. J Am Podiatr Med Assoc 72:535, 1982

27. Jenkin WM, Oloff LM: Implant arthroplasty in the rheumatoid arthritic patient. Clin Podiatr Med Surg 5:213, 1988

28. Nuzzo JJ, Ganio C: Intramedullary power broaching. J Am Podiatr Med Assoc 76:84, 1986

29. Arkin DB, Rubin DB, Tabb AJ: Use of closed drainage system in implant surgery. J Foot Surg 26:329, 1987

30. Landry J, Lowhorn MW, Black A, Kanat IO: Antibiotic prophylaxis in silastic joint implantation. J Am Podiatr Med Assoc 77:177, 1987

31. Vanore J, O'Keefe R, Pikscher I: Silastic implant arthroplasty: complications and their classifications. J Am Podiatr Med Assoc 74:423, 1984

32. Kneeland JB, Ryan DE, Carrera GE, et al: Failed temporomandibular joint prosthesis: MRI imaging. Radiology 165:179, 1987

33. Sollitto RJ, Shonkweiler W: Silicone shared formation: a product of implant arthroplasty. J Foot Surg 23:362, 1984

34. Verhaar J, Bulstra S, Walenkamp G: Silicone arthroplasty for hallux rigidus: implant wear and osteolysis. Acta Orthop Scand 60:30, 1989

35. Fortman D, Keating SE, DeVincentis AF: Prophylactic antibiotic usage in podiatric implant surgery of the 1st MPJ. J Foot Surg 27:66, 1988

36. Jacobs A, Oloff LM: Implants. p. 274. In Marcus SA (ed): Complications in Foot Surgery. Williams & Wilkins, Baltimore, 1984

37. Johnson JA, Christie MJ, Sander MP, et al: Detection of occult infection following total joint arthroplasty using sequential technetium-99 hpd bone scintigraphy and indium-111 wbc imaging. J Nucl Med 29:1347, 1988

38. Magnuson JE, Brown ML, Hauser MF, et al: In-111 labeled leukocyte scintigraphy in suspected orthopedic prosthesis infection: comparison with other imaging modalities. Radiology 168:235, 1988

39. Jacobs AM, Klein S, Oloff L, Tuccio MJ: Radionuclide evaluation of complications after metatarsal osteotomy and implant arthroplasty of the foot. J Foot Surg 23:86, 1984

40. Bakst RH, Kanat IO: Postoperative osteomyelitits following implant arthroplasty of the foot: diagnosis with indium-111 white blood cell scintigraphy. J Foot Surg 26:426, 1987

41. Rogers L, Longtine JA, Garnick MB, Pinkus GS: Silicone lymphadenopathy in a long distance runner: complication of a silastic prosthesis. Hum Pathol 19:1237, 1988

42. Digby JM: Malignant lymphoma with intranodal silicone rubber particles following metacarpophalangeal joint replacements. Br Soc Surg Hand 14:326, 1982

43. Corrigan G, Kanat IO: Modification of the total first metatarsophalangeal joint arthroplasty. J Foot Surg 28:295, 1989

44. Zeichner AM: Component first MPJ replacement. J Am Podiatr Med Assoc 75:254, 1985

45. Merkle P, Sculco TP: Prosthetic replacement of the 1st MPJ. Foot Ankle 9:267, 1989

# 25

# Review of First Metatarsophalangeal Joint Implants

*VINCENT J. HETHERINGTON*
*PAUL S. CWIKLA*
*MARIA MALONE*

Interest in the development of a functional first metatarsophalangeal joint prosthesis has gradually developed during the past several decades. The motivation for this interest is the recognition of the importance of first metatarsophalangeal joint in foot function and the significance of its proper functioning in achieving normal gait. Recent studies have focused on the shape, motion, and load-bearing characteristics of this joint. These efforts have been directed toward defining the range of motion required for normal function and the center of rotation and characteristics of motion.[1–4] An improved understanding concerning the osseous architecture of the joint will help to delineate joint shape and configuration and thereby define the osseous parameters to be replaced.[5–9] In addition, loading characteristics will clarify material and fixation needs.[10–13]

A classification of first metatarsophalangeal joint implants is presented in Table 25-1. This classification separates the implants into hemi-joints and total joints. The hemi joints are further categorized by materials, either metal or polymer. Total implants are classified as hinged, bipolar, or interpositional. The hinged implants are composed of a polymer, alone or as a composite; the total bipolar implants are constructed of a metal/polymer or ceramic.

This chapter presents a historical and contemporary view of implant arthroplasty designs of the first metatarsophalangeal joint. An effort has been made to be as thorough as possible; however, other first metatarsophalangeal joint designs may have been inadvertently omitted. All dates are approximate and are based on available literature sources.

## ENDLER (1951)

Endler[14] designed this custom implant using bone cement, acrylic methacrylate, to recreate the base of the proximal phalanx. This is the first reference in the literature specifically concerned with the first metatarsophalangeal joint.

## SWANSON HEMI-IMPLANT (1952)

The first Swanson-designed implant for the first metatarsophalangeal joint was a metal hemispherical cap with a tapered stem as a replacement of the first metatarsal head. Bone cement was not used. Swanson[15] stated that the implant was not successful because of the rigidity of the material.

## SEEBURGER (1964)

Seeburger[16] used Durallium to make a first metatarsal head prosthesis. His design had three modifications.

347

**Table 25-1.** Classification of Common and Some Experimental First Metatarsophalangeal Implants

Hemi-Joint implants
    Polymer
        Silastic great toe implant (Swanson design)[a]
        Silastic angled great toe implant (Swanson design), Weil modification[a]
    Metal
        Seeburger durallium[b]
        Swanson titanium great toe implant[a]
Total implants
    Hinge
        Polymer
            Silastic Swanson flexible hinge toe implant[a]
            Sutter hinged great toe metatarsophalangeal joint implant (Lawrence design)[c]
            Sutter hinged great toe metatarsophalangeal joint implant (Laporta design)[c]
            ZMR toe prosthesis[d]
            GAIT[e]
        Composite
            Cutter metatarsophalangeal prosthesis[f]
            Helal universal joint spacer[g]
    Bipolar
        Metal/polymer
            Richards total first metatarsophalangeal joint[b]
            Depuy first metatarsal phalangeal joint surface replacement[i]
            Biomet total toe system[j]
            Lubinus[k]
            Bio Action great toe implant[l]
            Wyss[m]
            Merkle
        Ceramics
            Pyrolytic carbon
            Alumina (Giannina and Moroni)
Interpositional (metals)
    Regnauld
    Barouk Spacer[n]

---

[a] Down Corning Wright, 5677 Airline Rd., Arkubgtibm TN 38002.
[b] Austen Co., New York, NY.
[c] Sutter Corp., 9425 Chesapeake Dr., San Diego, CA 92123.
[d] Zimmer, Warsaw, IN 46580.
[e] Sgarlato Lab. Inc., 100 O'Connor Dr., Suite 18, San Jose, CA 95128.
[f] Cutter Biomedical, San Diego, CA.
[g] Corin Medical LTD, Chesterton Lane, Cirencester, Gloucestersire, England GL7 1Y7.
[b] Richards Manufacturing Co. Inc., 1450 Brooks Rd., Memphis, TN 38116.
[i] Depuy, Warsaw, IN 46580.
[j] Biomet Ind., Warsaw, IN 46580.
[k] Waldemar Link GmbH & Co., Hamburg, Germany.
[l] Orthopaedic Biosystems LTD, 7725 E. Redfield Rd., #102, Scottsdale, AZ 85260.
[m] Questor Clinical Mechanics Group, Kingston, Ontario.
[n] ISI Manufacturing Inc., 1947 Ivahoe Dr., Irwin, PA 15642.

The first type was a complete metatarsal head prosthesis with a double flange, fabricated in 1962. This implant was designed to correct severe hallux valgus. The two flanges were used to fasten the implant onto the stump of the first metatarsal using two self-tapping screws.

The second type (Fig. 25-1) was a metatarsal cap of Durallium to replace the articular surface of the metatarsal head. The third type was a slight modification of the second (Fig. 25-2). Dacron was inserted into the

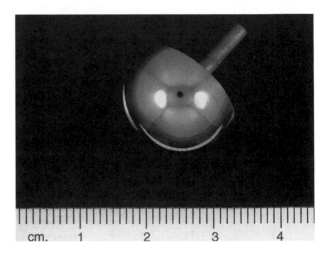

**Fig. 25-1.** Seeburger design, first metatarsal head cup.

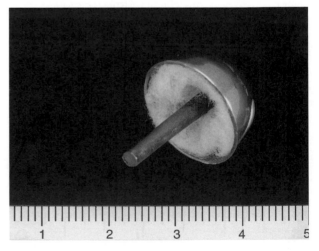

**Fig. 25-2.** Seeburger design, first metatarsal head cup with Dacron modification.

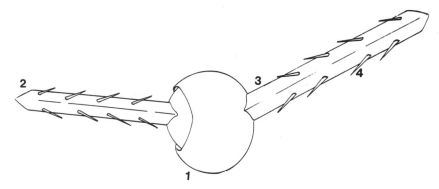

**Fig. 25-3.** Downey's proposed articulated ball-and-socket implant.

cap head in the hope that fibrous tissue would be deposited into the Dacron and secure the implant.

## JOPLIN (1964)

Joplin[17] discussed using noncemented Vitallium implants for the first metatarsophalangeal joint. One design was a single-stemmed prosthesis for the base of the proximal phalanx and the second a single-stemmed prosthesis for the metatarsal head.

## DOWNEY (1965)

Downey[18] proposed, but never constructed, a chromium alloy implant of a ball-and-socket design. Figure 25-3 illustrates this ball-and-socket implant with barbs on the medullary stems to secure the implant.

## SWANSON (1965)

This implant is similar to the implant designed by Swanson in 1952 with the exception that the implant was constructed using silicone.[15] The intramedullary stemmed implant was intended to replace the first metatarsal head.

## SILASTIC GREAT TOE IMPLANT (SWANSON DESIGN) (1967)

Swanson, with Dow Corning,[19] introduced a Silastic single-stemmed intramedullary prosthesis to replace the base of the proximal phalanx. The implant was designed to augment the Keller procedure by acting as a spacer and to preserve its weight-bearing function of the first metatarsophalangeal joint (Figure 25-4). The implant comes in five sizes (0 through 4), and each size has a smaller stem version.

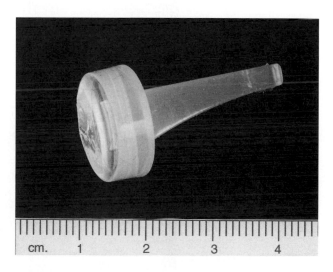

**Fig. 25-4.** Swanson design, silicon single-stemmed hemi-implant.

## CUTTER METATARSOPHALANGEAL PROSTHESIS (1971)

The Kampner-designed implant is a double-stemmed prosthesis with a central hinge. The implant was made from a silicone–polyester composite made by Cutter Biomedical. The first design contained polyester sleeves attached to the stems. It was hoped that the sleeves would allow for better fixation. One design had suture material to be used to increase initial stabilization of the implant (Fig. 25-5). The polyester sleeves were later dropped from the implant because Kampner[20] believed the sleeves caused the implant to be too rigid and constrained, thus causing too much stress across the joint hinge.

## SILASTIC SWANSON FLEXIBLE HINGE TOE IMPLANT (1974)

The Swanson Flexible Hinge Toe Implant was manufactured by Dow Corning. The implant consists of a proximal phalangeal tapered stem with a longer metatarsal tapered stem and a U-shaped crossbar (Fig. 25-6). The design of this implant is similar to a Swanson double-stemmed flexible finger implant from the mid-1960s. A discussion of this implant can be found in Swanson et al.[21] In 1985, Dow Corning introduced a titanium grommet (Fig. 25-7) to shield the Swanson hinged implant from bone damage.[22] The implant comes in 20 sizes that include two stem styles. A standard stem style is available along with a smaller style that requires less reaming of the intramedullary canal.

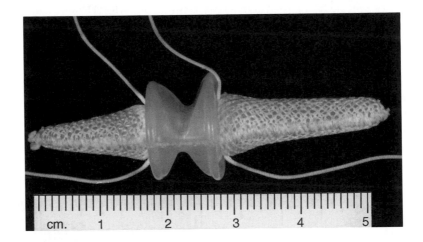

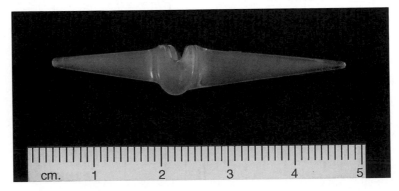

**Fig. 25-6.** Swanson design, silicon double-stemmed, hinged implant.

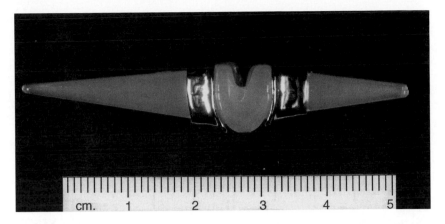

**Fig. 25-7.** Swanson design, hinged implant with titanium grommets.

Sizes are classified from 0 through 7 and 2-0 through 7-0. The smaller stem style is available in sizes 0 through 5. Sizes 0 through 7 and all small-stem implants are recommended for use in the great toe by Dow Corning.

## RICHARDS TOTAL FIRST METATARSOPHALANGEAL JOINT (1975)

Weil and Smith designed a total first arthroplasty system produced by Richards Manufacturing.[23] This two-piece implant had a phalangeal component made of ultrahigh molecular weight polyethylene (UHMWPE) and a metatarsal component of stainless steel (Fig. 25-8). The metatarsal component was designed for right and left components for hallux abductus valgus with an intermetatarsal angle between 12° and 16° and a neutral component for intermetatarsal angles below 12°. The implant was fixated using polymethylmethacrylate. Failure from recurrence of the abductus deformity and loosening were the main reason that use of this implant was discontinued.[23]

## REGNAULD (1975)

Regnuald[24] introduced a stainless steel cap used in interpositional cup arthroplasty. The cap is designed to be sutured into place between the head of the first metatarsal and proximal phalanx after a Keller arthroplasty for 1 year and then removed (Fig. 25-9). The cup was originally designed of polyethyline in 1968; the

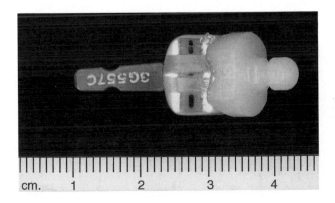

**Fig. 25-8.** Richards total implant.

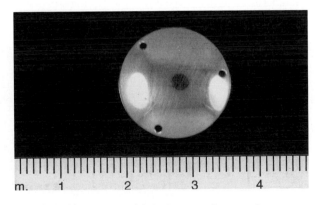

**Fig. 25-9.** Regnauld design, stainless steel cap.

purpose was to develop fibrocartilage on either side of the cup, which after removal of the cup would provide a pain-free mobile articulation.

bility, while the curvature of the collar was smaller to decrease the amount of articulation with the implant (Fig. 25-10).

## SILASTIC ANGLED GREAT TOE IMPLANT (SWANSON DESIGN), WEIL MODIFICATION (1977)

Weil noted an abductory drift of the hallux following resectional arthroplasty using the Swanson hemi-implant.[25] To correct this problem, the hemi-implant was given 15° of angulation so to offset an abnormal proximal articular facet angle. In addition, the stem was rectangular in an attempt to improve frontal plane sta-

## HELAL UNIVERSAL JOINT SPACER (1977)

This silicone elastomer implant reinforced with a Dacron core is a spacer with the central portion containing a spherical ball of silicone (Fig. 25-11).[26]

## DEPUY FIRST METATARSAL PHALANGEAL JOINT SURFACE REPLACEMENT (1981)

The DePuy First Metatarsal Phalangeal Joint Surface Replacement prosthesis is a two-component prosthesis fixed with methylmethacrylate. The metatarsal

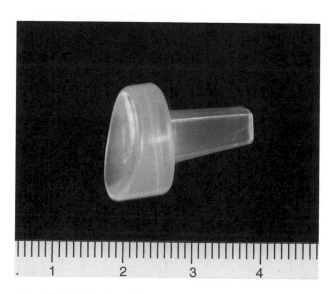

**Fig. 25-10.** Weil modification of Swanson hemi-implant.

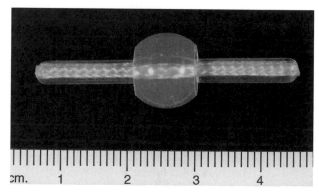

**Fig. 25-11.** Helal silicone spacer with Dacron core.

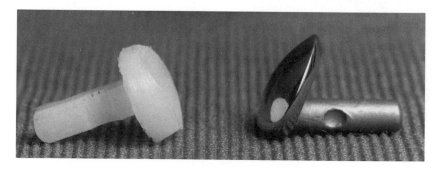

**Fig. 25-12.** DePuy two-component implant.

component is made from stainless steel and the phalangeal component from polyethylene (Fig. 25-12). Johnson and Buck[27] stated that the use of this implant should be limited to older patients with painful degenerative arthritis of the first metatarsophalangeal joint. The results reported were not better than resection arthroplasty.[28]

## SUTTER HINGED GREAT TOE METATARSOPHALANGEAL IMPLANT (LAWRENCE DESIGN) (1982)

The Lawrence-designed silicone intermedullary, double-stemmed, hinged implant is manufactured by Sutter Corporation Inc. The implant design consists of a stem angulated 15° in the sagittal plane (Fig. 25-13)

This angulation was designed to correspond with the metatarsal declination angle.[29] The phalangeal portion of the implant is modified to allow the flexor hallucis brevis tendon to remain attached to the base of the proximal phalanx. This preserves full flexor strength and normal sesamoid function. In addition, the implant has a broad collar for the separation of bone surfaces. The Lawrence-designed, double-stemmed implant is available in five sizes (10, 20, 30, 40, and 50).

## SUTTER HINGED GREAT TOE METATARSOPHALANGEAL IMPLANT (LaPORTA DESIGN) (1983)

The LaPorta-designed silicone intramedullary double-stemmed hinged total implant is manufactured by Sut-

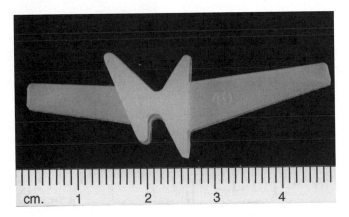

**Fig. 25-13.** Lawrence design, double-stemmed hinged implant.

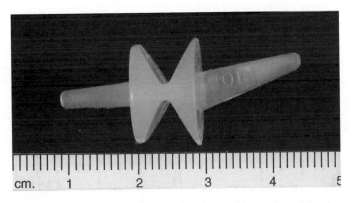

**Fig. 25-14.** LaPorta design, double-stemmed hinged total implant.

ter Corporation (Fig. 25-14). The metatarsal stem is angulated 15° in the sagittal plane to correspond to the normal metatarsal declination angle. In addition, the implant has broad collars to provide protection from cutting bone surfaces of the first metatarsal head and proximal phalanx. Dorsiflexion of the implant occurs in the hinge portion of the prosthesis. The Swanson implant, on the other hand,[30] relies on the viscoelastic properties of the silicone rubber for dorsiflexion. The LaPorta implant can have a 10° stem angulation built into the implant. Thus, the implant comes in right, left, or neutral forms. The LaPorta double-stemmed implant is available in four sizes (20, 30, 40, and 50), and each size has right, left, or straight forms.

## LUBINUS (1983)

This implant was designed to transfer the concept of the double-cup arthroplasty of the hip joint to the first metatarsophalangeal joint.[31] The implant consisted of a hemispheric metal cup made from cobalt chrome and a polyethelene socket that replaces the resected proximal phalanx. The proximal phalanx was cemented for wide osteoporotic canals. This implant was abandoned because of complications in 16 of 22 experimental cases (Hans H. Lubinus, M.D., personal communication to V.J.H.) that consisted of sclerosis and osteonecrosis of cancellous bone.

## ZMR TOE PROSTHESIS (1984)

This silicone elastomer hinged implant, known as the ZMR Toe Joint Implant, is a modification of the 1971 Kamper implant. Instead of the polyester sleeves over the stems, the ZMR toe implant has ribbed stems that allow some fibrous attachment for some stability yet also allow for slight pistoning within the medullary cavities.[31] The ZMR Toe Joint Implant was available in 48-mm, 57-mm, and 68-mm lengths.

## SWANSON TITANIUM GREAT TOE IMPLANT (1986)

Swanson designed this titanium hemi-joint as a intramedullary prosthesis for the base of the proximal pha-

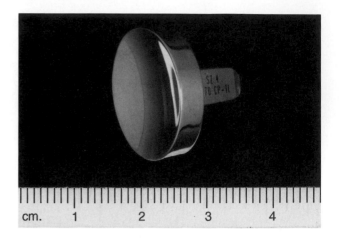

**Fig. 25-15.** Swanson design, titanium hemi-implant.

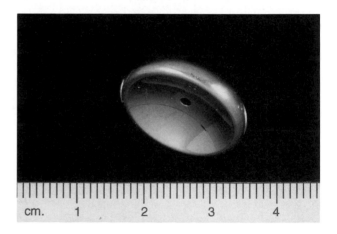

**Fig. 25-16.** Barouk stainless steel spacer cup.

lanx. The implant is manufactured by Dow Corning Wright (Fig. 25-15) and comes in five sizes (0, 1, 2, 3, and 4).

## BAROUK SPACER (1987)

Barouk designed a removable, stainless steel, Spacer cup used with a metatarsophalangeal resection (Fig. 25-16). The cups are to be used with K-wires for temporary fixation. They are made in six sizes and were designed for use in all five digits. This implant, known only from the promotional literature, is similar in

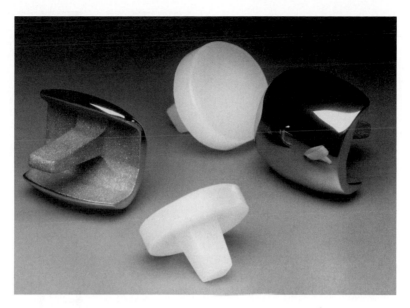

**Fig. 25-17.** Koenig total two-component implant.

function to the Regnauld implant. The implant was later designed using a ceramic material.

## BIOMET TOTAL TOE SYSTEM (1988)

The Koenig total great toe implant, manufactured by Biomet Inc., is a two-component, press-fitted implant that is not cemented.[33] The metatarsal component was initially made from a titanium alloy, while the phalangeal base component is made of UHMWPE or UHMWPE with a metal base (Fig. 25-17). Subsequent designs have resulted in a modification of the metatarsal component. The new component is constructed of cobalt-chrome with a titanium plasma sprayed coating of the stem and back of the articular surface. This design combines the superior wear properties of cobalt-chrome for articulation with the polyethylene material of the proximal phalanx and provides a surface of titanium to enhance fixation of implant. Future designs may consist of a metatarsal component manufactured of cobalt-chrome only (Richard Koenig, D.P.M., personal communication to V.J.A.) This implant, which has had limited clinical use, is available in small, medium, or large sizes.

## MERKLE (1989)

Merkle and Sculco[34] described a custom two-component, noncemented implant. The metal component was made from titanium alloy and the phalangeal component from titanium and UHMWPE. Implant loosening was observed in half of the implanted toes.

## WYSS (1989)

The proposed Wyss implant (Tray/Questor Clinical Mechanics Group, Kingston, Ontario, Canada) is a two-component, noncemented implant. The metatarsal component is titanium, and the phalangeal component is UHMWPE in a titanium tray.

## LU (1990)

Dr. Lu of the Arthritic Clinic and Research Center, People's Hospital, Beijing Medical University, Beijing, China, designed two types of implants (Fig. 25-18). The first design consists of a titanium cup for the metatarsal component and UHMWP for the phalangeal component. The second design resembled the first with notches on the stem for better fixation. In addi-

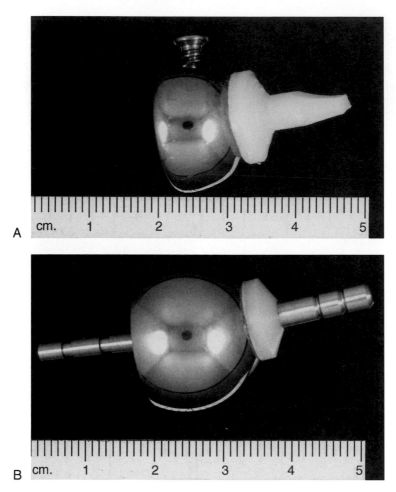

**Fig. 25-18.** Lu design, total two-component implant. (**A**) Type A; (**B**) type B.

tion, the second design used titanium for the stem of the phalangeal component.[35]

## BIO ACTION GREAT TOE IMPLANT (1990)

This two-piece, total joint system is inserted into the medullary canals. The metatarsal component is constructed from cobalt-chrome, while the phalangeal component is constructed from titanium, and polypropylene. This implant is purportedly available in small and large sizes and in right, left, and neutral forms.

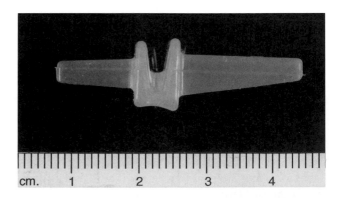

**Fig. 25-19.** GAIT double-stemmed silicone implant.

## PYROLYTIC CARBON (1991)

The proposed use of pyrolytic carbon as a joint replacement biomaterial for use in the foot was discussed by Hetherington et al.[36] in 1982. Kampner[32] in 1991 described short-term clinical results using a two-component pyrolytic carbon implant for the first metatarsophalangeal joint.

## GAIT (1991)

Sgarlato Labs, Inc. makes the GAIT (great toe arthroplasty implant technique) implant. The implant is a silicone, double-stemmed implant similar in design to the Swanson hinged implant and is stained to act as a spacer to augment a Keller arthroplasty (Fig. 25-19). The implant was designed to have a thicker hinge and to allow better toe purchase.

## GIANNINA AND MORONI (1991)

This implant was first described by Giannini and Moroni in 1991.[37] The prosthesis consists of a phalangeal and metatarsal component, both of which are composed of an inert biocompatible ceramic material called alumina. The implant design is based on an anatomic study of 20 cadaver first metatarsal phalangeal joints, resulting in three available sizes. Fixation is uncemented. Its only recorded use is in clinical trials. A report in 1993[38] documented poor performance of this implant with failure due to loosening and breakage of the implant.

## SUMMARY

Of the implants described, few have enjoyed the wide usage of the silicone implants. Recent concern regarding the longevity of the silicone implant and biocompatibility of particulate silicone has led to reassessment of their role in implant arthroplasty of the first metatarsophalangeal joint. The concept of temporary interpositional cup arthroplasty is primarily a European phenomena.

The recent designs have been predominantly nonconstrained bipolar designs with an articulation established between a metal metatarsal component of titanium or chromium and ultrahigh molecular weight polyethelene. To enhance its compatibility in bone, the polyethelene articulation is being secured to a titanium tray. Few data are currently available on the long-term performance of these implants. Ceramic material such as pyrolytic carbon may hold promise for future replacement designs of the first metatarsophalangeal joint.

## REFERENCES

1. Shereff MJ, Bejjani FJ, Kummer FJ: Kinematics of the first metatarsophalangeal joint range of motion. J Am Podiatr Med Assoc 78:439, 1988
2. Buel T, Green DR, Risser J: Measurement of the first metatarsophalangeal joint range of motion. J Am Podiatr Med Assoc 78:439, 1988
3. Hetherington VJ, Carnett J, Patterson BA: Motion of the first metatarsophalangeal joint. J Bone Joint Surg 68A:397, 1986
4. Hetherington VJ, Johnson RE, Albritton JS: Necessary dorsiflexion of the first metatarsophalangeal joint during gait. J Foot Surg 29:218, 1990
5. Yoshioka Y, Siu DW, Cooke DV, et al: Geometry of the first metatarsophalangeal joint. J Orthop Res 6:878, 1988
6. Wyss UP, Cooke TDV, Yoshioka Y, et al: Alignment of the first metatarsophalangeal joint: important criteria for a new joint replacement. J Biomed Eng 11:19, 1988
7. Christman RA, Ly P: Radiographic anatomy of the first metatarsal. J Am Podiatr Med Assoc 80:177, 1990
8. Cwikla PS, Hetherington VJ, Petek JM: Morphological considerations of the first metatarsophalangeal joint. J Foot Surg 31:3, 1992
9. Hetherington VJ, Cwikla PS, Malone M, et al: Sectional morphology of the first metatarsophalangeal joint. J Foot Ankle Surg 33:77, 1994
10. Stokes IAF, Hutton WC, Scott JRR: Forces acting on the metatarsals during normal walking. J Anat 9:579, 1979
11. Wyss UP, McBride I, Murphy L, Cooke TDV, Olhey ST: Joint reaction forces at the first MTP joint in a normal elderly population. J Biomech 23:977, 1990
12. McBride ID, Wyss UP, Cooke TDV et al: First metatarsophalangeal joint reaction forces during high heel gait. Foot Ankle, 11:282, 1991
13. Hetherington VJ, Chessman GW, Steuben C: Forces on the first metatarsophalangeal joint: a pilot study. J Foot Surg 31:450, 1992
14. Endler F: Zur entwicklung einer kuenstilichen arthroplasik des grosszenhengrudgel enke unde ihre bisheride indekation. Z Orthop 80:480, 1951

15. Swanson AB: Flexible Implant Resection Arthroplasty in the Hand and Extremities. CV Mosby, St. Louis, 1973

16. Seeburger RH: Surgical implants of alloyed metal in joints of the feet. J Am Podiatry Assoc 54:391, 1964

17. Joplin RJ: The proper digital nerve, vitallium stem arthroplasty, and some thoughts about foot surgery in general. Clin Orthop Relat Res 76:199, 1971

18. Downey MA: A ball and socket metal prosthetic joint replacement, as applied to the foot. J Am Podiatry Assoc 55:343, 1965

19. Kaplan EG, Kaplan GS, Kaplan DM, Kaplan RK: History of implants. Clin Podiatry 1:3, 1984

20. Kampner SL: Total joint prosthetic arthroplasty of the great toe—a twelve year experience. Foot Ankle 4:249, 1984

21. Swanson AB, Lumsden RM II, Swanson GD: Silicone implant arthroplasty of the great toe. Clin Orthop Relat Res 142:30, 1979

22. Swanson AB, Swanson G de G, Maupin BK, et al: The use of a grommet bone linear for flexible hinge implant arthroplasty of the great toe. Foot Ankle 12:149, 1991

23. Weil LS, Pollak RA, Goller WL: Total first joint replacement in hallux valgus and hallux rigidus, longterm results in 484 cases. Clin Podiatry 1:103, 1984

24. Regnauld B: The Foot, Pathology, Aetiology, Semiology, Clinical Investigation and Therapy. Springer-Verlag, New York, 1986

25. Arenson DJ: The angled great toe implant (Swanson design/Weil modification) in the surgical reconstruction of the first metatarsophalangeal joint. Clin Podiatry 1:89, 1984

26. Helal B, Chen SC: Arthroplastik des grosszehengrundgelenks mit einer neuen silastik—endoprothese. Orthopade 11:220, 1982

27. Johnson KA, Buck PG: Total replacement arthroplasty of the first metatarsophalangeal joint. Foot Ankle 1:307, 1981

28. Johnson KA: Dissatisfaction following hallux valgus surgery. p. 63. In Surgery of the Foot and Ankle, Raven, New York, 1989

29. Jarvis BD, Moats DB, Burns A, Gerbert J: Lawrence design first metatarsophalangeal joint prosthesis. J Am Podiatr Med Assoc 76:617, 1986

30. Hetherington VJ, Cuesta AL: Implant arthroplasty of the first metatarsophalangeal joint and alternatives. p. 1005. In Levy LA, Hetherington VJ (eds): Principles and Practice of Podiatric Medicine. Churchill Livingstone, New York, 1990

31. Lubinus H: Endoprothetischer ersatz des robzehengrundgelenkes. Arch Orthop Trauma Surg 121:89, 1983

32. Kampner SL: Implants and Biomaterials in the foot. p. 2688. In Jahss MH (ed): Disorder of the Foot and Ankle, Medical and Surgical Management. WB Saunders, Philadelphia, 1991

33. Koenig RD: Koenig total great toe implant, preliminary report. J Am Podiatr Med Assoc 80:462, 1990

34. Merkle PF, Sculco TP: Prosthetic replacement of the first metatarsophalangeal joint. Foot Ankle 9:267, 1989

35. Lu HS: Follow-up result in 14 cases of the 1st metatarsophalangeal joint arthroplasty with titanium total joint prostheses—introduction to two designs of titanium total MTP prosthesis (in Chinese). Chin J Orthop (submitted for publication)

36. Hetherington VJ, Kavros SJ, Conway F, et al: Pyrolytic carbon as a joint replacement in the foot, a preliminary report. J Foot Surg 21:160, 1982

37. Giannini S, Moroni A: Alumina total joint replacement of the first metatarsophalangeal joint. p. 39. In Bonfield W, Hastings GW, Tanner KE (eds): Bioceramics. Vol. 4. Butterworth-Heinemann, London, 1991

38. Giannini S. First metatarsal joint implant. Presented at the American College of Foot and Ankle Surgeons World Foot and Ankle Congress. October 21–23, 1993

# 26

# Surgical Management of Digital Deformities

## BONNIE J. NICKLAS

All too frequently, a painful and deformed digit may be diagnosed under the commonly used terminology of "hammer toe," when in fact it may not be a hammer toe at all. Digital deformities vary widely in their presentation, severity, and etiology. To choose the best possible surgical procedure for correction of the deformity, it is critical that certain aspects of the deformity be clearly identified.

Digital deformities involving the second, third, fourth, and fifth toes can be classified and described using a number of parameters (Fig. 26-1; Table 26-1). The deformities can occur on the sagittal, transverse, or frontal planes or any combination of these planes. They may be static or dynamic and may occur singularly or as part of a group in which all lesser digits display the abnormality. They may have no planal abnormalities, that is, display no contraction or rotation, yet exhibit painful pressure lesions. If contraction or rotation is present, the contraction may be flexible and reducible, or it may be rigid and nonreducible. Etiologies of digital deformities vary widely, and may be congenital or acquired, simple or complex, the result of surgical failure or naturally occurring.

The extensive history of digital surgery includes soft tissue procedures only, osseous procedures involving partial or total resection of bone, fusions and amputations, and an untold number of combinations of these.[1–8]

Soft tissue procedures include tendon releases and lengthenings, capsulotomies, extensor hood apparatus releases, ligament releases, and tendon transfers. Tenotomies with or without capsulotomies as isolated procedures are rarely indicated. Extensor and flexor tenotomy and capsulotomy find greatest application in the older patient in whom more definitive reconstructive surgery is not possible.[8]

Tendon transfers have been reported for a number of purposes. In 1928, Forrester-Brown used transfer of the long flexor tendon to the extensor tendons to replace lost intrinsic function to the hallux.[9] In 1942 Lapidus described transfer of the extensor tendon for correction of the overlapping fifth toe.[10] In 1947, Girdlestone transferred flexor digitorum longus tendons into dorsal expansions of the extensor tendons in the hope that intrinsic function that had been lost would be restored.[11] Sgarlato performed flexor tendon transfer to itself and to the extensor tendons for contracted digits.[12] In 1984, Barbari and Brevig performed the previously mentioned Girdlestone-Taylor with Parrish's modification.[13] In 1980, Kuwada and Dockery reported a modification of the flexor transfer in which the flexor tendon was brought through a drill hole in the anatomic neck of the proximal phalanx.[14] In 1988, Kuwada followed with a retrospective analysis of modification of the flexor tendon transfer for correction of hammer toe deformities, as a long-term look back at those performed previously.[15]

Osseous procedures include partial resection of phalanges,[1–5,16,17] total resections of phalanges, and digital amputations.[18,19] All parts of the phalanx have at one time or another been removed, including condyles, the head, the base, and the diaphyseal shaft. In 1910 Soule described the first arthrodesis procedure of the proximal interphalangeal joint (PIPJ).[20] Other modifications have included the "spike" and hole of Higgs in 1931[21] and the truncated cone-shaped design

359

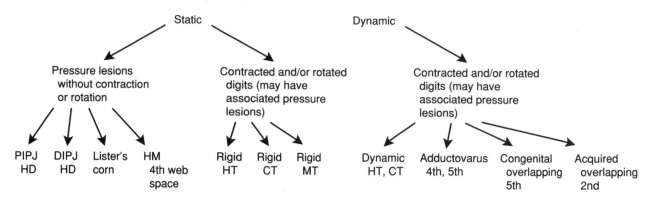

**Fig. 26-1.** Classification of lesser digital deformities.

**Table 26-1.** Classification of Digital Deformities

| Type of Deformity | Etiology | Procedure of Choice | Skin Incision |
|---|---|---|---|
| Static deformities | | | |
| Pressure lesions without contraction or rotation | | | |
| PIPJ HD | Enlarged or deformed proximal phalanx | Arthroplasty, proximal phalangeal head resection | Dorsal linear |
| PIPJ/DIPJ HD | Enlarged or deformed middle phalanx | Arthroplasty, middle phalangectomy | Dorsal linear[a] |
| Lister's corn | Enlarged lateral condyle, distal phalanx | Condylectomy, lateral aspect, distal phalanx | Lazy S |
| Mild to moderate HM, 4th web space | Pressure: head; proximal phalanx, 5th toe at base; proximal phalanx, 4th toe | Post procedure, 5th toe; lateral condylectomy, 4th toe | Dorsal linear 4/5 |
| Severe HM, 4th web space | Longstanding, recurrent, scar tissue | Syndactylization, 4th & 5th toes | Oval, diamond shaped |
| Pressure lesions with contraction | | | |
| Rigid hammer toe | Elongation, shoe gear influence, other | PIPJ arthroplasty, proximal phalanx head resection | Dorsal linear |
| Rigid claw toe | Elongation, shoe gear influence, other | DIPJ arthroplasty and possible middle phalangeal head resection | Dorsal linear |
| Rigid mallet toe | Elongation, shoe gear, fusion at PIPJ | DIPJ arthroplasty, middle phalangeal head resection | Transverse lenticular over DIPJ |
| Dynamic deformities with contraction and/or rotation | | | |
| Dynamic hammer toes or claw toes | Biomechanical: ext/flex subst, flex stab | PIPJ arthrodesis, 2, 3 PIPJ arthroplasty, 4, 5 with possible DIPJ arthroplasty with sequential reduction | Dorsal curvilinear extended over MPJ |
| Adductovarus 4th, 5th | Biomechanical: mechanical or congenital | PIPJ arthroplasty with derotational skin plasty | Oblique lenticular |
| Overlapping 5th | Congenital | Relocational arthroplasty | V–Y or Z-plasty |
| Overlapping 2nd | Acquired | Relocation/reduction with stabilization PIPJ arthroplasty or arthrodesis | Dorsal curvilinear |

*Abbreviations:* PIPJ, proximal interphalangeal joint; HD, heloma durum; DIPJ, distal interphalangeal joint; HM, heloma mollé.
[a] Over time, dynamic, flexible deformities can become static and rigid due to malignment of joints leading to articular damage.

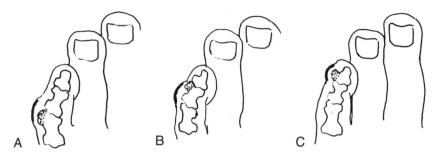

**Fig. 26-2.** (**A**) Proximal interphalangeal joint (heloma durum). (**B**) Distal interphalangeal joint (heloma durum). (**C**) Lateral nail fold (Lister's corn).

of Young in 1938.[22] Although spiked and pointed at the tip, Higgs' was the first peg-in-hole type of procedure. In 1980, Alvine and Garvin described a peg-and-dowel fusion of the PIPJ.[23] Although peg and dowel are synonymous terms, their procedure was similar to that described by Young.[22] Today the two most commonly performed fusion procedures include the end-to-end and peg-in-hole PIPJ arthrodesis.

This chapter formulates and puts into use a practical and workable classification system for the most commonly seen digital deformities, using as a general template the type, etiology, and apex of the deformity; this is followed by the procedure of choice for correction of all components of the deformity, including the skin incision, and technique of the procedure in a step-by-step fashion, and concludes with postoperative treatment plan designed around the specific needs of that procedure. Following classification of the deformity, description of appropriate surgical procedures, and followup care, the author provides a discussion and rationale for each of the plans undertaken.

# STATIC DEFORMITIES: PRESSURE LESIONS WITHOUT CONTRACTION OR ROTATION

## Heloma Dura

### Clinical Presentation and Etiology

When a patient presents with painful heloma dura on an otherwise normal-appearing toe, the apex can be the PIPJ (heloma durum) (Fig. 26-2A), the distal interphalangeal joint (DIPJ) (heloma durum) (Fig. 26-2B), or the lateral nail fold (Lister's corn) (Fig. 26-2C). The etiology is an enlarged or deformed proximal or middle phalanx, or an enlarged lateral condyle-distal phalanx.

### Procedure of Choice

The procedure of choice is the removal of the appropriate osseus segment. For an enlarged or deformed proximal phalanx, an arthroplasty and head resection of the proximal phalanx should be performed. For an enlarged or deformed middle phalanx, an arthroplasty and head resection of the middle phalanx or middle phalangectomy should be performed. A condylectomy should be performed for an enlarged lateral condyle of the distal phalanx.

### Technique

The incision for an arthroplasty and head resection of the proximal or middle phalanx is dorsal linear. A lazy S incision, which begins dorsally and curves distally and laterally, may be used for a condylectomy (Fig. 26-3).

Before surgery, hyperkeratotic tissue of the heloma durum is debrided, taking particular care not to "nick" or create abrasions in underlying healthy skin. Perform the appropriate skin incision, and dissect down through subcutaneous tissue to the level of the extensor digitorum longus tendon. Identify the appropriate joint and transect the tendon. Perform a capsulotomy and release collateral ligaments to free the bone of all soft tissue attachments. Using power or manual instrumentation, resect the head of the proximal or middle phalanx. When performing a middle phalangectomy, the middle phalanx must be carefully freed from all

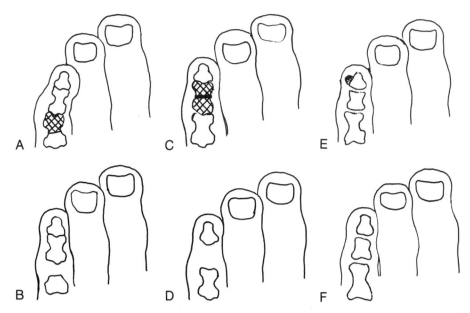

**Fig. 26-3.** (**A & B**) Arthroplasty involving head resection of proximal phalanx. (**C & D**) Arthroplasty involving head resection of middle phalanx or middle phalangectomy. (**E & F**) Condylectomy of lateral condyle of distal phalanx.

soft tissue attachments at both the PIPJ and DIPJ and removed en toto.

For digits that also display a callus formation at the lateral nail fold secondary to an enlarged lateral condyle of the distal phalanx, the dorsal linear incision can be curved distally, laterally, and plantarly to end over the lesion at the lateral nail fold. The incision is deepened, and careful dissection will expose the lateral condyle, which is resected.

The surgical sites are irrigated and tendon repair is performed with 3-0 absorbable suture material. Subcutaneous tissues that require approximation are repaired with 4-0 absorbable material, and skin closure is accomplished with 5-0 nylon or polypropylene on a plastic surgery tipped needle.

### Postoperative Management

Immediately after surgery the digit is splinted and a forefoot dressing is applied. Three to five days postoperatively, the dressing is changed and a new sterile dressing applied. The patient is seen in 1 week (10 to 12 days postoperative). The sutures are removed, and the digit is placed into splint or dressing. The patient is

seen again in 1 week (17 to 19 days postoperative), the dressings are discontinued and only splinting materials used. The patient is seen at 4 weeks and 6 weeks postoperative and splinting of the digit is continued. At 6 weeks postoperative, the surgical shoe may be changed to an athletic-type or walking shoe. Postoperative radiographs should be taken immediately after surgery and at 6 weeks, 3 months, and 6 months to evaluate alignment and osseous regrowth.

### Discussion and Rationale

Selective arthroplasty of the proximal or distal interphalangeal joints is a very successful and gratifying procedure for the patient with an uncomplicated, noncontracted or nonrotated digit. These painful digital deformities are the result of extrinsic pressure over a bony prominence, and have nothing to do with biomechanics or pathomechanics. Purely a pressure phenomenon, they respond well to removal of the offending osseous segment. Care must be taken in determining the apex of the deformity, and in deciding on the best course of action for that particular deformity or combination of deformities. Oftentimes a

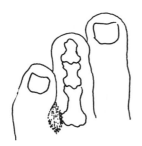

**Fig. 26-4.** Mild to moderate heloma mollé, fourth web space.

small, painful Lister's corn will accompany a larger, more proximal lesion, and care should be taken to ascertain each and every factor causing symptomatology in the digit and address each factor individually.

## Mild to Moderate Heloma Mollé

### Clinical Presentation and Etiology

The patient presents with a mild to moderate heloma mollé in the fourth web space (Fig. 26-4). The apex is a painful heloma mollé deepseated in the fourth web space, and a radiographic lesion marker may be needed. The lesion is pressure related, usually occurring between the head of the fifth proximal phalanx and the base of the fourth proximal phalanx.

### Procedure of Choice

The procedure of choice is a proximal phalangeal head resection of the fifth digit *and possible* lateral condylectomy of the base of the proximal phalanx of the fourth digit.

### Technique

A dorsal curvilinear incision is made over the fifth digit and extended proximally to the metatarsophalangeal joint (MPJ) (Fig. 26-5A). Perform a proximal phalangeal head resection of the fifth digit, as described for painful heloma durum and simple arthroplasty, over the PIPJ (Fig. 26-5B). Perform a lateral condylectomy of the base of the fourth proximal phalanx, which can usually be done through the same incision. Remodel, irrigate, and close the tissue layers as previ-

ously described for simple arthroplasty (Fig. 26-5C). Take postoperative radiographs to evaluate alignment and position (Fig. 26-5D).

### Postoperative Management

Postoperative management is the same as for simple arthroplasty; however, care is taken to splint both the fourth and fifth toes. The remainder of postoperative management is the same.

### Discussion and Rationale

The heloma mollé deformity is a very painful condition that responds well to properly selected surgical procedures.[24] A decision must be made regarding the necessity to remove the lateral condyle from the fourth proximal phalanx. This can usually be determined on the basis of the size and extent of the lesion preoperatively and by radiographic findings. When the lateral condyle is a contributing factor, generally there will be evidence of enlargement or abnormal contour on radiography, as well as a skin lesion that extends beyond the deep web space. It is as important as choosing the correct procedure that the surgical site should be carefully prepared, free of macerated, necrotic tissue, and the base should be carefully inspected for the presence of sinuses, drainage, or inflammation.

## Severe, Recurring Heloma Mollé

### Clinical Presentation and Etiology

When the patient presents with severe, recalcitrant, and recurring heloma mollé of the fourth web space, the apex is deep seated in the web space with additional lesions or extensions of lesions on the inside surface of the toes. The lesions are pressure related, with contributions from the fourth and fifth proximal phalanges. The lesions may be long standing and recurrent, with scar tissue buildup. The lesions may have been operated previously or have become previously infected.

### Procedure of Choice

The procedure of choice is syndactylization of the fourth and fifth toes.

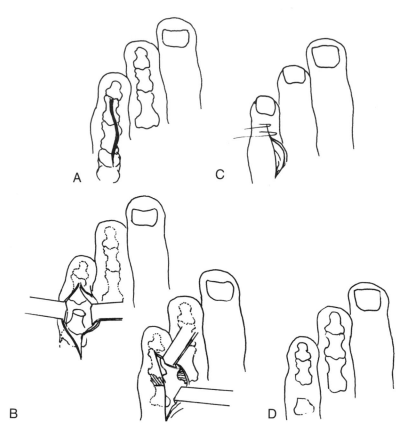

**Fig. 26-5.** (**A**) Dorsal curvilinear incision over the fifth digit; incision extended proximally to the metatarsophalangeal joint. (**B**) Proximal phalangeal head resection of the fifth digit, over the proximal interphalangeal joint. Lateral condylectomy performed at the base of the fourth proximal phalanx, using the same incision. (**C**) Remodeling, irrigation, and closure of tissue layers. (**D**) Final alignment and position.

## Technique

An interdigital, diamond-shaped or oval (double **U**) incision is made. Prepare the surgical site as described for the previous procedure. Using a sterile skin scribe, mark the area of skin flap removal on the inner surface of one of the digits. With the ink still wet, gently touch the two inner surfaces of the digits together, creating a mirror image on the opposite side (Fig. 26-6A). Using a #15 blade, circumscribe the area indicated by the ink, taking care not to skive the edges. Remove the entire flap of skin, taking care to remove only epidermis and dermis, leaving all subcutaneous tissue intact. From within the wound, carefully dissect to the level of bone, free up soft tissue attachments at the PIPJ, and remove an appropriate segment of bone (Fig. 26-6B)

As determined preoperatively, remove the lateral condyle from the base of the four proximal phalanx if appropriate. Following remodeling and irrigation as needed, place suture materials in skin, across the flap, but leave the flap in place until all sutures are placed. Using hand-tie methods, complete final square-knot ties with an assistant supporting the fifth toe in the proper position. All ties are completed, and tags are left longer than usual for easy removal (Fig. 26-6C). Take postoperative radiographs to evaluate alignment and position (Fig. 26-6D).

## Postoperative Management

The postoperative management is similar to that of the simple arthroplasty without significant variation.

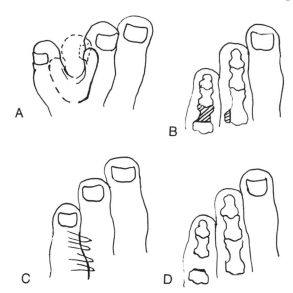

**Fig. 26-6. (A)** Area for skin flap removal marked using sterile scribe. With the ink still wet, the inner surfaces of the digits are gently touched together, creating a mirror image on the opposite sides. **(B)** Appropriate segment of bone removed. **(C)** Sutures are placed and completed using final square knots hand-tied with aid of assistant. **(D)** Final alignment and position.

### Discussion and Rationale

Although it may appear simple and harmless to a patient, a heloma mollé in any web space can become locally infected, and may undergo rapid progression into the deep plantar spaces of the foot; it is therefore particularly dangerous in the diabetic foot. This deformity should be carefully evaluated and aggressively treated, both conservatively and surgically. Some important points to remember when performing the procedure are precise mapping-out of the skin flap and careful removal of the skin, leaving all subcutaneous tissue intact for maximum healing potential. Additional comments include the specific technique used for skin closure, as difficulties have been encountered when a single suture is tied before placement of all other sutures. Placement across the skin flap, then hand-tying all sutures at once, avoids the difficulty encountered in passing a needle through tissue with the toe relocated.

Syndactylization is an excellent procedure for the severe, recalitrant heloma mollé that has been unre-

sponsive to conservative or surgical care.[25-30] It is also an excellent choice for the "flail toe" that may result from surgical failure, tissue loss from infection, or trauma.

## STATIC DEFORMITIES: PRESSURE LESIONS WITH CONTRACTION (SAGITTAL PLANE DEFORMITIES)

### Rigid Hammer Toe

#### Clinical Presentation and Etiology

When a patient presents with rigid hammer toe with a painful heloma durum, the apex is the PIPJ. By definition, there is dorsiflexion at the MPJ, plantar flexion at the PIPJ, and dorsiflexion at the DIPJ. The etiology can be an elongated digit, shoe gear pressure, or other extrinsic structures.

#### Procedure of Choice

The procedure of choice is arthroplasty with proximal phalangeal head resection.

#### Technique

A dorsal linear incision is made. The simple arthroplasty is performed in a similar fashion as previously described without significant variation (Fig. 26-7). Following resection of the proximal phalangeal head, the phalanx is evaluated to determine whether it is adequately relocated on the sagittal plane to the level of the adjacent digits.

#### Postoperative Management

The postoperative treatment plan is that described previously for the simple arthroplasty technique.

#### Discussion and Rationale

Arthroplasty via proximal phalangeal head resection is an excellent procedure for the simple, uncomplicated, rigid hammer toe deformity, and is usually very successful in alleviating the problem. As this is purely a sagittal plane contracture, the dorsal linear incision is adequate to provide exposure to vital areas of concern without damage to the neurovascular structures. Al-

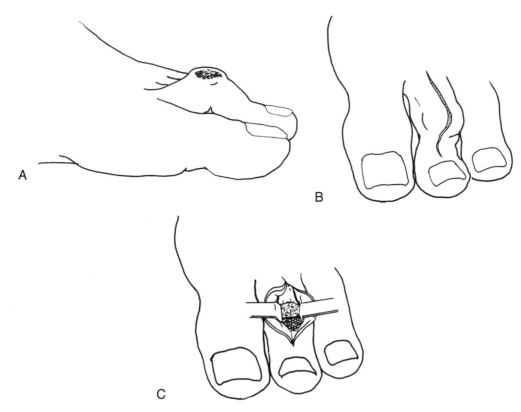

**Fig. 26-7.** (**A**) Isolated hammer toe deformity. (**B**) Skin incision. (**C**) Proximal phalangeal head resection.

though the digit is dorsiflexed at the MPJ, there is generally no need for additional procedures beyond resection of the proximal phalangeal head to relocate the digit. In most cases, reduction of the bone content by resection of the head provides the space necessary to correct the contracture. As this is a rigid deformity, one can often visualize degenerative changes in the joint, even to the degree that initial dissection into the joint for delivery of the head may be difficult because of partial fusion of the joint. If this procedure does not reduce the contraction at the MPJ, sequential reduction is performed.

## Rigid Claw Toe

### Clinical Presentation and Etiology

When the patient presents with rigid claw toe with painful heloma durum (Fig. 26-8), the apex is the PIPJ,

but the DIPJ may also be involved. By definition, there is dorsiflexion at the MPJ and plantar flexion at the PIPJ and DIPJ. There may be an associated distal clavus if clawing of the digit is severe. The etiology can be an elongated digit, shoe gear pressure, or neuropathy.

### Procedure of Choice

The procedure of choice is arthroplasty with proximal phalangeal head resection and possible middle phalangeal head resection.

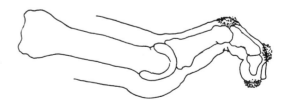

**Fig. 26-8.** Rigid claw toe with painful heloma durum.

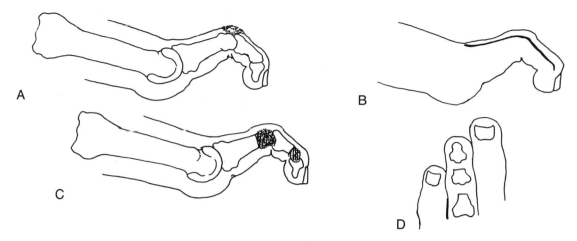

**Fig. 26-9.** (**A**) Rigid claw toe deformity. (**B**) Skin incision. (**C**) Appropriate sections of bone are resected. (**D**) Corrected digit.

### Technique

A simple arthroplasty (Fig. 26-9) is performed in a similar fashion as previously described without significant variation. Following this procedure, an intraoperative decision is made to perform a similar procedure at the level of the DIPJ. This is occasionally necessary.

### Postoperative Management

The postoperative treatment plan is that described previously for the simple arthroplasty procedure.

### Discussion and Rationale

Arthroplasty at the level of the PIPJ is an excellent procedure for the simple, uncomplicated rigid claw toe deformity, with results comparable to that of simple hammer toes. Occasionally deformity of plantar flexion may occur at the level of the DIPJ that is not reduced following the proximal procedure. In that case, arthroplasty at the level of the DIPJ may be necessary. Particular attention should be given to the plantar skin of a long-standing claw toe deformity, as it may exhibit shortening subsequent to contracture; this may disallow straightening of the digit without a larger amount of bone resection than was previously expected or additional skin plasty techniques for the purpose of lengthening the skin. Failure to address the

shortened plantar skin could result in damage to the soft tissue structures including nerves and vascular and lymphatic structures from excessive stretching, which could lead to loss of the digit.

## Rigid Mallet Toe

### Clinical Presentation and Etiology

When the patient presents with rigid mallet toe with painful distal clavus, the apex of the deformity is in the DIPJ, over which a heloma durum can form. However, the patient's chief complaint may be focused around a painful distal clavus that develops subsequent to the plantar flexion of the digit at the DIPJ, making it, by definition, a mallet toe contracture. The etiology can be an elongated digit or shoe gear pressure, or it may have developed secondary to PIPJ fusion.

### Procedure of Choice

The procedure of choice is arthroplasty with middle phalangeal head resection.

### Technique

A transverse lenticular or fusiform incision is made over the DIPJ (Fig. 26-10A). Utilizing a sterile skin scribe, the planned incisional approach is mapped out over the DIPJ. Using a #15 blade the incision is per-

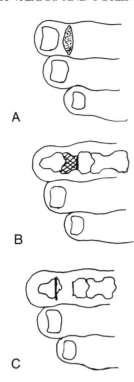

**Fig. 26-10.** (**A**) Transverse lenticular incision over distal interphalangeal joint. (**B**) Head of middle phalanx is resected and the remaining portion is remodeled. (**C**) Closure of the tendon, capsule, and skin are completed.

formed in the designated area, and the skin flap is removed, including all epidermis and dermis, leaving all subcutaneous tissue intact. Dissection is carried through the subcutaneous tissue to the level of the deep fascia and extensor tendon. The tendon is transected at the level of the DIPJ; capsulotomy is performed, collateral ligaments are transected, and the head of the middle phalanx is delivered through the operative site. The head of the middle phalanx is now resected using power or manual instrumentation (Fig. 26-10B). The remaining portion of the middle phalanx is remodeled, and after irrigation of the operative site, closure of the tendon, capsule, and skin are completed (Fig. 26-10C). Postoperative radiographs are taken to evaluate alignment and position.

### Postoperative Management

The postoperative treatment plan is the same as that described for the simple arthroplasty procedure.

### Discussion and Rationale

Arthroplasty at the level of the DIPJ via middle phalangeal head resection is an excellent procedure for correction of simple mallet toe contracture. Utilizing the transverse lenticular incision allows the surgeon direct access into the DIPJ for resection of the middle phalangeal head, and also allows dorsal relocation of the tip of the toe when skin closure is performed. Caution, however, should be taken to avoid damage to the dorsal medial and lateral neurovascular structures of the digit.

## DYNAMIC DEFORMITIES: DEFORMITIES WITH CONTRACTION OR ROTATION

### Clinical Presentation and Etiology

The patient with dynamic hammer toes or claw toes presents with MPJ dislocation with associated dorsal proximal or PIPJ irritations or calluses. The etiology is biomechanical, caused by extensor substitution, flexor substitution, or flexor stabilization.

### Procedure of Choice

The procedure of choice is digital relocation with stabilization via sequential reduction and digital arthroplasty/arthrodesis procedures.

### Technique

A dorsal curvilinear incision is centered over the digit, extending proximally to the level of the MPJ (Fig. 26-11A). Deepen the incision through the subcutaneous tissue using light brushing strokes to the level of the deep fascia and extensor hood apparatus. Perform a **Z**-plasty tendon-lengthening procedure on the extensor digitorum longus, reflecting one end proximally and the other end distally, and exposing the PIPJ of the digit (Fig. 26-11B). The tendon may be transected at the level of the PIPJ if the contracture is not severe enough to warrant **Z**-plasty lengthening.

Perform release of all soft tissue attachments and deliver the proximal phalangeal head through the surgical site. At this time, osseous procedures are performed (Fig. 26-11C).

*Arthroplasty.* If the procedure of choice is the arthroplasty, the proximal phalangeal head is now re-

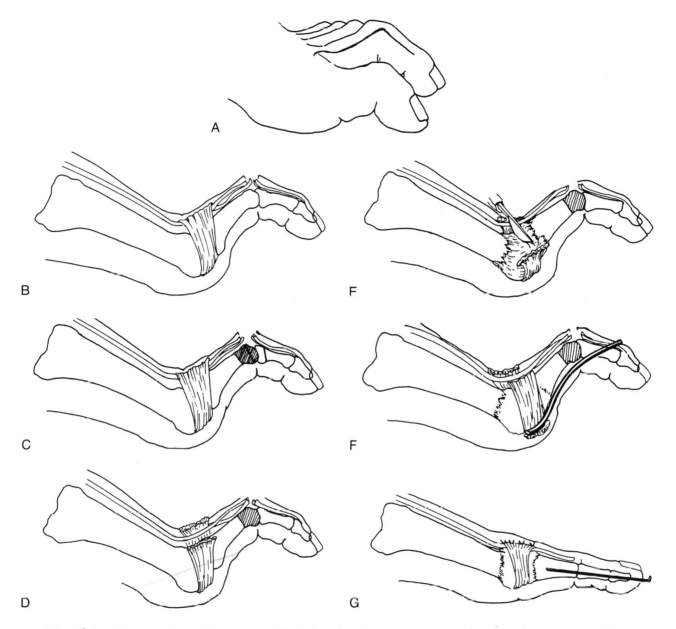

**Fig. 26-11.** (**A**) Dorsolinear skin incision. (**B**) Z-plasty lengthening of extensor digitorum longus tendon. (**C**) Head rsection (partial or total) of proximal phalanx. (**D**) Extensor hood recession. (**E**) Metatarsophalangeal joint capsulotomy. (**F**) Flexor plate release. (**G**) Kirschner-wire stabilization.

sected, whether by manual or power instrumentation. The remaining stump is remodeled and irrigated (Fig. 26-12A).

*Arthrodesis.* If the procedure of choice is the arthrodesis, the appropriate sections of bone are removed. For an end-to-end fusion, the cartilaginous surface of the proximal phalangeal head and middle phalangeal base are resected using manual and power instrumentation (Fig. 26-12B). If a peg-in-hole arthrodesis is being performed, the head of the proximal phalanx is

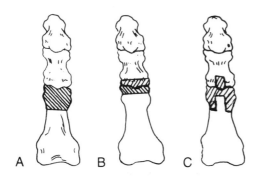

**Fig. 26-12.** (**A**) Arthroplasty of proximal phalangeal head resection. (**B**) End-to-end arthrodesis. (**C**) Peg-in-hole arthrodesis.

partially removed transversely with a power oscillating saw. The medial, lateral, and plantar cortical surfaces of the stump are removed. The dorsal cortex is left intact for stability and strength. A hole is then fashioned through the base of the middle phalanx, using a thin side-cutting burr initially, followed by a series of ball burrs of increasing size. The peg will be inserted into the hole as its final resting position following reduction of MPJ contracture (Fig. 26-12C).

Following osseous procedures, the "push-up" test as described by Kelikian is performed by directing upward pressure on the metatarsal head at the appropriate joint. If the phalanx remains elevated at the MPJ, the surgeon proceeds to the next step in the sequential reduction process.

The extensor hood recession is the next step in the sequential reduction process. To perform this, the proximal end of the extensor digitorum longus tendon is grasped and gently but firmly pulled in an upward direction. This maneuver places tension on the hood fibers, which become readily visible, exhibiting their perpendicular arrangement to the extensor tendon. The fibers of the hood are released in a sweeping-type motion using a #15 blade, keeping the scalpel blade parallel with the tendon. Particular care is taken to avoid penetration into the delicate tendon sheath, or damage to the periosteum of the metatarsal (Fig. 26-11D). This completes the extensor hood release. The Kelikian push-up test as previously described is again performed, and with persistent dorsiflexion of the proximal phalanx on the MPJ, the next step is undertaken, which is the MPJ capsulotomy.

With a #64 blade, the MPJ capsulotomy is performed on the dorsal, medial and lateral sides (see Fig. 26-11E). The plantar aspect of the joint capsule is left intact. The Kelikian push-up test is again performed, and if persistent elevation of the phalanx at the level of the MPJ is observed, the final soft tissue procedure in the sequential reduction is performed: the flexor plate release.

The flexor plate is released, using a metatarsal elevator, by gently yet firmly inserting the elevator under the metatarsal head and advancing it proximally (Fig. 26-11F). The flexor plate will be released, and the sequential reduction is completed.

The digits are stabilized using 0.045-in Kirschner wires (K-wires) in retrograde fashion first by inserting an unloaded 0.035-in K-wire into the proximal phalanx to establish location of the central canal. Next, a 0.045-in. wire is driven through the middle phalanx and out the end of the toe. The wire driver is relocated to the wire exiting the toe, the digit is repositioned into correct alignment, and the 0.045-in wire is driven into the canal previously established by the smaller wire. The 0.045-in K-wire is driven to the desired position, generally to the base of the proximal phalanx (Fig. 26-11G). If the digit were severely deformed preoperatively, the surgeon may elect to cross the MPJ with the wire for additional sagittal plane stability.

### Postoperative Management

The postoperative plan is basically the same as for other digital procedures previously mentioned; however, particular care and attention are given to pin management. The K-wires are left in place for 4 to 6 weeks, at which time they are removed with a pair of pliers. On weekly visits, the pin exit sites are carefully inspected for tuft blanching, inflammation, or drainage. They are cleansed at each visit, with a new application of antibiotic ointment placed at the base of the pin to seal the opening. Radiographs are taken immediately following surgery, then at 3 and 6 weeks postoperatively to monitor osseus healing. Light compression splints are utilized to avoid swelling of the digits as the patient's activity level increases and when the sutures and pins are removed. Occasionally, removal of the pins may cause mild temporary swelling of the toe.

## Discussion and Rationale

Contracted digits demonstrating dislocation at the level of the MPJ are a special circumstance in which all aspects of the deformity must be addressed or the surgery is doomed to failure. The chief complaint in these patients is often lesser metatarsalgia, and frequently submetatarsal calluses are observed. If the apex of the deformity, however, lies in the contracture of the digit at the level of the MPJ and IPJ(s), the surgeon must recognize the correct etiology and address the problem appropriately. Oftentimes the etiology is related to intrinsic muscle wasting (Fig. 26-13). In this case it would not be advisable to perform lesser metatarsal osteotomies before alleviating the symptoms through digital reduction and stabilization. Generally this is all that is required to successfully convert the very painful, unstable forefoot into a nonpainful, stable forefoot. It is essential that the physician recognize which symptoms are primary and which are secondary so that the correct surgical procedures may be selected. The arthroplasty is generally performed on those digits where flexibility at the PIPJ is necessary. The end-to-end arthrodesis is generally performed in those digits that are mildly contracted, have some dynamic component, and are of normal length. The peg-in-hole procedure is generally performed on those digits that are severely contracted, have a significant dynamic component, and are excessively long. The peg-in-hole procedure provides significant shortening capabilities by its design. Sequential reduction will correct all the soft tissue contractures that are significant deforming forces proximally, and allow the digit to be returned to proper alignment in the sagittal plane. K-wire stabilization will provide the temporary support necessary to allow for healing in the corrected position.

When this procedure is performed correctly, it is very successful and very gratifying to the patient. This type of severe digital deformity is typically very painful and may even be disabling. Stabilizing the digits through this complex repair restores some of the stability that has been lost, allowing improved function of the digits, better propulsion in gait, and improved alignment of the metatarsal heads in the sagittal plane individually and the transverse plane collectively. When all the lesser toes are addressed as a group, the second and third toes are generally arthrodesed, while

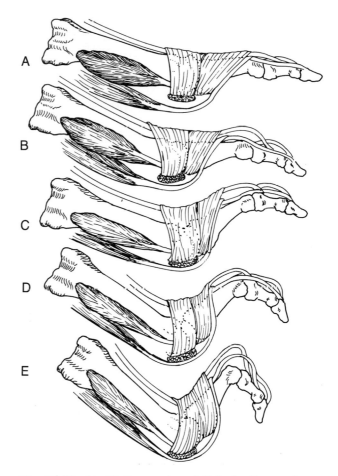

**Fig. 26-13.** (A–E) Contraction of digits leading to plantar flexion of metatarsal heads. Note wasting of intrinsic musculature.

the fourth and fifth toes undergo arthroplasty procedures. The fifth toe is never arthrodesed.

The sequential reduction of complex claw toe and hammer toe deformities, described by Jimenez et al., is an excellent method for reducing several digital contractures and often eliminates accompanying metatarsalgia secondary to digital dislocation.[31,32]

## Adductovarus Deformity of the Fifth Toe

### Clinical Presentation and Etiology

When a patient presents with adductovarus deformity of the fifth toe, the apex is the proximal IPJ, and occasionally the distal IPJ as well. The etiology can be bio-

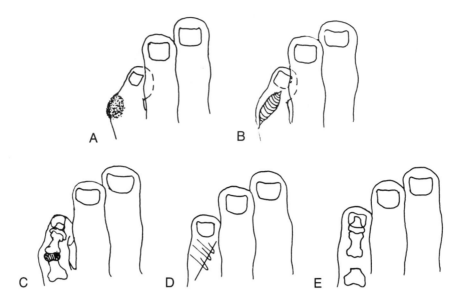

**Fig. 26-14.** (**A**) Debridement of hyperkeratotic tissue of the heloma durum. (**B**) Lenticular skin incision. (**C**) Arthroplasty via proximal head resection. (**D**) Skin closure with digit supported in corrected position. (**E**) Final alignment and position.

mechanical, caused by the quadratus plantae losing its normal vector pull on the digits associated with pronation of the foot. The direction of pull is shifted medially, creating a varus and adductus pull on the fifth toe. The fourth toe may also develop the same deformity. The etiology can also be mechanical because of extrinsic pressure from shoe gear influencing malalignment of the digit. Some authors believe there are also congenital factors.

### Procedure of Choice

The procedure of choice is the PIPJ arthroplasty with head resection using derotational skin plasty technique.

### Technique

An oblique lenticular or fusiform incision is made. Carefully debride hyperkeratotic tissue of the heloma durum to determine the extent of the lesion (Fig. 26-14A), using caution not to nick or abrade the skin. Before drawing the intended incision with a sterile skin scribe, gently derotate the digit and lightly pinch the skin in the area of the skin incision. In performing

this maneuver, the surgeon can visualize the dimensions of the skin ellipse to be removed.

Using a sterile skin scribe, mark the skin ellipse to be removed. The skin incisions will be two converging semielliptical incisions placed in a proximal-lateral to distal-medial direction over the lesion (Fig. 26-14B). This "lenticular" incision will result in derotation of the digit as the skin flap is removed and skin edges are reapproximated. Important considerations are to remove all epidermis and dermis and leave intact all subcutaneous tissue for vascular supply to the skin, to maximize healing potential and maintain a 3 : 1 length-to-width ratio of dimensions for the flap.

Following removal of the skin flap, dissection is carried down to the level of the deep fascia and extensor tendon, and an arthroplasty via proximal head resection is performed in the manner previously described (Fig. 26-14C).

The tendon and capsule are repaired in the usual fashion, and skin closure is then accomplished with an assistant supporting the digit in the corrected position (Fig. 26-14D). On closure of the skin, the digit should be derotated and rest in an upright position with its alignment restored. Postoperative radiographs are taken to evaluate alignment position (Fig. 26-14E).

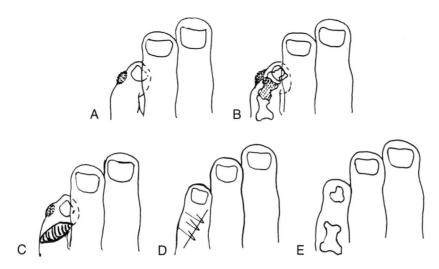

**Fig. 26-15.** (**A**) Adductovarus digit with apex at the middle phalanx. (**B**) Middle phalangectomy. (**C**) Lenticular incision centered over the apex. (**D**) Skin closure with digit supported in corrected position. (**E**) Alignment and final position.

### Postoperative Management

The postoperative management is the same as that described for the simple arthroplasty; however, particular care is taken to maintain the digit in a derotated position using dressings and splints.

### Discussion and Rationale

The adducto varus deformity of the fifth toe, and less often of the fourth toe, is very common. Because of its position, extrinsic shoe pressure frequently leads to hyperkeratotic tissue formation in the form of heloma dura, over the dorsal or dorsolateral aspect of the digit. The fifth toe is particularly subject to this type of repetitive trauma because of its location and size. The derotational arthroplasty is an excellent way to achieve precise realignment of the digit and removal of underlying bony prominences.[33] The same deformity can occur in the fourth digit if medial vector forces are strong enough. Preoperative radiographic lesion markers are excellent in assisting the surgeon to precisely identify the apex of the deformity if it is unclear on clinical examination.

## Middle Phalangectomy

A modification of this procedure can be performed if the apex of the deformity is actually in the middle phalanx (Fig. 26-15A), rather than the proximal phalanx, as is usually the case.[4,5] In this situation the middle phalanx is generally enlarged or abnormal in contour and shape, and may be removed in toto (Fig. 26-15B).

### Technique

The procedure is identical to that previously described with the following exceptions. The skin ellipse is performed slightly distal to that previously mentioned, as the apex of the deformity is now in the middle phalanx (Fig. 26-15C). The dissection is carried to the level of the deep fascia and extensor tendon, at which the capsulotomy of the PIPJ is performed. The middle phalanx is freed of all soft tissue attachments by sharp dissection, and it is removed. The remainder of the procedure is similar to that of the aforementioned procedure, and postoperative management treatment plans are similar as well (Fig. 26-15D and E).

### Discussion and Rationale

Middle phalangectomy is an excellent procedure for the adductovarus deformity of the fourth or fifth digit where the apex of the deformity is clearly at the level of the middle phalanx. Careful preoperative evaluation of the radiographs in such a situation will usually demonstrate a middle phalanx that is enlarged or ab-

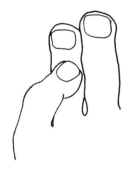

**Fig. 26-16.** Congenital overlapping fifth toe.

normally contoured. It is interesting to note that the section of bone removed when removing an entire middle phalanx is generally approximately the same as the amount of bone removed with the head of the proximal phalanx.

## Congenital Overlapping Fifth Toe

### Clinical Presentation and Etiology

In patients who present with congenital overlapping fifth toe (Fig. 26-16), the apex is the fifth MPJ. The etiology is congenital, however, the deformity can worsen over time.

### Procedure of Choice

The procedure of choice is relocation of the digit via complete reduction of the contracture and reduction of bone content in the toe.

### Technique

Perform a **V–Y** skin plasty technique over the MPJ in line with the contracture (Fig. 26-17A). Create a flap, dissect down through the subcutaneous tissue to the level of the deep fascia, and locate the extensor digitorum longus tendon. Perform **Z**-plasty lengthening, then reflect the tendon ends, one distally and one

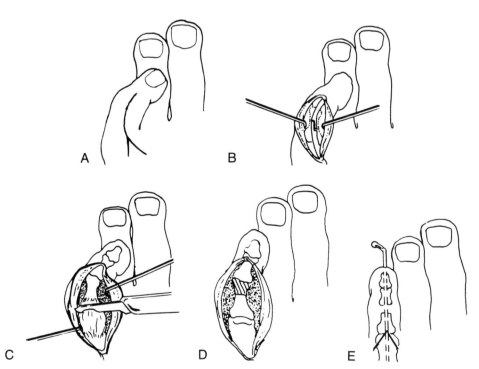

**Fig. 26-17.** (**A**) V–Y skin plasty over the metatarsophalangeal joint. (**B**) Z-plasty, lengthening the extensor digitorum longus tendon. (**C**) Capsulotomy of the fifth metatarsophalangeal joint. (**D**) Arthroplasty via proximal phalangeal joint. (**E**) Postoperative Alignment and final position.

proximally (Fig. 26-17B). Locate the fifth MPJ. Using a #64 blade, perform a medial, dorsal, and if necessary, lateral, capsulotomy of the MPJ (Fig. 26-17C).

Perform a dorsal linear incision, either separately, or by extending the arm of the V to Y (short Y to long Y), centered over the fifth digit. In the fashion previously described, perform an arthroplasty technique via proximal phalangeal head resection (Fig. 26-17D). Irrigate the surgical site, and complete the procedure with K-wire stabilization by retrograde fashion across the MPJ. Closure of soft tissue structures and skin is now accomplished in the usual fashion. Postoperative radiographs are taken to evaluate alignment and position (Fig. 26-17E). Note: alternative incisional approach includes dorsal linear over the digit and Z-plasty to lengthen skin contracture.

### Postoperative Management

The postoperative treatment plan for relocation of the congenital overlapping fifth toe is essentially the same as for that of any digital procedure in which K-wires are exiting the digits. The pin may be removed from across the MPJ at 3 to 6 weeks, and is usually left in place in the digit for 4 to 6 weeks.

### Discussion and Rationale

Because of significant malalignment, the overlapping fifth toe is particularly prone to injury and trauma, which may result in callus or ulcer formation. Historically, many procedures have been designed and modified to address this deformity with incomplete success.[10,18,34–41] Failure was most likely attributed to a series of incomplete approaches because not all components of the deformity (i.e., shortened dorsal skin, shortened extensor digitorum longus tendon, contracted MPJ capsule, and normal bone content) were addressed. Rather, each attempt was only partially complete and resulted in only partial success. It is also interesting to note that, although the digit itself is relatively normal with the exception of its malaligned position at the MPJ, it must have some bone removed; in other words, it is necessary to decrease the internal cubic content of bone to relocate the digit. Failure to do this will most likely place an excessive amount of tension on the digit and stretch the delicate neurovascular structures beyond their capacity for survival.

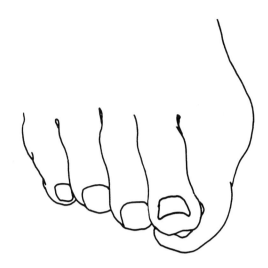

**Fig. 26-18.** Acquired overlapping second digit.

## Acquired Overlapping Second Digit

### Clinical Presentation and Etiology

For a patient presenting with an acquired overlapping second digit (Fig. 26-18), the apex is the MPJ <u>and</u> IPJs of the digit. The etiology is variable. If may originate in the digit itself, or it may be the result of other space-occupying structures taking its place (e.g., the hallux).

### Procedure of Choice

The procedure of choice is relocation of the digit via sequential reduction at the MPJ, realignment and stabilization at the digital interphalangeal joints, and stabilization of periarticular structures around the MPJ.

### Technique

A dorsal curvilinear incision is centered over the digit and extended proximally to curve over the MPJ (Fig. 26-19A). The procedure is as previously described for relocation and stabilization of severe hammer toe and claw toe deformities with the following additional procedures.

Following completion of the usual reduction of the digit, attention is directed to the flexor structures in an attempt to realign the flexor tendon sheath back into normal position under the metatarsal head (Fig. 26-19B). It is well accepted by most authorities that the adductus component is caused by a shift of the flexor

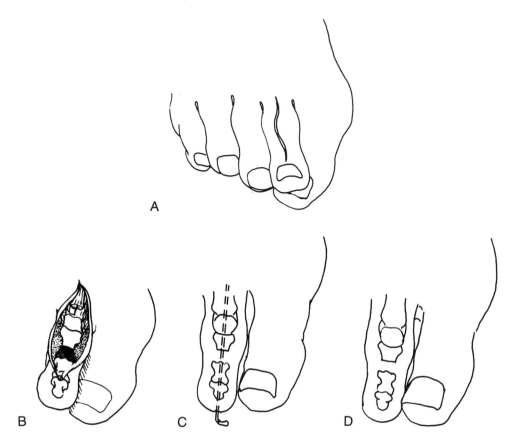

**Fig. 26-19.** (**A**) Dorsal curvilinear skin incision. (**B**) Realignment of flexor tendon sheath below the metatarsal head. (**C**) K-wire stabilization. (**D**) Postoperative alignment.

structures in addition to the sagittal plane contracture of the digit; this has been shown by flexor tenogram technique. The goal, then, is to realign and stabilize these flexor structures, or it is likely that the digit will not maintain a corrected position in the long term. K-wire stabilization is performed by retrograde technique (Fig. 26-19C).

### Postoperative Management

The postoperative treatment plan is essentially the same for this procedure as for the complex hammer toe repair previously described. It is likely that the K-wire will be placed in retrograde fashion, extending across the MPJ. Following removal, the digit is evaluated as to its sagittal plane and transverse plane stability (Fig. 26-19D).

### Discussion and Rationale

Rationale for this procedure is similar in philosophy, success, and repair to that for complex hammer toes. The challenging component and least predictable outcome of the procedure is the long-term stability of the adductus component of the deformity.

## REFERENCES

1. Sorto LA: Surgical correction of hammer toes, a five year postoperative study. J Am Podiatry Assoc 64:930, 1974
2. Johnson CP, Hugar DW: A literature review of congenital digiti quinti varus: clinical description and treatment. J Foot Surg 22:116, 1983
3. Sokoloff HM: Soft tissue digital procedures. Clin Pod Med Surg 3:23, 1986

4. Jenkin WM: Arthroplasty via intermediate phalangectomy. Clin Pod Med Surg 3:41, 1986

5. Dobbs BM: Arthroplasty of the fifth digit. Clin Pod Med Surg 3:29, 1986

6. Monson DK, Buell TR, Scurran BL: Lesser digital arthrodesis. Clin Pod Med Surg 3: 1986

7. McGlamry ED, Jimenez AL, Green DR: Lesser ray deformities. p. 341. In McGlamry ED (ed): Comprehensive Textbook of Foot Surgery. 2nd Ed. Williams & Wilkins, Baltimore, 1992

8. McGlamry ED: Lesser ray deformities. Comprehensive Textbook of Foot Surgery. 2nd Ed. Williams & WIlkins, Baltimore, 1992

9. Forrester-Brown MF: Tendon transplantation for clawing of the great toe. J Bone Joint Surg 20:57, 1938

10. Lapidus PW: Transplantation of the extensor tendon for correction of the overlapping fifth toe. J Bone Jont Surg 24:555, 1942

11. Girdlstone GR: Physiology for the foot and hand. J Bone Joint Surg 29:167, 1947

12. Sgarlato TE: Transplantation of the flexor digitorum longus muscle tendon in hammer toes. J Am Podiatry Assoc 60:383, 1970

13. Barbari SG, Brevig K: Correction of clawtoes by the Girdlestone-Taylor flexor-extensor transfer procedure. Foot Ankle 5:67, 1984

14. Kuwada GT, Dockery GL: Modification of the flexor tendon transfer procedure for the correction of flexible hammertoes. J Foot Surg 19:38, 1980

15. Kuwada GT: A retrospective analysis of modification of the flexor tendon transfer for correction of hammer toe. 27:57, 1988

16. Post AC: Hallux valgus with displacement of the smaller toes. Med Rec NY 22:120, 1882

17. Terrier: Orteils en marteau avec durillons et bourses sereuses sousjacentes enflammees. Resection des deux Cotes, et dans la meme seance, de l'articulation phalango phalangeinne. Bull Mem Soc Chir 14:624, 1888

18. Kelikian H: Hallux Valgus, Allied Deformities of the Forefoot and Metatarsalgia. p 327. WB Saunders, Philadelphia, 1965

19. Friend G: Correction of elongated underlapping lesser toes by middle phalangectomy and skin plasty. J Foot Surg 23:470, 1984

20. Soule RE: Operation for the cure of hammer toe. New York Med J pp 649–650, March 26, 1910

21. Higgs SL: Hammer-toe. Med Press 131:473, 1931

22. Young CS: An operation for the correction of hammer-toe and claw-toe. J Bone Joint Surg 20:715, 1938

23. Alvine FG, Garvin KL: Peg and dowel fusion of the proximal interphalangeal joint. Foot Ankle 1:90, 1980

24. Zeringue GN, Harkless LB: Evaluation and management of the web corn involving the fourth interdigital space. J Am Pod Med Assoc 76:210, 1986

25. Strach EH, Cornah MS: Syndactylopoiesis: a simple operation for interdigital soft corn. J Bone Joint Surg 54:530, 1972

26. Kurtz CM, Guthrie JD: Syndactylization: a surgical approach to heloma molle. J Foot Surg 23:407, 1984

27. Hoffman GA: Plastic web reconstruction for soft corn of fourth interspace. J Nat Assoc Chirop 39:22, 1949

28. Bottnick S: Surgical syndactylizm for heloma molle, a case report. J Am Pod Assoc 54:411, 1964

29. Kelikian H, Clayton, L, Loseff H: Surgical syndactylia of the toes. Clin Orthop 19:219, 1961

30. Bernback E: A surgical procedure to syndactylize. J Am Pod Assoc 46:447, 1956

31. McGlamry ED: Lesser ray deformities. p. 349. In: Comprehensive Textbook of Foot Surgery. 2nd Ed. Williams and Wilkins, Baltimore, 1992

32. Nicklas BJ: Prophylactic surgery in the diabetic foot. p. 526. In Frykberg R (ed): The High Risk Foot in Diabetes Mellitus. Churchill Livingstone, New York, 1991

33. McGlamry ED, Lesser ray deformities. p. 354. In: Comprehensive Textbook of Foot Surgery. 2nd Ed. Williams and Wilkins, Baltimore, 1992

34. Anderson BV: Combination surgery for overlapping fifth digit. J Am Pod Assoc 61:137, 1971

35. Cockin J: Butler's operation for an overriding fifth toe. J Bone Joint Surg Br 50:78, 1968

36. Du Vries HL: Surgery of the Foot. CV Mosby, St. Louis, 1959

37. Goodwin FC, Swisher FM: The treatment of congenital hyperextension of the fifth toe. J Bone Jont Surg 25:193, 1943

38. Jahss MH: Diaphysectomy for severe acquired overlapping fifth toe and advanced fixed hammering of the small toes. p. 211. In Bateman JR (ed): Foot Science. WB Saunders, Philadelphia, 1976

39. Kaplan EG: A new approach to the surgical correction of overlapping toes. J Foot Surg 3:24, 1964

40. Lantzounis LA. Congenital subluxation of the fifth toe and its correction by a periosteocapsuloplasty and tendon transplantation. J Bone Joint Surg 22:147, 1940

41. Wilson JN: V-Y correction for varus deformity of the fifth toe. Br J Surg 41:133, 1953

42. Coughlin MJ: Crossover second toe deformity. Foot Ankle 8:29, 1987

43. Branch HE: Pathologic dislocation of the second toe. J Bone Joint Surg 19:978, 1937

44. Johnson JB, Price IV TW: Crossover second toe deformity: etiology and treatment. J Foot Surg 28:417, 1989

# 27

# Orthodigital Evaluation and Therapeutic Management of Digital Deformity

*KENDRICK A. WHITNEY*

The definition of orthodigita might imply a conservative nonoperative approach to the correction and control of digital malalignments and associated lesions. A better concept, however, might include the combined orthopedic and judicious surgical management of digital deformities where indicated. The decision as to which approach, whether conservative, surgical, or combined, would be most beneficial for the patient should be based on clear principles and findings. It is paramount that the examination determine the precise type, degree, and reducibility of a presented deformity. The most important and perhaps most often overlooked factors are the various orthopedic influences that may contribute directly or indirectly to the development of the digital deformity and which will most certainly help determine the most appropriate type of treatment.

Before selecting and performing any digital procedure, it is essential that the practitioner have an appreciable understanding of the presenting problem or complaint. The nature and developmental sequence of the digital deformity must be ascertained through a careful and thorough history and physical examination. Only then should the practitioner proceed with a specific treatment plan based on clear and sound principles rather than on financial gain, technical ease, or short-term cosmetic results. further, it is generally not only the severity of the deformation that should determine the therapeutic procedure to be performed. In most cases, the success of treatment will

depend greatly on the recognition and classification of the relative resistance to manual corrective digital realignment. It is thus the author's hope that a systematic approach to the evaluation and treatment of digital deformities may help to deter some of the indiscriminate digital surgery leading to long-term disfigurement and dysfunctional results.

## ORTHODIGIAL EVALUATION PROCEDURE
### Patient History

A detailed patient narrative should be taken, which may often provide valuable insight to an overall understanding of the nature and developmental sequence of the presented digital problem. Previous treatments received and the negative or positive results obtained may yield clues as to the best therapeutic direction. This becomes increasingly important when the treatment received was related to a secondary orthopedic complaint. Certainly the functional demands imposed by the patient's vocational and avocational needs will also play a significant role in the treatment program selected.

The limiting factor to successful orthodigital management is, very often, the patient's shoe gear. It is extremely important to ascertain whether the patient's shoe style has contributed to the progression or worsening of the problem. Foot abuse from improper shoe style with respect to the last, toe box room, and the heel height are significant contributors to digital malposition and associated lesions that must not be taken lightly. Careful shoe inspection and patient education with respect to a favorable shoe type for the digital condition can make the difference between failure and successful orthodigital management.

The past medical history should include a clear understanding of the patient's current health with an emphasis on circulation, injuries, operations, and allergies in terms of potential digital surgery needs.

## Overall Evaluation

The orthodigital exam should be considered a vital portion of the generalized lower extremity exam as the two are inevitably linked. The examiner should refrain from immediately addressing the digital complaint (often to the patient's chagrin) while an overall perception is formed as to the nature of the digital complaint and its probable development. This lower extremity preorthodigital evaluation should allow the practitioner to distinguish between the purely positional, chronically adapted, and structural congenital digital deformity.

## Visual Evaluation

With the patient comfortably seated and the knees placed in a slightly flexed attitude the examiner should observe the foot and toes in the relaxed state, noting both the location and plane of deformity while also observing skin tensions, lesional characteristics, tendinous contractures, and joint abnormalities that may be present (Fig. 27-1).

## Manual Evaluation

Following the visual inspection a manual appraisal will help further determine the nature, extent, and therapeutic prognosis of the digital deformity while palpable pain and associated arthritic changes are noted. Passive and active range of motion (ROM) and muscle testing should be performed on all digits (Fig. 27-2). Metatarsophalangeal malalignments are specifically charted with reference to their degree, taxicity, subluxation, or frank luxation (Fig. 27-3). A simple test used to determine subluxation potential at the meta-

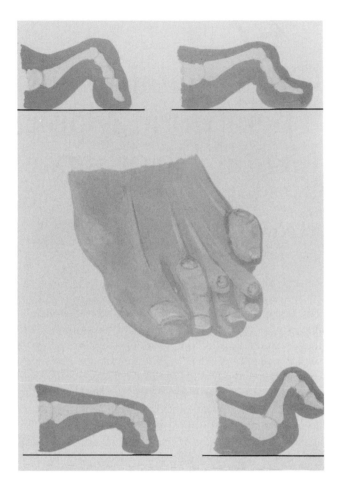

**Fig. 27-1.** Visual foot and digital evaluation.

tarsophalangeal joint level involves the application of resistance over the distal aspect of the toe by the examiner while the patient actively extends the digits (Fig. 27-4). If a subluxation tendency exists, the proximal phalangeal base can be observed to sublux proximally over its metatarsal head.

## FUNCTIONAL ORTHODIGITAL EVALUATION
### Taxicity Testing

To help the examiner determine the taxic (reducible) from the nontaxic digital elements, the author has de-

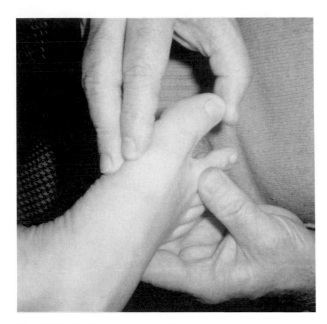

**Fig. 27-2.** Resistive testing of the extensor digitorum brevis muscle.

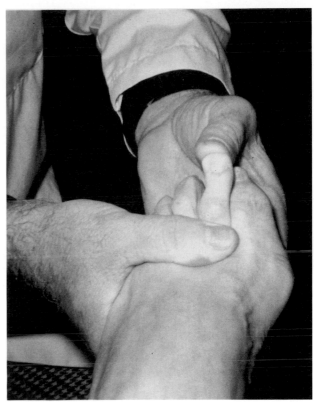

**Fig. 27-4.** Testing metatarsophalangeal joint subluxation potential.

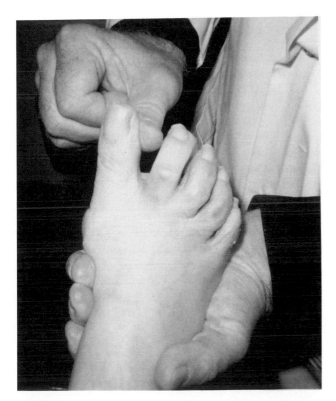

**Fig. 27-3.** Passive hallux motion and resistance testing.

vised a taxicity resistance scale (Table 27-1) in which the resistance to manual reduction of digital deformity is measured on a scale of 1 to 5. This test procedure, which measures the ease of digital realignment by the practitioner, is performed with the patient both sitting and standing. The information derived from this test is utilized for determining the most appropriate therapeutic measures and probable prognosis. Lesser digital deformities, which have taxicity resistance values

**Table 27-1.** Taxicity Resistance Scale

|  | At Rest | During Stance |
|---|---|---|
| 1(+) | Easily reducible | Reducible |
| 2(++) | Reducible | Mild resistance |
| 3(+++) | Mild resistance | Moderate resistance |
| 4(++++) | Moderate resistance | Incomplete reduction |
| 5(+++++) | Nonreducible | Nonreducible |

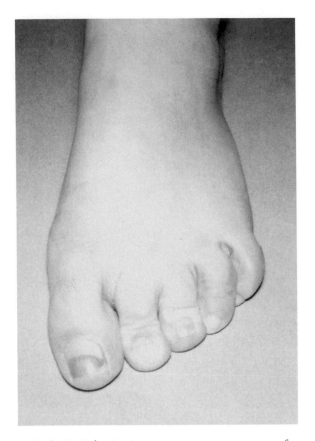

**Fig. 27-5.** Digital gripping response to compensate forefoot varus deformity.

between 1 and 3 and are secondary to functional imbalance rather than tendinous malinsertion or progressive neurologic deformities, will generally respond favorably to aggressive conservative orthodigital therapy. Deformities falling within a 3 to 4 taxic resistance range while still manually reducible will generally require some type of soft tissue release or osseous surgical procedure in conjunction with retentive orthodigital measures to prevent recurrence. Grade 5 nontaxic deformities are totally nonreducible and will require either surgical reconstructive techniques or protective orthodigital shielding.

## Positional Digital Malalignment

Digital deformities generally representing the lower end of the taxicity resistance scale display the easiest manual reduction and are usually secondary to an underlying foot defect whereby the digits will grip or claw to compensate or counterbalance the underlying deficiency (Fig. 27-5). These easily reducible deformities will generally respond well to conservative orthopedic measures via mechanical accommodation. Other orthopedic influences that may contribute to these functional digital patterns include the patient's occupational and avocational demands, weight, posture, gait patterns, foot gear, and general health. Without an appreciation or clear understanding of the underlying foot–limb imbalance responsible for these digital deformities, surgical intervention will inevitably produce greater long-term problems than the initial presenting complaint. The role of the practitioner should then be to determine which of these functional/orthopedic influences may be contributing to the presenting digital malalignment and then to act on those influences.

## Sway Balance Testing

To help determine the nature and source of imbalance in the foot responsible for the digital deformation forces during stance and gait, the sway balance technique[1] may be employed. With the patient standing in the relaxed angle and base of gait, we first need to observe the static appearance of the digits with respect to digital alignment and abnormal tensions. Next we have the patient go through a series of specified motions while we observe and note any accentuation or relaxation of digital gripping or retraction patterns. In this manner one can determine if the foot/leg vector of imbalance is anterior, posterior, medial, lateral, or a combination of these orientations. The motions described include an axial limb motion wherein the patient's pelvis is rotated in both a clockwise and counterclockwise direction (Fig. 27-6). Another motion pattern has the patient lean from side to side in the frontal plane (Fig. 27-7). Perhaps the most revealing motion, with respect to the influence on compensatory digital patterns, involves the patient leaning forward and backward (Fig. 27-8), which reflects the influence of underlying sagittal plane foot defects on the toes. As the patient moves in the direction of the foot imbalance, the digital counterbalancing is exacerbated, revealing the nature and extent of the underlying foot imbalance. The practitioner may then attempt

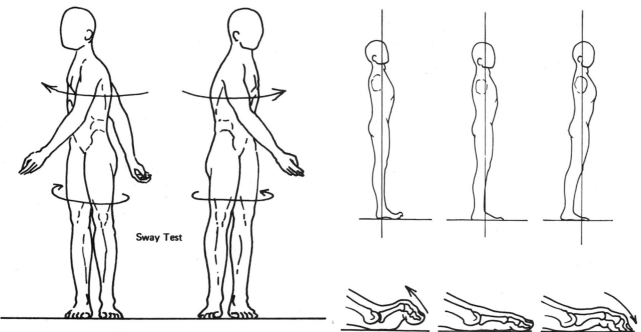

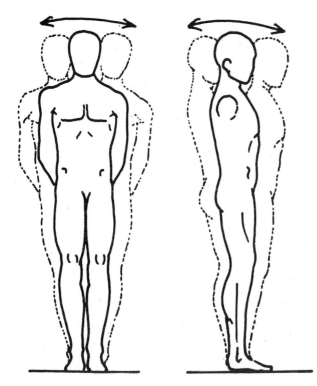

**Fig. 27-6.** Sway rotation testing.

**Fig. 27-7.** Side-to-side and front-to-back sway testing.

**Fig. 27-8.** Digital response to front-to-back sway testing.

corrective test rebalance of the suspected foot defect with test blocks or wedges.

## Block Balance Technique

After the suspected area of foot insufficiency has been identified, blocks and wedges of a semirigid nature are placed under that area or region to neutralize the situation (Fig. 27-9).[2] When the appropriate block or wedge has been selected, the digits should attain a more relaxed normal alignment attitude (Fig. 27-10). The extent of corrective digital reduction usually depend on the degree of functional involvement and chronicity of deformity. When the deformity is purely positional in nature and no adaptive changes have taken place, complete correction is often achieved with functional foot rebalance utilizing initial test balance pad therapy[3] followed by orthosis control. In situations in which adaptive digital changes have already occurred and that demonstrate a moderate to high taxicity resistance grading, a more aggressive orthodigital approach and a surgical solution may be required.

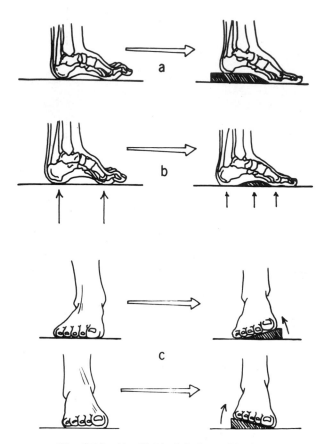

**Fig. 27-9.** (**A–C**) Block balance Testing.

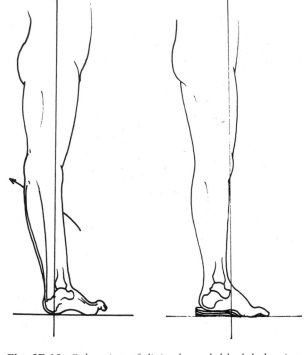

**Fig. 27-10.** Relaxation of digits through block balancing.

# STRUCTURAL ORTHODIGITAL EVALUATION

## Radiographic Digital Assessment

Radiographs should be considered an integral part of the orthodigital assessment to help gain an overall understanding of the presented digital problem. In the evaluation, the digital deformities should be straightened with assistive measures, if necessary, before obtaining the radiographs to detect the presence of structural digital anomalies and to help ascertain the nature, location, and extent of deformity (Fig. 27-11). Care must be taken not to overexpose the radiograph as this will obscure distal forefoot detail and hinder an essential portion of the digital evaluation (Fig. 27-12).

## Digital Line-Up Technique

Although the manual reduction of a digital deformity may indicate a functional developmental influence, the examiner should be careful not to overlook an underlying structural anomaly that may be hidden. To determine if a structural component is present we use the digital line-up technique[2] to uncover masked digital deformities (Fig. 27-13). It is not uncommon for long digits secondary to hyperphalangism to attain an apparently normal digital length pattern by retreating to the common line of gripping. To detect the presence of these camouflaged digits the examiner must straighten all the toes, preferably with the patient standing, noting any irregularities in size, shape, length, and contour as they relate to each other, the hallux, and the normal digital parabola. While these structural deformities are obviously best suited to surgical intervention, the operative approach will cer-

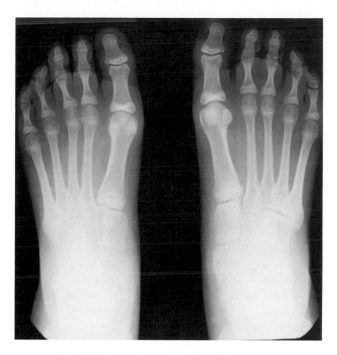

**Fig. 27-11.** Radiographic digital assessment.

tainly be influenced by the discovery of hidden digital deformities. The surgical implications are extremely important, because the long digit, which may present as a hammer toe deformity, will require an osseous modification procedure rather than a soft tissue procedure (i.e., tenotomy) even though it may have a low taxicity resistance grading (Fig. 27-14).

## Acquired Digital Deformity

Positional deformities of a long-standing nature will tend to become chronically adapted at the affected joint of deformation. These adaptive arthropathic changes are not conducive to conservative corrective measures and will usually require invasive operative procedures to restore a more normal digital alignment. Digital deformities that have attained a nontaxic state must now be relegated to the same status as the structural or congenital digital anomaly and should be treated in the same fashion.

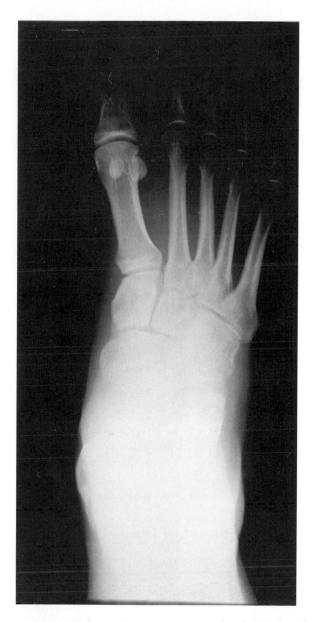

**Fig. 27-12.** Radiographic overexposure hindering digital evaluation.

## THERAPEUTIC DIGITAL MANAGEMENT
### Relief and Preliminary Care Phase

Once the digital malalignment or deformity has been recognized and classified, the preventive, corrective, and retentive steps of orthodigital therapy can be

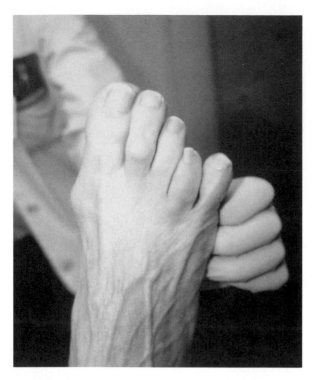

**Fig. 27-13.** Digital line-up technique.

addressed. Following the initial lower extremity and orthodigital evaluation the patient will generally require and desire some type of immediate attention for the presented digital complaints. Initial treatment may include lesional reduction, protective shielding, trial

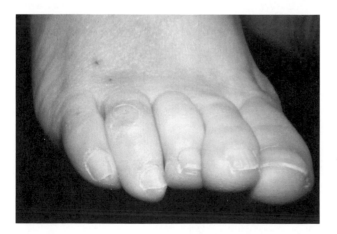

**Fig. 27-14.** Long fourth digit revealed through a poorly advised tenotomy procedure.

splinting, and test realignment and rebalance with selected functional foot balance pads.

Following lesional debridement, the deformity should be protected against further shoe irritation via precise digital shielding. The skin should be cleansed and prepped with an adherent before padding to provide better contact and, most importantly, to help prevent irritation, maceration, or fungal infection. Sound principles of digital pad design and application should be followed when optimal protective padding qualities are desired. The padding material should be firm enough to shield the lesion or prominence from the offending shoe pressures while not being so firm as to create new direct pad irritations. For this reason the selection of felt materials is generally preferred over softer compressible foam rubber materials.

The size and shape of the pad should be commensurate with the protective need for which it is intended (Fig. 27-15). All pad edges should be beveled and any sharp or abrupt corners are to be avoided to prevent potential irritation. The thickness of the pad is extremely important in that a pad which is either too soft or too shallow will not adequately protect or shield the prominence for which it was designed. A common misconception is that the aperture that is designed to subtract focal pressure should be exactly the same size as the prominence or lesion to be protected. While it is true that an aperture that is too remote will fail to protect, the aperture which is too small may cause irritation of the sensitive area surrounding the lesion. Along these same lines, it is also important to bevel the inner walls of the aperture to prevent excessive edge pressure and irritation (Fig. 27-16).

The first step to achieving long-term success in the management of functionally induced digital deformity is through the recognition and control of the underlying imbalance responsible for the development of the deformity. Toward this goal, the use of functional in-shoe temporary test padding may reduce or eliminate the necessity of further protective or corrective orthodigital measures (Fig. 27-17). Selection of appropriate test pad elements should improve digital function and alignment as lower extremity and foot imbalances are controlled. This padding system also serves to provide valuable information as to the individual patient response to the proposed correction and thus the need for orthotic control. The versatile and highly specific

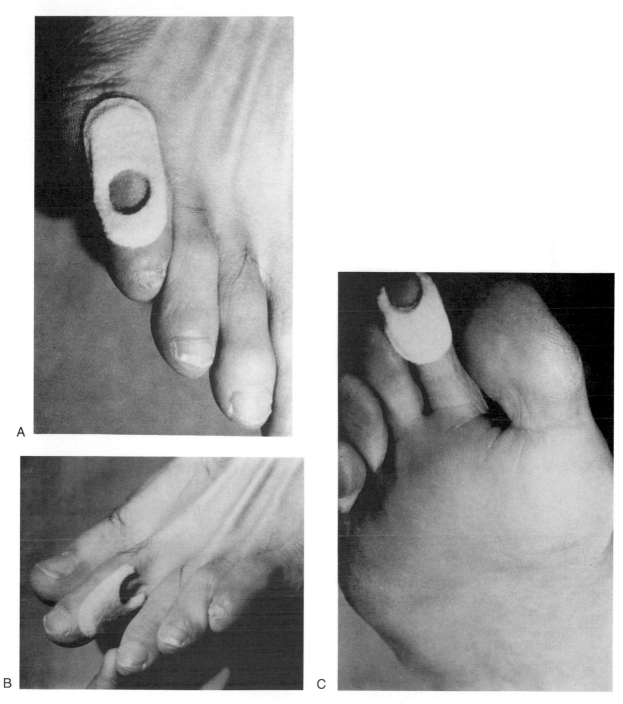

**Fig. 27-15.** (**A–F**) Selected digital and metatarsal shields. (*Figure continues*).

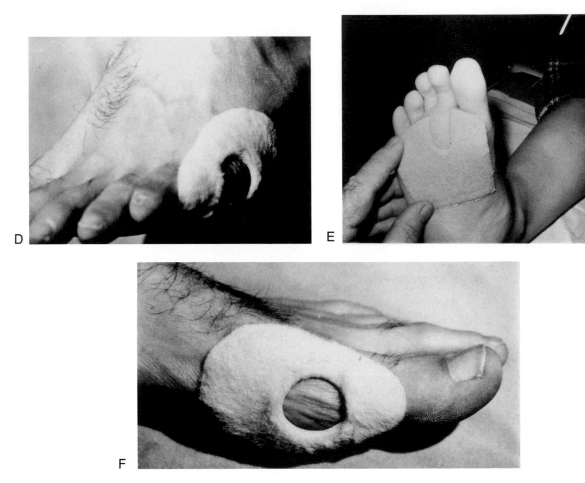

**Fig. 27-15** (*Continued*).

nature of the test padding system may be realized with the use of the "varus" test pad to which a Morton's platform or bunion flange may be added as needed (Fig. 27-18).

Additionally, stress reduction through weight management, occupational/avocational trends, postural habits, and general health also have contributory roles. The greatest factor, however, has to be the role of the patient's foot gear as either beneficial or detrimental with respect to the foot and digital problems.

## Foot Gear Survey

A careful survey of both the inner and outer shoe should be considered essential for the determination of proper shoe fit and appropriate alterations as well as education as to future shoe selection. Whenever possible, an attempt should be made to help patients select shoes in accordance with their particular foot type. The shoe taper, last, and width are all important considerations in selecting the appropriate shoe style

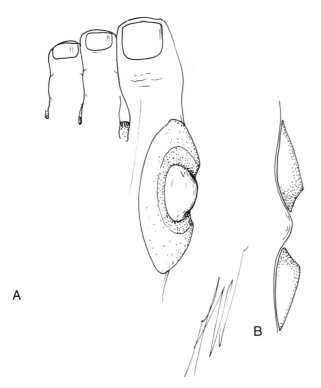

**Fig. 27-16.** Protective padding of prominences. (**A**) Full view; (**B**) profile view.

(Fig. 27–19): I have devised a technique that has proved useful for patient education by demonstrating how existing pressure lesions resulting from shoe–foot conflict can be identified and resolved with a proper shoe selection. An outline of the patient's shoe is traced on transparent acetate film and then placed over a dorsoplantar x-ray projection. This technique is highly graphic in visually demonstrating to the patient the effect of shoe crowding and poor fit on specific anatomic landmarks.

## Realignment Phase

Digital deformities that are easily reduced manually will generally respond favorably to conservative orthopedic and orthodigital treatment approaches. Digital malpositions secondary to foot or lower extremity defects must be addressed before any direct digital therapy. Once the underlying imbalance has been re-solved through corrective foot bracing and support, any remaining digital malalignment can be effectively addressed. The lower the taxicity resistance grading, the easier the corrective task when coupled with the appropriate orthodigital therapy. Orthodigital techniques such as urethane mold therapy,[4] splinting, tractive therapy,[5] hallux exercise, and other home digital exercise techniques should ensure lasting correction and prevention of recurrence so long as the underlying deforming forces are controlled.

The urethane mold orthosis (UMO) technique as described by Whitney is an extremely versatile orthodigital technique that can be effectively utilized for both corrective and retentive digital alignment needs as well as for protective and prosthetic applications. The UMO device is easily fashioned from blocks of polyurethane foam, being cut to the desired shape with a skiving knife and cork boring punches. Once the device has been properly fitted over the patient's toes, a water-based latex (vultex) is mixed with the foam until it is saturated. The activated mold is then placed back on the foot and covered with a plastic bag; the patient is instructed to wear the device for several hours until the urethane mold orthosis becomes functionally molded within the shoe confines (Fig. (27-20).

Digital traction therapy is another orthodigital technique that has proved extremely useful over the years as a rehabilitative measure for overcoming joint stiffness and adaptive changes secondary to positional imbalance. The original tractive device described and utilized by Budin some 50 years ago has since been refined by Whitney into a lightweight, simple, chairside technique (Fig. 27-21). With a series of office visits the patient may expect to gradually reduce the extent of digital deformity or help to restore motion lost through injury and functional disuse.

A digital band splint may be used for isolated digital deformities that are manually reducible but which still require external assistance to help overcome postural, congenital, or postsurgical malpositional influences (Fig. 27-22).

Motivated and enlightened patients may wish to take an active role in their treatment plan to help ensure success in the shortest possible time. Home exercises, which may include making toe fists, picking up marbles with the toes, and single foot balancing will often help the patient gain the flexibility and strength to

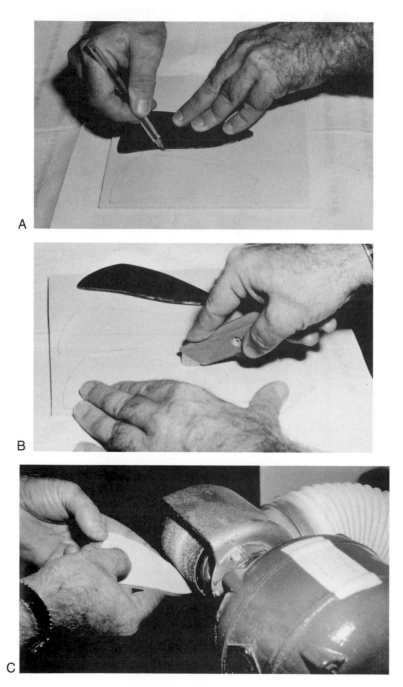

**Fig. 27-17.** In-shoe temporary test pad technique. (**A**) Tracing pad design; (**B**) cutting out pad; (**C**) bevel grinding pad edges. (*Figure continues.*)

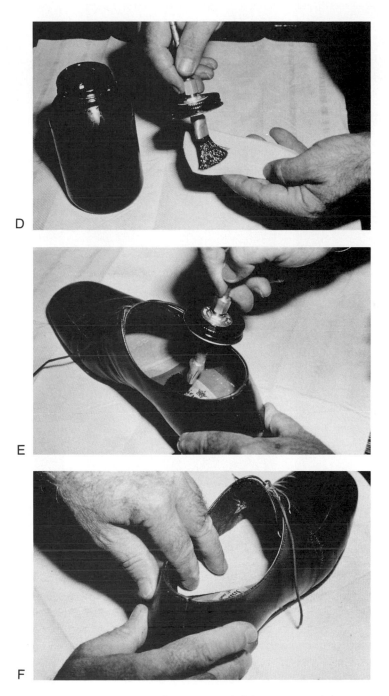

**Fig. 27-17** (*Continued*). (**D**) Rubber cement application to pad; (**E**) cement application to shoe; (**F**) pad placement in shoe.

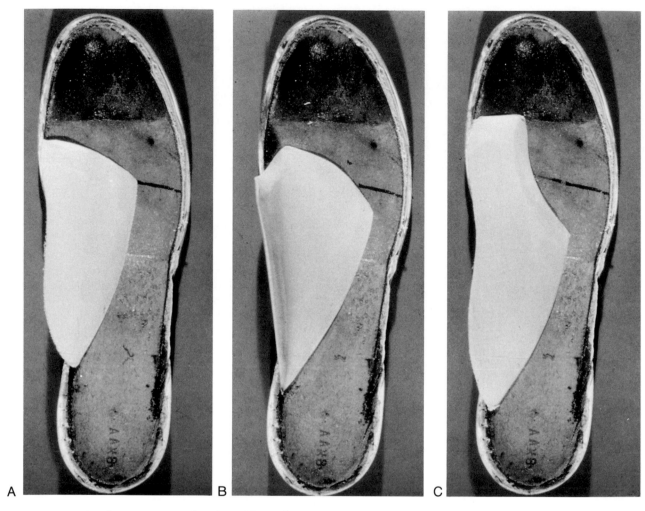

**Fig. 27-18.** The varus test pad and modifying elements. (**A**) Varus pad; (**B**) varus bunion flange pad; (**C**) varus Morton's extension pad.

overcome digital malpositions more quickly. One such exercise device designed for home use is the "Hallexorcist," which can dramatically reduce the realignment phase of the hallux abductus deformity especially when coupled with retentive and night splint therapy (Fig. 27-23).

## Repair Phase

Surgical intervention for structural or chronically adapted digits of a nontaxic nature will generally require a combination of soft tissue release and osseous procedures to render successful realignment and symptomatic relief. Digital deformities with a taxicity resistance grading between 3 and 4, yielding moderate to severe resistance to manual reduction, will usually require tenotomy and capsulotomy procedures in conjunction with conservative orthodigital techniques. Digital deformities that are completely nontaxic or which are only partially reduced with pain (grade 4–5) will require a combination of soft tissue and osseous reconstruction procedures.

Another therapeutic consideration involves the use of conservative protective or accommodative mea-

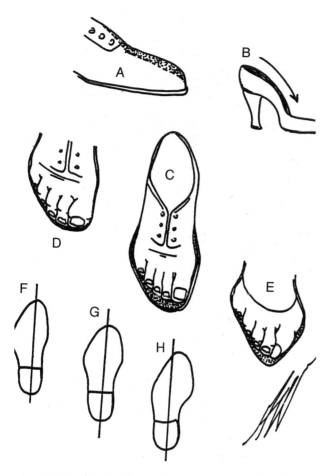

**Fig. 27-19. (A–H)** Shoe influences and considerations.

sures, which may be preferred when the digital deformity is so advanced that improved digital function will not be achieved through surgical intervention (Fig. 27-24).

## Hallux Abducto Valgus Management

Evaluation and treatment of the hallux abducto valgus (HAV) deformity based on the pattern, degree, and taxicity testing offers an enlightening overview of the therapeutic approach to be selected.

The mild or incipient HAV deformity that is minimally deviated with an HAV angle of 15° to 25°) and which is easily reducible with a taxicity resistance grading of 2 or less may be treated conservatively. The

use of a dry urethane mold hallux ram crest or silicone spacer is often effective in maintaining the desired hallux position, together with a hallux retention strap and metatarsal elastic binder. The etiologic and aggravating factors must be identified and negated with orthosis application and optimal shoe selection. The use of a hallux night splint (Fig. 27-25) and home digital exercises will also help to hasten the correction process.

Treatment of the moderate HAV deformity demonstrating a malalignment angle of 25° to 35°, mild subluxation, and a taxicity resistance grading between 2 and 4 will generally require a combined orthodigital and surgical approach to effectively treat and correct the problem. Preliminary foot and shoe control must first be achieved with appropriate foot rebalancing and shoe selection. Depending on the relative resistance to manual realignment, a decision involving aggressive digital traction therapy versus selective soft tissue procedures, which may include adductor release-capsulotomy and or a medial capsulorraphy, is determined. The use of a urethane mold ram crest and night splints will help to attain and maintain correction.[6]

Advanced to severe HAV malalignments of 35° or greater with a nonreducible dislocated first metatarsophalangeal joint (Fig. 27-26C) will usually require soft tissue and osseous reconstructive techniques, followed by orthosis control and retentive orthodigital measures to help maintain the correction and to prevent future recurrence. Severely dislocated and rigidly fixed HAV deformities may be best treated with protective orthodigital measures rather than radical surgical intervention. As a general rule, when operative procedures cannot improve digital function, conservative treatment including accommodative shoe prescription, urethane mold shielding, and surgical removal of symptomatic prominences is the preferred approach.

## Case Control and Evaluation

The periodic inspection and evaluation of the digital correction and treatment is essential to ensure continued success and maintenance of digital function and correction. Follow-up radiographic studies, models, and photos are extremely useful as reference documents for treatment progress. Foot orthoses should be adjusted or replaced if recurrence of deformity or loss

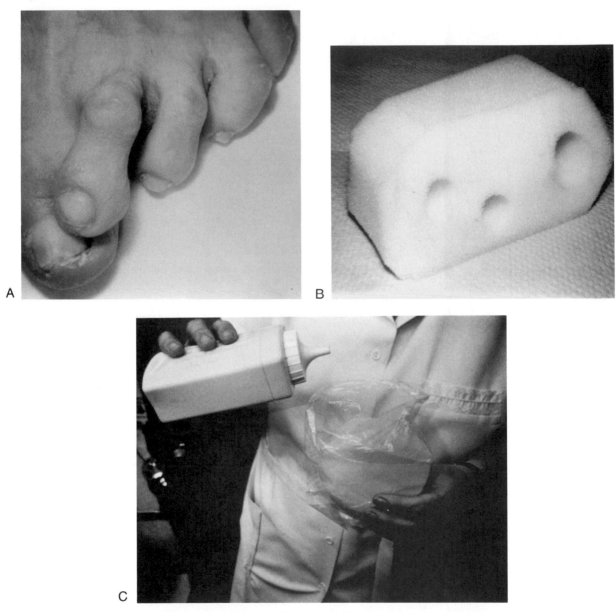

**Fig. 27-20.** Urethane mold orthosis technique. (**A**) Digital deformity to be corrected; (**B**) apertured foam block; (**C**) adding vultex solution to dry foam. (*Figure continues.*)

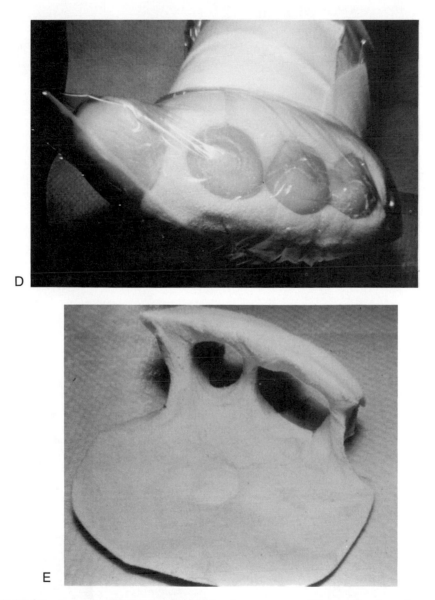

**Fig. 27-20** (*Continued*). (**D**) Saturated mold in place over toes; (**E**) completed urethane mold.

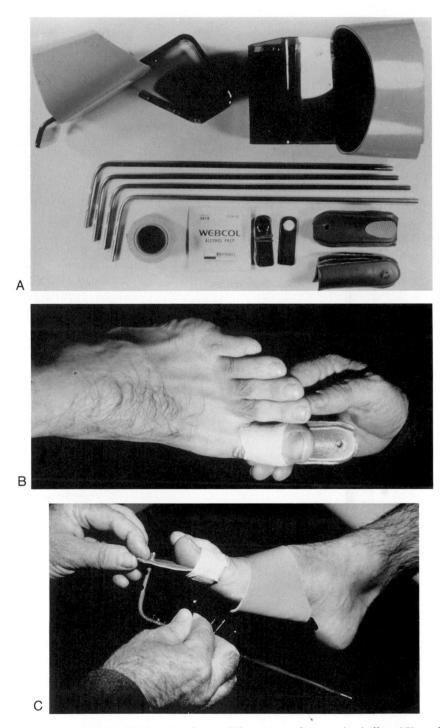

**Fig. 27-21.** Digital traction technique. (**A**) Traction device; (**B**) traction splint taped to hallux; (**C**) applying tractive force to first MPJ.

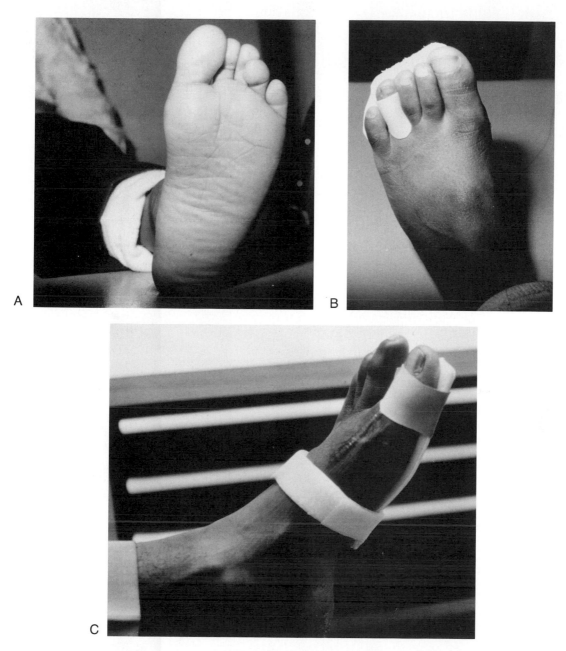

**Fig. 27-22.** Digital band splint technique. (**A**) Underlapping fourth toe; (**B**) realigned toe with splint; (**C**) post-surgical splint for hallux extensus.

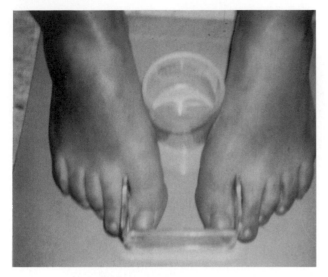

**Fig. 27-23.** The Hallexercist hallux home exercise device.

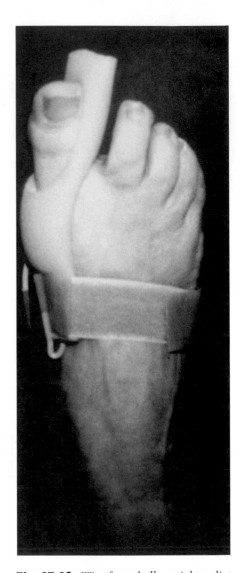

**Fig. 27-25.** Wire-foam hallux night splint.

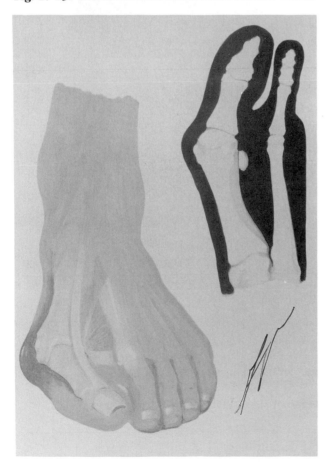

**Fig. 27-24.** Hallux abductor valgus deformity.

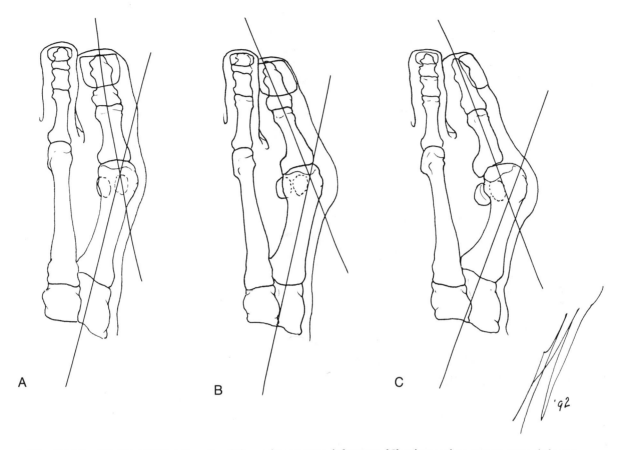

**Fig. 27-26. (A)** Mild HAV deformity; **(B)** moderate HAV deformity; **(C)** advanced to severe HAV deformity.

of digital function is noted. Any digital retainers being used should be inspected and replaced as necessary. The patient's current foot gear should be inspected and discussed with regard to any alterations in style, fit, and heel elevation. Digital stretching or strengthening exercises if still beneficial should also be prescribed or reviewed with the patient.

## CONCLUSION

Therapeutic shortcuts may produce disastrous results, but a thorough orthodigital evaluation leading to the most appropriate treatment should ensure gratifying results. Perhaps the most important assurance of long-term success is the patient's comprehension of the proposed treatment program. Through understand-ing, sustained patient motivation and cooperation are ensured.

## REFERENCES

1. Whitney AK: OrthoPodiatric Examination Procedure. Pennsylvania College of Podiatric Medicine, Philadelphia, 1973
2. Whitney KA, Whitney AK: Orthodigita Techniques, Principles and Practice of Podiatric Medicine. Churchill Livingstone, New York, 1990
3. Whitney AK: Biomechanical Footwear Balancing. Pennsylvania College of Podiatric Medicine, Philadelphia, 1979
4. Whitney AK: Urethane mould therapy. N Engl J Podiatry 42:17, 1963
5. Budin HA: Principles and Practice of Orthodigita. Strathmore Press, New York, 1941
6. McGlamery ED: Postoperative use of urethane moulds. J Am Podiatry Assoc 58:169, 1968

# 28

# Entrapment Neuropathies

*STEPHEN J. MILLER*

## DEFINITIONS

*Peripheral neuropathy* is defined as deranged function and structure of peripheral, motor, sensory, and autonomic neurons, involving either the entire neuron or selected levels.[1,2] The major categories of peripheral neuropathies are seen in Table 28-1. Because this chapter is concerned with nerve problems seen in the foot that are most amenable to local treatment, only the last four categories are considered.

A true *neuroma* consists of an unorganized mass of ensheathed nerve fibers embedded in scar tissue that originate from the proximal end of a transected peripheral nerve.[3] Neuromas are always the result of trauma. When the injury is incomplete (partial laceration, traction) or the result of blunt trauma the lesion will form within the epineurium and produce a fusiform or eccentric nodular swelling termed "neuroma-in-continuity."[4] In either case, the axonal elements are disrupted such that they are arranged in a somewhat haphazard fashion.

Morton's neuroma, the interdigital or intermetatarsal lesion accurately described initially by the English chiropodist Louis Durlacher,[5] is actually a misnomer. It is neither a true neuroma nor a neoplasm. Rather, it is best defined as a mechanical neuropathy with compression, stretching, and entrapment components in its etiology. Pathologically, this lesion is a progressive degenerative, and at times regenerative, process in which early and late changes may be found. Characteristic histologic findings support this etiology (Table 28-2). As a result, Morton's neuroma might be more accurately termed a perineural fibroma.[6,7]

Mechanical peripheral neuropathies are caused by local or extrinsic compression phenomena or impingement by an anatomic neighbor causing a localized entrapment.[8] Entrapment may also be caused by scarring or fibrosis from local trauma, bleeding, or traction that tends to bind the nerve down, thus restricting normal mobility within the tissues.

Traumatic neuropathies are the result of either closed injuries or open injuries to peripheral nerves. Early treatment usually involves prophylaxis and repair, while later attention is directed toward the painful neuromas or nerve entrapments that result from the body's healing processes.

Nerve sheath tumors are named according to their structure derivation. They can be benign or malignant. Nerve sheath tumors fall under another general category known as parenchymatous disorders because they can involve excessive growth of specific neural elements: neuron or axon, Schwann cell, perineurial cell, and endoneurial fibroblast. This is in contrast to the lesions described previously, termed interstitial disorders, in which external factors cause the derangements.[1,2]

## ANATOMY

Neuralgic pain in the foot and ankle can be traced to problems with the peripheral nerves. When the presenting symptoms—burning, tingling, numbness and other paresthesias—sound as though there is nerve involvement, it is important to exclude proximal and systemic causes of neuropathy. Examples include radiculopathy, compression syndromes, entrapment neuropathies, autonomic dysfunction, diabetes mellitus, ischemia, pernicious anemia, polycythemia vera,

**Table 28-1.** Peripheral Neuropathies

Vascular-ischemic
Metabolic
Nutritional
Infectious
Toxic
Hereditary
Inflammatory demyelinating
Mechanical
    Compression
    Entrapment
Traumatic
    Closed injuries
    Open injuries
Painful neuromas
Nerve sheath tumors

**Table 28-3.** Motor Innervation to the Leg and Foot

| Muscle | Peripheral Nerve | Spinal Level |
|---|---|---|
| Tibialis anterior | Deep peroneal | $L_{4,5}$ |
| Extensor digitorum longus | Deep peroneal | $L_{4,5}$ |
| Extensor hallucis longus | Deep peroneal | $L_{4,5}$ |
| Peroneus tertius | Deep peroneal | $L_{4,5}$ |
| Gastrocnemius | Tibial | $S_{1,2}$ |
| Soleus | Tibial | $S_{1,2}$ |
| Plantaris | Tibial | $S_{1,2}$ |
| Popliteus | Tibial | $L_{4,5}S_1$ |
| Flexor hallucis longus | Tibial | $S_{2,3}$ |
| Flexor digitorum longus | Tibial | $S_{2,3}$ |
| Tibialis posterior | Tibial | $L_{4,5}$ |
| Peroneus longus | Superficial peroneal | $L_5S_{1,2}$ |
| Peroneus brevis | Superficial peroneal | $L_5, S_{1,2}$ |
| Extensor digitorum brevis | Deep peroneal | $S_{1,2}$ |
| Abductor hallucis | Medial plantar | $S_{2,3}$ |
| Flexor digitorum brevis | Medial plantar | $S_{2,3}$ |
| First lumbricalis | Medial plantar | $S_{2,3}$ |
| Flexor hallucis brevis | Medial plantar | $S_{2,3}$ |
| Abductor digiti quinti brevis | Lateral plantar | $S_{2,3}$ |
| Quadratus plantae | Lateral plantar | $S_{2,3}$ |
| Second, third, fourth lumbricales | Lateral plantar | $S_{2,3}$ |
| Adductor hallucis | Lateral plantar | $S_{2,3}$ |
| Flexor digiti quinti brevis | Lateral plantar | $S_{2,3}$ |
| Plantar interossei | Lateral plantar | $S_{2,3}$ |
| Dorsal interossei First, second | Deep peroneal, lateral plantar | $S_{1,2,3}$ |
| Third, fourth | Lateral plantar | $S_{2,3}$ |

hypothyroidism, erythromelalgia, and alcoholism and other systemic diseases.

To further isolate problems within the nerves of the foot, a thorough understanding of the peripheral neuroanatomy and cord level innervation is essential. Six nerves cross the ankle joint into the foot: the saphenous nerve, the medial dorsal cutaneous nerve, the intermediate dorsal cutaneous nerve, the deep peroneal nerve, the posterior tibial nerve, and the lateral dorsal cutaneous nerve or sural nerve[9] (Figs. 28-1 through 28-4).

There can be anatomic variations of all the peripheral nerves, deviating somewhat from these descriptions. However, the basic pattern must be understood and applied in the clinical setting. Also required is a thorough knowledge of the neurodermatomes (Table 28-3; Figure 28-5) and muscle innervation by peripheral nerve and spinal cord level. This battery of information is essential so that the clinician can isolate and locate peripheral nerve pathology in the foot, ankle, and leg.

**Table 28-2.** Histopathology of Morton's Neuroma (Perineural Fibroma)

Venous congestion (early stages)
Endoneural and neural edema (early stages).
Perineural, epineural, and endoneural fibrosis and hypertrophy (late stages)
Renaut's body formation (evidence of local pressure damage)
Hyalinization of the walls of endoneurial blood vessels.
Subintimal and perivascular fibrosis that may lead to occlusion of local blood vessels (resembling healed vasculitis)
Mucinous changes endoneurially and perineurally
Demyelination with axonal loss

## PERIPHERAL NERVE ANATOMY

A peripheral nerve is composed of many nerve fibers, which may vary in length from 0.5 mm to 1 m or more.[10,11] Each nerve fiber consists of the *axon,* with its thin outer layer or *axolemma* surrounding the viscous *axoplasm,* the *Schwann cell,* and *Schwann cell sheath* with or without myelin (Fig. 28-6A). Myelinated nerves have one axon per Schwann cell, while unmyelinated fibers have several axons surrounded by a single Schwann cell (Fig. 28-6B). It should be noted, as conduction rates are directly related to fiber size, that the larger myelinated fibers conduct at a more rapid rate than unmyelinated axons.

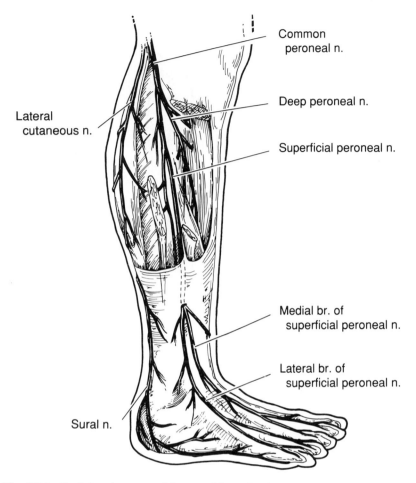

**Fig. 28-1.** Peripheral nerves of front and lateral side of leg and dorsum of foot.

Each nerve fiber is surrounded by an endoneurial sheath (*endoneurium*), which includes the basal membrane of the Schwann cell outside the myelin sheath as well as the reticular and collagen fibers that provide the supporting framework (Fig. 28-7).

Within a peripheral nerve is a *fascicle,* a unit consisting of a group of nerve fibers surrounded by the *perineurium.* This perineurial sheath is composed of epithelial-like cells as an inner layer and collagen connective tissue as an outer layer (Fig. 28-7).

Finally, a single fascicle or group of fascicles will make up the peripheral nerve itself. The collagenous connective support tissue surrounding these fascicles is known as the *epineurium,* which may be external or interfascicular. It is this tissue that can become bound

with local scar tissue in certain entrapment neuropathies.

## DIAGNOSIS OF NERVE INJURIES AND ENTRAPMENTS

Patients afflicted with nerve injuries or compression problems tend to experience pain and paresthesia typical of nerves. Sometimes these are enhanced with bizarre symptoms, especially when the patient has an overly anxious or hysterical personality. The pain is characteristically of a sharp or burning nature, localized over the sensory distribution of the involved nerve. The extent of the area involved will depend on

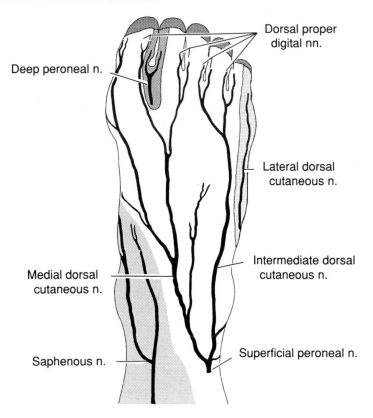

**Fig. 28-2.** Peripheral nerves on dorsum of foot.

what portion of the nerve trunk is damaged or impinged.

Early in the entrapment process the patient may experience muscle cramps or a feeling of tight, heavy, or swollen feet. Dysesthesia, hyperesthesia, and hypesthesia can be extremely uncomfortable. The pain may then progress to altered sensations of tingling, burning, or numbness that are often present at rest and may increase in severity at night, causing restlessness. It is aggravated by increased extremity movement and activity; proximal radiation is common. Altogether, the symptoms can be very exasperating and debilitating, to the point of causing complete disability. They may further precipitate a reflex sympathetic dystrophy syndrome.

When a motor nerve is primarily involved, the symptoms are less well defined as to distribution. Motor nerve pain is characteristically dull and aching in nature, affecting the muscle or muscles innervated by the affected nerve. Local joints will also hurt, especially

proximally. As the neuropathy persists over time, muscle tenderness can be found, leading eventually to paresis and disuse atrophy.

Sensorimotor examination is central to objective evaluation. Decreased two-point tactile discrimination greater than 6 mm is an early sign. When the nerve is accessible, deep palpation may reveal enlargement or elicit tenderness and paresthesia; often, it will reproduce the patient's symptoms. Percussion of the nerve causing distal radiation or paresthesia is a positive Tinel's sign while proximal and distal radiation indicates a positive Valleix phenomenon. Both are indicative of traumatic or compression damage.

Diagnostic nerve blocks, selectively anesthetizing the suspected nerve with lidocaine or bupivicaine, will result in dramatic relief when there is a nerve entrapment. This helps identify the nerve trunk and localize nerve branches to further isolate the problem. Perineural infiltration with steroid at the site of entrapment can also remarkably decrease symptoms by re-

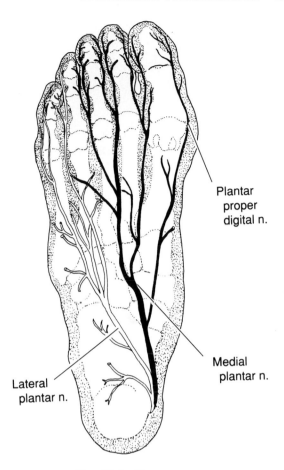

**Fig. 28-4.** Plantar nerves.

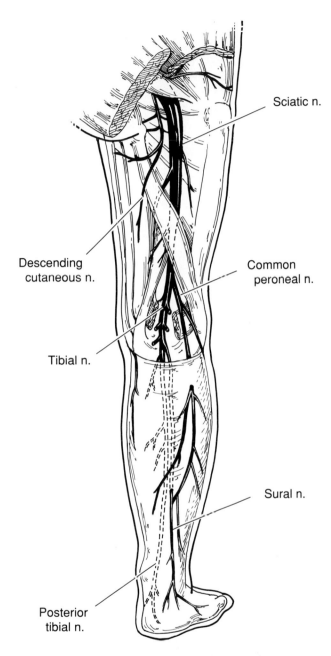

**Fig. 28-3.** Nerves of posterior lower limb.

ducing inflammation and fibrosis, another good diagnostic aid.

Nerve conduction velocity is decreased in most cases of nerve entrapment, although normal findings do not rule out impingement. Electromyographic studies are less helpful unless there is virtually complete nerve conduction blockade.

Magnetic resonance imaging (MRI) has provided some rather striking visualizations of nerve entrapments, although diagnostic value relative to cost must be considered because it is an expensive test. It can give good contrasts in soft tissue density.

## TARSAL TUNNEL SYNDROME

The symptom complex caused by entrapment of the posterior tibial nerve was first described by Pollock and Davis in 1933,[12] then named by Keck in 1962[13] and later by Lam.[14] Entrapment may result from recent weight gain, posttraumatic fibrosis, chronic compres-

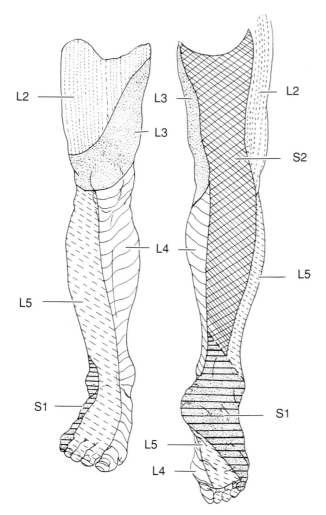

**Fig. 28-5.** Dermatome mapping of lumbar and sacral nerve roots.

at night when the patient is in bed. Patients may also relate a feeling of "fullness" or "tightness" in the arch, while others complain of a sensation of impending arch cramps.[18] The onset of the neuropathy is usually spontaneous or slow and insidious and may be mistakenly diagnosed as intermetatarsal neuromas.[19]

There is rarely any motor weakness detectable, although electromyograph (EMG) studies often demonstrate abnormal fibrillation potentials within the intrinsic muscles. Prolonged latency in the conduction of impulses along the medial and plantar nerves greater than 6.1 ms and 6.7 ms, respectively, help confirm the presence of a compression neuropathy.[20] Percussion of the posterior tibial nerve will almost always elicit a positive Tinel's sign as well as Valleix phenomenon. Turk's test, performed by inflating a thigh cuff to just below the systolic blood pressure, can exacerbate symptoms as the venae comitantes become engorged within the tarsal tunnel.[21]

Conservative measures include control of excess pronation, NSAIDs, massage, ultrasound, and the injection of steroid preparations or large volumes of local anesthetic into the third canal of the tarsal tunnel. If symptoms persist, then surgical decompression is indicated. The laciniate ligament must be incised over the third canal, followed by careful neurolysis, first proximally and then distally where the porta pedis is dilated as the nerve passes beneath the abductor hallucis muscle belly into the plantar vault. Tortuous veins in the area are excised and ligated. Only the superficial fascia is sutured, leaving the laciniate ligament open. A compression dressing is applied and the patient kept non-weight-bearing for no longer than 2 weeks so as to mobilize the tissues early. Postoperative Tinel's sign will usually diminish with time.[22]

With symptoms generally the same, an extension of the tarsal tunnel syndrome involves entrapment or compression of the plantar nerves at the level of the abductor hallucis on entering the foot or beneath the midtarsus in the severely collapsed flatfoot. In the latter case, the patient may actually be placing full weight on the nerve through the bones of the tarsus. This is an extremely difficult condition to treat successfully. Conservative care involves using soft orthoses to distribute the weight away from the nerve. Surgery, when necessary, must not only free the nerve tissue but create some form of arch architecture through arthrodesing procedures to get the weight-bearing pressure off the nerve.

sion from fascial bands, restriction within the laciniate canal, and entrapment by the abductor hallucis muscle[15] (Fig. 28-8). It has also been postulated to occur in association with os trigonum syndrome.[16] Goodman and Kehr[17] reported 27 cases of bilateral tarsal tunnel syndrome, suggesting that it is more common than previously believed.

Symptoms consist primarily of sharp or burning paresthesia radiating into the plantar aspect of the foot aggravated by activity and relieved somewhat by rest and removing shoewear. Proximal radiation is not uncommon, although not past the knee. Pain may occur

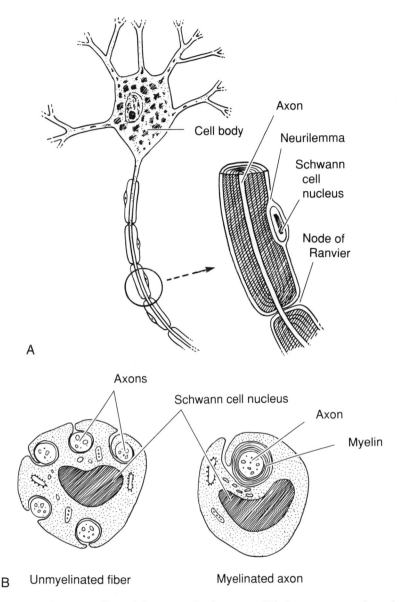

**Fig. 28-6.** Microanatomy of a nerve fiber. (**A**) Longitudinal section. (**B**) Cross section of myelinated axon and unmyelinated fiber with several unmyelinated axons enveloped by a single Schwann cell.

## INFERIOR CALCANEAL NERVE ENTRAPMENT

Heel involvement has been reported as part of the tarsal tunnel syndrome,[15,23] but generally this area is spared. However, patients with recalcitrant heel pain, with or without calcaneal spurs, have been shown to have good relief from decompression and neurolysis of the inferior calcaneal nerve, the mixed sensorimotor branch to the proximal abductor digiti quinti muscle.[24-26]

The most common origin of the inferior calcaneal nerve is from the lateral plantar nerve, where it is also known as the "first branch." The lateral plantar nerve gives off the first branch within or distal to the tunnel.[27]

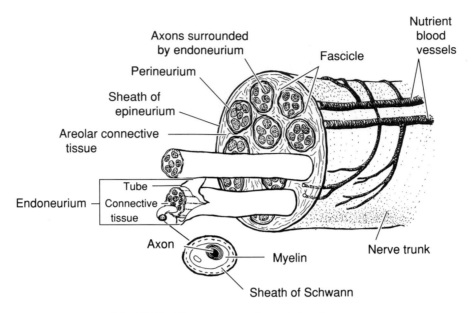

**Fig. 28-7.** Microanatomy of a peripheral nerve.

Except when involved in tarsal tunnel syndrome, entrapment of the inferior calcaneal nerve branch to the abductor digiti quinti muscle can cause severe and disabling heel pain. The nerve can be traumatized and compressed primarily at two sites: the firm fascial edge of the abductor hallucis muscle,[28,29] and the me-

dial edge of the calcaneus where the nerve traverses either beneath the medial tuberosity or along the origin of the flexor brevis muscle and plantar fascia.[26]

The symptoms usually differ from those of plantar fasciitis in that they include sharp, burning pain that often radiates up the posteromedial leg. It can be re-

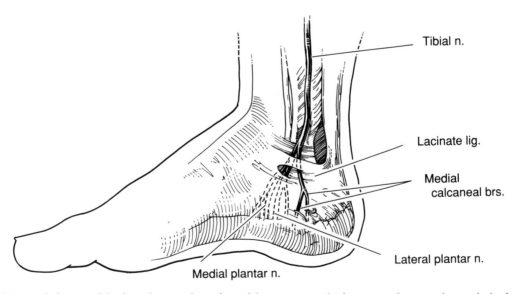

**Fig. 28-8.** Medial view of the foot showing branches of the posterior tibial nerve as they pass beneath the lacinate ligament through the third compatment of the tarsal canal.

produced by deep compression just medial or distal to the medial tuberosity. Patients frequently fail to experience the pain on weight-bearing after rest (poststatic dyskinesia) that is almost pathognomonic of the plantar fasciitis enthesopathy.

Pronation can be a great contributor to this entrapment but the syndrome also occurs in feet with normal or supinated architecture. Affected patients are commonly athletes or people whose occupations require long hours of standing or walking on concrete or other unforgiving surfaces. They characteristically do not respond to the variety of conservative therapeutic measures used to treat heel pain including rest, tape strapping, steroid injections, shoe adjustments, orthotic devices, ultrasound, and massage. In fact, many of these therapies tend only to aggravate the condition.

Surgery begins with a medial incision to access the nerve at or distal to the medial tuberosity of the calcaneus. The deep fascia of the abductor hallucis muscle is released. The nerve is then freed along its course distal and deep to the medial tuberosity as it approaches the abductor digiti quinti muscle. The medial plantar fascia should be incised, and only a small portion of heel spur removed when present and only if it appears to be contributing to the entrapment. Results are often in the form of dramatic relief the next day. Patients should be kept non-weight-bearing for 2 weeks with a gradual return to full activity.

## SURAL NERVE ENTRAPMENT

Entrapment of the sural nerve will cause sensory alterations and pain locally at the site of entrapment or all the way along its courses laterally to the fifth toe. Local trauma, surgical iatrogenic injury, and long-term chronic tendonitis of the tendo Achilles are the leading etiologies of this compression syndrome.[22]

If symptoms are unresponsive to the usual conservative approaches, surgical intervention is frequently necessary. Neurolysis is the first choice for release but because the sural nerve is totally sensory, sectioning and excising the nerve are commonly necessary to alleviate the pain. Care must be taken to allow the nerve to retract into the shelter of soft tissues to prevent sensitive stump neuroma formation.

## DORSAL FOREFOOT NERVE INJURY AND ENTRAPMENT

In addition to entrapment of the deep peroneal nerve on the dorsum of the foot, compression of the superficial peroneal nerve as it exits the deep fascia in the lower leg can cause painful symptoms. This nerve can also be trapped against dorsal exostoses along the course of its branches or can be injured by trauma.

Because many surgical approaches are via the dorsal foot, surgical trauma can result in painful sensory neuromas in that area. In one study, 19 of 25 (76 percent) of the neuromas occurred within the medial two-thirds of the dorsal midfoot, an area termed the neuromatous or N-zone (Fig. 28-9). Although nerves

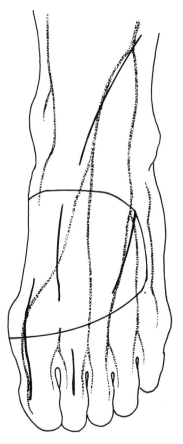

**Fig. 28-9.** Neuromatous or N-zone where incisions are more likely to lead to symptomatic neuromas. (Adapted from Kenzora,[30] with permission.)

are frequently damaged in bunion surgery, they are seldom symptomatic. In addition, toe surgery rarely results in painful neuromas or nerve injuries.[30]

Once identified, nerves trapped in scar tissue can be treated by injection therapy using enzyme mixtures, sclerosing solutions,[31] steroid preparations, or volume injection adhesiotomy techniques.[32] If they remain painful, they are best treated by neurolysis and excision. This is a technically difficult and often painful approach that can yield up to 26% unsatisfactory results.[33] The conclusion is that it is much easier to prevent a sensory neuroma by careful surgical technique than to treat a highly symptomatic neuroma. This requires thoughtful planning for the location of the incision, gentle tissue separation and retraction, identification and visualization of peripheral nerves, and judicious suturing technique.

Symptoms can also occur on the dorsal foot when the superficial peroneal nerve suffers a traction injury, as in an ankle sprain, or entrapment at the fibular neck[34,35] or where it exits the deep fascia in the anterior lower leg.[36] Local injury can occur from contusions, fractures, or midfoot exostoses, or by compression from adjacent soft tissue masses such as ganglia.

## ENTRAPMENT NEUROPATHY OF THE DEEP PERONEAL NERVE

Compression neuropathy involving the anterior tibial or deep peroneal nerve has been described as "anterior tarsal tunnel syndrome."[37] It may be an entrapment of the nerve at the inferior extensor retinaculum[38,39] (Fig. 28-10). It can also be caused by traction, trauma, local exostoses, edema, or shoe pressure. Altered sensation in the first web space is the hallmark diagnostic sign.[40] EMG studies may reveal distal latency in the deep peroneal nerve, and there may be signs of denervation in the extensor digitorum brevis muscle.

Treatment includes avoidance of shoe pressure, steroid injections, and pads to disburse direct pressure on the nerve. If conservative therapy fails, surgical intervention for relief of symptoms includes exostectomy, neurolysis, or retinacular release. In one study where entrapment release was performed on 20 nerves in 18 patients followed for a mean of 25.9

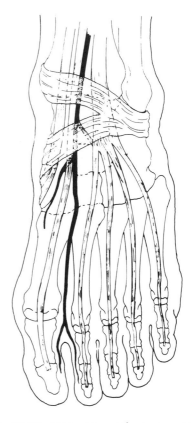

**Fig. 28-10.** Deep peroneal nerve anatomy.

months, operative results were excellent in 60 percent, good in 20 percent, and not improved in 20 percent.[41]

## ENTRAPMENT NEUROPATHY ABOUT THE FIRST METATARSOPHALANGEAL JOINT

There are four nerve branches crossing the first metatarsophalangeal joint, corresponding roughly to the four corners of the hallux. The dorsolateral surface is supplied by the deep peroneal nerve; its pathology is described elsewhere.

Joplin[42] described a perineural fibrosis of the proper digital nerve as it coursed along the plantome-

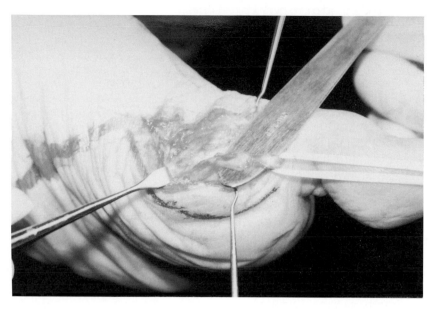

**Fig. 28-11.** Example of a Joplin's neuroma dissected from beneath the medial edge of a bunion.

dial first metatarsal head. He reported the removal of 265 of these entities.[42] The nerve either displaces laterally from its usual anatomic position or, in the course of the development of hallux valgus deformity, the metatarsal head drifts medially to bear weight directly on top of the nerve. Pronatory forces that concentrate body weight through the medial foot provide further compressive forces that stimulate perineural edema and fibrosis, axon degeneration, and Renaut body formation. The result is pain, paresthesia, and numbness.

Treatment with pads and orthotics to redistribute body weight will help relieve pressure on the nerve. Steroid injections can be helpful and anesthetic infiltration diagnostic. Surgery is the curative treatment by means of a neurectomy through a medial approach at the junction of the dorsal and plantar skin. Clean transection of the proximal nerve trunk under tension will allow the nerve end to retract into the abductor hallucis muscle belly for protection[43] (Fig. 28-11).

Another location for entrapment compression neuropathy is the dorsomedial first metatarsophalangeal joint.[44] The most medial branch of the medial dorsal cutaneous nerve becomes compressed between an enlarged medial eminence and the shoe, and very little enlargement is necessary to develop the problem. Avoidance of shoe pressure, padding, injection therapy, and bunionectomy will all help alleviate the pressure. At times nerve excision is necessary to relieve painful paresthesia unresponsive to other forms of treatment. Similar neuromas can be found in association with tailor's bunions where treatment is generally the same.[45]

Intermetatarsal plantar neuromas are rarely found between the first and second metatarsal heads, only 3.9 percent in one study.[46] Such a painful lesion can remain after corrective bunion surgery, having been overseen as contributing to the patient's symptoms preoperatively. Hypermobility is part of the cause of intermittent nerve compression, but a contributing factor can be the laterally displaced fibular sesamoid impinging the nerve against the second metatarsal head. Neuralgic symptoms are the result.

Failure of conservative treatment requires surgical excision through a dorsal or plantar approach, or a fibular sesamoidectomy. Again, the nerve trunk must be sharply divided and allowed to retract into the intrinsic muscle bellies. The patient must be made aware of the areas of anesthesia that will result.

# INTERMETATARSAL NEUROMA SYNDROME: MORTON'S NEUROMA

## Definition and Anatomy

Morton's neuroma is a misnomer used to describe a painful pedal neuropathy that most commonly appears as a benign enlargement of the third common digital branch of the medial plantar nerve located between, and often distal to, the third and fourth metatarsal heads. The lesion, also known as a *perineural fibroma,* is usually supplied by a communicating branch from the lateral plantar nerve[7] (Fig. 28-12).

Classically, the involved nerve passes plantar to the deep transverse intermetatarsal ligament. The only additional structures traversing this immediate area are the third plantar metatarsal artery with its accompanying vein or veins, and the tendon slip from the third lumbrical muscle that inserts into the extensor hood apparatus on the medial aspect of the fourth toe. This perineural fibroma is separated from the sole by the subcutaneous fat pad, plantar fascial slips, and connective tissue compartments (Fig. 28-13). Frequently, there is found, either alone or in close association with Morton's neuroma, an intermetatarsal bursa that

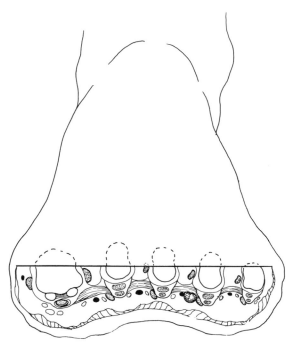

**Fig. 28-13.** Cross section through the forefoot at the level of the metatarsophalangeal joints.

is deep and usually distal to the deep transverse intermetatarsal ligament (Fig. 28-14).[47–50]

Interestingly, this is also the area in which pacinian corpuscles are normally found in the subcutaneous tissues,[51] and it is common to find multiple sensory branches diving plantarly from the nerve trunk and/or neuroma at the time of dissection. As an observation, these usually are found in the patients with the greater neuralgic symptoms causing the metatarsalgia.

## Histopathology

Summarized in Table 28-2 is the microscopic pathology of Morton's neuromas.[52–61] Many of these findings are also found in "normal" plantar nerves after years of wear and tear; endoneural edema, exceptional fibrosis and demyelination are diagnostic of Morton's neuroma[62,63] (Fig. 28-15). Serial section analysis has revealed that these degenerative nerve changes are usually found distal to the deep transverse intermetatarsal ligament.[64]

Investigators have found that a neuroma does not have to be particularly large or be present for a long

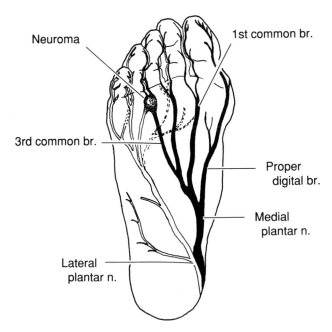

**Fig. 28-12.** Classic site of Morton's neuroma in relationship to the plantar nerves.

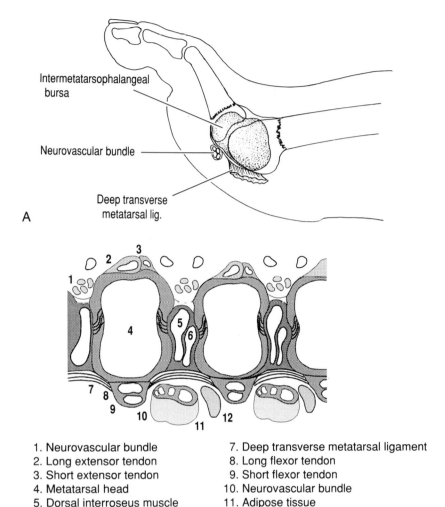

1. Neurovascular bundle
2. Long extensor tendon
3. Short extensor tendon
4. Metatarsal head
5. Dorsal interroseus muscle
6. Plantar interroseus muscle

7. Deep transverse metatarsal ligament
8. Long flexor tendon
9. Short flexor tendon
10. Neurovascular bundle
11. Adipose tissue
12. Lumbrical

**Fig. 28-14.** (**A**) Longitudinal section through third intermetatarsal space. (**B**) Frontal section through bases of proximal phalanges. There is no bursa in the lateral web space.

time to undergo pathologic changes and cause painful symptoms.[58,65,66] Except for Reed and Bliss[47] and Hauser,[67] no researchers have found any histologic evidence of inflammation in a neuroma.[58,60,68]

## Etiology and Biomechanics

Recent published information leaves little doubt that the syndrome of intermetatarsal neuroma is indeed a mechanical entrapment neuropathy[52,63,64,69] with degenerative changes that are largely the result of both stretch and compression forces. In reference to the

development of fibrosis within nerve support structures, Goldman[53] suggested that the epineurium responds to mechanical compression whereas the perineurium responds to stretch.

The next question is what is the source of these mechanical forces. A common observation is that the majority of intermetatarsal neuromas occur in the pronated foot,[65,70–72] where there are not only excessive stretch forces imposed on the interdigital nerves but also compressive and shearing forces from adjacent hypermobile metatarsal heads.[73–75]

Observing that the medial and lateral plantar nerves

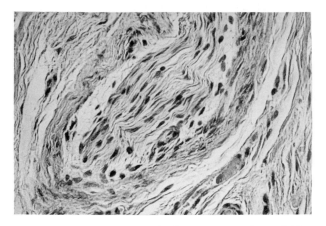

**Fig. 28-15.** Photomicrograph of cross section through Morton's neuroma (H & E, ×100.)

pass down the posteromedial side of the foot and dive plantarly under the arch, it is easy to visualize the stretch placed on these nerves during prolonged midstance pronation as the foot is everted, abducted, and dorsiflexed. Tension is increased as the nerves pass

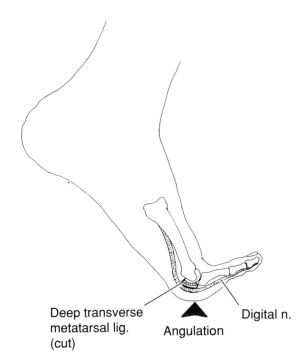

Deep transverse
metatarsal lig.    Angulation    Digital n.
(cut)

**Fig. 28-16.** Toe hyperextension causes stretch of interdigital nerves and tension against deep transverse metatarsal ligaments.

**Table 28-4.** Intermetatarsal Neuromas: Distribution by Sex

| Study | Male | Female | n |
|---|---|---|---|
| Bradley et al. (1976)[81] | 14 (16%) | 71 (84%) | 85 |
| Gauthier (1979)[82] | 19 ( 9%) | 187 (91%) | 206 |
| Mann and Reynolds (1983)[83] | 3 ( 5%) | 53 (95%) | 56 |
| Wachter et al. (1984)[80] | ? (17%) | ? (83%) | ? |
| Gudas and Mattana (1986)[84] | 7 (16%) | 36 (84%) | 43 |
| Addante et al. (1986)[46] | 27 (20%) | 109 (80%) | 136 |
| Johnson (1989)[122] | ? (22%) | ? (78%) | 124 |
| Average | 15% | 85% | |

around the flexor digitorum brevis "sling"[76] and are drawn up tightly against the plantar and anterior edge of the unyielding deep transverse intermetatarsal ligament. Further tension and compression will occur at this ligament when the toes hyperextend or dorsiflex at the metatarsophalangeal joint.[8,64,66,76–80] Occupations requiring toe hyperextension can therefore result in the development of an intermetatarsal neuroma, regardless of foot type (Fig. 28-16).

Pointed-toe or narrow shoes can definitely add compressive forces toward the development of intermetatarsal neuromas.[76,78] High-heeled shoes will not only throw weight forward onto the ball of the foot, jamming it into the narrow toe box, but will also force the toes into hyperextension and thus contribute to the entrapment etiology.

## Diagnosis

Morton's neuroma is classically and most commonly found in the third intermetatarsal space in females (Table 28-4). Otherwise known as an intermetatarsal neuroma, it also develops frequently in the second intermetatarsal space but rarely in the first or fourth (Table 28-5). Although it usually presents as a single

**Table 28-5.** Intermetatarsal Neuromas: Location

| Study | 1st (%) | 2nd (%) | 3rd (%) | 4th (%) | Other (%) |
|---|---|---|---|---|---|
| Wachter et al. (1984)[80] | — | 43 | 57 | — | — |
| Gudas and Mattana (1986)[84] | — | 5.1 | 86.4 | 8.5 | — |
| Addante et al. (1986)[46] | 3.9 | 17.8 | 66.4 | 2.6 | 9.2 |
| Johnson (1989)[122] | — | 16 | 84 | — | — |

**Table 28-6.** Intermetatarsal Neuromas: Occurrence

| Study | Single (%) | Double (%) | Bilateral (%) | Repeat (%) | (n) |
|---|---|---|---|---|---|
| Bradley et al. (1976)[81] | 63 | 4 | 27 | 6 | 85 |
| Gauthier (1979)[82] | 42 | 23 | 35 | — | 304 |
| Mann and Reynolds (1983)[83] | 61 | — | 39 | 15 | 76 |
| Gudas and Mattana (1986)[84] | 63 | 11 | 26 | — | 43 |
| Johnson (1989) | 82 | 2 | 14 | | 149 |
| Average | 62 | 10 | 28 | 11 | — |

entity, more than one intermetatarsal neuroma may develop in the same foot or both feet[80–85] (Table 28-6). The lesion is most commonly diagnosed between the fourth and sixth decades and the patient is likely to be overweight.[51,72] Symptoms may be present from a few weeks to several years.

The patient may initially describe a sensation as if walking on a wrinkle in her stocking or a lump in her shoe. In more advanced cases, the pain may be sharp, dull, or throbbing, but classically presents as paroxysmal burning "like walking on a hot pebble" or "having a hot poker thrust between the toes."

The pain is most often localized to the region of the third and fourth metatarsal heads and may radiate distally into adjacent toes, especially the fourth, or proximally up the leg to the knee. Numbness in the third and fourth toes may be the presenting symptom; however, there is seldom a sensory deficit. Sometimes, patients describe a "cramping" sensation in the arch or toes but there is no physical evidence of cramping[83,86] (Table 28-7).

The pain is greatly aggravated by walking in shoe gear and is relieved somewhat by rest. Pathognomonic is the overwhelming desire to remove the shoe, massage the forefoot, and flex the toes although relief is only transient. Occasionally, the pain persists at rest and at night the patient might even find that pressure from the bedsheets is intolerable.

In many cases, acute pain symptoms appear after an incident of trauma. Examples include stepping on a rock, twisting an ankle, jamming the foot into the floorboard in a motor vehicle accident, or simply changing into a pair of new shoes and doing an extraordinary amount of walking. Narrow or tight-fitting shoes can both instigate and aggravate pain symptoms. Occupations that mandate repetitive foot stress, such as working a pedal, walking on concrete, or squatting, can incite neuroma pain.

The intermetatarsal spaces are often tender to direct plantar palpation. A thickened nerve cord can frequently be rolled against a thumb over the distal metatarsal heads in the plantar sulcus when the toes are dorsiflexed. This may reproduce a varying amount of pain.

Dorsoplantar palpation of the affected intermetatarsal space with simultaneous side-to-side compression of the metatarsal heads (the "lateral squeeze test") can reproduce the pain by directly trapping the neuroma with pressure (Fig. 28-17). When lateral compression of the metatarsal heads elicits a silent, palpable, and sometimes painful "click," Mulder's sign is said to be positive.[87] However, the intermetatarsal bursa can also be responsible for the click.[88]

Electrodiagnostic techniques for evaluating Mor-

**Table 28-7.** Preoperative Symptoms of Morton's Neuroma

| Symptoms | Neuromas [n = 65 (%)] | | Recurrent Neuromas [n = 11 (%)] | |
|---|---|---|---|---|
| Pain radiating to toes | 40 | 62 | 4 | 36 |
| Burning pain | 35 | 54 | 4 | 36 |
| Aching or sharp pain | 26 | 40 | 7 | 63 |
| Pain up foot or leg | 22 | 34 | 2 | 18 |
| Relief by removing shoe | 46 | 70 | 6 | 54 |
| Relief by rest | 58 | 89 | 11 | 100 |
| Cramping sensation | 22 | 34 | 0 | 0 |
| Pain increased with walking | 59 | 91 | 11 | 100 |
| Plantar pain | 50 | 77 | 11 | 100 |
| History of associated injuries | 10 | 15 | 1 | 9 |
| Numbness into toes or foot | 26 | 40 | 2 | 18 |

(From Mann and Reynolds,[83] with permission.)

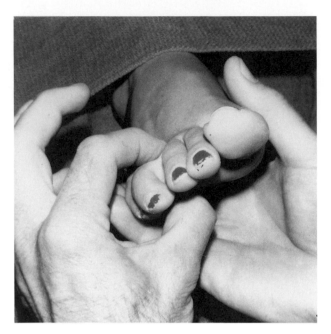

**Fig. 28-17.** The "lateral squeeze test" is positive when the maneuver reproduces pain symptoms.

ton's neuroma are not precise because of the difficulty in isolating a single interdigital nerve with an electrode to measure sensory conduction velocity.[63] However, in one such study the diagnosis was confirmed by electrophysiologic testing of five patients. Positive results were characterized by an "abnormal dip phenomenon," a relatively normal nerve conduction velocity, and normal duration of the sensory compound nerve action potential. These findings are the hallmarks of a neuropathy with predominantly axonal degeneration.[89]

The differential diagnosis of Morton's neuroma includes metatarsal stress fractures, tarsal tunnel syndrome, nerve root compression syndromes, metabolic peripheral neuropathy, localized vasculitis, ischemic pain, intermetatarsal bursitis, rheumatoid arthritis, and osteochondritis dissecans of metatarsal heads.

Weight-bearing radiographs should be taken to rule out other pathology. However, the neuroma itself is not visible on x-ray films or xeroradiographs. Morton's neuroma can be defined using MRI. Because this is a costly test, it should be ordered judiciously for difficult cases.[90] Neuromas have also been visualized in high-resolution ultrasound studies.[91]

## Conservative Management

Initial measures for treatment should be directed toward reducing or preventing irritation of the neuroma. Wider shoes with good arch support and adequate toe room provide the simplest approach. Avoiding high heels can be helpful but most patients have already discovered this. Toe crests sometimes provide relief. Metatarsal pads set at the proximal edges of metatarsal heads two, three, and four will help splay the bones and draw the weight proximally off the neuroma (Fig. 28-18). Several padding techniques have been described,[92–97] which can be com-

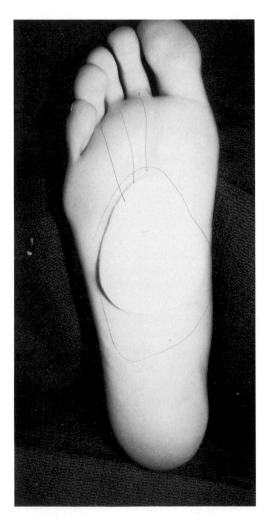

**Fig. 28-18.** Placement of a metatarsal pad to treat Morton's neuroma.

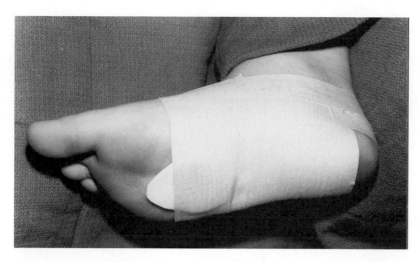

**Fig. 28-19.** Low-dye strapping with metatarsal pad to relieve metatarsalgia.

bined with a low-Dye strapping to add more support (Fig. 28-19). If pads and strappings are successful, then cast-fitted neutral position orthoses can be helpful. The goal is to limit pronation and hypermobility of the forefoot, both of which cause painful irritation of the neuroma.[98–101]

Using proper techniques, injection therapy can provide a measure of relief.[31] Vitamin B$_{12}$ or cyanocobalamin infiltration, advocated by one author,[102] resulted in some success although the relief may have been due to the sclerosing effects of the preserving agent, 1 percent benzoyl alcohol.

The use of a local anesthetic by itself acting as a nerve block is rarely therapeutic, but can give helpful diagnostic information. It is especially useful for differentiating more proximal neuropathies such as spinal radiculopathies.

Injection therapy has been described by several writers using various steroid preparations combined with local anesthetic agents.[103–105] Starting dorsally, infiltration should be directed between the metatarsal heads, injecting before and after penetration of the deep transverse intermetatarsal ligament, then distally into the sulcus area (Fig. 28-20). The patient should be cautioned that the symptoms may even get worse for 1 or 2 days before the desired effects are obtained. This so-called "steroid flare" is seen especially when less soluble steroid salts are utilized. Pain may also be accentuated if there is direct injury to the nerve tissue by the needle.

Finally, infiltration with a dilute 4 percent alcohol solution can be effective when the neuroma has a chronic history, using approximately 1 ml per infiltration to provide the necessary sclerosing effect. This solution is made by withdrawing 2 ml from a 50-ml vial of 2 percent lidocaine and replacing it with 2 ml alcohol USP (ethanol, ethyl alcohol). Care must be taken when increasing the percent alcohol strength because the infiltration of pure alcohol has led to disastrous results, including sloughing of the skin and intervening tissues.[106]

## Surgical Management

### Indications

When conservative measures fail and painful symptoms persist, surgical excision becomes the treatment of choice.[6,7,48,50,60,77,78,86,87,96,101,107–110] Although no well-controlled studies have been reported analyzing and comparing the conservative approaches to intermetatarsal neuromas, except for mixed results from injection therapy, it is the general experience that only 20 to 30 percent of symptomatic patients respond to nonoperative measures. Patients should be made aware of this early in their management program, because the majority will likely elect surgical resection for relief of their painful symptoms. Even with surgical intervention, however, as many as 24 percent of the patients will have unsatisfactory results.[81–84]

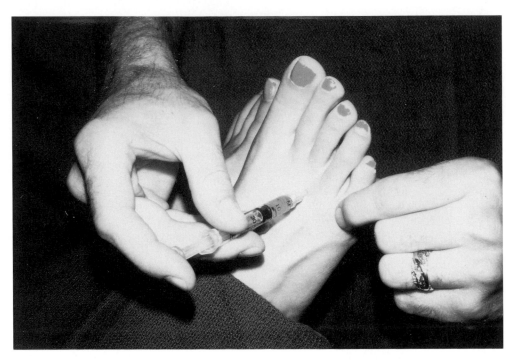

**Fig. 28-20.** Injection therapy for treatment of intermetatarsal neuroma.

Surgery is usually performed in an outpatient setting under general, regional, or local anesthesia. When excised under local anesthesia, field infiltration should be augmented with a posterior tibial nerve block to prevent the lancinating pain that can occur when the proximal nerve trunk is sharply severed.

Four approaches have been described for access to the intermetatarsal neuroma; plantar longitudinal,[76,77,87,111] plantar transverse,[55,111] web-splitting,[78,102] and dorsal[112,113] (Fig. 28-21): all have advantages and disadvantages. The two most frequently used techniques are described here.

### Plantar Approach

The second most common approach is via plantar longitudinal incision. This approach provides the best exposure to the neuroma and leaves the deep transverse intermetatarsal ligament intact. The disadvantage is the potential for a painful plantar scar on the weight-bearing surface. Prophylaxis against this includes careful placement of the incision between the metatarsal heads as well as 3 weeks of absolutely no weight-bearing postoperatively.[7] Excision via plantar approach has achieved a 93 percent success rate in one study.[114]

Once the plantar incision is made and hemostasis achieved, minimal dissection will expose the entire neuroma. Vascular structures are easily identified and preserved, and the deep transverse intermetatarsal ligament is left undisturbed because the neuroma lies plantar to it. The digital branches are isolated and clearly transected, followed by the proximal nerve trunk and, if present, accessory branches. Using vertical mattress sutures, deep closure is made with little or no dead space (Fig. 28-22).

### Dorsal Approach

The more common dorsal approach has the advantage of allowing early ambulation because the incision is on a non-weight-bearing surface (Fig. 28-23). There is some disadvantage in the initial awkwardness of dissecting deep between the metatarsal heads as well as having to severe the deep transverse intermetatarsal ligament. These tasks are facilitated with the use of the

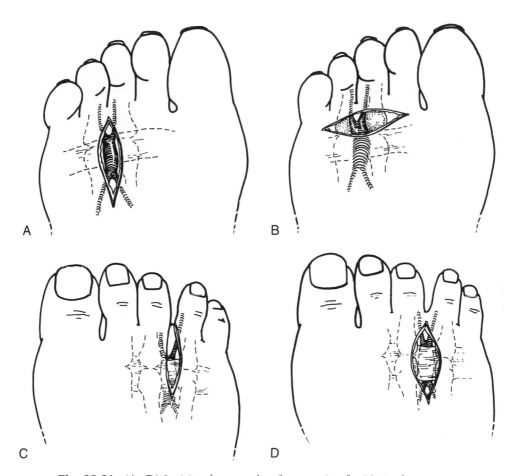

**Fig. 28-21.** (**A–D**) Incisional approaches for resection for Morton's neuroma.

Schink metatarsal spreader (Fig. 28-24). There is also greater potential for dead space.[7]

After the initial dorsal incision over the intermetatarsal space, blunt dissection is carried down to the deep transverse intermetatarsal ligament, which is sharply incised. The metatarsal spreader is inserted for maximum exposure. Gentle finger pressure on the plantar sulcus will deliver the fusiform neuroma into the wound so the digital branches can be isolated, clamped, and cut distally (Fig. 28-25). Vascular structures must be identified and divided for hemostasis only when necessary. The neuroma is then dissected as far proximal as possible, placed under tension, and cleanly transected along with any other communicating branches present (Fig. 28-26). Keeping the blade "coaxial" to the neuroma will help preserve local vas-

cular and tendon structures. Routine closure should include a large over-and-over suture through adjacent capsules to bring the metatarsal heads close together and allow healing of the deep transverse intermetatarsal ligament. A closed suction drain can be inserted if necessary.

### Deep Transverse Intermetatarsal Ligament

The role of the deep transverse intermetatarsal ligament has raised some interesting issues. Gauthier[82] achieved an 83 percent overall success rate by simply transecting the ligament (which he identified as plantar fascia) and then performing microscopic epineural neurolysis. Bradley et al.[81] achieved better results when the neurectomy was combined with percuta-

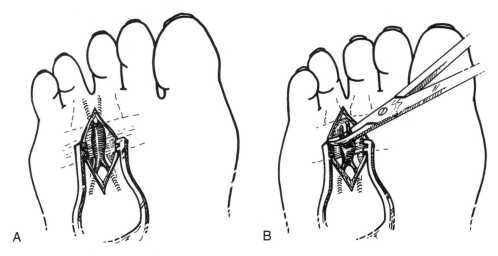

**Fig. 28-22.** Plantar approach for resection of Morton's neuroma.

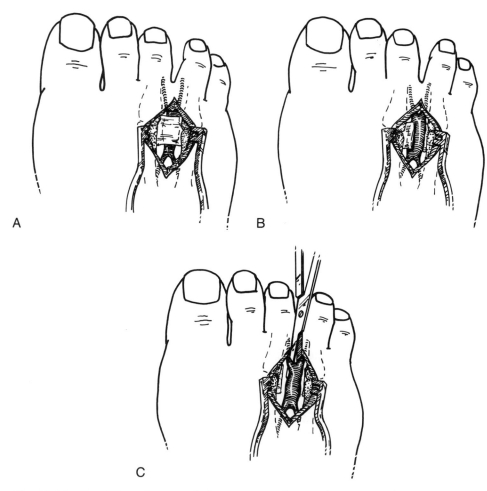

**Fig. 28-23.** (**A–C**) Dorsal approach for resection of Morton's neuroma. (*Figure continues.*)

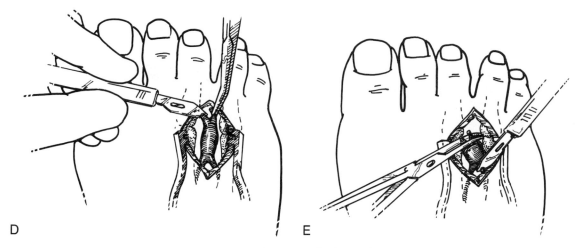

D                                                                E

**Fig. 28-23** (*Continued*). (**D & E**).

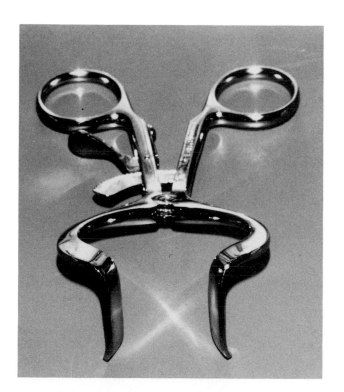

**Fig. 28-24.** Schink metatarsal spreader. Strong, thin blades allow ease of introduction into the surgical site to spread the metatarsal for less traumatic access to the proximal trunk for the neuromas. (Courtesy of Miltex Instrument Company, Inc., 6 Ohio Drive, Lake Success, NY, 11042; instrument number 40-1235.)

neous fasciotomy: 83 percent as compared to 66 percent without combining. Gudas and Mattana[84] reported good to excellent results in 79 percent of their series in which the neuromas were excised via dorsal approach leaving the said ligament intact.

It is important to preserve the function of the deep transverse ligament as it provides a fulcrum around which the lumbrical tendon stabilizes the lesser toes. When this tendon loses its functional ability, the affected lesser toe begins a dorsal contracture at the proximal phalanx until the extensor tendon and hood apparatus acquire function. The result is a full hammer toe deformity. Suturing the adjacent capsules will bring the metatarsal heads close enough for the ligament to heal. In reoperating on recurrent neuromas, Mann and Reynolds[83] noted complete reconstitution of the deep transverse intermetatarsal ligament that had been sectioned at the initial surgery.

## Adjacent Interspaces

Because neuromas can occur in adjacent intermetatarsal spaces, excision of both neuromas simultaneously adds to the risk of vascular embarrassment. Separate incisions should be kept as far apart as possible to avoid necrosis of the intervening skin. When using a single incision, the incorporation of curves will make allowance for scar contracture and help prevent digital

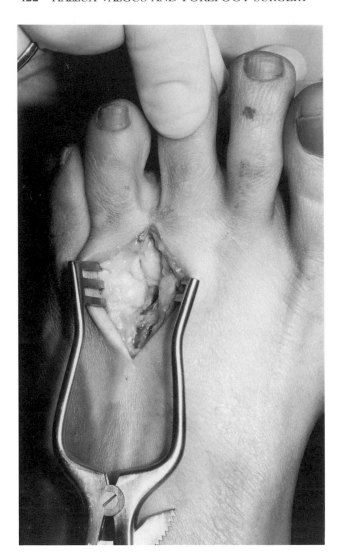

**Fig. 28-25.** Dissection for dorsal excision of Morton's neuroma.

## Surgical Complications

Whatever approach is made for intermetatarsal neuroma surgery, observance of several principles will minimize complications.[7] These include the following:

1. Gentle handling of tissues at all times.
2. Meticulous hemostasis. A cuff or tourniquet is not necessary.
3. Identification of the digital branches before completing the resection.
4. Removal of the neuroma without damaging the intermetatarsal artery or the local tendon from the lumbrical muscle.
5. Clean transection of the nerve trunk far enough proximally to prevent irritation or adhesions to the stump.
6. Intraneural injection of the proximal nerve trunk before transection, with one or two drops of steroid solution to impede scar adhesions and sensitive axon sprouts at the nerve end.

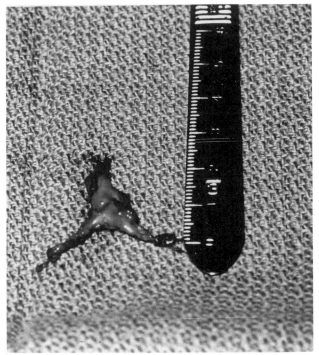

**Fig. 28-26.** Gross neuroma specimen exhibiting digital branches.

deformities. When a single incision is utilized, it is necessary to ensure dissection is carried down to a level below the subcutaneous tissue that contains the vascular structures before undermining into either intermetatarsal space. When circulation is identified as marginal, the more painful neuroma should be excised first and the adjacent intermetatarsal neuroma resected 1 to 2 months after the primary incision has healed.[7]

7. Closure of dead space as necessary. When this is not possible a closed suction drain should be inserted.
8. Use of a firm, even compression dressing, which is essential to help prevent postoperative hematoma formation.

*Hematoma* can form in the dead space following a neuroma resection as a result of blood and serum accumulation. Not only will this intensely prolong the initial inflammatory phase of healing, with added pain and frustration, but it is also an excellent medium for bacteria proliferation. Prophylactic antibiotics, expression of the hematoma, compression dressings, needle aspiration, and surgical removal of the clot are approaches to treatment.

*Vascular ischemia* of the toes results from interruption of arterial supply, vasospasm, and congestion from postoperative edema. Early recognition should lead to prompt treatment including the following: loosening of any tight dressings, removal of ice, reflex heat, sympathetic nerve blocks, reversal of epinephrine effects using local infiltration with phentolamine (Regitine), abstinence from caffeine and nicotine, and warming up the surrounding environment. In emergency situations, 5 to 10 mg of isoxuprine (Vasodilan) intramuscularly or 10 mg of nifedipine (Procardia) orally should stimulate effective vasodilation. Unchecked, a cyanotic toe can progress to frank gangrene with subsequent amputation.

The most troublesome complication probably is the painful *stump neuroma* or *recurrent neuroma* formation. Actually, a true bulbous stump neuroma is a rare finding at secondary operation. In most instances, recurrent neuromas presented with adhesions to the plantar joint capsule of a metatarsal head; the pain appeared to be the result of traction/impingement forces causing mechanosensitivity at the transected nerve ending.[83,115] The same authors[83] identified, in one-third of their reoperated cases, an accessory nerve trunk passing under the deep transverse intermetatarsal ligament. It appeared to have developed into a "recurrent neuroma," having been damaged at the time of the primary surgery.[69]

Recurrent neuroma is identified by sharp, often lancinating, or burning paresthesia aggravated by weight-bearing or point pressure and persisting well after

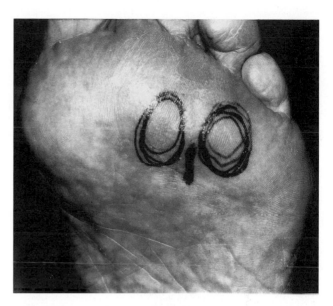

**Fig. 28-27.** Usual point of maximum tenderness following excision of Morton's neuroma.

local tissues have healed (Fig. 28-27), Symptoms can even be similar to those experienced before the initial surgery. Treatment is initially conservative using various padding and injection techniques. Triamcinolone acetonide infiltration is thought to soften the scar tissue adhering the nerve end to surrounding tissue, thus providing a measure of release.[116]

Surgical reentry must be via a plantar incision to provide good visualization plus access to the more proximal nerve trunks (Fig. 28-28). The goal is neurolysis to free the nerve plus a clean transection of the nerve more proximally with the nerve under tension. The end should then withdraw into the intrinsic muscle bellies away from weight-bearing areas for protection. Implementation of several prophylactic measures will help minimize further adhesions or stump neuroma formations. Intraneural steroid injection, 4 percent alcohol sclerosing solution, and a metal ligation clamp help discourage neurite formation.[7] Containment of the axon sprouts and protection against adhesions is the goal of silicone caps, which can be applied to the end of the nerve to isolate it.[117–119] Unfortunately, there are no good controlled studies to examine the efficacy of such treatment.

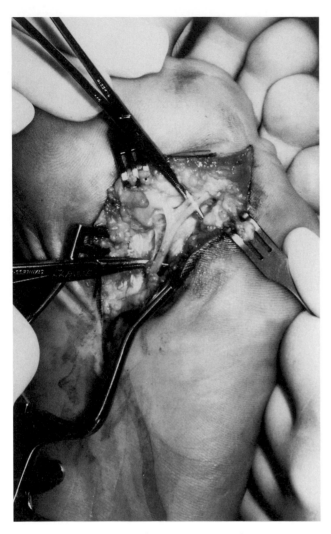

**Fig. 28-28.** Adherence of nerve stump to adjacent metatarsal head capsular tissue as seen on reentry (plantar approach).

## Results of Surgery

Several studies have shown that satisfactory results occur in an average of 84 percent of the patients who undergo neurectomy surgery[81–84,122] (Table 28-8). A good portion of these will still have some uncomfortable yet tolerable sensations lingering. Results are better when the third intermetatarsal space alone is involved and decrease dramatically when it is dissected bilaterally or when the second or others are involved.[84,122]

Beskin and Baxter[120] identified two clinical groups of patients who experience pain following neurectomy: those that remain symptomatic after neurectomy and those that recur after a period of quiescence. Identifying patients preoperatively who are at risk for recurrent neuroma formation is virtually impossible, although it is a goal worthy of pursuing.

Actually, what remains after neurectomy is a severed nerve, the same as when a limb is amputated. Spontaneous firing starts the day the nerve is cut and has two peaks of activity: the first occurs at about the third day and the second occurs within the third week.[123] For some people this is a much more sensitive phenomenon than for others, perhaps moderated or enhanced by neighboring sympathetic fibers.[124,125] Ectopic neural discharge can be suppressed by intraneural injection of corticosteroid preparations before severance of the nerve.[126]

As the end of the nerve degenerates, immature axon "sprouts" form. These can be quite sensitive, especially to mechanical pressure. The axons will extrude with unlimited growth potential seeking to connect with the distal axons. When blocked by local tissues or scar, the axons can convolute into a painful stump

Results of reoperation for intermetatarsal neuromas vary widely. Bradley and associates[81] found unsatisfactory results in four of five patients reexplored while Mann and Reynolds[83] reported significant improvement in nine of eleven patients (81 percent), and Beskin and Baxter[120] achieved 50 percent or greater improvement in 33 of 38 patients (87 percent). Nelms et al.[121] were able to obtain good to excellent results in 24 of 27 patients (89 percent) by tucking the nerve end into a drill hole in an adjacent metatarsal.

**Table 28-8.** Unsatisfactory Results of Neuroma Surgery

| Study | Percentage |
| --- | --- |
| Bradley et al. (1976)[86] | 13 (34.3) |
| Gauthier (1979)[82] | 17 |
| Mann and Reynolds (1983)[83] | 20 |
| Gudas and Mattana (1986)[84] | 21 |
| Karges (1988)[114] | 7 |
| Johnson (1989)[122] | 19 |
| Average | 16 |

neuroma. Simultaneously, the fibroblasts within the supporting perineurium and epineurium are forming scar tissue that can bind down the end of the nerve and place it under traction tension or compression.

In conclusion, excision of the intermetatarsal neuroma is a procedure not to be undertaken without a thorough patient workup and meticulous surgical technique. Honest patient rapport and responsible postoperative management will lead to a cooperative relationship when complications arise.

# REFERENCES

1. Dyck PJ: The causes, classification and treatment of peripheral neuropathy. New Engl J Med, 307:283, 1982
2. McQuarrie IG: Peripheral nerve surgery—today and looking ahead. Clin Plast Surg 13:255, 1986
3. Fisher GT, Boswick JA: Neuroma formation following digital amputations. J Trauma 23:136, 1983
4. Matthews GJ, Osterholm JL: Painful traumatic neuromas. Surg Clin N Am 51:1313, 1972
5. Durlacher L: A Treatise on Corns, Bunions, the Diseases of Nails and the General Management of the Feet. p. 52. Simkin, Marshall, London, 1845
6. Miller SJ: Surgical technique for resection of Morton's neuroma. J Am Podiatry Assoc 71:181, 1981
7. Miller SJ: Morton's neuroma: a syndrome. p. 38. In McGlamry ED, McGlamry R (eds): Textbook on Foot Surgery, Vol. 1. Williams & Wilkins, Baltimore, 1987
8. Kravette MA: Peripheral nerve entrapment syndromes in the foot. J Am Podiatry Assoc 61:457, 1971
9. Sarafian SK: Anatomy of the Foot and Ankle: Descriptive, Topographic and Functional, p. 317. JB Lippincott, Philadelphia, 1983
10. Millesi H, Terzis J: Nomenclature in peripheral nerve surgery. Committee report of the International Society of Reconstructive Microsurgery. Clin Plast Surg 11:3, 1984
11. Battista AF, Lusskin R: The anatomy and physiology of the peripheral nerve. Foot Ankle 7:65, 1986
12. Pollock LJ, Davis L: Peripheral Nerve Injuries, p. 484. Hoeber, New York, 1933
13. Keck C: The tarsal tunnel syndrome. J Bone Joint Surg Am 44:180, 1962
14. Lam SJS: The tarsal tunnel syndrome. J Bone Joint Surg Br 49:87, 1967
15. Edwards WG, Lincoln CR, Bassett FH, Goldner JL: The tarsal tunnel syndrome: diagnosis and treatment. JAMA 207:716, 1969
16. Havens RT, Kaloogian H, Thul JR, Hoffman S: A correlation between os trigonum syndrome and tarsal tunnel syndrome. J Am Podiatr Med Assoc 76:450, 1986
17. Goodman CR, Kehr LE: Bilateral tarsal tunnel syndrome: a correlative perspective. J Am Podiatr Med Assoc 78:292, 1988
18. Radin EL: Tarsal tunnel syndrome. Clin Orthop Relat Res 181:167, 1983
19. Mann RA: Tarsal tunnel syndrome. Orthop Clin N Am 5:109, 1974
20. Johnson EW, Ortiz PR: Electrodiagnosis of tarsal tunnel syndrome. Arch Phys Med 45:548, 1964
21. Gilliat RW, Wilson TG: A pneumatic tourniquet test in carpal tunnel syndrome. Lancet 2:595, 1953
22. Malay DS, McGlamry ED, Nava CA Jr: Entrapment neuropathies of the lower extremities. In Textbook on Foot Surgery, Vol. II, p. 668. Williams & Wilkins, Baltimore, 1987
23. Dellon AL, MacKinon SE: Tibial nerve branching in the tarsal tunnel. Arch Neurol 41:645, 1984
24. Przylucki H, Jones CL: Entrapment neuropathy of muscle branch of lateral plantar nerve: a cause of heel pain. J Am Podiatry Assoc 71:119, 1981
25. Henricson AS, Westlin NE: Chronic calcaneal pain in atheletes: entrapment of the calcaneal nerve. Am J Sports Med 12:152, 1984
26. Baxter DE, Thigpen CM: Heel pain—operative results. Foot Ankle 5:16, 1984
27. Havel PE, Ebraheim NA, Clark SE, Jackson WT, DiDio L: Tibial branching in the tarsal tunnel. Foot Ankle 9:117, 1988
28. Kopel HP, Thompson AL: Peripheral entrapment neuropathy of the lower extremity. N Engl J Med 262:56, 1960
29. Rask ME: Medial plantar neuroparaxia (jogger's foot): report of three cases. Clin Orthop 154:193, 1978
30. Kenzora JE: Symptomatic incisional neuromas on the dorsum of the foot. Foot Ankle 5:2, 1984
31. Dockery GL, Nilson RV: Intralesional injections. Clin Podiatr Med Surg 3:473, 1986
32. Edwards WG, Lincoln CR, Bassett FH, Goldner JL: The tarsal tunnel syndrome: diagnosis and treatment. JAMA 207:716, 1969
33. Kenzora JE: Sensory nerve neuromas—leading to failed foot surgery. Foot Ankle 7:110, 1986
34. Meals RA: Peroneal nerve palsy complicating ankle sprain. J Bone Joint Surg Am 59:966, 1977
35. Vasamaki M: Decompression for peroneal nerve entrapment. Acta Orthop Scand 57:551, 1986

36. Lemont H, Hernandez A: Recalcitrant pain syndromes of the foot and ankle: evaluation of the lateral dorsal cutaneous nerve. J Am Podiatry Assoc 62:331, 1972
37. Krause KH, Witt T, Ross A: Anterior tarsal tunnel syndrome. J Neurol 217:67, 1977
38. Borges LF, Hallett M, Selkoe DJ, Welch K: The anterior tarsal tunnel syndrome. Report of two cases. J Neurosurg 54:89, 1981
39. Gessini L, Jandolo B, Pietrangeli A: The anterior tarsal syndrome: Report of four cases. J Bone Joint Surg Am 66:786, 1984
40. Adelman KA, Wilson G, Wolf JA: Anterior tarsal tunnel syndrome. J Foot Surg 27:299, 1988
41. Dellon AL: Deep peroneal nerve entrapment on the dorsum of the foot. Foot Ankle 11:73, 1990
42. Joplin RJ: The proper digital nerve, vitallium stem arthroplasty, and some thoughts about foot surgery in general. Clin Orthop Relat Res 76:199, 1971
43. Merritt GN, Subotnick SI: Medial plantar digital proper nerve syndrome (Joplin's neuroma): typical presentation. J Foot Surg 21:166, 1982
44. Lee B, Crowhurst JA: Entrapment neuropathy of the first metatarsophalangeal joint: two case reports. J Am Podiatr Med Assoc 77:657, 1987
45. Thul JR, Hoffman SJ: Neuromas associated with tailor's bunion. J Foot Surg 24:342, 1985
46. Addante JB, Peicott PS, Wong KY, Brooks DL: Interdigital neuromas: results of surgical excision of 152 neuromas. J Am Podiatric Med Assoc, 76:493, 1986
47. Reed RJ, Bliss BO: Morton's neuroma: Regressive and productive intermetatarsal elastofibrositis. Arch Pathol, 95:123, 1973
48. Sheperd E: Intermetatarsophalangeal bursitis in the causation of Morton's metatarsalgia. J Bone Joint Surg Br 57:115, 1975
49. Bossley CJ, Cairney PC: The metatarsophalangeal bursa—its significance in Morton's metatarsalgia. J Bone Joint Surg Br 62:184, 1980
50. Burns AE, Stewart WP: Morton's neuroma, J Am Podiatry Assoc 72:135, 1982
51. Goldman F, Gardner, R: Pacinian corpuscles as a cause for metatarsalgia. J Am Podiatry Assoc 70:561, 1980
52. Ochoa J: The primary nerve fibrepathology of plantar neuromas. J Neuropathol Exp Neurol 35:370, 1976
53. Goldman F: Intermetatarsal neuroma: Light microscopic observations. J Am Podiatry Assoc 69:317, 1979
54. King LS: Note on the pathology of Morton's metatarsalgia. Am J Clin Pathol 16:124, 1946
55. Nissen KI: Plantar digital neuritis. J Bone Joint Surg Br 30:84, 1948
56. Scott TM: The lesion of Morton's metatarsalgia (Morton's toe). Arch Pathol 63:91, 1957
57. Lassmann G, Machacek J: Clinical features and histology of Morton's metatarsalgia. Wien Klin Wochenschr 81:55, 1969
58. Meachim G, Aberton JJ: Histological findings in Morton's metatarsalgia. J Pathol 103:209, 1971
59. Lassmann G, Lassmann H, Stockinger L: Morton's metatarsalgia. Light and electron microscopic observations and their relation to entrapment neuropathies. Virchows Arch Pathol Anat 370:307, 1976
60. Lassmann G: Morton's toe: clinical, light, and electron microscopic investigations in 133 cases. Clin Orthop 142:73, 1979
61. Goldman F: Intermetatarsal neuromas—light and electron microscopic observations. J Am Podiatry Assoc 70:265, 1980
62. Ringzertz N, Unander-Scharin ML: Morton's disease: a clinical and patho-anatomical study. Acta Orhtop Scand 19:327, 1950
63. Guiloff RJ, Scadding JW, Klenerman L: Morton's metatarsalgia: clinical, electrophysiological, and histological observations. J Bone Joint Surg Br 66:586, 1984
64. Graham CE, Graham DM: Morton's neuromas: a microscopic evaluation. Foot Ankle 5:150, 1984
65. Tate RO, Rusin JJ: Morton's neuroma: its ultrastructural anatomy and biomechanical etiology. J Am Podiatry Assoc 68:797, 1978
66. Baker LD, Kuhn MH: Morton's metatarsalgia: localized degenerative fibrosis with neuromatous proliferation of the fourth plantar nerve. South Med J 37:123, 1944
67. Hauser EDW: Neurofibroma of the foot. JAMA 121:1217, 1943
68. Viladot A, Moragas A: Entermedad de Morton. Podologica 5:233, 1966
69. Alexander IJ, Johnson KA, Parr JW: Morton's neuroma: a review of recent concepts. Orthopedics 10:103, 1987
70. Gilbey VP: The non-operative treatment of metatarsalgia. J New Ment Health Dis 19:589, 1894
71. Pincus A: Intractable Morton's toe (neuroma). Review of the literature and report of cases. J Am Podiatry Assoc 40:19, 1950
72. Bartolomei FJ, Wertheimer SJ: Intermetatarsal neuromas: distribution and etiologic factors. J Foot Surg 22:279, 1983
73. Carrier PA, et al: Morton's neuroma: a possible contributing etiology. J Am Podiatry Assoc 65:315, 1975
74. Sgarlato TE: Compendium of Podiatric Biomechanics. California College of Podiatric Medicine, San Francisco, 1971
75. Root ML, Orien WF, Weed JM: Normal and abnormal function of the foot. In Clinical Biomechanics, Vol. 2, pp. 112, 296, 322. Clinical Biomechanics Corp., Los Angeles, 1977

76. Bickel VH, Dockerty MB: Plantar neuromas, Morton's toe. Surg Gynecol Obstet 84:111, 1947

77. Betts LO: Morton's metatarsalgia. Med J Aust 1:514, 1940

78. McElvenny RT: The etiology and surgical treatment of intractable pain about the fourth metatarsophalangeal joint (Morton's toe). J Bone Joint Surg 25:675, 1943

79. Denny-Brown D, Doherty MM: Effects of transient stretching of peripheral nerve. Arch Neurol Psychol 54:116, 1945

80. Wachter S, Nilson RZ, Thul JR: The relationship between foot structure and intermetatarsal neuromas. J Foot Surg 23:436, 1984

81. Bradley N, Miller WA, Evans JP: Plantar neuroma: analysis of results following surgical excision in 145 patients. South Med J 69:853, 1976

82. Gauthier G: Thomas Morton's disease: a nerve entrapment syndrome. A new surgical technique. Clin Orthop Relal Res 142:90, 1979

83. Mann RA, Reynolds JC: Interdigital neuroma—a critical analysis. Foot Ankle 3:248, 1983

84. Gudas CJ, Mattana GM: Retrospective analysis of intermetatarsal neuroma excision with preservation of the transverse metatarsal ligament. J Am Podiatr Med Assoc, 25:459, 1986

85. Addante JB, Peicott PS, Wong KY, Broods DL: Interdigital neuromas: results of surgical excision of 152 neuromas. J Am Podiatry Assoc 52:746, 1962

86. Pincus A: The syndrome of plantar metatarsal neuritis. J Am Podiatry Assoc 52:746, 1962

87. Mulder JD: The causative mechanism in Morton's metatarsalgia. J Bone Joint Surg 33B:94, 1951

88. Berlin SJ, Donick I, Block LD, Costa AL: Nerve tumors of the foot: diagnosis and treatment. J Am Podiatry Assoc 65:157, 1975

89. Oh SJ, Kim HS, Ahmed BK: Electrophysiological diagnosis of interdigital neuropathy of the foot. Muscle Nerve 7:218, 1984

90. Sartoris DJ, Brozinsky S, Resnick D: Magnetic resonance images. J Foot Surg 28:78, 1989

91. Redd PA, Peters VJ, Emery SP, Bunch HM, Rifkin MD: Morton neuroma: sonographic evaluation. Radiology 171:415, 1989

92. Schreiber LJ: Method of padding for Morton's neuralgia. J Am Podiatry Assoc 29:5, 1939

93. Polokoff MM: The treatment of Morton's metatarsalgia. J Am Podiatry Assoc 38:27, 1948

94. Brohner MD: Morton's toe or Morton's neuralgia. J Am Podiatry Assoc 39:18, 1969

95. Silvermann LJ: Old principles and new ideas. J Am Podiatry Assoc 31:7, 1941

96. Milgram JE: Morton's neuritis and management of post-neurectomy pain. p. 203. In Omer GE, Spinner M (eds): Management of Peripheral Nerve Problems. WB Saunders, Philadelphia, 1980

97. Milgram JE: Office methods for the relief of the painful foot. J Bone Joint Surg Am 49:1099, 1964

98. Withman R: Anterior metatarsalgia. Trans Am Orthop Assoc 11:34, 1898

99. Hohmann G: Uber die Mortonsche neuralgie am fuss Bietrage. Orthopade 13:649, 1966

100. Silverman LJ: Morton's toe or Morton's neuralgia. J Am Podiatry Assoc 66:749, 1976

101. Milgram JE: Design and use of pads and strappings for office relief of the painful foot. p. 95. In Kiene RH, Johnson KA (eds): Symposium on the Foot and Ankle. CV Mosby, St. Louis, 1983

102. Steinberg MD: The use of vitamin B-12 in Morton's neuralgia. J Am Podiatry Assoc 45:41, 1955

103. Wright EW: Injection therapy in Morton's neuralgia. J Am Podiatry Assoc 45:566, 1955

104. Cozen L: Neuroma of plantar digital nerve. p. 224. In Clinical Orthopedics, Vol. 2. JB Lippincott, Philadelphia, 1958

105. Greenfield J, Rea J, Ilfeld FW: Morton's interdigital neuroma: indications for treatment by local injections versus surgery. Clin Orthop Relat Res 185:142, 1985

106. Lapidus PW, Wilson MJ: Morton's metatarsalgia. Bull NY Med Coll 12:34, 1969

107. Giannestras NJ: Foot Disorders, Medical and Surgical Management, p. 494. Lea & Febiger, Philadelphia, 1967

108. May VR Jr: The enigma of Morton's neuroma. p. 222. In Bateman JE (ed): Foot Science. WB Saunders, Philadelphia, 1976

109. Joplin RJ: Some common foot disorders amenable to surgery. AAOS Instructional Course Lectures 15:144, 1958

110. Kelikian H: Hallux Valgus, Allied Deformities of the Forefoot, Metatarsalgia, p. 359. WB Saunders, Philadelphia, 1965

111. Kaplan EB: Surgical approach to the plantar digital nerves. Bull Hosp Joint Dis Orthop Inst, 1:96, 1950

112. McKeever DC: Surgical approach for neuroma of plantar digital nerve (Morton's metatarsalgia). J Bone Joint Surg 34A:490, 1952

113. Kitting RW, McGlamry ED: Removal of an intermetatarsal neuroma. J Am Podiatry Assoc 63:274, 1973

114. Karges DE: Plantar excision of primary interdigital neuromas. Foot Ankle 9:120, 1988

115. Nelms BA, Bishop JO, Tullos HS: Surgical treatment of recurrent Morton's neuroma. Orthopedics 7:1708, 1984

116. Smith JR, Gomez NH: Local injection therapy of neuro-mata of the hand with triamcinalone acetonide. J Bone Joint Surg 52:71, 1970

117. Swanson AB, Boeve NR, Lumsden RM: The prevention and treatment of amputation neuromata by silicone capping. J Hand Surg 2:70, 1977

118. Burke BR: A preliminary report in the use of silastic nerve caps in conjunction with neuroma surgery. J Foot Surg 17:53, 1978

119. Midenberg ML, Kirshcenbaum SE: Utilization of silastic nerve caps in conjunction with neuroma surgery. J Foot Surg 17:53, 1978

120. Beskin JL, Baxter DE: Recurrent pain following inter-digital neurectomy—a plantar approach. Foot Ankle 9:34, 1988

121. Nelms BA, Bishop JO, Tullos HS: Surgical treatment of recurrent Morton's neuroma. Orthaopedics 7:1708, 1984

122. Johnson KA: Surgery of the Foot and Ankle, p. 69. Raven Press, New York, 1989

123. Scadding JW: Development of ongoing activity, me-chanosensitivity, and adrenaline sensitivity in severed peripheral nerve axons. Exp Neurol 73:345, 1981

124. Devor M, Janig W: Activation of myelinated afferents ending in a neuroma by stimulation of the sympathetic supply in the rat. Neurosci Lett 24:43, 1981

125. Wall PD, Gutnick M: Ongoing activity in peripheral nerves: the physiology and pharmacology of impulses originating from a neuroma. Exp Neurol 43:580, 1974

126. Devor M, Govrin-Lippmann R, Raber P: Corticosteroids suppress ectopic neural discharge originating in ex-perimental neuromas. Pain 22:127, 1985

# 29

# Metatarsalgia and Lesser Metatarsal Surgery

## VINCENT J. HETHERINGTON

Metatarsalgia is defined as pain localized to the forepart of the foot. Although the definition is simple enough, it describes only a symptom: metatarsalgia can be a complex clinical problem. Pain under the metatarsals may be a reflection of systemic disease, a result of biomechanical imbalances, or local foot pathology.

## CLASSIFICATION

Several authors have attempted to classify metatarsalgia. Helal[1] classified metatarsalgia into primary, secondary, and unrelated to weight distribution. Primary metatarsalgia is defined as pain across the area of the metatarsophalangeal joints associated with plantar keratoses. It may be a result of functional problems such as wearing a high-heeled shoe or structural problems associated with, for example, a short first metatarsal, limb length discrepancies, or pes cavus. Also included by Helal as primary metatarsalgia were Freiberg's disease, hallux valgus, hallux rigidus, and problems of iatrogenic and traumatic origin. Secondary metatarsalgia was caused by systemic disease such as rheumatoid arthritis. Metatarsalgias attributed to tarsal tunnel and vascular insufficiency are those types of metatarsalgia unrelated to load distribution.

Regnauld[2] defined metatarsalgia into diffuse, localized, subcutaneous soft tissue, and cutaneous metatarsalgia. Diffuse metatarsalgia is an example of an acquired mechanical disorder, such as functional disorders, abnormalities of the ankle such as ankle equinus, overload of the metatarsals, and metatarsalgia

from high-heeled shoes. Localized metatarsalgia results from an osseous disorder such as a long metatarsal, large metatarsal, or aplasia of a metatarsal. Subcutaneous soft metatarsalgia includes pain from intermetatarsal neuroma, articular synovial cysts, and bursa. Cutaneous metatarsalgia is a result of plantar calluses, verruca, or ulcerations of the skin Viladot[3] describes metatarsalgia in two categories: first, overload of anterior support as a result of high-heeled shoes, an equinus or cavus foot in which support is by the heel, and the metatarsal heads only, resulting in subluxation of the toes, a change in load, and change in cadence of gait. The second aspect of this classification is irregular distribution of mechanical load, as evidenced by the following symptoms:

First-ray insufficiency syndrome, examples of which are a short first metatarsal and hypermobility of the first ray. It may also be result iatrogenically following ostotomy of the metatarsal or Keller resection.

First-ray overload syndrome, which may be a result of chronic overload, plantar flexion of the first metatarsal, an index plus, or excessively long first metatarsal or first ray.

Central ray insufficiency syndrome, which may arise from congenital, iatrogenic, or neurogenic causes.

Central ray overload syndrome, attributed to long metatarsal or plantar-flexed metatarsals.

Scranton[4] described metatarsalgia as primary, secondary, and pain under the forepart of the foot. Primary metatarsalgia included hallux rigidus, a long first ray, Freiberg's disease, hallux valgus, and postsurgical

429

deformities. Secondary metatarsalgia was attributed to rheumatoid arthritis, neurogenic disorders, gout, limb length discrepancies, stress fractures, and sesamoditis. Pain under the forefoot included diagnosis of Morton's neuroma, plantar fascitis tarsal tunnel syndrome, tumors, Friberg's disease and plantar warts.

It is readily apparent that it is difficult to classify metatarsalgia; however, certain themes run through these classifications. These include evidence of systemic involvement, metatarsalgia as result of disturbances within the foot itself or of the biomechanics and function of the foot, and those unrelated to problems in weight-bearing.

# ETIOLOGY

Complaints of pain and parasthesias in the forefoot may also accompany neurologic processes such as nerve impingement syndromes, low back problems, and peripheral neuropathy. Peripheral neuropathy may be associated with diabetes and other systemic diseases. Dyck[5] has reported that burning in the forefoot may be one of the first signs indicating peripheral neuropathy. Rheumatoid arthritis is another form of systemic disease that results in painful disturbances of the forefoot. Metatarsalgia may also occur as a result of vascular insufficiency.

Metatarsalgia may be result from cutaneous soft tissue and osseous pathology. Cutaneous causes of metatarsalgia include plantar hyperkeratoses, inclusion cysts, foreign-body reactions, porokeratosis, and plantar verruca. Manifestations of inherited palmar plantar diskeratoses should also be considered in the differential diagnosis of metatarsalgia associated with plantar lesions. Plantar hyperkeratotic lesions presents with a varied clinical picture (Fig. 29-1). They may be diffuse in nature, involving an area plantar to several metatarsal heads, or they may be isolated under discrete metatarsal heads or appear as punctuate-type keratotic lesions.

Subotnik[6] described two types of plantar calluses, one caused by friction and other caused by shearing forces. Frictional calluses are superficial and nonnucleated. It was theorized that they occur as a superficial portion of the skin moves along with the metatarsal heads against a resistant force. Frictional keratosis may surround the localized shearing lesion. This type

of callus may be more ameanable to biomechanical or orthotic treatment. Shearing calluses on the other hand are a result of the skin being stabilized with the supporting surface and the metatarsal heads moving such that shear occurs within the soft tissues on the weight-bearing surface of the foot. Shearing results in fibrosis and scarring of the soft tissues and causes more symptoms than the frictional callus. These types of lesions are believed to result from a structural component to the deformity and may benefit from surgical intervention. Several types of shearing calluses were identified, including the following[6]:

Superficial shearing callus
Superficial fibrous shearing callus
Nucleated shearing callus
Fibrous nucleated callus
Multinucleated fiberous shearing callus
Neurovascular fiber shearing callus.

The degree of fibrous scarring, as well as the prognosis, worsens as one moves from the superficial shearing callus to the fibrous nucleated callus. In the superficial shearing callus there may be a small shallow hyperkeratitic nucleus with a surrounding frictional-type callus. As the condition worsens with the fibrous nucleated shearing callus, a deep fibrous base is present that is easily and well differentiated from the surrounding margins. The multinucleated fibrous shearing callus and the neurovascular shearing callus are uncommon. The neurovascular shearing callus with its extended neurovascular filaments may be confused with a plantar verruca. However, the lesion is extremely painful, which helps distinguish it from that of the plantar verruca.

In evaluations of patients with plantar hyperkeratosis, the existence of an inherited palmer and plantar diskeratosis should be kept in mind. Examples of such conditions are keratosis punctata[7] and Unna-Thost[8]-type palmer plantar keratoderma. Mechanically induced plantar hyperkeratotic lesions can be distinguished histologically from nonmechanical keratoses. As pointed out by Lemont,[9] pressure-induced histologic changes are not limited to the epidermis but involve the dermas and fatty tissue as well. In contrast, nonmechanical keratoses, even if located on weight-bearing surfaces, usually do not exhibit epidermal, dermal, or fat changes seen in those with mechanical

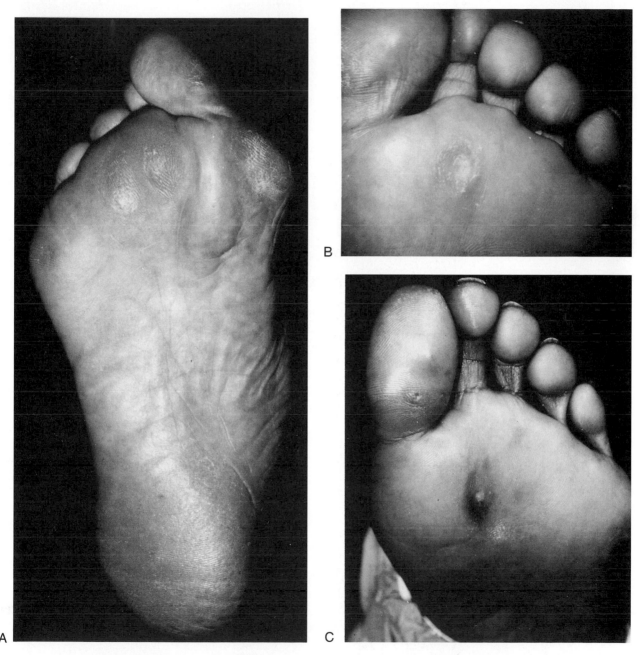

**Fig. 29-1.** Examples of plantar keratotic lesions. (**A**) Frictional hyperkeratosis in a patient with multiple digital contractions and hallux valgus plantar and dorsal view (flat triangular forefoot syndrome). (**B**) Nucleated plantar keratosis. (**C**) Porokeratosis plantaris discreta diagnosis (confirmed by biopsy). (*Figure continues.*)

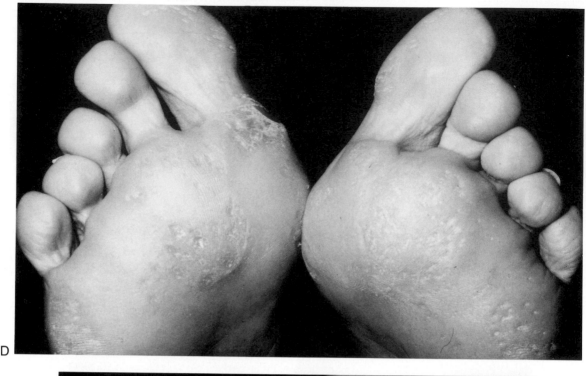

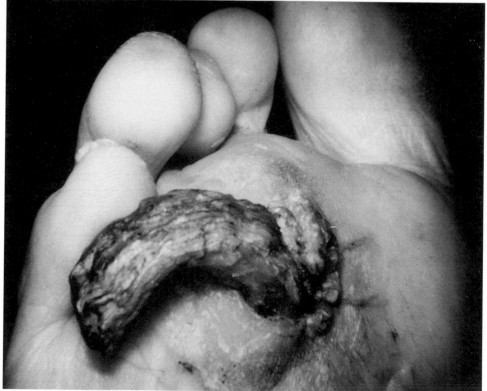

**Fig. 29-1** (*Continued*). (**D**) Plantar lesions in a patient with an inherited palmar-plantar dyskeratosis. (**E**) An atypical presentation of a plantar wart (confirmed by biopsy) in an older patient with neglected general health and foot care.

causes. The characteristic features in nonmechanically induced keratosis of the sole include a thick stratum cornium with a normal underlying stratum malpighii. The dermis also remains normal.

Foreign-body reactions may also demonstrate small hyperkeratotic lesions as part of the clinical reaction. Inclusion cysts or epidermal inclusion cysts[10] may also be a cause of metatarsalgia. They can usually be palpated as cystic lesions and may have an overlying hyperkeratosis dependent on the location of the lesion itself. Another keratotic lesion, originally described by Taub and Steinberg,[11,12] is the porokeratosis plantaris discreta, which has come under some challenge as to whether it exists as a lesion discrete from other mechanically induced keratoses.[13] The term porokeratosis plantaris discreta was originally used to described a plugged sweat duct. The lesion is clinically described as a sharply marginated, cone-shaped, wide-based callus surface of a rubbery consistency. The keratotic plug is easily separated by blunt dissection, and an opaque material may be obtained.[12]

The verruca plantaris or plantar wart is a viral-induced lesion that has a tendency to occur in the nonmechanical portions or areas of the foot. The lesion is caused by the human papova virus. Single or multiple lesions may appear on the plantar surface of the foot as well-delineated, circumscribed lesions that are most painful on palpation by lateral pressure. The overlying hyperkeratotic tissue may be hard; it gives way to the softer verrucous tissue. The lesions are characterized by pinpoint bleeding. A plantar verruca on an area of the foot other than the plantar surface may not be associated with an overlying keratosis. As mentioned previously, verruca may occur singly, in small groups, or in a mosaic lesion pattern.

There is a wide variety of treatment for warts, including applications of liquid nitrogen, electrodesiccation and curretage, topical acid preparations, and the carbon dioxide laser.[14] Surgical excision may also be performed. The depth of the excision has been reported to be to the level of the dermoepidermal junction or as recommended by Lemont and Parekh[15] to the level of the superficial fascia.

Other soft tissue lesions contributing to the development of the metatarsalgia may include the intermetatarsal neuroma, intermetatarsal bursitis,[16] and degeneration of the accessory plantar ligament.[17] Displacement of the plantar fat pad, as reported by

Hlavac and Schoenhaus,[18] is associated with digital deformities. Atrophy of the plantar fat pad, which may result after trauma, surgical intervention, or with the natural aging process, may also result in a painful metatarsalgia. Wasting or atrophy of the plantar fat pad interferes with the ability of the foot to absorb shock and dissipate heat, resulting in these energies being transferred to the underlying osseous structures. Treatment of this type of metatarsalgia is best handled by the use of a orthotic device to augment and replace the loss of the dysfunctional area of the skin.

Plantar calluses, especially those of the shearing type, may occur with either structural or mechanical problems in foot functions. Structural considerations for isolated plantar lesions have been divided into stance-phase and propulsive-phase lesions. These for the most part have been described as follows: stance-phase lesions are related to patient history as being lesions more painful with prolonged standing, as opposed to the propulsive-phase lesions, which the patient may complain cause more pain with active ambulation.

The stance-phase lesion is believed to be caused by a structurally plantar-flexed metatarsal. These may be detected on clinical examination by palpation of the relative position of one metatarsal head to the other while the foot is held in neutral position, and may be identified in axial radiography of the forefoot. The lesion is palpated and observed to be present directly beneath the head of the metatarsal. An elevating osteotomy is the treatment of choice for this type of lesion. The propulsive-phase lesions are clinically located distal to the metatarsal head, and an abnormality in the length of one or more metatarsals may be seen in the dorsoplantar view. This is essentially a focal abnormality of the metatarsal parabola. Other causes of isolated plantar lesions may be an (a) enlarged metatarsal heads, as a result of trauma or degenerative changes, or (b) as secondary to the retrograde instability of the metatarsophalangeal joint associated with a hammer toe or other digital deformity (Figs. 29-2 and 29-3). Variation and alteration in the location and severity of clinical lesions may result from differences in the relative motion of the lesser metatarsals. The degree of mobility available to the second and third metatarsals is limited and increases for the fourth, fifth, and first metatarsals. The degree of mobility may allow the more mobile elements to avoid participation in load-

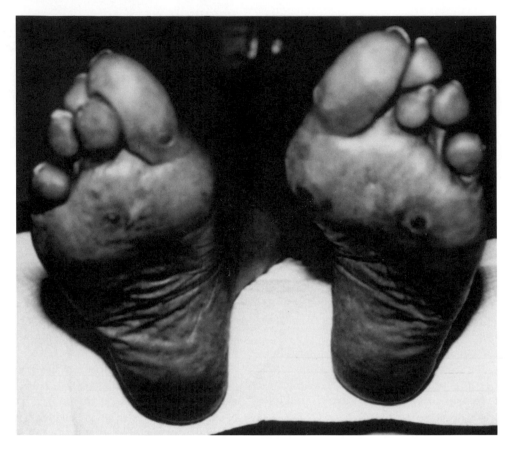

**Fig. 29-2.** A patient with multiple painful plantar lesion resulting from pes planus, hypermobility of the first ray, and multiple digital deformities.

bearing, increasing the load on the less mobile metatarsal. Pressure over time (duration) may be as important as direct vertical load in the development and clinical symptomatology of plantar lesions.

Metatarsalgia may be associated with localized arthritic problems such as degenerative joint disease and Freiberg's disease (Fig. 29-4), which is discussed in a separate chapter. The sesamoids of the forefoot may also be actively involved in a patient with metatarsalgia and this is also addressed separately. Metatarsal stress fractures are a cause of metatarsalgia; pain can be repetitively elicited by a palpation of the metatarsal shaft. Initially no radiographic changes may be found; however, radiographic follow-up will reveal the development of a periosteal callus.

Compensation for functional or biomechanical disorders of the foot may also lead to the development of plantar lesions. These plantar lesions results from alterations in the mechanical function of the foot and interfere with its ability to distribute the loads placed on it by the mechanics of walking. These are illustrated by the development of the sub-second-metatarsal lesions seen with hypermobility of the first metatarsal that result in hallux valgus, hallux rigidus and digital deformity. Digital deformity such as hammer and claw toe deformities are a principal cause of painful plantar lesions. These dynamically produced deformities cause retrograde instability of the metatarsophalangeal joint, which results in an inability to distribute the forces in gait effectively, producing areas of overload culminating in a painful plantar lesion. The role that digital deformities play in the etiology of painful plantar lesions should not be underestimated. The assessment and management of digital deformity is discussed in Chapter 26.

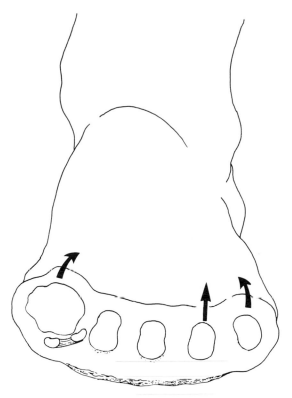

**Fig. 29-3.** Diagram illustrating the potential for overload of the second and third metatarsals resulting from excessive pronation, causing hypermobility of the first ray and, as a result of increased mobility at the metatarsal-cuboid articulation, loss of participation by the fourth and fifth metatarsals in distribution of forefoot load.

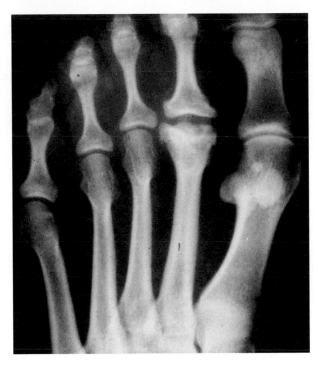

**Fig. 29-4.** Freiberg's disease of the second metatarsal.

Another osseous problem in metatarsalgia is abnormalities of the metatarsal parabola, which may be reflected as a long first metatarsal, short first metatarsal, and insufficiency of the central metatarsals or brachymetatarsia. These types of deformity may have a congenital, acquired, or iatrogenic basis. A normal metatarsal parabola has been defined by the formula of $1 < 2 > 3 > 4 > 5$; various abnormalities in the length pattern of the metatarsals can be described according to Whitney[19] (Fig. 29-5) as follows.

A short first metatarsal segment, at times referred to as Morton's syndrome, by itself, as reported by Whitney,[19] may not represent a potential first-ray insufficiency but when combined with other defects and pronatory stresses must be regarded as significant (Fig. 29-5B). The short great toe mentioned previously as part of insufficiency of the first ray results in an improper distribution of the weight load of the first ray, allowing a displacement of the vertical component of force more laterally and causing greater load to be borne underneath the lesser metatarsals. It is important to note that insufficiency of the first ray may be acquired as in an iatrogenically short first metatarsal or from procedures involving resection of the base of the proximal phalanx. In high-heeled shoes, the abnormally short first metatarsal leads to an adjacent metatarsal overload.

A long third ray may lead to overload of that metatarsal (Fig. 29-5C). A long first segment or a long first ray (Fig. 29-5D) leads to direct trauma of the hallux, dynamic functional overload of the first metatarsophalangeal joint leading into hallux rigidus. Brachymetatarsia, more commonly of the fourth metatarsal, may involved any of the central metatarsals. Brachymetatarsia (Fig. 29-5 E and F) may have either a congenital, acquired, or iatrogenic basis.

A recent concept in the function and alignment of the forefoot and their relationship to metatarsalgia is that of the forefoot syndromes. Regnauld[2] describes the central metatarsals as a functional unit. He further

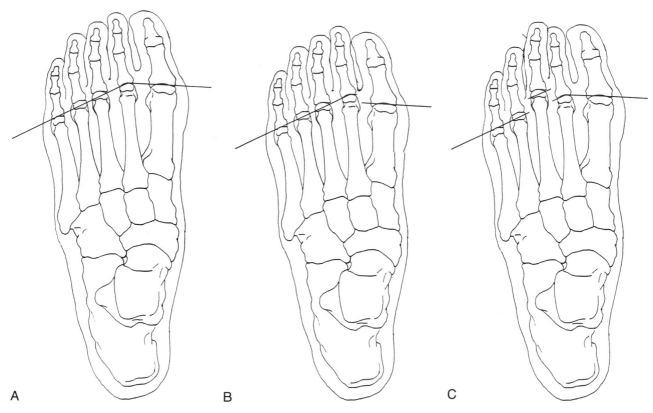

**Fig. 29-5.** (**A**) Normal metatarsal alignment (parabola). (**B**) Short first segment. (**C**) Long third metatarsal. (*Figure continues.*)

states that any "disadvantageous configuration" in the alignment of the metatarsal heads cannot be compensated for by a intrinsic or extrinsic muscular control. Conversely, however, activity of plantar flexors especially of the first and fifth rays result in a cavus foot and weakness of these plantar flexors causes central metatarsal overload. Inability of the first and fifth rays to compensate for forefoot loading, may be regarded as the main influence in protecting the weight-bearing function of the ball of the foot.[2] Failure of this mechanism is an important cause of painful syndromes of the forefoot (Fig. 29-6). The anterior or frontal plane configuration of the Lisfranc's joint is influenced by the load generated by body weight acting through the talus. This is reflected by a change in the convexity of Lisfranc's joint that controls the relative position of the metatarsals and results in four forefoot syndromes:

1. The flat triangular forefoot with frontal protrusion of the second, third, and fourth metatarsals without equinus of the metatarsals with all metatarsals on the same plane (see Fig. 29-1A);

2. Simple convex forefoot with frontal protrusion of the second, third, and fourth metatarsals associated with the equinus of those metatarsals. The horizontal position of the first and fifth metatarsals is normal. One of the more difficult of these forefoot conditions to manage is convex forefoot with insufficiency of the first ray;

3. The convex triangular forefoot, in which the augmentation of the frontal convexity of Lisfranc's joint occurs with equinus of the second, third, and fourth metatarsals and divergence of the first and fifth metatarsals;

4. The cavus forefoot, in which metatarsals one or five are lower or relatively shortened in relationship to the central metatarsals.

Regnauld[2] recommends management of these disorders address realignment of the metatarsal formula to

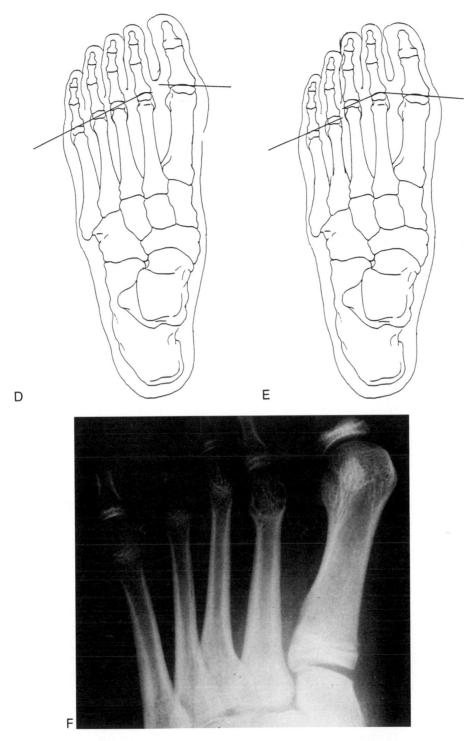

**Fig. 29-5** (*Continued*). (**D**) Long first ray. (**E**) Brachymetatarsia. (**F**) Brachymetatarsia, second metatarsal.

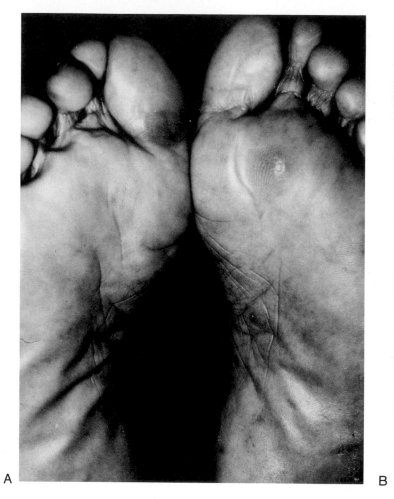
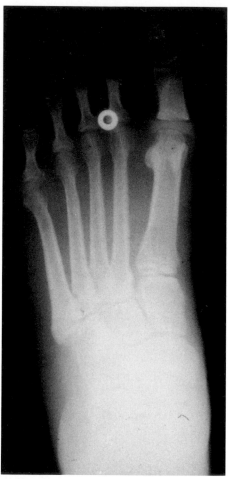

A

B

**Fig. 29-6.** (**A & B**) Example of insufficiency of the great toe. The patient underwent implant arthroplasty of the left first metatarsophalangeal joint with a silicone hemi-implant. The right foot was not operated. Postoperatively, a plantar keratosis developed beneath the second metatarsal as a result of the inability of the hallux to participate in weight-bearing because of loss of intrinsic muscle stability of the great toe.

a correct position and preservation of the metatarsophalangeal joint (Fig. 29-7).

If one considers the alignment of the metatarsals, two axes of function have been described by Bojsen-Moller.[20] He described a transverse axis consisting of the first and second metatarsals and an oblique axis consisting of the second through the fifth metatarsals (Fig. 29-8). The transverse was considered to be a high-speed axis and the oblique axis a low-speed axis. These are similar to the axis of propulsion and axis of balance as described by Whitney.[19] The second metatarsal participates in both axes and represents the key or fulcrum of the forefoot.

Painful conditions of the first-ray, for example, hallux valgus and hallux rigidus, will force the patient to use the low-speed or oblique axis. The foot of the patient with hallux valgus is prevented by the deformity of the toe and the hypermobility of the first ray from using the long lever arm or transverse axis. The fourth and fifth metatarsals with their greater freedom of mobility than the second or third and can yield dorsally so that the brunt of pressure may be then carried by the second or third metatarsals. Abnormalities of metatarsal length may aggravate the situation.

Radiographic assessment of plantar lesions should include dorsoplantar, oblique, forefoot, axial, and lat-

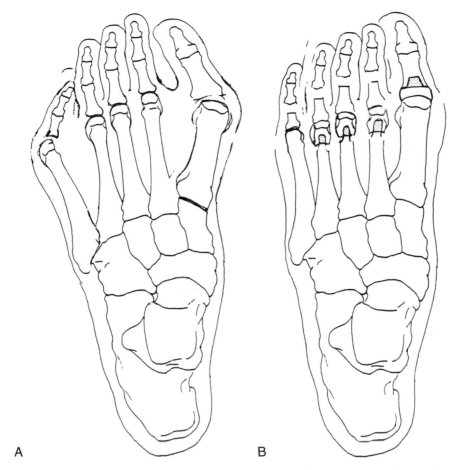

A                                    B

**Fig. 29-7. (A & B)** Pronated or pes planus foot type, which will develop, depending on the severity and composition of the rearfoot deformity, a flat triangular or convex triangular forefoot. In this instance, a flat triangular forefoot is demonstrated. As a result of the change in the decrease in height of the longitudinal arch, as well as the transverse height of the foot, Lisfranc's joint projects distally, increasing its frontal convexity and resulting in splaying of the forefoot and protrusion and prominence of the central metatarsals. This will be accompanied by digital deformity, hallux valgus, and possibly a tailor's bunion. Treatment may include correction of the first-ray pathology and central metatarsal shaft-head enclavement to restore the metatarsal alignment. At the other end of the spectrum, supination reflected by an increase in the longitudinal arch and transverse height of the foot may result in a simple convex forefoot or cavus forefoot. This foot type is described as frontal protrusion the central metatarsals with equinus of those metatarsals as a result of upward displacement of the cuneiforms, causing overload. This overload will be associated by insufficiency of the first and fifth rays. The cavus forefoot results from continued displacement of the cuneiforms and relative equines of the first and fifth metatarsals. Treatment may include enclavement, osteotomy, or a combination to restore metatarsal alignment with other procedures of the first ray as indicated.[2]

eral views of the foot. The dorsoplantar or anteroposterior view allows assessment of metatarsophalangeal joint pathology as well as assessment of metatarsal length patterns. The axial view of the forefoot may identify plantar-flexed metatarsals and plantar prominences, and is especially useful in the evaluation of

patients following metatarsal osteotomy or those with transfer lesions. This view has limited value in preoperative patient assessment for it rarely demonstrates that a plantar-flexed metatarsal. The reason for this is probably that the presence of a true structurally plantar-flexed metatarsal is uncommon and most lesions

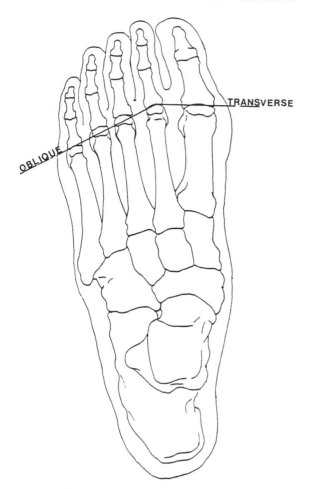

**Fig. 29-8.** The transverse and oblique axes of the metatarsals as described by Bojsen-Möller.

result from biomechanical imbalances often associated with hallux valgus, hallux rigidus, digital deformity or other dynamic imbalances. Oblique views can reveal abnormalities in the relationship of lesser metatarsals by loss of the normal colinear relationship of the lesser metatarsals. Lateral views may serve as a baseline for future comparisons (Fig. 29-9).

## MANAGEMENT

Several procedures have been described for the management of lesser metatarsal lesions (Fig. 29-10). These include the following:

Metatarsal head resection, including both total and
    partial head resection

Condylectomy
Osteoclasis
Distal metaphaseal osteotomy
Tilt-up osteotomy
Distal V osteotomy
Proximal wedge osteotomy
Proximal V osteotomy
Collectomy-type procedures
Metatarsal head recession or enclavement.

### Metatarsal Head Resection

Metatarsal head resection for the management of plantar lesions has been advocated by several authors.[21–23] Rutledge and Green[21] in 1957 reported on the removal of the metatarsal head and one-third of the shaft of the metatarsal. They described their results as excellent in a study involving 30 plantar "corns." They described recession of the toe as a complication and did not observe transfer lesions; 18 months was the longest follow-up in their series. Perhaps the most aggressive form of resection is that of Dickson,[24] who advocated total ray resection for the management of intractable plantar warts. He reported as results as uniformly successful in 25 cases.

Metatarsal head resection is not a commonly indicated procedure in the management of isolated plantar lesions. It is primarily associated with complications of dorsal and posterior retraction of the digit, as well as developments of transfer lesions. Metatarsal head resection is reserved for those cases associated with advanced degenerative disease of the metatarsophalangeal joint, including prolonged subluxation of the digit, and in certain cases for the management of plantar ulcerations. Metatarsal head resection is indicated in the management of tumors of the metatarsal heads. Multiple metatarsal head resections or panmetatarsal head resections play as an important role in the management of the rheumatoid patient, as well as other patients with chronic disabling arthritic processes involving all the metatarsophalangeal joints. Isolated metatarsal head resections have less application.

### Condylectomy

Condylectomy, originally described by DuVries,[25] involves the resection of the plantar condyles of the metatarsal head and is usually reserved for those pa-

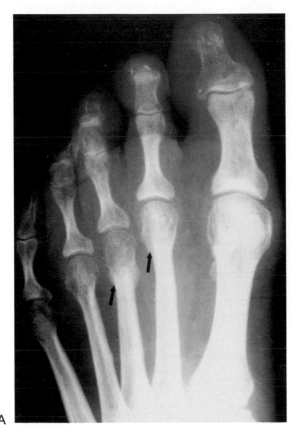
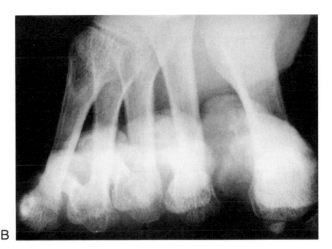

**Fig. 29-9.** Radiographs of a patient who underwent several lesser metatarsal osteotomies. (**A**) The dorsoplantar view reveals the osteotomies with the metatarsal parabola intact; (**B**) the axial view, however, demonstrates the reasons for the patient's continued complaints of metatarsalgia.

tients in whom prominent condyles can be ascertained preoperatively. DuVries[25] and Mann and DuVries[26] have reported success in the management of intractable plantar keratosis by this technique. In the study by Mann and DuVries, a 93 percent patient satisfaction rate was reported. Complications reported by them with this procedure were fracture of the metatarsal head, avascular necrosis of the metatarsal head, cocked-up deformity of the toe, and occasionally medial or laterally drifting in the position of the toe. They also reported recurrent and transfer lesions and that a number of patients required a second procedure because a lesion occurred adjacent to the original site. Anderson[27] described the use of condylectomy in association with a plantar rotational flap for the management of "intractable plantar warts." The modification of the plantar condylectomy using a min-

imal incision approach, called plantar metatarsal head reduction, was also reported by Brown.[28]

## Osteoclasis

Osteoclasis is a procedure attributed to Dr. Joseph Addante[29,30] in which a bone-cutting forceps or rongeur is utilized to create an osteotomy in the neck of a lesser metatarsal for the management of plantar keratosis. Addante reported an 85 percent success rate in his experiences in more than 1,000 cases. A transfer lesion incidence of 15 percent occurred, but there was no report of delayed union or nonunion. Osteoclasis is a simple technique that is usually managed immediately postoperatively by weight-bearing; it is however a rather unstable osteotomy and may cause shortening of the metatarsal.

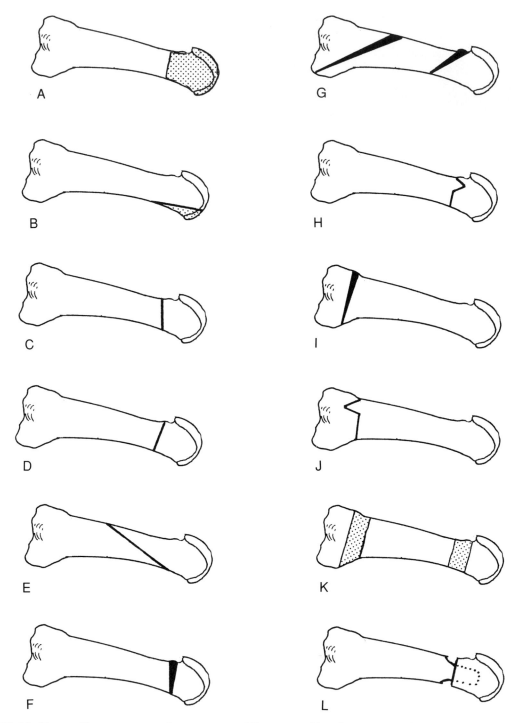

**Fig. 29-10.** Types of lesser metatarsal osteotomies. (**A**) Metatarsal head resection. (**B**) Condylectomy. (**C**) Osteoclaisis. (**D**) Distal metaphyseal osteotomy. (**E**) Helal. (**F & G**) Tilt-up osteotomy. (**H**) Distal V osteotomy. (**I**) Proximal dorsiflexory wedge osteotomy. (**J**) Proximal V osteotomy. (**K**) Collectomy procedure. (**L**) Metatarsal head recession (enclavement).

## Distal Metaphyseal Osteotomies

Distal metaphyseal osteotomies have been reported by several authors. The procedure is usually a transverse or oblique osteotomy performed in the distal metaphaseal area of the metatarsal. Variations in technique relate to the angle of orientation of the osteotomy to the bone itself. Sullivan and O'Donnell[31] performed the osteotomy in an oblique fashion and reported on a study of 75 patients and 150 procedures. The follow-up range was 4 months to 2.5 years. They reported uniform resolution of the chief complaint and minimal evidence of transfer lesions. The osteotomy was performed in an oblique fashion from distal-dorsal to plantar-proximal to limit the amount of dorsal excursion of the metatarsal head. Pedowitz[32] performed an osteotomy in the distal metaphaseal area with the osteotomy perpendicular to the supporting surface. He reported on 69 distal osteotomies with an average follow-up time from 8 months to 8 years (average, 16 months). The overall results were reported as 83 percent good, with a good rating consisting of no complaints of pain, unrestricted shoe wear, no limitation of activity, and no transfer or asymptomatic calluses. Six patients had loss of the weight-bearing function of the toe on the involved rays and three patients developed transfer lesions. Use of a postoperative shoe and immediate weight-bearing was encouraged.

A modification of the distal metaphaseal osteotomy called the percutaneous metaphyseal osteotomy was described by Smith[33]; in this technique the metatarsal neck ws cut perpendicular to the long axis 2 to 4 mm proximal to the capsular attachments through a percutaneous approach without visualization.

A modification of the distal metaphaseal reported by Helal[34] was initially described to include both distal diaphaseal and metaphaseal bone. The technique as described by Helal is a distal oblique osteotomy in the distal one-half of the metatarsal shaft. The osteotomy is angled 45 degrees plantar and distally. In this procedure it is important that the distal fragment slide upward but that it is not angled. The prominent dorsal tip of the distal fragment is remodeled. The purpose of the osteotomy was to allow for soft tissue relaxation to realign deformed toes and reposition the metatarsal fat pad. In long-term follow-up, Helal and Greiss[35] have reported an overall 88.4 percent success rate.

Primary indication for the procedure is for the management of "pressure metatarsalgia." The procedure is also indicated for the management of patients with rheumatoid arthritis, and it is not uncommon for the procedure to be performed simultaneously on all three metatarsals. Postoperatively the patients are managed by immediate postoperative weight-bearing. Other authors have also reported uniformly successful results. Reikeras,[36] in a comparison between a proximal wedge resection dorsiflexed osteotomy and a distal oblique osteotomy, reported the distal oblique to be preferred over the more proximal osteotomy.

An osteotomy similar to that of Helal was performed by Turan and Lindgren[37] using a distal oblique osteotomy with internal screw fixation. They thought that the internal fixation in this instance ensured metatarsal head symmetry and provided for more predictable results. Winson[38] and others reported that better results were obtained in the Helal procedure when plaster and immobilization was not used postoperatively. Further details of the Helal osteotomy are described by a subsequent chapter by Steinbock.

## Tilt-Up Osteotomy

One of the more common osteotomies in recent years is the tilt-up osteotomy, which has been described several authors. Although it is more commonly performed in the area of the distal metaphysis of the metatarsal, Meisenbach[39] in 1916 described this type of osteotomy to be performed 3 cm from the metatarsal phalangeal joint. Other authors have referred to the tilt-up osteotomy as a V-type osteotomy (not to be confused with the distal metaphaseal V osteotomy, which is discussed later). This reference is to a wedge osteotomy with a dorsal base and a plantar apex. Wolf[40] described this as a V-shaped notch made in the metatarsal down to but not including the plantar cortex of the metatarsal shaft. He reported 35 of 42 osteotomies were completed with excellent results. Four were fair, because of the remaining callous tissue, and 3 were poor because the callus recurred.

Thomas[41] also used a tilt-up osteotomy similar to that of Meisenbach and reported a 90 percent success rate as judged by of relief of pain in 73 patients, of whom 39 were rheumatoid; the average follow-up was

4 years. Indications were for painful prominent metatarsals with only moderate toe deformity. He recommended in his paper that if an adjacent metatarsal feels prominent after osteotomy of the prominent metatarsal then that metatarsal should be osteotomized as well. Complications included transfer lesions in 4 patients that were treated by osteotomy of the adjacent metatarsal. Kuwada et al.[42] described a dorsiflexory distal tilt-up osteotomy for painful plantar lesions. The plantar cortex was left intact, and a rongeur was used to perform the bone cut; in some instances the plantar lesion was excised. They reported no incidence of painful scars, and no transfer lesions, and managed the patient non-weight-bearing for the first 3 weeks postoperative. Berkun et al.[43] reported on 14 patients and 25 osteotomies managed by the tilt-up osteotomy. Their overall objective rating was 65 percent excellent, 35 percent good, determined by the appearance of a transfer lesion, and 8 percent poor where there was a painful recurrence and painful transfer lesion. Subjectively, all but 1 patient had a good or excellent result; patients satisfaction was 92.5 percent. There was no reports of nonunion, and only minimal bone callous tissue formed. They also noted toe purchase remained active in 23 of 25 digits.

Leventen and Pearson[44] described an osteotomy, similar to that of Kuwada et al., as a simple V-shaped osteotomy cut transverse to the shaft with a small longer cut close to the metatarsal head and reported an overall success rate of 86 percent. They noticed that the key to the procedure is early weight-bearing to maintain adequate elevation of the metatarsal head. Dannels[45] advocated the use of distal fixated tilt-up osteotomy in the management of preulcers in a diabetic population. Another osteotomy described by Schwartz et al.,[46] is a double oblique lesser metatarsal osteotomy. This osteotomy in the metaphaseal diaphaseal area of the distal metatarsal is performed in an oblique manner and fixated by a simple Kirschner wire (K-wire). For a long metatarsal, the plantar cortex may be osteotomized and shortened. This osteotomy is also readily fixated by screw fixation (interfragmentary compression). Jimenez et al.[47] described a similar osteotomy called a transverse V-osteotomy, an oblique wedge resection osteotomy that again is amenable to screw fixation and may be performed at the distal metaphysis or as a base osteotomy in the proximal metaphysis.

## Distal V Osteotomy

The distal V osteotomy in the podiatric profession has been attributed to Jacoby.[48] In the initial report, a V osteotomy was performed in the distal metaphaseal area of the metatarsal neck. The osteotomy did not extend through the plantar cortex. Two dorsal cuts were made and the bone impacted. The osteotomy was further elaborated on by Reese,[49] who also described the use of the osteotomy for shortening by performing a chevron resection including plantar cortical bone. Young and Hugar[50] reported on their study of the distal V osteotomy of lesser metatarsals in 66 patients. The procedures were uniformly performed with osteotomy completed through the plantar cortex. They reported excellent results to be obtained in 87.5 percent of 56 patients during a 2-year period. The osteotomy was performed at a 45° angle with impaction of the fragments onto the shaft. Graver[51] also reported on a distal V osteotomy that is oriented with the apex proximal, opposite of that described by Jacoby (Fig. 29-11).

# PROXIMAL DORSIFLEXORY OSTEOTOMY

Proximal dorsiflexory wedge osteotomy has been described by Sgarlato,[52] and consists of a dorsal wedge resection in the proximal metaphysis of a lesser metatarsal. Proximal metatarsal osteotomy, because of the nature and location of the osteotomy, makes a correction possible with minimal bone resection. The osteotomy usually requires internal fixation and cast mobilization postoperatively. A similar osteotomy was described by Thomas.[53]

## Proximal V Osteotomy

A proximal V osteotomy performed with the apex proximally has also been described by Aiello[54] and by Sclamberg and Lorenz.[55] They reported that the advantages of this osteotomy is that the V-shape osteotomy provides an excellent fit of the fragments and affords good postoperative stability. They reported a 89.4 percent rate of satisfaction. Sclamberg and Lorenz[55] reported the procedure to be effective with no transfer

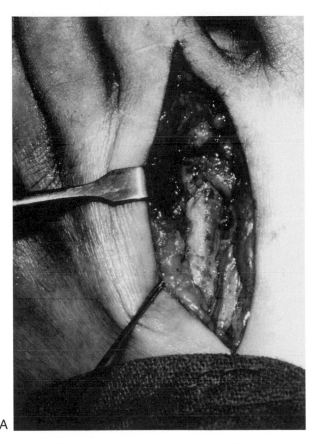
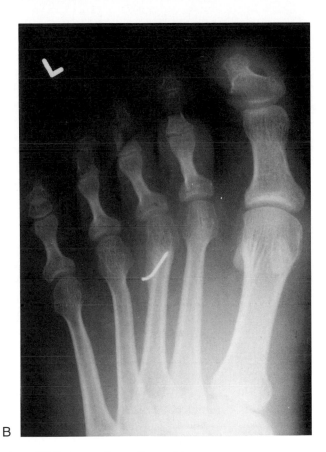

A                                                                      B

**Fig. 29-11.** Distal **V** osteotomy. (**A**) Intraoperative view. (**B**) Postoperative radiographic appearance.

lesions and no subjective complaints voiced by the patients at a 6-month follow-up.

## COLLECTOMY

A resection of part of the metatarsal was described by Allen Whitney from the Pennsylvania College of Podiatric Medicine. Levine[56] reported on the use of collectomy or cylindrical resection of bone of the metatarsal neck in three cases. The cylindrical resection of proximal metatarsal bone 0.5 cm in length was described by Spence et al.[57] The osteotomy or resection was performed by 54 patients (70 metatarsals) with a 6-year follow-up; the results were 89 percent good. Transfers developed in 18 percent; transfers were 23 percent associated with patients undergoing concurrent hallux valgus correction and 12 percent in isolated proce-

dures. The rate of recurrence was reported as 7 percent.

In this author's opinion, the two osteotomies more commonly used today are the distal **V** osteotomy as described by Jacoby and a variation of the tilt-up osteotomy. The distal **V** osteotomy is usually performed with an anglation of the arms of the **V** at 45 to 60 degrees. Minimal dorsal displacement is allowed, and fixation with a K-wire or other simple fixation may be utilized. Weight-bearing in the immediate postoperative phase is usually in a postoperative wooden shoe. The advantages of this osteotomy are the ease of performance and the frontal and transverse plane stability afforded by the configuration of the osteotomy. Because it is a dorsal displacement osteotomy, if unfixated it may exhibit varying degrees of instability in the sagittal plane and result in a floating toe syndrome. Minimal periarticular dissection will reduce the amount of postoperative limitation of motion of the metatarsal phalangeal joint. The transverse V or tilt-up osteotomy allows one to use interfragment compression and in most cases no wedge of bone is removed.

Studies on the outcomes of surgical correction of interactable plantar keratosis have been reported. Hatcher et al.[58] reported on 238 surgical procedures of the central metatarsals with an average follow-up of 2 years and 2 months. The types of procedures evaluated in this study were the percutaneous metaphyseal osteotomy, distal V osteotomy, partial metatarsal head resection, total metatarsal head resection, osteoclasis, extension osteotomy, and extension osteoarthrotomy. One hundred patients representing a total of 238 lesser metatarsal osteotomies were studied. Although the paper did not support one procedure over another, certain conclusions were drawn. The authors reported a 18 percent rate of recurrence of symptomatic lesions and an instance of transfer lesions in 39 percent. This included both symptomatic and asymptotic transfer lesions. That number dropped to 27 percent when only symptomatic transfer lesions are included. The overall success rate for proximal osteotomies was 46 percent, for distal osteotomies, 61 percent, and for joint arthroplastic procedures, partial head or total head resection, it was 53 percent. They did report, however, that based on the studies' criteria for an acceptable result that patients' satisfaction levels were considerably higher than the clinically observed satisfaction level. These authors recommended, in light of the low success rate of proximal osteotomies, that these osteotomies not be recommended as a primary procedure. The authors also believed that the arthroplastic procedure should not be performed unless pathology at the metatarsophalangeal joint such as arthritic changes is distinctly present. They concluded that distal osteotomies are the preferred procedure based on their findings.

The authors[58] reported an increasing number of acceptable results with multiple osteotomies. They indicated that consideration should be given to osteotomizing adjacent metatarsal heads if there is evidence of a lesion beginning adjacent to the primary lesion. The authors also reported better results were obtained for patients of older age and attributed this to the possibility of decreased physical activity in the older age patients.

Hatcher et al. also reported that there was a lack of toe purchase in those cases in which the metatarsophalangeal joint demonstrated limited plantar flexion postoperatively; however, this problem was not believed to affect the overall outcome of the surgery. They reported the distal V osteotomy to be associated with the greatest lack of plantar flexion and lack of toe purchase when compared with the other osteotomies. Extensor tendon tenotomy did not seem to improve the results or enhance toe purchase postoperatively. The overall decrease in metatarsal length for each individual procedure was also reported. The least amount of shortening was associated with the proximal osteotomies and the greatest amount of shortening with total metatarsal head resection. Almost half their osteotomies were of the second metatarsal, and the remainder was divided between the third and fourth metatarsals. There was no reported difference between the success rates when evaluating the individual metatarsals. Overall the average success rate for lesser metatarsal surgery was 56.5 percent, with patient satisfaction being considerably higher.

In another study by Goforth et al.[59] an overall success rate of 78 percent was reported for 119 osteotomies in 94 patients; 74 osteotomies were performed on the second, third, and fourth metatarsals. The distal osteotomies on these metatarsals were nonfixated distal V osteotomies or simple transverse metaphyseal osteotomies. Follow-up time in this study for the patients averaged 16.9 months. The overall results for osteotomies of the second, third, and fourth metatarsals were approximately 67 percent success. Recurrent or transfer lesions were reported as complications.

Young and Hugar[50] discussed the evaluation of the V osteotomy for the intractable plantar keratosis. They reported on 56 patients over a 2-year period, and on the basis of their clinical observations and patient satisfaction, 75 percent excellent results were obtained. This was defined as resolution of the original lesion with no transfer lesion. Seven patients were reported as good. Three symptomatic transfer lesions and four asymptomatic transfer lesions occurred, and 7 patients were described as having an unacceptable result. Complications included transfer lesions, lack of toe plantar flexion and purchase, and dorsal bone callus associated with the nonfixated osteotomy. They also reported that the diminished range of motion in the

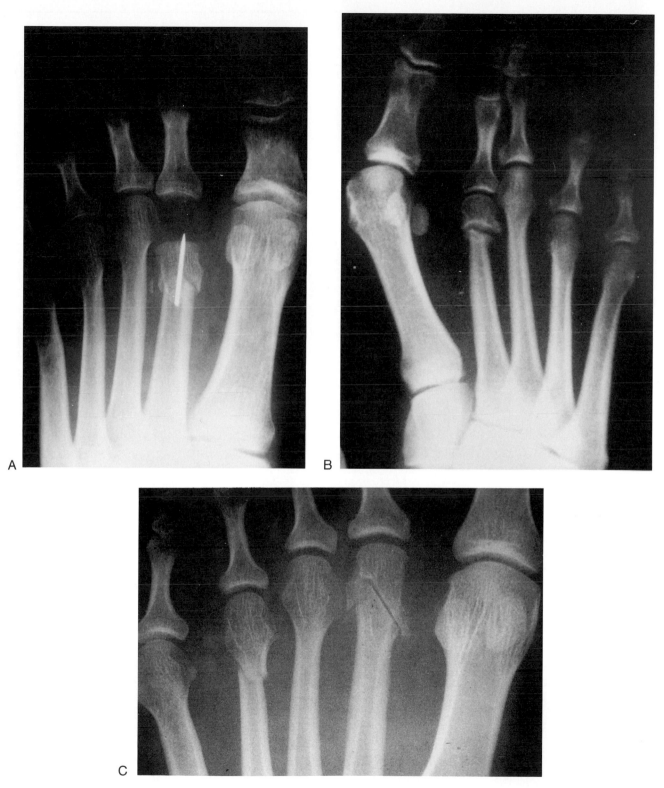

**Fig. 29-12.** Complications of lesser metatarsal osteotomy. (**A**) Excessive shortening. (**B**) Excessive shortening with atrophic nonunion. (**C**) Poor osteotomy placement. (*Figure continues.*)

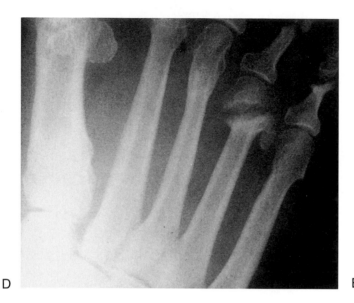

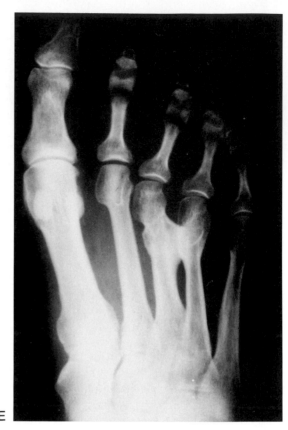

D                                                 E

**Fig. 29-12** (*Continued* ). (**D**) Poor osteotomy placement. (**E**) Osseous coalition of adjacent metatarsals.

digit was proportional to the amount of elevation of the distal fragment.

Reinherz and Toren[60] reviewed 32 patients with simultaneous adjacent metatarsal osteotomies to determine the effect of surgical location on postoperative healing. They concluded that the placement of simultaneous adjacent metatarsal osteotomies does indeed influence postoperative healing. A significant high incidence of bone callus was found when adjacent osteotomies were performed in the metatarsal neck as compared to those performed in the neck and adjacent metatarsal base. They also suggested that greater prolonged postoperative edema occurs when adjacent osteotomies are performed at the metatarsal base. It was their conclusion and recommendation that, when two adjacent osteotomies are to be performed, one should be performed in the surgical neck and the other in the metaphyseal area of the base to reduce

the possibility and consequences of the prolonged postoperative healing. Hart and Hart[61] reported on a case of an iatrogenic osseous coalition between two adjacent metatarsals having undergone simultaneous osteotomy; this is an unusual occurrence.

Schweitzer et al.[62] reported on metatarsal shortening following osteotomy and its clinical significance. Some degree of shortening may accompany different metatarsal osteotomies. Comparing the dorsoflexory wedge, osteoclasis, V distal metaphyseal, crescentic, and percutaneous metaphyseal osteotomies, the authors demonstrated that the osteotomies which produced the least amount of shortening were the cresentic followed by the percutaneous metaphyseal osteotomy and distal metaphyseal osteotomy. The greatest amount of shortening resulted with the osteoclasis procedure. The amount of shortening for the distal V osteotomy and the proximal base osteotomy were found to be similar, falling between that of the osteoclasis and the cresentic osteotomies. The percutaneous metaphyseal, distal metaphyseal, and cresentic osteotomies revealed less than 0.2 cm of shortening; the proximal base osteotomy and V osteotomy more than about 0.2 cm of shortening, and the osteoclasis had slightly more than 0.3 cm. McGlamry[63] reported that the most common cause of the floating toe in a lesser ray is overcorrection following metatarsal osteotomy.

## COMPLICATIONS

Complications of lesser metatarsal surgery (Fig. 29-12) include the following[64]:

1. Recurrence of lesion and symptoms
2. Development of transfer lesions to a adjacent metatarsals because of too much elevation or shortening of the metatarsal
3. Loss of digital function as evidenced by lack of toe purchase and floating toe syndrome seen clinically
4. Loss of metatarsophalangeal joint range of motion as a result of excessive elevation of the metatarsal and of secondary degenerative changes occurring as a result of osteotomy placement or osteonecrosis[65]
5. Disordered bone healing resulting in the development of malunion (abnormal alignment of a metatarsal head), delayed union, and nonunion
6. Contraction of the metatarsophalangeal joint.

Fixation of osteotomies has always been left to the surgeon's preference. Fixation of lesser metatarsal osteotomies is readily achieved by a variety of simple fixation techniques including K-wire and absorbable fixation. In cases where a nonfixated osteotomy is anticipated, consideration need be given to the type of osteotomy and the compliance of the patient in the immediate postoperative period. Complications are best avoided by careful preoperative planning and assessment. Isolated metatarsal and multiple osteotomies should be performed only in the presence of the demonstrative criteria.

Prophylactic osteotomies and the management of plantar lesions associated with biomechanical problems such as hallux valgus and hallux rigidus should be avoided because it does not address the primary etiology and thus only in the most recalcitrant lesions should this be considered as a option. With regards to the surgical management of postoperative transfer lesions, the goal is to establish normal weight-bearing relationship function and of the metatarsal heads. Management of transfer lesions may require plantarflexory or lengthening osteotomies with or without bone grafting and, in some instances, osteotomy of the adjacent metatarsals. Panmetatarsal head resection may be indicated as a end-stage salvage procedure. The cause and treatment of metatarsalgia associated with mechanical as well as structural deformities of the foot and leg is an area ripe for continuing study and research as evidenced by the diversity in classifications and treatment methods. Advances in the use of force plate analysis for the distribution of plantar pressures combined with biomechanical assessment hold promise for a better understanding of forefoot pathology in the future.

## REFERENCES

1. Thomas N, Nissen KI, Helal B: Disorders of the lesser ray. p. 486. In Helal B, Wilson D (eds): The Foot. Churchill Livingstone, New York, 1988
2. Regnauld B: The Foot. Springer-Verlag, Berlin, 1986
3. Viladot A: Metatarsalgia due to biomechanic alterations of the forefoot. Orthop Clin North Am 4:165, 1973
4. Scranton PE: Metatarsalgia diagnosis and treatment. J Bone Joint Surg 62:723, 1980
5. Dyck PJ, Low PA, Stevens JC: Burning feet as the only manifestation of dominantly inherited sensory neuropathy. Mayo Clin Proc 58:426, 1983
6. Subotnick S: Observations and discussion of plantar calluses. Arch Podiatr Med Foot Surg 1.329, 1974
7. Todoroff S, Sanders LJ: Keratosis punctata. J Am Podiatr Med Assoc 76:13, 1986
8. Tomassi F, Comerford J, Ransom RA: Unna-Thost-type palmoplantar keratoderma. J Am Podiatr Med Assoc 77:150, 1987
9. Lemont H: Histologic differentiation of mechanical and nonmechanical keratoses of the sole. Clin Dermatol 1:44, 1983
10. Fisher BK, MacPherson M, Epidermoid cyst of the sole. J Am Acad Dermatol 15:1127, 1986
11. Taub J, Steinberg MD: Porokeratosis plantaris discreta; Int J Dermatol 9:83, 1970
12. Mandojana RM, Katz R, Rodman OG: Porokeratosis plantaris discreta. Acad Dermatol 10:679, 1984

13. Yanklowitz B, Harkless L: Porokeratosis plantaris discreta; a misnomer. J Am Podiatr Med Assoc 80:381, 1990
14. Mancuso JE, Abranmow SP, Dimichino BR, Landsman MJ: Carbon dioxide laser management of plantar verruca: a 6-year follow-up survey. J Foot Surg 30:238, 1991
15. Lemont H, Parekh V: Superficial fascia: an appropriate anatomic boundary for excising warts on the foot. J Dermatol Surg Oncol 15:710, 1987
16. Bossley CJ, Cairney PC: The intermetatarsal bursa; its significance in Morton's metatarsalgia. J Bone Joint Surg 62:1984, 1980
17. Fitton J, Swinburne L: Degenerative lesions of the accessory plantar ligament. Int Orthop 4:295, 1981
18. Hlavac H, Schoenhaus H: The plantar fat pad and some related problems. J Am Podiatr Med Assoc 60:151, 1970
19. Whitney AK: Triplane Taxonomy of Foot and Limb Deformity. Lecture notes, Pennsylvania College of Podiatric Medicine
20. Bojsen-Moller F: Anatomy of the forefoot, normal and pathologic. Clin Orthop Relat Res 142:10, 1979
21. Rutledge A, Green AL: Surgical treatment of plantar corns. US Armed Forces Med J 8:219, 1957
22. Margo MK: Surgical treatment of conditions of the forepart of the foot. J Bone Joint Surg, 49:1665, 1967
23. Joplin RJ: Surgery of the forefoot in the rheumatoid arthritic patient. Surg Clin North Am 49:847, 1969
24. Dickson JA: Surgical treatment of intractable plantar warts. J Bone Joint Surg 30A:757, 1948
25. DuVries HL: New approach to the treatment of intractable verruca plantaris (plantar wart). JAMA 152:1203, 1953
26. Mann A, DuVries L: Intractable plantar keratosis. Orthop Clin North Am 4:67, 1973
27. Anderson R: The treatment of intractable plantar warts. Plast Reconstr Surg 19:384, 1957
28. Brown R: Curr Podiatry 26:9, 1977
29. Addante B: Metatarsal osteotomy as a surgical approach for elimination of plantar keratosis. J Foot Surg 8:36, 1969
30. Addante JB, Kaufmann D: The metatarsal osteotomy: a ten-year follow-up on the second, third, and fourth metatarsal osteotomies and a new approach to the fifth metatarsal osteotomy. J Foot Surg 16:92, 1977
31. Sullivan JD, O'Donnell JE: The dorsal displacement floating metatarsal subcapital osteotomy. J Foot Surg 14:62, 1975
32. Pedowitz WJ: Distal oblique osteotomy for intractable plantar keratosis of the middle three metatarsals. Foot Ankle 9:7, 1988
33. Smith D: Percutaneous metaphyseal osteotomy. Annu J Acad Ambulat Foot Surgeons 1980
34. Helal B: Metatarsal osteotomy for metatarsalgia. J Bone Joint Surg 57:187, 1975
35. Helal B, Greiss M: Telescoping osteotomy for pressure metatarsalgia. J Bone Joint Surg, 66:213, 1984
36. Reikeras O: Metatarsal osteotomy for relief of metatarsalgia. Arch Orthop Traum Surg 101:177, 1983
37. Turan I, Lindgren U: Metatarsal osteotomy using internal fixation with compression screws. J Foot Surg 28:116, 1989
38. Winson IG, Rawlinson J, Broughton NS: Treatment of metatarsalgia by sliding distal metatarsal osteotmy. Foot Ankle 9:2, 1988
39. Meisenbach RO: Painful anterior arch of the foot and operation for its relief by means of raising the arch. Am J Orthop Surg 14:206, 1916
40. Wolf M: Metatarsal osteotomy for relief of painful metatarsal. J Bone Joint Surg 55:1750, 1973
41. Thomas WH: Metatarsal osteotomy. Surg Clin 49:879, 1969
42. Kuwada GT, Dockery GL, Schuberth JM: The resistant painful plantar lesion; a surgical approach. Foot Surg 22:29, 1983
43. Berkun RN, Devincentis A, Goller WL: The tilt-up osteotomy for correction of intractable plantar keratosis. J Foot Surg 23:52, 1984
44. Leventen O, Pearson W: Distal metatarsal osteotomy for intractable plantar Keratosis. Foot Ankle 10:247, 1990
45. Dannels EG: A preventive metatarsal osteotomy for healing pre-ulcers in American Indian Diabetes. J Am Podiatr Med Assoc 76:33, 1986
46. Schwartz N, Williams JE, Marcinko DE: Double oblique less metatarsal osteotomy. J Am Podiatr Med Assoc 73:218, 1983
47. Jimenez AL, Martin DE, Phillips AJ: Lesser metatarsalgia evaluation and treatment. Clin Podiatr Med Surg 7:597, 1990
48. Jacob RP: "V" Osteoplasty for correction of intractable plantar keratosis. J Foot Surg 12:10, 1973
49. Reese HW: Surgical treatment of intractable plantar keratosis. J Foot Surg 12:92, 1973
50. Young E, Hugar W: Evaluation of the V-osteotomy as a procedure to alleviate the intractable planter keratoma. J Foot Surg 19:187, 1980
51. Graver H: Angular metatarsal osteotomy: a preliminary report. J Am Podiatry Assoc 63:96, 1973
52. Sgarlato TE: A compendium of podiatric biomechanics. California College of Podiatric Medicine, San Francisco, 1971
53. Thomas F: Levelling the tread: (elevation of the dropped metatarsal head by metatarsal osteotomy). J Bone Joint Surg 56B:314, 1974
54. Aiello CL: Surgical treatment of metatarsalgia. Int Orthop, 5:107, 1981
55. Sclamberg EL, Lorenz MA: A dorsal wedge "V" osteotomy for painful plantar callosities. Foot Ankle 4:30, 1983

56. Levine LA: Modern therapeutic approaches to foot problems. Futura Publishing, Mt. Kisco, NY, 1975.

57. Spence KF, O'Connell SJ, Kenzora JE: Proximal metatarsal segmental resection: a treatment for intractable plantar keratoses. Orthopedics 13:741, 1990

58. Hatcher RM, Goller WL, Weil LS: Intractable planter keratoses. J Am Podiatr Med Assoc 68:366, 1978

59. Goforth PW, Karlin JW, DeValentines S, et al: Distal metatarsal osteotomy (retrospective study). J Am Podiatr Med Assoc 74:402, 1984

60. Reinherz RP, Toren DJ: Bone healing after adjacent metatarsal osteotomies. J Foot Surg 20:198, 1981

61. Hart DJ, Hart TJ: Iatrogenic metatarsal coalition: a post-operative complication of adjacent V-osteotomies. Foot Surg 24:205, 1985

62. Schweitzer DA, Lew J, Morgan J: Central metatarsal shortening following osteotomy and its clinical significance. J Am Podiatry Assoc 72:6, 1982

63. McGlamry ED: Floating toe syndrome. J Am Podiatr Med Assoc 72:561, 1982

64. Weinstock RE: Surgical judgement in metatarsal surgery for the elimination of intractable plantar keratoses. J Am Podiatr Med Assoc 65:979, 1975

65. Bayliss NC, Kleneman L: Avascular necrosis of lesser metatarsals heads following forefoot surgery. Foot Ankle 10:124, 1989

# 30

# Freiberg's Disease

T.W.D. SMITH
D.N. KREIBICH

Infraction of the second metatarsal bone was first described by Cincinnati surgeon Albert Freiberg in 1914.[1] In much of the English-speaking world the condition retains his name, although following a later report in 1924, on the continent of Europe it is referred to as Kohler's second disease.[2] Since then, the medical literature has contained few reports on the disease although there remains much controversy about its etiology and treatment.

Freiberg's disease is generally agreed to represent an avascular necrosis of the metatarsal head. Although recognized as primarily a disorder of the second metatarsal, it has been reported to affect the other metatarsals, but rarely the first.[3] The pathologic process characteristically begins on the dorsal surface of the metatarsal head, and Gauthier[4] described the disease evolution in terms of five stages: stage 0, a subchondral bone march fracture with normal radiographic appearances; stage 1, osteonecrosis without deformation; stage 2, deformation caused by subchondral bone collapse; stage 3, cartilaginous tearing and thus gradual detachment of the segment of abnormal bone; and stage 4, arthrosis of the joint.

Although it is reported in boys,[5] this is predominantly a condition affecting teenaged girls. Pain, both at rest and on exercise, is the predominant clinical feature, although the patients often also complain of local swelling and tenderness that make the wearing of fashionable shoes difficult. The diagnosis is made by a combination of clinical suspicion and plain films. The radiographic appearance is typical with flattening of the subchondral bone of the metatarsal head progressing to increased bone density, fragmentation, and intra-articular loose body formation (Fig. 30-1). According to Hoskinson,[5] the radiographic projection that most reliably demonstrates the early lesion is a 45° oblique of the forefoot.

## ETIOLOGY

The etiology of the condition is not very clear. According to Crock,[6] the metatarsal head is penetrated by radial arteries from either side that unite to form a centrally placed arterial network in the bone from which branches are given off to the subchondral area. The metatarsal head, like the femoral head, the capitellum, and the scaphoid, would seem to be particularly susceptible to avascular necrosis. Its vulnerability, like these other sites, presumably occurs because the subchondral bone is compromised by being enclosed as it is by a convex surface of avascular hyaline cartilage. Further, until the age of 17 to 20 years when the metatarsal epiphysis fuses,[7] the subchondral bone circulation may be further isolated by the presence of the growth plate. What predisposes the head to the development of avascular necrosis is uncertain although certain risk factors have been reported.

## TRAUMA

In Freiberg's original report of six patients, three gave a definite history of trauma, leading him to implicate trauma as being of prime importance in the development of the condition. In 1926, however, he revised this viewpoint acknowledging that "simple trauma was not a satisfying explanation of the clinical and roentgenographic phenomena."[8] Although this view was supported by Kohler,[2] authors have since reverted to a

453

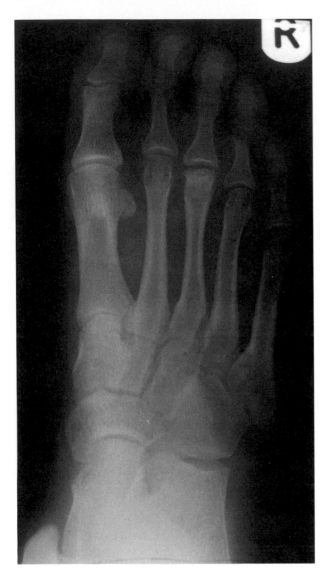

**Fig. 30-1.** Anteroposterior radiograph showing typical appearance of Freiberg's disease involving the third metatarsal head.

traumatic etiology either as an acute event or, as Smillie[9] postulated, the result of repeated minor trauma.

To investigate this further, Braddock[10] studied the effect of axially applied forces on cadaveric articulated phalanges and metatarsals from patients of different ages. He noted that the phalanx fractured in all the specimens except those two in which the stage of epiphyseal maturation corresponded closely to that

seen in early Freiberg's disease. He thus was able to conclude that there is a period of development during which the metatarsal head is particularly sensitive to trauma, resulting in the development of Freiberg's disease. In a series of 33 cases reported by Stanley et al.,[11] only 5 patients (15 percent), all of whom were girls, gave a definite history of trauma. It might be argued that if trauma were an important factor, the condition would occur more commonly in boys who are much more likely to injure themselves playing ball sports, and this clearly is not the case.

## METATARSAL LENGTH AND MOBILITY

It has not gone unnoticed by previous authors that the metatarsal that is most commonly affected is both the longest and least mobile. Gauthier[4] noted that this predisposed it to repeated traumatic stresses. However, in his series of 88 cases the longest metatarsal was affected in only 28 (32 percent) of cases. This was in marked contrast to the experience of Stanley et al.,[11] who measured the metatarsal lengths in both feet of 33 patients who had unilateral Freiberg's disease. The second metatarsal was the longest in 31 (94 percent) of cases and was the seat of the pathology in 30 (91 percent), the remaining 3 cases being Freiberg's disease of the third metatarsal head. There was however no significant difference between the lengths of the metatarsals of the affected feet and the unaffected feet, and thus while there is no doubting that the disease process has a predeliction for the second metatarsal, which also happens to be the longest, there is no firm evidence to correlate this with the development of the disease process.

## PLANTAR PRESSURE

Betts et al.[12] have investigated the importance of local plantar pressure in the development of the disorder. Using the Dynamic Pedobarograph they showed that in only 15 percent of their cases was there evidence of abnormally high pressure under the affected metatarsal head. In addition they reported no differences in pressure distribution between the affected and unaffected feet, concluding that there was little evidence to support the theory that Freiberg's disease was related to increased plantar pressures during walking.

## TREATMENT

Conservative therapy is said to be adequate in most cases. This may take the form of rest, crutches, and even a plaster cast support during the acute phase of symptoms. Once the acute symptoms have subsided, an orthosis in the form of a metatarsal bar support affords a degree of comfort and support.

If conservative therapy fails, a number of surgical techniques have been described that either attempt to modify the disease process or to salvage the situation once the metatarsol phalangeal joint develops signs of degenerate change (Table 30-1 and Fig. 30-2).

In his original series, Freiberg[1] stressed the significance of the presence of loose bodies in the joint, stating that they may be the reason for a failure of conservative treatment. He performed arthrotomies on two of the three patients with intra-articular loose bodies with an excellent relief of symptoms. Hoskinson[5] agreed with this approach although Trott[13] cautioned that it did not relieve the symptoms in all cases, and Stanley et al.[14] found that the presence of loose bodies was not an important predictor of final outcome whatever form of treatment the patient underwent.

Smillie[9] proposed a technique of exploring the metatarsophalangeal joint, elevating the depressed segment of metatarsal head, the buttressing the repair with cancellous bone graft. His procedure was indicated so long as the depressed fragment remained attached by a rim of hyaline cartilage, and although his results demonstrated almost perfect restoration of the articular surface he makes no comment as to the functional outcome of these cases.

Gauthier[4] recommended a similar philosophy of reconstructing the metatarsal head. Based on his obser-

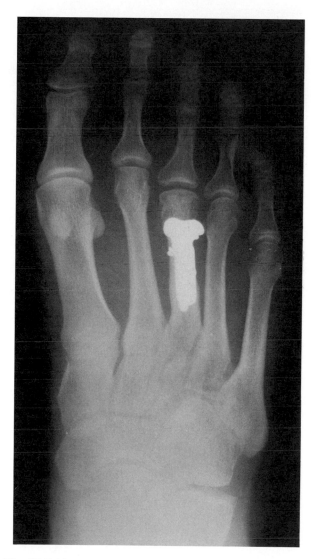

**Fig. 30-2.** Same patient as in Figure 30-1 treated by metatarsal osteotomy.

vation that the lesion was situated on the plantar aspect of the metatarsal head, he performed a dorsiflexion osteotomy of the metatarsal head excising the abnormal segment; 52 of his 53 cases obtained a good result with this procedure. However, in common with Smillie's aforementioned technique it may be a technically difficult procedure that may further damage the already compromised metatarsal head.

The policy on our unit has been to offer surgery to all those patients receiving no lasting benefit from a 6-

**Table 30-1.** Surgical Treatment of Freiberg's Disease

Excision of loose bodies (Freiberg)
Elevation of depressed metatarsal head (Smillie)
Dorsiflexion osteotomy of metatarsal head (Gauthier)
Metatarsal shortening osteotomy (Smith)
Excision base of proximal phalanx (Trott)
Metarsal head excision (Giannestras)

month trial of conservative therapy. A shortening oste- otomy of the metatarsal is then performed, excising approximately 4 mm the metatarsal neck.[15] The osteot- omy is stabilized by a small T-shaped plate, and the patient is immobilized in a below-knee plaster cast for 4 weeks. Of the 18 patients treated in this way, all but 1 were satisfied with the outcome. Further, in 3 cases we have seen apparent remodeling of the metatarsal head and improved congruity with the proximal phalanx following surgery (Fig. 30-3). The rationale for this

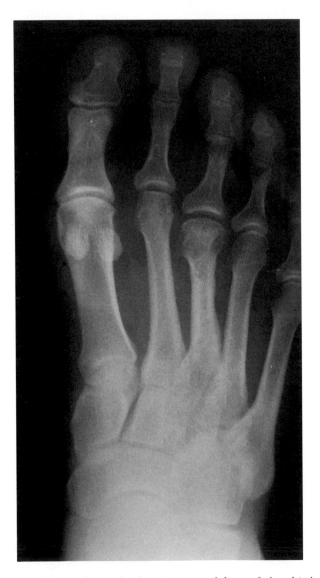

**Fig. 30-3.** Radiograph showing remodeling of the third metatarsal head after removal of the plate.

approach is that it decompresses the joint allowing repair of the subchondral bone; it does not involve an arthrotomy, and therefore the potential to do further damage to the joint is minimized; and it is a technically simple procedure.

It is clear that the disease process may progress to such an extent that such reconstructive procedures are inappropriate. In this situation, Trott's[13] technique of partial resection of the proximal phalanx with syndac- tylization of the second to the third toe may be appro- priate. The disadvantage of this procedure, at least in theory, is that surgery is directed toward normal anat- omy and does not address the underlying pathologic process. Despite this, Trott claims that the procedure provides relief of symptoms and a reasonable cos- metic result.

Giannestras[16] suggested that metatarsal head resec- tion was appropriate for severe disease. Although we have no experience of this technique, we feel that there is a risk such surgery will result in load transfer- ence and pain under the adjacent metatarsals. In addi- tion, Hoskinson[5] reported unsatisfactory results with this procedure.

## PROGNOSIS

Little is known of the long-term outcome of patients with Freiberg's disease, irrespective of method of treatment. Patients are rarely seen in adult orthopedic clinics, suggesting that symptoms resolve with time. Hoskinson's series[5] of 28 patients reviewed for a mean of 12 years following diagnosis is the longest in the literature. Of the 16 patients who had been treated conservatively, 11 remained asymptomatic with only 2 complaining of persistent aching. The remaining 12 patients had been treated by a variety of surgical meth- ods, and 8 of them continued to complain of trouble- some residual symptoms. In our series of 30 patients, with a mean follow-up of 7 years,[17] the patients were initially treated conservatively followed by a shorten- ing osteotomy if they were still symptomatic 6 months later. Of the conservatively treated group 58 percent of patients described their pain as less than at the time of presentation, 33 percent said it was the same, and 9 percent said it was worse. Those patients who re- quired surgery fared better, with 89% saying their pain was better, 11% the same, and no patients saying their

**Table 30-2.** Long-Term Results of Conservative and Surgical Treatment

| Treatment | Symptoms Compared to Presentation (%) | | |
|---|---|---|---|
| | Better | Same | Worse |
| Conservative | 58 | 33 | 9 |
| Surgical | 89 | 11 | 0 |

(From Kreibich et al.,[17] with permission.)

pain was worse than on presentation (Table 30-2). While the two groups are not comparable it is interesting to note that those patients whose symptoms were initially bad enough to require surgery were actually less symptomatic than those treated purely conservatively. However, it must be added that there is a group of patients in whom the disorder escapes the attention of the orthopedic surgeon until the foot may be radiographed for a totally different reason.

There is still much to be learned about the etiology and treatment of this condition. When several different operations are described for the treatment of a disorder, it is often a sign that the results have been unsatisfactory. Because the condition is relatively rare, different forms of treatment have never been subjected to a prospective randomized trial. In addition, the timing of surgery may be vital. Repair and remodeling of the metatarsal head undoubtedly occurs in some patients, and there may be a crucial period in the progression of the disease when surgery would be more likely to be successful.

# REFERENCES

1. Freiberg AH: Infraction of the second metatarsal bone. A typical Injury. Surg Gynecol Obstet 19:191, 1914

2. Kohler A: Grenzen des Normalen und Anfange des Pathologischen. p. 77. In Rontgenbilde. LucasGrafe and Sillem, Hamburg, 1924

3. Wagner A: Isolated aseptic necrosis in the epiphysis of the first metatarsal bone. Acta Radiol 11:80, 1930

4. Gauthier G, Elbaz R: Freiberg's infraction: a subchondral bone fracture. A new surgical treatment. Clin Orthop 142:93, 1979

5. Hoskinson J: Freiberg's disease: A review of the long term results. Proc R Soc Med 67:10, 1974

6. Crock HV: The Blood Supply of the Lower Limb Bones in Man. Livingstone Ltd., Edinburgh and London, 1967

7. Sutton D (ed): A Textbook of Radiology and Imaging. Vol. 2. 3rd Ed. Churchill Livingstone, New York, 1980

8. Freiberg AH: The so-called infraction of the second metatarsal Bone. J Bone Joint Surg 8:257, 1926

9. Smillie IS: Freiberg's infraction (Kohler's second disease). J Bone Joint Surg 39B:580, 1957

10. Braddock GTF: Experimental epiphyseal injury and Freiberg's disease. J Bone Joint Surg 41B:154, 1959

11. Stanley D, Betts RP, Rowley DI, Smith TWD: Assessment of the aetiological factors in the development of Freiberg's disease. J Foot Surg 29:444, 1990

12. Betts RP, Stanley D, Smith TWD: Foot pressure studies in Freiberg's disease. Foot 1:21, 1991

13. Trott AW: Developmental disorders. In Jahss MH (ed): Disorders of the Foot, WB Saunders, Philadelphia, 1982

14. Stanley D, Smith TWD, Rowley DI: The conservative and surgical management of Freiberg's disease. Foot 1:97, 1991

15. Smith TWD, Stanley D, Rowley DI: Treatment of Freiberg's disease. A new operative technique. J Bone Joint Surg 73B:129, 1991

16. Giannestras NJ: Foot Disorders: Medical and Surgical Management. 2nd Ed. Lea & Febiger, Philadelphia, 1973

17. Kreibich DN, Stanely D, Smith TWD: The aetiology and treatment of Freiberg's disease. Presented to the British Association of Children's Orthopaedic Surgery, Glasgow, 1992

# 31

# Tailor's Bunion Deformity

*JANIS E. LEHTINEN*

*Tailor's bunion* or *bunionette* is a term applied to an enlargement of the lateral aspect of the fifth metatarsal head that produces various degrees of pain, swelling, and tenderness. This enlargement of the lateral aspect of the fifth metatarsal head may present as either hypertrophy of soft tissue overlying the fifth metatarsal, a congenitally enlarged or dumbbell-shaped fifth metatarsal head, an abnormal lateral angulation of the fifth metatarsal shaft, or a combination of these conditions. The deformity is located at the dorsolateral or lateral aspect of the fifth metatarsophalangeal joint. Commonly, a splayfoot deformity is associated with a Tailor's bunion deformity.

## ETIOLOGY

Various causes are attributed to the development of a Tailor's bunion deformity. The various factors may occur alone or in combination to produce the deformity and may be divided into structural and functional causes.

In review of the literature, the following authors describe the structural etiology of this deformity. Davies[1] attributes the deformity to persistent embryonic splaying of the fifth metatarsal caused by incomplete or imperfect development of the transverse intermetatarsal ligament. Gray states that failure of the transverse pedis muscle to insert at the fifth metatarsophalangeal joint between the fourth and fifth metatarsal heads results in a loss of contractural support. Leliévre[2] attributes the development of a Tailor's bunion deformity to one of three mechanisms: (1) a supernumerary bone that attaches to the lateral aspect of the fourth metatarsal head, forcing the fifth metatarsal

head laterally; (2) spreading of the metatarsals resulting in a wide intermetatarsal angle; (3) pressure on the lateral side of the fifth metatarsal head caused by sitting with crossed legs. DuVries[3] states that hypertrophy of the soft tissue overlying the fifth metatarsophalangeal joint, a congenitally wide, dumbbell-shaped fifth metatarsal head, and lateral deviation of the fifth metatarsal shaft or head whether singly or a combination of these three conditions will produce the deformity. Frankel et al. stated that a medially dislocated fifth metatarsophalangeal joint will cause the symptoms associated with this deformity.

The functional etiologies of a Tailor's bunion deformity are attributed to abnormal biomechanics.[4] The fifth ray consists of the fifth metatarsal only. It moves in supination and pronation about a triplane axis, and has mainly sagittal plane dominance. The axis of motion lies in an angle of approximately 20° from the transverse plane and 35° from the sagittal plane.[5] Clinically, there is equal dorsiflexion and plantar flexion of the fifth ray. The functional etiology of a Tailor's bunion deformity consists of four factors: (1) excessive subtalar joint pronation; (2) uncompensated varus position of the forefoot or rearfoot in a fully pronated subtalar joint; (3) a congenitally plantar-flexed fifth metatarsal; and (4) idiopathically, an absence of the transverse pedis muscle or an enlarged fifth metatarsal head.

Subtalar joint pronation alone will not cause a Tailor's bunion deformity. With excessive subtalar joint pronation, the midtarsal joint unlocks, subsequently unlocking the fifth ray and causing dorsiflexion with weight-bearing. This excessive dorsiflexion causes eversion of the fifth metatarsal. The deep transverse intermetatarsal ligament through its attachment to the

459

flexor cap of the hypermobile fifth metatarsal, combined with the stable fourth metatarsal, causes a medial pull of the flexor cap. This causes frontal plane deformity at the metatarsophalangeal joint while the long flexor and extensor tendons bowstring across the joint. The abductor digiti minimi migrates plantarly, which causes the lateral capsule to stretch while the medial capsule contracts. Retrograde forces will therefore accentuate this deformity.

An uncompensated varus deformity in a fully pronated foot will produce subluxation and pronation of the fifth ray. With this varus deformity of the foot, the total number of degrees of varus deformity must exceed the potential degrees of calcaneal eversion that can be produced by maximal subtalar joint pronation. Thus, with the fifth ray plantar to the central three rays, with weight-bearing the fifth metatarsal will dorsiflex and evert, causing a Tailor's bunion deformity.

Idiopathic causes of Tailor's bunion deformity are either osseous or soft tissue in nature. The absence of attachment of the transverse pedis muscle is a soft tissue abnormality described as causing idiopathic Tailor's bunion deformity. A congenitally enlarged or dumbbell-shaped metatarsal head is an osseous idiopathic cause of a Tailor's bunion deformity. In either case (soft tissue or osseous), the idiopathic cause of the deformity is not common, but should be considered in cases without subtalar joint pronatory conditions.

## CLINICAL EVALUATION

When evaluating the fifth metatarsophalangeal joint, clinical evaluation should involve gross inspection of the entire foot. Deformities should be noted. The patient's complaints will vary with the degree of deformity, but usually pain or discomfort over the lateral, dorsolateral, or plantar-lateral aspect of the fifth metatarsophalangeal joint is the chief complaint. Lesion patterns, whether purely lateral, plantar-lateral, or plantar, and mild to diffuse hyperkeratosis should be noted. These lesion patterns will afford the evaluator a clue as whether the deformity has a structural or functional cause. An adventitious bursa may be palpated in the area. The skin overlying the joint may be erythematous as a result of friction, pressure, or local trauma caused by shoe gear. Mild to moderate pain may be

palpable in this area. The pain is alleviated by ambulating barefoot, in sandals, or even in jogging shoes.

Range of motion of the fifth metatarsal and its relationship to the axis of the three central metatarsals should be evaluated. Quite commonly, an adducto varus deformity of the fifth digit is found. The foot is also evaluated in the relaxed calcaneal stance position and neutral calcaneal stance position (both weight-bearing and non-weight-bearing). With weight-bearing, the increased degree of deformity is noted. Following this, the subtalar joint is put in the neutral position with the patient standing, and the amount of improvement in the Tailor's bunion is observed. This should give one an idea of the amount of control to expect of the fifth ray with control of the subtalar joint. The foot is finally observed during the gait cycle in comparison with the other foot.

## RADIOGRAPHIC EVALUATION

Radiographs are taken with the patient in the angle and base of gait. The areas to specifically evaluate in association with a Tailor's bunion deformity are (1) rotation of the entire fifth metatarsal, making the lateral plantar tubercle and the styloid process of the fifth metatarsal more prominent; (2) an increased intermetatarsal angle between the fourth and fifth metatarsals; (3) an increased lateral deviation angle; (4) hypertrophy of the fifth metatarsal head; and (5) arthritic changes of the fifth metatarsal head. The specific angles used to evaluate a Tailor's bunion include the intermetatarsal angle and the lateral deviation angle.

Schoenhaus[6] tried to determine the intermetatarsal angle between the fourth and fifth rays and the second and fifth rays. The results showed that the normal intermetatarsal angle between the second and fifth rays is approximately $16° \pm 2°$, and the normal intermetatarsal angle between the fourth and fifth rays is approximately 8°. Angles greater than these were considered pathologic. Fallat and Buckholz[7] in 1980 presented a more comprehensive study to accurately assess the intermetatarsal angle between the fourth and fifth metatarsals, taking into account anatomic variations. They also determined the effect of supinatory and pronatory positions on the intermetatarsal angle and on lateral bowing of the fifth metatarsal. The intermetatarsal angle is measured by comparing the long longitudinal bisection of the fourth metatarsal with a line that is tangent to the proximal one-half of the medial cortex of the fifth metatarsal (Fig. 31-1A). In measuring the proximal one-half of the medial cortex of the fifth metatarsal, the bowing often found at the fifth metatarsal neck does not influence the findings. They reported an average normal of approximately 6.5° with an increase to approximately 8° to 9° in patients with Tailor's bunion deformities.

Lateral bowing of the fifth metatarsal head becomes another factor in radiographic assessment of a Tailor's bunion deformity on the dorsiplantar views. This lateral bowing is usually seen at the distal one-third, or

neck, of the metatarsal, but may arise at the midshaft region of the fifth ray. The lateral deviation angle as described by Fallat and Buckholz is formed by a line bisecting the head and neck of the fifth metatarsal with the line measuring the proximal one-half of the medial cortex of the fifth metatarsal (Fig. 31-1B). The average normal lateral deviation angle was measured at approximately 2.5°, whereas an average value of approximately 8° was noted in the pathologic foot. An angle of 5° warranted an osteotomy at the neck of the fifth metatarsal.

With radiographic evaluation, the deformity will either lie in one or more of the following areas: (1) the

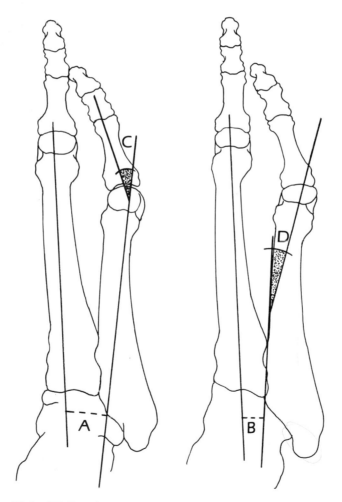

**Fig. 31-1.** (**A**) Fourth intermetatarsal angle; (**B**) lateral deviation angle.

fifth metatarsal base, (2) the fifth metatarsal neck, (3) the lateral condyle of the fifth metatarsal, or (4) the entire articulating surface of the fifth metatarsal.

## SURGICAL RECOMMENDATIONS AND CONSIDERATIONS

Ideally, when considering and planning fifth metatarsal surgical correction of a Tailor's bunion deformity, It is important to identify the deformity, perform stable osteotomies with appropriate fixation, follow logical postoperative care, and recognize problems that arise and have the flexibility to alter management.

Historically, Davies[1] in 1949 described a simple lateral exostectomy (Fig. 31-2). Others copied him and later did partial exostectomies or exostectomies combined with soft tissue procedures. The soft tissue procedures included a medial vertical ligament release, freeing the flexor cap, performing an inverted L capsulotomy with ellipses, and an abductor digiti minimi transfer to help achieve and maintain correction and decrease recurrence or dislocation of the Tailor's bunion deformity. Lelievre[2] described an adaptation of the Keller arthroplasty (Fig. 31-3) that increased tone and function of the medial periarticular structures; this caused further varus or adducto varus of the fifth toe with an increase in retrograde forces on the fifth metatarsal head.

Weisberg[8] and Amberry[9] described a fifth metatarsal head resection with a lateroplantar condylectomy of the proximal phalanx of the fifth toe (Fig. 31-4). The indications for performing a fifth metatarsophalangeal joint arthroplasty were a dumbbell-shaped metatarsal head with no other pathology noted. The usefulness of an arthroplasty as an isolated procedure is rather limited. Undercorrection, recurrence, loss of congruity, or dislocation at the fifth metatarsophalangeal joint are relatively common sequelae of this procedure. These are explained when one understands that there is a dynamic imbalance of the joint secondary to these procedures which increases the deformity. The lateral capsular structures are weakened, and recurrence is facilitated. When joint destruction is obvious on radiography, a complete or hemi-head resection is performed on the fifth metatarsal head. An effort is made to draw as much capsule as possible together in the center of the joint through a pursestring suture. This helps to maintain the digit in a proper position postoperatively. Implant arthroplasty has been performed in this area; however, it is not recommended because of the extreme range of motion of the fifth ray during gait.

When one is planning an osteotomy of the fifth metatarsal for correction of a Tailor's bunion deformity, principles of fixation, bone healing, and the degree of deformity need to be addressed. Stability of the osteotomy site is required for optimal healing. Fixation must stabilize fragments until bone healing has occurred after 5 to 6 weeks. This is especially true for diaphyseal bone in which the blood supply is decreased and nonunion and malunion are common. Floating osteotomies are less than optimal. The ex-

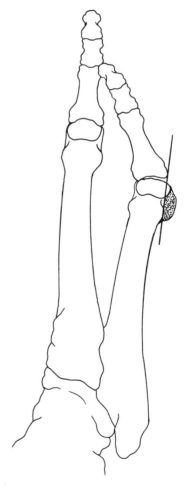

**Fig. 31-2.** Lateral exostectomy.

treme independent range of motion of the fifth meta-tarsal makes an osteotomy of the fifth metatarsal in this area nearly impossible to heal without fixation.

Use of a fifth metatarsal neck osteotomy is indicated when the apex of the deformity is at the fifth metatarsal neck. Neck osteotomies are performed quite frequently today. In a study by Keating[10], patients stated that they were extremely satisfied with neck osteotomies, but the recurrence of the deformity was approximately 12 percent and the occurrence of transfer lesions approximately 76 percent. Of the 76 percent transfer lesions present, 36 percent were very symptomatic. The success rates of neck osteotomies to correct Tailor's bunion deformities averaged approxi-

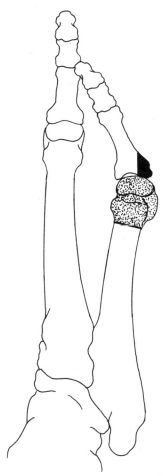

**Fig. 31-4.** Fifth metatarsal head resection with lateral plantar condylectomy of the proximal phalanx of the fifth toe as described by Weisberg and Amberry.

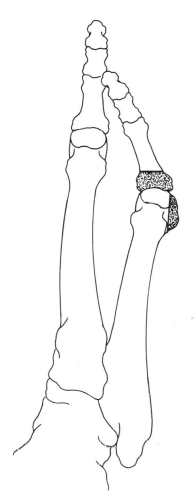

**Fig. 31-3.** Adaption of Keller arthroplasty as described by Lelievre.

mately 56 percent. Therefore, it is imperative to recognize the apex of the deformity when planning surgical correction. In 1951, Hohmann[11] described a single transverse osteotomy at the level of the metatarsal neck with medial displacement of the capital fragment toward the fourth metatarsal (Fig. 31-5). This is usually fixated with a single Kirschner wire (K-wire). A Wilson-type displacement osteotomy, or rather reverse Wilson osteotomy, is described as an oblique osteotomy from distal lateral to proximal medial with displacement of the capital fragment medially (Fig. 31-6). The osteotomy is orientated in a perpendicular relationship to the long axis of the fifth metatarsal when viewed laterally. Shortening is noted to occur

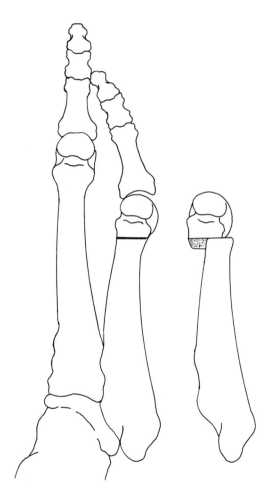

**Fig. 31-5.** Hohmann osteotomy.

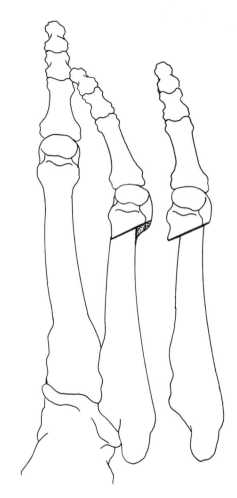

**Fig. 31-6.** Wilson-type displacement osteotomy.

with this osteotomy. A distal oblique osteotomy described by Helal[12] in 1975 was orientated in a dorsal-proximal to plantar-distal direction with respect to the fifth metatarsal. This was to be perpendicular to the weight-bearing surface of the foot. Complications of this procedure encouraged telescoping of the fragments.

The Mitchell displacement osteotomy as described by Leach[13] in 1974 was advocated in patients with intermetatarsal angles greater than 9° between the fourth and fifth metatarsals (Fig. 31-7). The reverse Austin or sagittal plane **V** sliding osteotomy allows for displacement of the head of the fifth metatarsal medi-

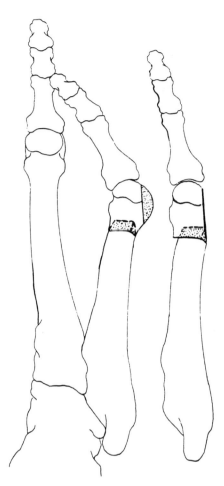

**Fig. 31-8.** Reverse Austin/sagittal plane **V** sliding osteotomy.

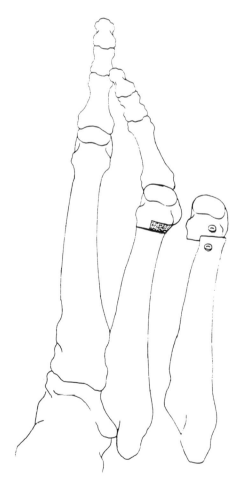

**Fig. 31-7.** Mitchell displacement osteotomy.

ally 2 mm with resection of a small amount of bone from the lateral aspect of the fifth metatarsal head (Fig. 31-8). This corrected only in the transverse plane, and is usually fixated with K-wires. Closing wedge osteotomies have been described by Mercado,[14] Gerbert,[15] and Buchbinder[16] (Fig. 31-9). Mercado[14] advocated a medially based closing wedge osteotomy at the neck of the fifth metatarsal, which was performed at the point of greatest deviation of the shaft of the fifth metatarsal and was fixated with K-wire or an intramedullary cortical bone plug graft. Yancy[17] described a closing base wedge osteotomy at the junction of the middle and distal one-third of the metatarsal that was fixated performing a distal oblique wedge osteotomy for the correction of a Tailor's bunion deformity is that the primary level of the deformity is the lateral bowing in the distal portion of the metatarsal. This procedure involves two oblique cuts with an appropriate wedge resection removed. Key conceptual factors involve the distal cut, which should be placed at approximately 60° to the long axis of the fifth metatarsal, and the proximal cut, which will vary with the degree of the deformity. The lateral hinge should be preserved, and this osteotomy must be fixated. Potential complications of this procedure include proximal lateral cortical hinge fracture, fracture displacement, excessive wedge resection, and recurrence of the lateral exostosis.

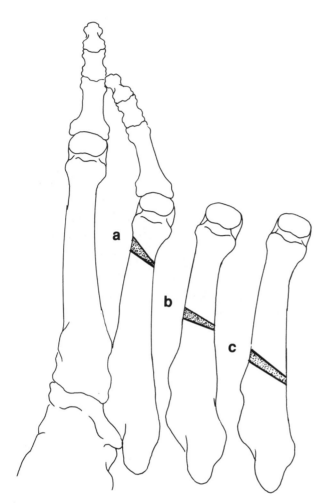

**Fig. 31-9.** Closing wedge osteotomies as described by (**A**) Mercado, (**B**) Yancey, and (**C**) Gerbert.

with K-wire (Fig. 31-10). This procedure must be fixated, and there must be good bone-to-bone contact, or delayed union, nonunion, or pseudoarthrosis may result.

A closing base wedge osteotomy is performed when the apex of the deformity is at the metatarsal base. This type of oblique wedge osteotomy is fixated according to AO/ASIF protocol, whereas a transverse/arcuate osteotomy has been fixated with K-wire or monofilament wire. Buchbinder[16] described a derotational angular transpositional osteotomy that involved a small resection of bone perpendicular to the fifth metatarsal and 2 to 3 cm distal to its base. The key indicator to

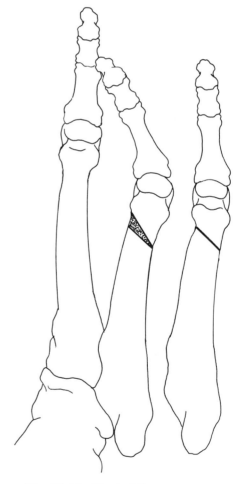

**Fig. 31-10.** Distal oblique osteotomy.

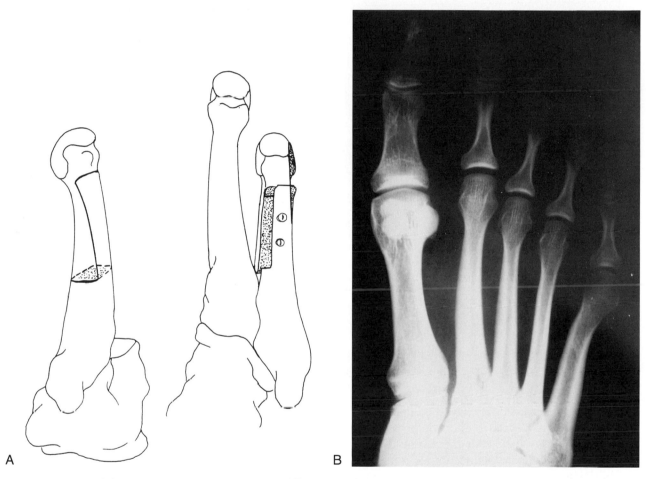

**Fig. 31-11.** (**A**) Diagram depicting transpositional **Z** osteotomy; (**B**) preoperative radiograph; (*Figure continues.*)

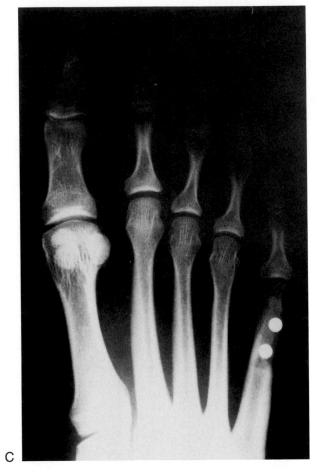

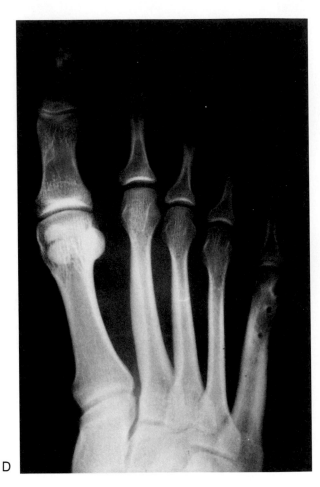

**Fig. 31-11** (*Continued*). (**C**) postoperative radiograph; (**D**) postoperative radiograph after screw removal.

Many surgical procedures have been described for correction of the Tailor's bunion deformity, encompassing all levels of the fifth metatarsal. It becomes readily apparent that no one technique is adequate in treating all forms of fifth metatarsal pathology. Complications are well documented, including delayed union or nonunion, floating fifth digit, transfer lesions to adjacent metatarsals, and recurrence of the deformity. The selection of the surgical procedure is most accurate when based on the preoperative radiographic findings as advocated by Fallat and Buckholz.[7] With a significantly increased intermetatarsal angle, the procedure of choice may be a base wedge osteotomy. The more proximal axis allows a longer radius arm so that greater medial displacement of the fifth metatarsal

head can be achieved with every degree of wedge resected. Procedures done at the base, however, demand excellent reduction with internal fixation as well as strict non-weight-bearing postoperatively.

When the primary focus of the deformity is lateral bowing of the distal metatarsal, the surgical osteotomy should be directed at this level. When the main focus of the deformity is at the distal neck of the fifth metatarsal, or the intermetatarsal angle is mild to moderate, neck osteotomies can be quite satisfactory. With a significantly increased intermetatarsal angle and significant bowing of the distal metatarsal, the author would recommend a transpositional **Z** osteotomy with 2.0 screw fixation (Fig. 31-11). This horizontally directed **Z** osteotomy as described by Gudas and Zygmunt

(1983–1990, University of Chicago) for correction of hallux valgus allows for a potentially longer radius arm so that greater medial displacement of the fifth metatarsal head can be effected. The importance of adequate internal fixation cannot be stressed enough with this procedure. Complications of this technique include fracture through the shaft distal to the proximal cut as well as those previously mentioned.

## CONCLUSION

A comprehensive literature review and logical approach to the treatment of a symptomatic Tailor's bunion deformity has been introduced. As one can deduce, no state-of-the-art procedure can be presented for the correction of this fifth ray deformity. The etiologic factors, preoperative assessment, and focus of the deformity should be thoroughly assessed to achieve a successful outcome.

## REFERENCES

1. Davies H: Metatarsus quintus valgus. Br Med J 1:664, 1949
2. Leliévre J: Exostosis of the head of the fifth metatarsal bone. Concours Med 78:4815, 1956
3. DuVries HL: Surgery of the Foot. 3rd Ed. CV Mosby, St. Louis, 1973
4. Sgarlato TE: Compendium of Podiatric Biomechanics. California College of Podiatric Medicine, San Francisco, 1971
5. Root ML, Orien WP, Weed JH: Normal and Abnormal Function of the Foot. Clinical Biomechanics, Los Angeles, 1977
6. Schoenhaus H, Rotman S, Meshon AL: A review of normal intermetatarsal angles. J Am Podiatry Assoc 63:88, 1973
7. Fallat L, Buckholz J: An analysis of the tailors bunion by radiographic and anatomic display. J Am Podiatry Assoc 70:597, 1980
8. Weisberg MH: Resection of the fifth metatarsal head in lateral segment problems. J Am Podiatry Assoc 57:374, 1967
9. Amberry TR: Foot surgery. p. 168. In Weinstein F (ed): Principles and Practice of Podiatry. Lea & Febiger, Philadelphia, 1967
10. Keating S: Oblique fifth metatarsal osteotomy: a follow-up study. J Foot Surg 21:104, 1982
11. Hohmann G: Fuss and Bein. JF Bergmann, Muenchen, 1951
12. Helal B: Metatarsal osteotomy for metatarsalgia. J Bone Joint Surg Br 57:187, 1975
13. Leach RE, Igou R: Metatarsal osteotomy for bunionette deformity. Clin Orthop Relat Res 100:171, 1974
14. Mercado OA: An Atlas of Foot Surgery. Vol. 1. Carlando Press, Oak Park, 1979
15. Gerbert J, Sgarlato TE, Subotnick SI: Preliminary study of a closing wedge osteotomy of the fifth metatarsal for correction of a tailors bunion deformity. J Am Podiatry Assoc 62:212, 1972
16. Buchbinder IJ: Drato procedure for tailors bunion. J Foot Surg 21:177, 1982
17. Yancey HA: Congenital lateral bowing of the fifth metatarsal. Clin Orthop Relat Res 62:203, 1969

# 32

# Amputation of the Foot

*EDWARD L. CHAIRMAN*

With the increasing success rate of various treatments for dysvascular limbs, partial amputations of the foot are becoming much more frequent. Peripheral vascular disease, neuropathy, severe infection, diabetes, and trauma do not require a patient to undergo a below-knee or above-knee amputation as often as in the past. More aggressive vascular surgery, plastic reconstructive surgery (i.e., flaps), and medication allow the physician to improve the chance of success for a partial amputation of the foot.

With the increased use of partial amputations, surgeons have developed many modifications of old standard procedures. These modifications have improved the chance of long-term viability and decreased secondary breakdown from friction, imbalance, and other medical and surgical complications.

In addition to the causes just noted, amputation is also used to treat trauma, malignancies, congenital and acquired deformities, and even cosmesis.[1]

Amputation should be considered a treatment. It is a method of increasing the patient's ability to ambulate. If the patient has no chance of ambulating with a partial amputation, then a more proximal amputation should be considered. Every consideration should be given to maximizing the function of the remaining portion of the extremity while considering, at the same time, its viability. The level of the foot amputation is dependent upon many variables. Invasive and noninvasive vascular testing along with the surgeon's subjective and objective clinical evaluation of other factors such as neuropathy, infection, necrosis, malignancy, function, and rehabilitation determine the most appropriate level of amputation and necessary modifications.

All amputations should be approached with the knowledge that a more proximal amputation may be necessary once the surgical intervention begins. Surprises are not uncommon. Devitalized necrotic tissue may be hidden by a superficial flap that appears viable. At this point, the surgical experience and creativity of the surgeon is put to a test. All nonviable tissue must be removed. As the surgery proceeds, modifications and various plastic revisions are designed to overcome problems of atypical anatomy.

In the following descriptions of various types of amputations, certain rules are common to all. In general, the more distal the site of amputation the more functional the foot remains.

Skin flaps should not be undermined layer by layer. They should be dissected from the bone as one thick combination layer of skin, subcutaneous tissue, and muscle. Nonviable tissue obviously has to be dissected from the flap. Flaps should be as broad based as possible to avoid compromising the blood supply. Although they are full thickness, the edges should not be bulky or redundant.[2]

Tension at the incision line must be avoided at all costs. The incision must be sutured with nonabsorbable material (e.g., prolene, ethilon). Vertical mattress alternating with simple sutures have proven to be very successful. A distance of approximately 1 cm between the sutures allows for drainage postoperatively. "Pretty" repairs are not necessarily advantageous to the healing of an amputation site. Drains are generally used when the surgeon believes it is necessary. The amount of drainage and seepage in the surgical site is easily determined if the surgeon does not use a tourniquet for the procedure.

All nerves should be cut at a site well proximal to the incision and preferably in a well-cushioned soft tissue mass. This helps avoid irritation by pressure from the prosthesis or other shoe gear. Traction neuropathy can be avoided by not pulling on the nerves when dissecting.[2] All bone edges left in the surgical site should be rounded off and rasped smooth. Bone wax should be avoided on bone edges to avoid any chance of a foreign body reaction.[2]

Dressings of an amputation site should provide mild to moderate compression but no proximal constriction. Ice and elevation are used postoperatively only if the leg is not ischemic. Early weight-bearing will negate the best surgical technique. However, range-of-motion exercises and muscle strengthening can be started at an early stage.

It should be noted that not all amputations can be finished with primary closure. At times, the wound must be packed open and a second or third surgery will be necessary to debride infected and nonviable tissue before closure. When this is the case, the original flaps should be approximately 20 percent longer than would be used to cover the stump in primary closure; this allows for shrinkage of the flaps.[3]

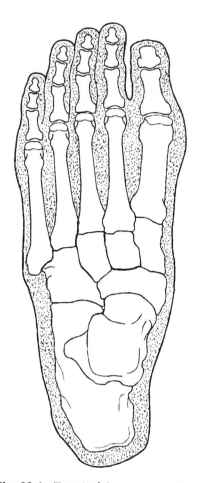

**Fig. 32-1.** Terminal Symes amputation.

## SYME TERMINAL AMPUTATION

The Syme terminal amputation has been used by many surgeons to overcome an onychauxic or mycotic and ingrown nail. The procedure includes the radical excision of the matrix, nail, and nailbed along with the distal half of the distal phalanx (Fig. 32-1).

### Technique

The plantar incision is distal to the more proximal dorsal skin flap, which is made at the level of the intended bone resection. Using a power saw, a transverse osteotomy is performed at the junction of the proximal and middle one-third of the phalanx. The osteotomy is performed so that the plantar surface is more proximal than the dorsal surface. All edges are contoured and rasped smooth. The area is flushed copiously with sterile saline and antibiotic irrigant. The plantar flap is then brought dorsally and trimmed to the proper length allowing closure without tension. Vertical mattress or simple sutures are used to approximate the incision line. Betadine-soaked sterile dressings followed by dry sterile fluff and mild compression are used to dress the wound.[4]

Although this procedure is still in vogue, many plastic procedures can be used to overcome the onychauxic nail with the hypertrophied tuft. Amputation of the distal portion of the toe is not necessarily the best approach to overcome a cosmetic problem but works well to eliminate an ulcerated or nonviable area where the proximal tissue is still viable.

# LESSER TOE AMPUTATION

When lesser toes are individually amputated, several techniques may be applied. The significant fact to remember is that any closure of the amputated stump should be tension free. Whether one uses a plantar flap, a dorsal flap, variations of side flaps, or elliptical incisions, lack of tension is the most significant technical requirement for success in an amputation where all other preoperative criteria were fulfilled.

The technical approach to the amputation varies with the incision line. The optimal site for a digital amputation is at the level of the metatarsophalangeal joint. The choice of incision depends on the anatomy of the forefoot. Whether the incision is elliptical or flap, the surgical approach after the incision is basically the same.

My preference is to perform this amputation with a tear-shaped incision in the web around the toe (Fig. 32-2). The apex of the incision is dorsal. The dorsal part of the incision is carried proximally over the metatarsophalangeal joint. With sharp and blunt dissection, the surrounding skin and subcutaneous tissue are reflected aside. All bleeders are cauticated. The extensor and flexor tendons are pulled distally and severed at their most proximal portion in the wound. The capsule is then incised, allowing the surgeon to remove the toe in toto. If dead space is a concern, the base of the proximal phalanx may be left intact.

If there is redundant subcutaneous tissue, it is dissected out of the wound. However, in most cases this is not the fact. Nonviable tissue is removed. If it is determined that the nonviable tissue continues proximally, a more radical amputation (i.e., ray amputation or possibly transmetatarsal amputation) should be considered at this time. If all nonviable tissue is adequately removed from the wound, the subcutaneous tissue can be approximated over the metatarsal head with absorbable sutures. This acts as a cushion. It is my preference to leave the cartilage on the metatarsal head intact; I only remove the cartilage when it shows signs of nonviability. The skin is approximated with a nonabsorbable suture (i.e., prolene or ethilon). Vertical mattress sutures interspersed with single interrupted sutures allow for an adequate closure without tension.

The wound is then dressed with betadine-soaked sterile dressings followed by dry sterile fluff and mild

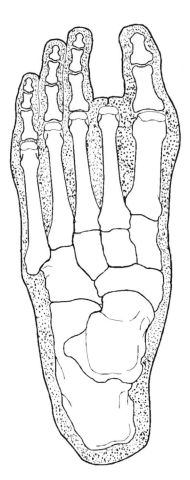

**Fig. 32-2.** Lesser toe amputation.

compression. No Ace bandage is used. Depending on the viability and circulation of the remaining limb, surgeons should use their judgment in recommending ice or elevation. I do not find it necessary to use a drain in digital amputations. However, if in one's judgment a drain is needed, it should be inserted at the most plantar aspect of the incision, allowing for gravity drainage.

There should be no rush to remove the sutures postoperatively. Most patients who require amputations of any sort usually require more time for healing. It is not uncommon to allow sutures to remain for more than 30 days if the surgeon judges this to be necessary.

Prostheses for amputated toes are as varied as surgical approaches to amputation. Whatever material is used, a prosthesis is to act as a spacer between the remaining toes. If a second toe is being amputated and a hallux valgus already exists, it is not necessary to provide any spacer. However, if no hallux valgus exists, it is very likely that one will develop if the second toe is amputated.[5] A spacer slows down the progression of the hallux valgus but does not stop it. In addition to the consideration of a spacer, the surgeon should prescribe a metatarsal bar behind the metatarsal heads to allowing for toe-off without increased stress on the affected metatarsal head.

Amputation of two or more lesser toes modifies the initial incision and approach somewhat. The toes can be removed individually as previously noted, or a combined incision around the affected toes can be considered. Curvilinear incisions made on the dorsal and plantar aspect of the affected toes meet at the medial and lateral aspects (Fig. 32-3). The affected toes are then removed in similar fashion to that used for individual toes. The plantar flap is pulled dorsally to meet the dorsal incision. Vertical mattress and simple interrupted sutures are used to approximate the wound.

## AMPUTATION OF THE HALLUX

The anatomy of the hallux requires us to approach its amputation differently than we would that of a lesser toe. Because the base of the proximal phalanx is used for the insertion of various tendons, an attempt is made to save it.

If the plantar flap is viable, a more distal transverse curilinear incision is made at the level of the midproximal phalanx. A corresponding dorsal curvilinear incision is made over the base of the proximal phalanx. Both incisions meet on the medial and lateral aspect of the toe. It has been my practice to place my initial incisions as distal as possible allowing modification of flaps at closure.

After the incision is made, sharp and blunt dissection separates the subcutaneous tissue from the bone. The dorsal and plantar flaps are retracted proximally allowing the surgeon to expose the dorsum of the base of the proximal phalanx. The extensor hallucis longus and flexor hallucis longus tendons are severed, and depending on the viability of the limb and the patient may be sutured into the capsule of the metatar-

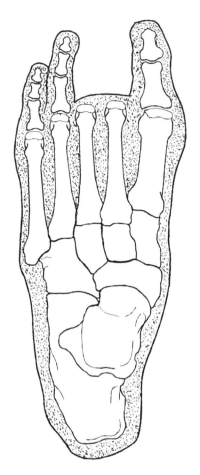

**Fig. 32-3.** Adjacent toe amputation.

sal phalangeal joint. A transverse osteotomy is performed at the junction of the proximal and middle thirds of the proximal phalanx. The osteotomy should be slightly more proximal on its plantar aspect. The remaining edges of the proximal phalanx are rasped smooth with a bone rasp followed by copious flushing with sterile saline and an antibiotic solution. With the hallux removed the plantar flap should be approximated dorsally over the base of the proximal phalanx. Keep in mind that the plantar circulation is usually better than the dorsal circulation. All excess skin and subcutaneous tissue can be removed when remodeling the flap.

Ideally, the base of the proximal phalanx should be saved,[6] but this is not always practicable. Variations of hallux amputation include the removal of the proximal and distal phalanx allowing the metatarsal head to remain. Attempts should be made to suture the flexor hallucis brevis tendon into the distal portion of the capsule of the metatarsal phalangeal joint. This will allow the patient to maintain the sesamoids in a proper position. Additional attempts should be made to suture the flexor and extensor hallucis longus tendons together, allowing good function at this level. Plantar flaps are ideal for this type of amputation. However, medial plantar flaps may be more practical, depending on the remaining tissue viability.

In practice, I find it necessary to remove the first metatarsal head when it is necessary to do a full hallux amputation. My experience indicates that this prevents breakdown at the medioplantar and plantar aspects of the first metatarsal head postoperatively. The surgical technique for this procedure is modified to allow for a plantar medial flap to close the wound. The skin should not be underscored superficially. Full thickness separation of bone from subcutaneous tissue is done with adequate blunt and sharp dissection.

The osteotomy is performed approximately at the level of the junction of the middle and distal one-thirds of the first metatarsal. The osteotomy is performed from dorsal to plantar in an oblique fashion allowing the dorsolateral aspect to be distal while the medial plantar aspect is proximal. The plantar edge of the remaining shaft of the metatarsal should be rasped smooth. No spurs or rough edges should be allowed. The area is copiously flushed with saline and antibiotic irrigant. The plantar medial flap is approximated over the remaining metatarsal and remodeled to close without tension. When suturing the flap, care should be taken to ensure that the lateral sutures do not ligate any of the vasculature leading to the second toe. The sutures should be placed approximately 1 cm apart allowing for drainage postoperatively.

If a drain is warranted, it should be placed at the most proximal plantar portion of the wound allowing for gravity drainage. A betadine-soaked sterile dressing followed by dry sterile fluff and gauze is applied to the wound with mild compression. The surgeon's judgment is needed to determine whether application of an Ace bandage is appropriate or whether ice and elevation are required postoperatively (Fig. 32-4).

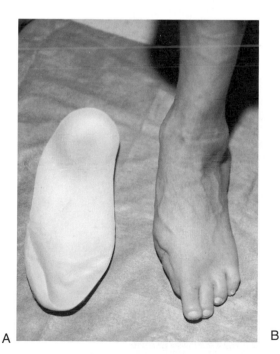 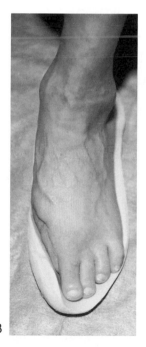 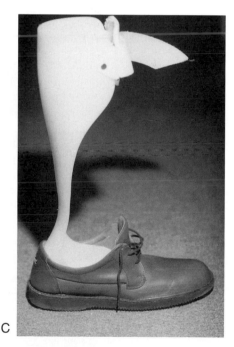

A        B        C

**Fig. 32-4.** (**A & B**) A plastasote molded insole to accommodate altered weight-bearing of the foot following hallux amputation with partial first ray resection. (**C**) Function can further be enhanced by the use of appropriate shoe and orthotic devices, for example, a posterior foot-ankle orthosis.

## METATARSAL RAY RESECTION

Metatarsal ray resection is used in cosmesis (removing a supernumerary ray) and in excision of devitalized tissue. The procedure is an excellent method in removing the cause of chronic ulcerations (Fig. 32-5). Technique and postoperative care must be altered for various ray resections. Again, tension in the flap must be avoided. Removal of one or more of the metatarsals causes a shift in the weight-bearing of the remaining metatarsals. Compensation must be considered in postoperative orthosis and gait training.

## Technique

It is advantageous to do this procedure without a tourniquet. However, this is left to the judgment of the surgeon. The incision varies from a racket type around the base of the toe, with an elongated handle dorsally allowing exposure of much of the metatarsal shaft, to elliptical incisions around the base of the toe and ulceration with a dorsal extension. Again, the surgeon's judgment is necessary in planning the actual incision that will allow for good exposure, avoidance of dead space, and no tension on the incision line. Once the incision is made, sharp and blunt dissection are used to separate the metatarsal from the surrounding tissue. Using a power saw, the proximal portion of the metatarsal shaft should be transected in an oblique manner allowing the plantar surface of the remaining stump to be more proximal than the dorsal surface. The edges of the remaining stump should be rasped smooth. The area should be flushed copiously with sterile saline and antibiotic irrigant. All devitalized tissue should be

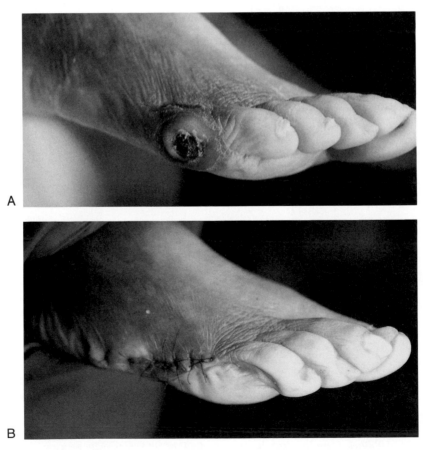

**Fig. 32-5.** Chronic ulceration of the area of the fifth metatarsal head managed by resection of the toe and part of the metatarsal. (**A**) Preoperative; (**B**) postoperative.

removed. Extensor and flexor tendons inserting into the affected ray should be dissected proximally and if possible reinserted into a more proximal position at the base of the affected metatarsal.

Drains should be used when excessive bleeding or oozing is noted or infection is present. In fact, the surgeon may decide to leave the incision open and pack it if infection is present.

When the first or fifth rays are to be amputated, the incision should be made in such a way as to allow as much of the plantar medial or plantar lateral flap to be brought up and approximated dorsally. When the first and second rays are removed, postoperative ambulation causes increased weight-bearing on the lesser metatarsals and a medial shifting of the lesser digits. This shift in weight-bearing and position then cause additional ulcerations that ultimately lead to further amputation.

Although I personally have been successful in first and second metatarsal amputations, it is my opinion in general that a transmetatarsal amputation will be more successful. Patients may find amputation of the first and second ray easier to accept but with proper instruction can realize they have a better chance statistically by choosing a transmetatarsal amputation.

# TRANSMETATARSAL AMPUTATION

In my experience, transmetatarsal amputations are very successful (Figs. 32-6 and 32-7). Certain criteria are required for this statement to be valid. It is obvious that circulatory viability is a must. If gangrene is present, it must be well demarcated distal to the amputation site. The plantar flap must be viable for successful closure. Infection, if present, must be under control.

Transmetatarsal amputations may necessarily be performed in two phases. However, the following technique is described as if one surgery is being done.

## Technique

Although some surgeons make their initial dorsal incision at the level of the amputation site desired, it is my preference to make both the plantar and dorsal incisions as distal as possible allowing remodeling of the

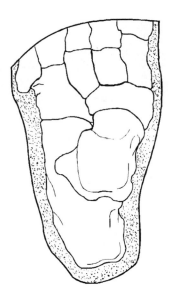

**Fig. 32-6.** Transmetatarsal amputation.

flap at closure. It is not uncommon to require a two-step surgical approach to transmetatarsal and more proximal amputations. Thus, as stated previously, the dorsal and plantar flaps should be approximately 20 percent longer than will be necessary to close over the stump in a second surgery. This allows for the normal shrinkage of the flaps between the primary and secondary operations.[3]

The actual level of the transmetatarsal amputation varies from just proximal to the metatarsal head to just distal of the bases of the metatarsals. The choice of the level of transmetatarsal amputation depends on the amount of viable tissue needed to allow soft tissue closure without tension plus the viability and function of the remaining stump.

The plantar and dorsal incisions are transverse curvilinear. They meet more proximally at a sharp point on the medial and lateral sides of the foot. Dissection is carried down to bone without dissecting planes. The skin, subcutaneous tissue, muscle, and other tissues are dissected in toto and separated from the bone. The transverse osteotomy of the metatarsals is done in a parabolic fashion allowing for medial and lateral beveling on the first and fifth metatarsals, respectively.

The osteotomy of all five bones should be done in such a fashion that the cut should be from dorsal distal to plantar proximal. This will ultimately allow ambula-

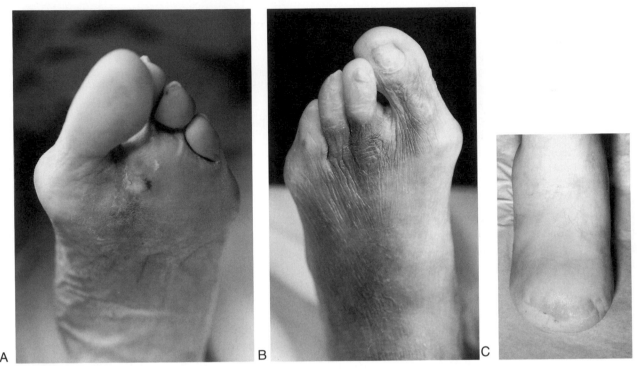

**Fig. 32-7.** (**A & B**) Preoperative views of recurrent plantar ulceration in a patient with insensitivity who underwent prior amputation of the second digit. The patient's ulceration was managed by transmetatarsal amputation. (**C**) A well-healed transmetatarsal amputation.

tion without causing irritation or friction on the plantar-distal aspect of the foot. Care should be taken to dissect and sever all nerves proximal to the actual osteotomy site. Tendons should be pulled distally and severed proximally, allowing them to then retract out of the amputation site.

When the surgeon is confident that all the nonviable tissue has been dissected out, it is time to revise the plantar and dorsal flap in such a manner that the ultimate repair is on the dorsum of the metatarsals. Dog ears in the corners are avoided by bringing the original plantar and dorsal incisions to a sharp corner on the medial and lateral aspect.

Care is taken to close the incision with no tension. Number 2-0 vertical mattress sutures are used to approximate the skin and subcutaneous tissue. All sutures should be at least 1 cm apart. Drains are used if the surgeon judges they are necessary for removal of

exudate and blood. I have found that repair of the incision with sutures 1 cm apart often eliminates the need for a drain. The gapping of the incision allows drainage along the total incision line. Betadine-soaked sterile dressings followed by dry sterile fluff and mild compression work well to minimize edema and dehiscence.

Sutures are left in for at least 3 to 4 weeks and sometimes longer. Early ambulation is absolutely contraindicated. I have found that any weight-bearing stresses the incision line and should be avoided for at least 1 month. Range-of-motion exercise at the ankle level can be started immediately after surgery but no weight-bearing is permitted. Earlier ambulation can be successful if a short leg walking cast is used. However, my preference is to keep a full range of motion at the ankle level and eliminate all weight-bearing for 4 weeks.

## LISFRANC AMPUTATION

The Lisfranc amputation is defined as a tarsal metatarsal disarticulation (Fig. 32-8). We should not lose sight of the fact that amputations are varied to suit the remaining viability of the extremity. All the contributing factors that have been discussed in previous amputations are relevant here.

Although a Lisfranc amputation is a disarticulation at the tarsal metatarsal joint, it should be noted that this amputation must be modified to increase its chance of success. Initial incisions through the dorsal and plantar surface are similar to those described for the transmetatarsal amputation. The incisions are made as distal as the viability of the tissue will allow. The plantar and dorsal incisions are transverse curvilinear, meeting at the medial and lateral borders of the foot in a sharp point. Planes are not dissected. All tissue surrounding the bone is separated from the bone and flapped proximally. The tarsal metatarsal joints are incised dorsally and plantarly and disarticulated.

The distal surface of the medial cuneiform protrudes distally in front of the other distal tarsal bones. With this in mind, an attempt should be made to remodel the medial cuneiform in such a way that the medial and plantar aspects are beveled proximally and the anterior aspect should be even with the middle cuneiform. The plantar edge of the middle and lateral cuneiforms as well as the lateral and plantar edges of the cuboid should be beveled in such a manner as to avoid friction on ambulation.

All nerves should be severed proximal to the incision. Tendons should be pulled distally and severed at their most proximal exposure and then allowed to retract out of the amputation site. Ulcers and nonviable tissue should be removed from the surgical site. The dorsal and plantar flap can then be revised in the best possible manner allowing for the final repair to be performed dorsally. As before, dog ears are avoided by bringing the dorsal and plantar incisions together on the medial and lateral aspect in a sharp corner.

No tension should be allowed at the incision site. Number 2-0 nonabsorbable (ethilon, prolene) vertical mattress sutures should be used to approximate the skin and subcutaneous tissue. All sutures should be placed approximately 1 cm apart. As before, I use drains only when I judge that it is necessary for the removal of exudate and blood. The 1-cm gapping between sutures allows for most drainage to be eliminated throughout the incision line. The wound is dressed with betadine-soaked sterile dressings followed by dry sterile fluff and mild compression.

Early ambulation is prohibited. The sutures remain intact for at least 4 weeks. Ambulation is allowed only after the sutures are removed and the incision line is intact. Exercises are permitted for range of motion at the ankle level while the extremity is elevated.

Postoperatively, complications have occurred with this type of disarticulation. Equinovarus is a common post-operative problem leading to ulcers and tyloma on the distal aspect of the foot and the incision line.[7] This has been overcome quite adequately with the reinsertion of the extensor tendons and the peroneal tendons at a more proximal site. Some surgeons perform an achilles tendon lengthening when they think that an equinovarus is probable.[1]

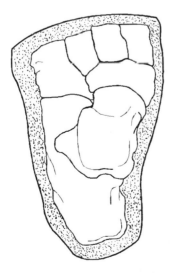

**Fig. 32-8.** Modified Lisfranc amputation.

## CHOPART AMPUTATION

The Chopart amputation (Fig. 32-9) is a disarticulation through the talonavicular and calcaneocuboid joints. The procedure is not commonly performed because of postoperative problems.

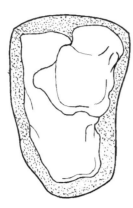

**Fig. 32-9.** Modified Chopart amputation.

The technique is essentially the same as that of a Lisfranc amputation. The dorsal and plantar incision meet more proximally on the medial and lateral border. Dissection of the subcutaneous tissue and muscle down to bone is carried out in a manner similar to the Lisfranc and transmetatarsal procedures. The disarticulation is done at the midtarsal joint. The distal-dorsal and distal-plantar surfaces of the talus and calcaneus, respectively, are beveled in such a manner as to reduce friction on the anterior aspect of the stump. The extensor tendons and tibialis anterior must be reimplanted in the dorsum of the talar head.

Closure of the wound is carried out in the manner already described for the Lisfranc amputation. The dressing is applied with betadine-soaked sterile dressings followed by dry sterile fluff and compression. However, a posterior rigid splint should be used to prevent an equinus deformity. In addition to non-weight-bearing for at least 1 month, the posterior splint must be worn for the same time.

# PIROGOFF, BOYD, AND SYME AMPUTATIONS

More proximal partial foot amputations include the Pirogoff amputation and Boyd amputation. Both amputations are attempts to keep the full length of the extremity and allow weight-bearing using a portion of the calcaneus as an end-bearing stump. The Syme amputation is an actual disarticulation at the ankle joint but a retention of the heel flap for cushioning of the stump.

These more proximal amputations are rarely used. Historically, they present many postoperative complications and difficulty with ambulation. They are mentioned here only as a reference to additional possibilities.

# REFERENCES

1. Wagner WF: Amputations of the foot and ankle. p. 93. In Moore WS (ed). Lower Extremity Amputation. 1st Ed. WB Saunders, Philadelphia, 1989
2. Berardi RS, Keomny: Amputations in peripheral vascular occlusive disease. Am J Surg 135:231, 1978
3. Roach JJ, Deutsch A, McFarlane DS: Resurrection of the amputations of Lisfranc and Choparts for diabetic gangrene. Arch Surg 122:931, 1987
4. Sanders LJ: Amputations in the diabetic foot. Podiatr Med Surg 4:481, 1987
5. Turek SL: Amputations. p. 1487. In Orthopaedics. 3rd Ed. JB Lippincott, Philadelphia, 1977
6. Bohne WH: Toe amputation. p. 37. In Atlas of Amputation Surgery. 1st Ed. Thieme Medical, New York, 1987
7. Greene WB, Cary JM: Partial foot amputations in children. J Bone Joint Surg [AM] 6:438, 1982

# 33

# Nail Surgery

*JOHN E. LACO*

Nail surgery can be divided into two basic categories: excision of the pathologic or undesirable tissue by use of sharp instrumentation, or destruction of the pathologic tissue by physical means such as chemicals, freezing, electrogalvanism, burring, or lasering. Currently, the procedures most popular and most regularly performed are chemical. However, laser surgery is gaining popularity because the public currently perceives laser surgery as being in vogue.

## ANATOMY

It is important to understand the standard terminology used when examining the nail and performing nail surgery. Most terms are fairly common and easy to understand[1] (Fig. 33-1). When reviewing the literature, discrepancies are seen in the exact location of the nail matrix, which is a pivotal point in the success or failure of certain procedures. There seems however to be a general agreement as to the posterior location of the matrix.[1–7]

As depicted[1] (see Fig. 33-1), some authors describe the nail matrix as having a "wrap-around characteristic"[7] and therefore being located dorsal and plantar to the nail root. Others have depicted the nail matrix as being plantar or plantar and proximal to the nail root only. Anatomy text descriptions of the exact location of the nail matrix seem vague and nonspecific. It is suggested at this time that the low recurrence rate of chemical matrixectomies may be attributed to the fact that the nail matrix dorsal to the nail is destroyed by the nature of the procedure, which would lend support to the idea of a wrap-around characteristic of the nail matrix. Further studies specifically designed to

identify the exact location of the nail matrix and its nail borders must be performed.

## DIRECT TRAUMA TO THE NAIL

Direct trauma to the nail from stubbing the toe or a falling object may lead to formation of a subungual hematoma. The subungual hematoma should be evacuated to relieve any pressure that may be being applied to the nail bed and causing the patient pain, as well as relieving any deforming force the hematoma may be applying to the nail itself. Wee and Shieber described using a red-hot paper clip to burn through the nail and decompress the hematoma, thus avoiding use of anesthetics and unnecessary discomfort to the patient.[8] Palamarchuk and Kerzner[9] describe using a hand-held cautery device for evacuation of subungual hematoma. If the podiatric physician has access to a laser, a small, precise portal of evacuation for the subungual hematoma can be created but this will require anesthesia because of the surrounding heat created.

I prefer using a large-bore needle in a rotating fashion to evacuate the hematoma. Minimal pressure is required to penetrate the nail, and anesthesia is usually not necessary. In cases of old subungual hematoma where coagulation has already occurred, a sterile burr may be used to deroof a portion of the nail over the hematoma so that a sterile currette or other instrument can be used to evacuate the coagulated tissue.

Direct trauma may also result in partial lysis or separation of the nail from the nail bed. Usually any type of pressure such as the upper of a shoe will cause excruciating pain. It is recommended that a total nail avulsion be performed to relieve discomfort, prevent fur-

481

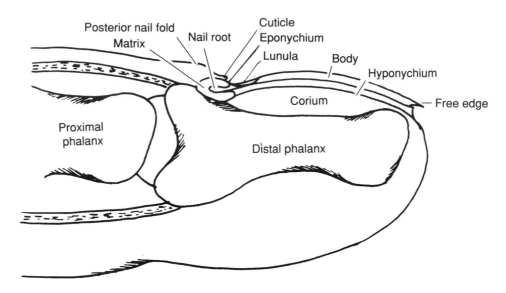

**Fig. 33-1.** Common terminology of nail anatomy. (Illustration by Marlene Burns.) (From Burns et al.,[1] with permission.)

ther traumatic onycholysis, and prevent infection, because a lysed nail is no longer an effective barrier against microbes. Several techniques can be used to perform a total nail avulsion. After suitable prepping and anesthesia, a periosteal elevator or a flat spatula is used to separate the nail from the nail bed, as well as the nail plate from its dorsal attachments to the posterior nail fold. The nail may be avulsed with a hemostat. Forcefully removing the nail from the toe may fragment the nail and unnecessarily traumatize the nail bed and nail matrix. Therefore, adequate separation must be achieved before removal.

Albom recommends using a #24 or #24A dental spatula to separate the nail plate from the nail bed.[10] Scher describes using a dental spatula and avulsing the nail in a proximal to distal manner.[11] Other variations include splitting the toenail in half with an English nail anvil and a #62 blade and avulsing the halves separately. Some clinicians prefer inserting a curved hemostat proximally between the nail plate and the soft tissue underneath the opening the jaws of the hemostat to avulse the nail. After avulsion of the toenail by any means, adequate care should be taken of the exposed area until healing is evident. A long-term follow-up appointment should be made to monitor regrowth of the new nail and prevent "shoveling" (Fig. 33-2).

# ONYCHOCRYPTOSIS
## Etiology

There are many theories on the etiology of onychocryptosis. Many authors believe improper debridement by the patient can lead to ingrown nails.[12–15] Ill-fitting shoes may also be a causative factor.[12,13,16,17] The presence of a subungual exostosis has been stated to be the pathogenesis,[18] and excess soft tissue or soft tissue growing in excess has also been blamed as the etiologic factor for ingrown toenails.[12,14,19–22] Hypermobility of the first metatarsal segment and hallux valgus have been indicated as etiologies of onycho-

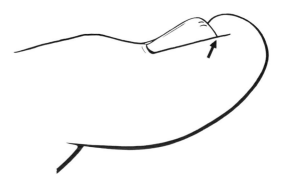

**Fig. 33-2.** "Shoveling" of distal aspect of nail.

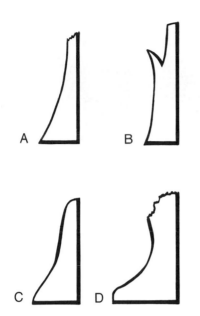

**Fig. 33-3.** Resected ingrown nail borders. (**A**) Wedged; (**B**) spiculated; (**C**) extended nail route; (**D**) combination.

cryptosis.[23] Other causes may be trauma to the nail matrix or nail bed, with a resultant dystrophic nail. Onychomycosis may allow the nail to thicken and grow abnormally, which may result in a cryptotic border. Probably one of the most common causes of paronychia from a cryptotic border is iatrogenic in nature (i.e., bathroom surgery).

## Classifications

Cryptotic nails have been classified into types[24] or stages.[12] However, the ingrown nail is either symptomatic or asymptomatic and is either infected or noninfected. There are certain border presentations that vary from patient to patient, but treatments do not (Fig. 33-3).

The arc of the nail has much to do with symptomatology and infection, as the pathology probably increases with an increasing frontal plane arc of a nail (Fig. 33-4).

## Paronychia

A paronychia is described as a local soft tissue infection surrounding the nail.[25] Onychocryptosis, if severe, will eventually puncture the skin and lead to soft tissue infection. If mistreated long enough, a local cellulitis may progress to systemic involvement with red streaks, swollen lymph glands, fever, and sepsis. Another sequela may be osteomyelitis of the distal phalanx, which will then require debridement and long-term antibiosis. Therefore, it is imperative that a swift and decisive treatment be performed immediately. Antibiotics and foot soaks alone are not adequate treatment to resolve the paronychia. The offending nail that has punctured the skin must be extracted through a partial or total nail avulsion.

A general guideline for treatment of paronychia is as follows. A total nail avulsion should be performed in the most extreme and chronic cases of paronychia,

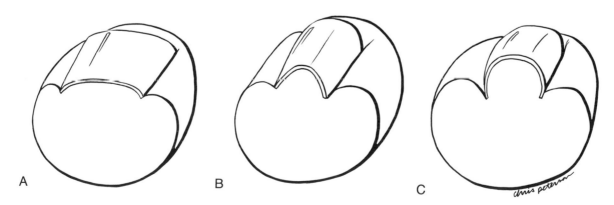

**Fig. 33-4.** Frontal plane arc of nails. (**A**) Normal arc; (**B**) moderate arc; (**C**) severe arc.

especially if the paronychia is of long-term duration. It may also be necessary to perform a total nail avulsion if the nail is dystrophic. Antibiotics in this case are required, along with local care in the form of antiseptic soaks, antiseptic creams, or both. If only one border is involved and inflammation and drainage is evident around the eponychium, an adequate strip of nail that includes the proximal aspect of the nail should be removed. Again, appropriate antibiotics and antiseptic local care are required. However, on the other hand, if paronychia is localized to the nail spicule itself and the nail spicule can e isolated, a partial oblique excision of the nail may be performed. Usually, local antiseptic care without systemic antibiotics will resolve this problem.

A radiographic study is indicated in chronic paronychia of long-term duration to rule out bony involvement, especially if the foregoing measures do not resolve the problem in a reasonable length of time. Also, a chronic unresolving paronychia may not be caused by an ingrown nail exclusively. A case in point is a young woman who presented to the office with inflammation to the distal one-half of the hallux for 2 years. The patient had seen many physicians, but none had taken radiographs. A foreign body was discovered of which the patient was unaware (Fig. 33-5).

At the time of the initial visit, the patient should be informed that there is a high probability of recurrence of the ingrown nail several months after resolution of the paronychia and that a permanent nail removal procedure is recommended in the future. The high recurrence rate for ingrown nails after avulsion is well documented in the literature.[13,26,27]

The permanent removal of an ingrown nail should not be performed unless the paronychia is resolved. Many authors agree that the infection should be eliminated before performing a permanent nail procedure.[2,17,27,28] In fact, postoperative sepis has been reported as a complication when performing surgery on infected toes.[2,28]

Another consideration in the resolution of paronychia is the health status of the patient. Prolonged recovery from a paronychia, high recurrence of paronychia, or multiple occurrences of paronychia may indicate an underlying disease process such as anemia, diabetes, or malnutrition. Of curiosity is the apparent increased rate of paronychia in women after pregnancy. Possible reasons for this may be anemias, edema, tight-fitting shoes, and "crash" diets.

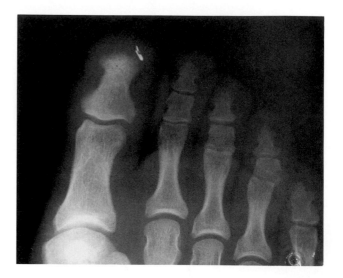

**Fig. 33-5.** Subungal foreign body of hallux.

## Physical Modalities for Permanent Correction of Onychocryptosis

There are several methods using different physical modalities to destroy the nail matrix and correct onychocryptosis. Perrone reported using a high-speed, low-torque air motor with a Busch burr to "erase" the nail matrix.[29] This can be performed for partial or total eradication of nails. Silverman in 1984 described using a liquid nitrogen cryoprobe to destroy the germinal matrix after the nail border was removed.[30] Electrosurgery to treat ingrown nail pathology has been described by many authors.[5,23,31–33] Interestingly enough, one of the mechanisms of destruction is by the production of sodium hydroxide.[5,33] Although one postoperative study seemed to have promising results,[33] electrosurgery for treatment of ingrown nails is not performed on a widespread basis.

Devices and tools have been designed for treatment of onychocryptosis. In 1954, the Steinberg trephine was introduced for surgery of ingrown toenails.[28] A multitude of devices have been described, ranging from a toenail splint[34] to a surgically inserted nail plate[22] to a wire brace[35] to a Teflon plastic strip glued to the toenail.[36] In 1979, the "gutter treatment" was described for treatment of ingrown toenails.[37] Unfortunately, the ease and success of other procedures have overshadowed such devices completely and most have fallen by the wayside.

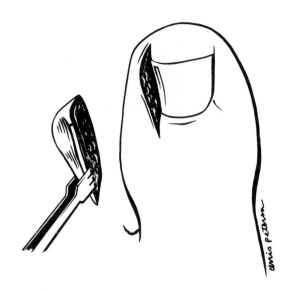

**Fig. 33-6.** Winograd procedure. A pie-wedge incision is used to resect the offending nail plate, nail bed, nail lip, and nail matrix. (From Mercado,[38] with permission.)

## Wedge Resections for Permanent Treatment of Onychocryptosis

### Winograd Procedure

The current concept of the Winograd procedure in podiatry is a wedge resection that includes the nail lip[25,38] and is indicated for onychocryptosis along with a hypertrophied or overlapping ungualabia.[1] In the original procedure described by Winograd, the soft tissue around the margin of the ingrown nail is retracted and preserved.[39,40] A current description of the Winograd procedure is that the nail is split longitudinally and an incision is made down to the bone through the split that extends proximal to the eponychium and distal to the nail itself.[38] A second incision is performed that is semielliptical and is deepened to bone. A wedge resection is then performed. Elements of the wedge are therefore nail plate, nail bed, nail lip, and nail matrix. The periosteum is removed by rasping and the nail lip remodeled before closure (Fig. 33-6).[38]

### Frost Procedure

Although the original Frost procedure was described in 1950,[17] it still maintains a high degree of popularity. The description of the Frost technique from 1950 and 1957 is as follows.[17,24] The entire nail is split at the point where the incurvated nail begins its arc. A vertical incision is then made down to but not into the phalanx and extending beyond either edge of the nail. The inverted L is created by making an incision 90° to the proximal end of the first incision. This incision should be through the dermis but not into adipose tissue. A flap is then underscored and created, taking care not to include any white, fibrous, glistening soft tissue, because this may indicate the nail root. A third incision is made parallel to the first, starting under the flap and extending distally. This incision becomes semielliptical as its courses to join the first incision at the distal aspect of the toe. The section of the nail, nail bed, and root is excised. Care is taken not to damage the periosteum. The area is inspected for white, glistening fibers, which are excised before the flap is replaced. No suturing is recommended, according to Frost (Fig. 33-7).

The indications for a Frost procedure are onychocryptosis; some clinicians do not advocate its use with a concurrent hypertrophic nail lip[38] while others do.[1]

## Phenol and Alcohol Partial Nail Matrixectomy

The most popular and widely used permanent correction of onychocryptosis in the United States is the phenol and alcohol partial nail matrixectomy.

The advantages of this procedure far outweigh its disadvantages of the advantages of other permanent partial nail corrections. The most obvious advantage is the success rate. Gallocher reports a success rate of 98.5 percent.[41] Suppan and Ritchlin report a success rate of 98.7 percent,[42] while Robb and Murray report a recurrence rate of 5 percent. Another advantage is lack of postoperative discomfort.[43–45] Most patients do not require a prescription for postoperative pain, and if discomfort is experienced over-the-counter headache medication will usually suffice. Surgical excision procedures, on the other hand, usually require narcotic analgesics. It has been suggested that the neurolytic action of phenol is responsible for the decreased postoperative pain.[45] One major advantage is lack of disability after the procedure. A patient can usually return to work the same day without losing time from the job. Another advantage is cosmesis. There are no incisions into the skin and therefore no scarring occurs. The

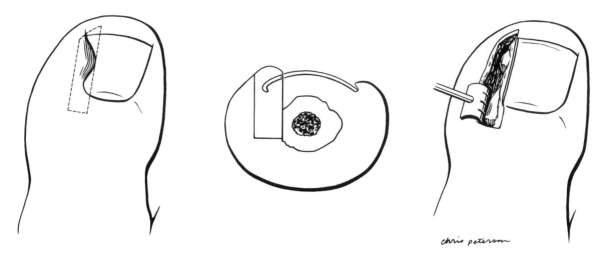

**Fig. 33-7.** Frost nail procedure. (From Frost,[24] with permission.)

procedure is easily performed in an office setting with basic podiatric instruments.

One major disadvantage of this procedure is prolonged healing time[46] and therefore prolonged postoperative care. The phenol is a weak acid and therefore produces a burn. The normal process of healing is an immediate inflammatory reaction and a wound that must drain adequately before final healing occurs. Another disadvantage is that if a patient has a hypertrophic nail lip, plastic remodeling is not part of the procedure. Some clinicians have stated that the procedure is indicated where there is no significant or gross hypertrophy of the ungualabia.[1,42] Some authors believe that a thin, cornified, epidermoid layer secreted by the nail bed after nail matrix destruction may be mistaken for nail plate,[2,12] and this is in fact sometimes observed after phenol and alcohol matrixectomy procedures.

### Description of Procedure

The phenol and alcohol partial matrixectomy procedure has been described on several occasions.[42,43,46–48] After suitable prepping and anesthesia, a penrose drain is applied around the digits for hemostasis. Used here to prevent excessive bleeding and dilution of the phenol, which may cause a recurrence, a penrose drain must always be used with discretion as it is contraindicated in patients with impaired circulation. The nail is split where desired with a nail nipper and onychotome or an English nail anvil. The nail is split under the eponychium with a #61 or #62 blade along the longitudinal striations of the nail. This is a very important point as the nail grows in this direction and if the nail split is not parallel to the striations of the nail, an excessive regrowth of nail may occur that is not anticipated (Fig. 33-8). Note that an English nail anvil will leave a perfectly straight edge of nail but if applied to the nail too far proximally will allow a separation of the nail plate from the nail bed or nail matrix on the desired new nail border. This occurs because of the wedged shape of the lower jaw. This can allow phenol to penetrate into the new nail border bed and matrix areas and create irregularities in the nail border that appear months later.

After the nail is split completely, a spatula or periosteal elevator is used to undermine the nail section to be removed. Once again, it is advised to undermine the nail after the nail is split so that unnecessary undermining of the new nail border is not performed. This is to avoid phenol penetration in those areas and unnecessary damage to the new matrix or nail bed, which may lead to unnecessary border irregularities or lysis of a nail plate, respectively.

A hemostat is used to grasp the nail completely and under the eponychium. The nail is removed by rolling the hemostat to the center of the nail. Removal of the nail should not be forced with the hemostat. Undermining procedures should be repeated again as tear-

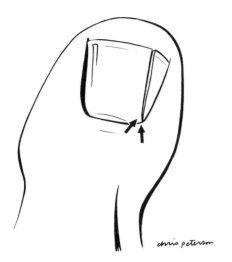

**Fig. 33-8.** Improper splitting of nail for phenol and alcohol matrixectomy. Arrows depict nail matrix not destroyed by phenol. Original border will return.

ing the nail spicule out may fragment the nail spicule and cause unnecessary recurrences. If care is used, an eponychial envelope will be created and the phenol will be applied exactly to the desired areas of destruction. Fibrous tissues are then resected with a currette and tissue nippers, and 85 percent phenol is applied by cotton-tipped applicators, cotton pellets, or with cotton rolled on toothpicks. A handmade toothpick applicator is usually applied for 30 seconds; this is repeated two times. Variations within this time will occur as different applicators vary in the amount of phenol delivered to the desired area of destruction.

Many experienced clinicians will apply phenol by sight as it will burn the tissues and appear white. Many clinicians will also coat the eponychium with a cream or ointment to prevent phenol burn; however, if phenol is applied meticulously, only small amounts of phenol will contaminate the eponychium. The small amounts of phenol contamination can be removed with a sterile gauze. If the phenol applicator is indiscriminately contaminated with ointment or cream, the medication may enter into the nail matrix area, prevent destruction of the nail matrix by the phenol, and therefore provide another reason for recurrence.

After phenol application, the area is flushed with alcohol, the tourniquet released, and appropriate sterile dressings applied, usually after antiseptic applica-

tion of the clinician's choice. Unfortunately, as pointed out be Greenwald and Robbins, no chemical reaction occurs between isopropyl alcohol and phenol under the condition of a matrixectomy and therefore neutralization refers to a physical or mechanical dilution.[49]

### Complications

Complications are recurrence of the nail spicule. As seen from the previous discussion, poor technique may result in recurrence. It should be stressed that phenol does have an expiration date and therefore the date should be checked as this in itself may cause a recurrence. Other complications include losing the whole toenail when performing a bilateral nail border resection. This is especially true with indiscriminate use of the English nail anvil, unnecessary trauma or poor technique, or if the nail is thickened and dystrophic.

A patient may have an acute reaction to the phenol with resulting phenol burn. According to Yale, careless application may result in Beau's lines.[48] Phenol should never be manipulated near the patient as splattering droplets of phenol may burn the integument.

Formation of an abscess may occur after the phenol and alcohol matrixectomy procedure. It is not an infection per se, but emulates an infection because of increased inflammation and expression of purulent drainage on currettement. The abscess is usually very painful. It is postulated that the distal eponychial border forms an eschar and does not allow proper drainage of the phenol burn from an eponychial envelope proximal to it. It is recommended on postoperative visits that a currette or spatula be inserted in the area of the destroyed nail matrix to ensure adequate drainage. Also, during soaking, the patient may massage the eponychial dorsally to prevent premature closure of the eponychium border. These abscesses usually resolve within a few days after debridement and adequate soaking.

### Postoperative Care

Postoperative care varies from clinician to clinician. A straw-colored exudate is expected to drain from the operative site[43,44] and may persist for several weeks. The immediate postoperative response is one of intense inflammation that can certainly have the appearance of an infection. Debridement of the area is a key point to prevent infection. The necrotic, sloughing tissue should be removed on a regular basis to prevent a medium for microbial growth. Also, as mentioned earlier, the eponychial envelope should be cleared of debris to allow for proper draining. If debridement is not performed regularly, a plug of escharotic tissue and callus may form in the nail groove and be as painful as the initial ingrown nail.

Many topical agents have been studied to treat the postoperative phenol and alcohol partial matrixectomy procedure. Some agents that have been reported in the literature are Debrisan,[46] Chymar,[50] and Travase.[51] Combinations such as aqueous Zephiran 1 : 750 solution, metiderm aerosal, and Elase ointment[52] for use immediately after surgery have been reported. Other favorites in this country include Cortisporin otic solution,[53] Silvadene, Neosporin powder and cream, Furacin, and betadine. As noted by Greenwald and Robbins, postoperative creams may be more beneficial than ointments[49] because creams do not inhibit drainage as do petroleum-based waterproof ointments. It is suggested here that if topicals are applied by the physician or patient, probably the most beneficial is a combination of antibiotic cream with an anti-inflammatory steroidal agent. This will provide prophylaxis as well as decrease the intense inflammatory response elicited by the phenol.

More important than topical agents used by the patient are foot soaks. Various agents include normal saline, Domeboros soaks, Epsom salts, tea soaks, betadine and water, vinegar and water, Pedi-boro soaks, and warm soapy water. These soaks will form an ionic solution that should assist in the drainage process. I personally prefer to have the patient begin with betadine soaks; the article by Ranaldi et al. specifically points out reduction in bacterial proliferation after matrixectomy using topical betadine microbicides.[54] After the initial inflammatory reaction has occurred, the patient is switched to a household product such as warm soapy water to enhance patient compliance as well as avoid irritation of the skin from betadine. It should be noted that the detergent Dreft be suggested to the patient if advising soapy water soaks. Because Dreft is specifically designed for laundering baby diapers, many allergenic agents found in other soaps are purposely avoided in the manufacture of this product.

## Nail Spiculectomy

Many patients present to the office with nail spicules or remnants from previous attempts at total nail ablation or a permanent partial removal of the onychocryptosis. These nail spicules may be especially bothersome as they may project superior and become irritated by the uppers of shoes.

These spicules are easily addressed by following the same basic procedure of a phenol and chemical matrixectomy. After suitable prepping and anesthesia, the nail spicule is separated completely from soft tissue using a spatula. Careful separation will identify the "pocket" of residual nail matrix cells. After the nail matrix cells have been delineated, a phenol and alcohol chemical matrixectomy may be performed.

Postoperative visits are important to prevent early closure of the eponychium and abscess formation, as discussed earlier. Most patients are pleased with the results and the procedure itself, as many nail spicules are the results of inadequate sharp tissue resection and can be performed in the office with minimal postoperative pain.

## Partial Phenol and Alcohol Matrixectomy for an Intractable Calloused Nail Groove

Of special interest is the use of a phenol and alcohol partial chemical matrixectomy for treatment of a heloma durum on the lateral nail border of an adducto varus fifth digit (Fig. 33-9).

With such a deformity, it is possible to remove a portion of the nail and prevent recurrence of the heloma dura. However, radiographs should be taken to rule out a bony exostosis on the distal phalanx as a cause of the heloma durum, and a clinical evaluation and discussion with the patient should occur regarding possible derotation of the fifth digit. Admittedly, a derotation of the fifth digit may be advisable, but the patient may not desire that extent of surgery or be able to afford time away from work or any debilitation whatsoever during recovery. It should be pointed out that the patient's chief complaint is the heloma dura on the lateral aspect of the fifth nail and not the abducto varus twist of the fifth digit. This procedure has been performed several times, and the patients seem to be pleased with the results.

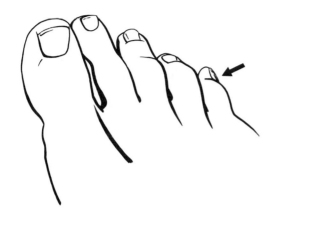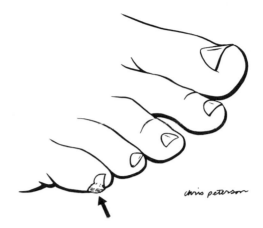

**Fig. 33-9.** Heloma durum lateral nail groove of adducto varus fifth digit.

## Sodium Hydroxide Chemical Matrixectomy

The sodium hydroxide chemical matrixectomy is performed in essentially the same manner as the phenol and alcohol matrixectomy procedure, but sodium hydroxide is used instead of phenol and acetic acid rather than alcohol. Destruction occurs by liquification necrosis[4] and a true chemical neutralization takes place.[49]

Brown applies a 10 percent sodium hydroxide solution with a thinned out cotton-tipped applicator two times for a total of 20 to 25 seconds using pressure for hemostasis and neutralizing with a 3% solution of acetic acid.[55] Travers and Ammon obtain hemostasis with Lidocaine with Epinephrine 1:200,000 or 1:300,000 which allows visualization of the capillaries as they coagulate.[4] They apply cotton pellets with 10% sodium hydroxide solution for 3 seconds to 3 minutes, "until the capillaries of the nail bed visually coagulate." They use a 5% acetic acid solution for neutralization. Sodium hydroxide chemical matrixectomy would probably be more common if the phenol and alcohol matrixectomy were not already an established and popular procedure.

### Advantages

The advantages of the sodium hydroxide chemical matrixectomy over the phenol and alcohol chemical matrixectomy procedure are decreased drainage and therefore decreased recovery time. Also, there seems to be less chance of a violent reaction using sodium hydroxide as opposed to using the phenol (personal communication, Dr. Tom Silver).

## Laser Treatment for Ingrown Nails

The use of the laser for ingrown toenails has received a lot of public attention. The $CO_2$ laser produces an infrared light that is selectively absorbed by water and tissues, and the tissue is vaporized as the light is converted into heat energy.[56] Borovoy et al.[57] report the advantages of a laser as being precise control of depth and extent of the surgical site, as well as sterilization and cauterization.

The problem with laser surgery for onychocryptosis is that the laser beam itself is a straight line and adequate exposure of the matrix is difficult as it is not completely visualized with resection of the nail strip. This may lead to unnecessary destruction of the periosteum and "burning of the bone." Some clinicians will laser the eponychium over the matrix, which again leads to unnecessary destruction. Also, the laser beam will produce a zone of necrosis as the cells adjacent to the vaporized cells are heated to high temperatures. One possible suggestion is to make a small incision in the eponychium so retraction and visualization of the matrix can be attained without unnecessary destruction of soft tissue and bone.

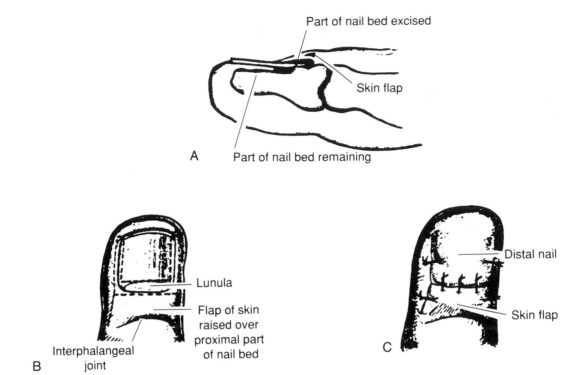

**Fig. 33-10.** (A–C) Zadik procedure. (From Zadik,[3] with permission.)

## Permanent Total Nail Removal

Permanent total nail removal may be advocated in onychogryphosis, onychomycosis, dystrophic nails, and continually recurring cryptotic borders. Trauma to the nail specifically may result in a need for a permanent total nail removal. A deformed nail may be caused by damage to the nail bed or nail matrix.[7] Many partial permanent nail removals discussed earlier may also be used in total nail ablation, including onychotripsy,[29] $CO_2$ surgical laser,[57] phenol and alcohol chemical matrixectomy, and sodium hydroxide chemical matrixectomy. It should be stated once again that a proper and extensive patient history and physical examination be performed to identify high-risk patients such as the vascularly impaired, or the patient who presents with decreased peripheral sensation, relates a history of healing slowly, and then reveals a random blood sugar that is abnormally high. Unfortunately, repeated palliation may be the only choice of treatment. Urea ointment formulations for nonsurgical avulsion of nail dystrophies[58] may also be an option. A double scrub before and after nail avulsion to decontaminate subungual tissues has been suggested,[59] and may be prudent, especially if sharp matrix excision is performed.

### Zadik Procedure

A true Zadik procedure involves creating a skin flap, avulsing the nail, and resecting the nail bed proximal to the border of the lunula.[3] The flap is advanced and sutured to the nail bed without tension. According to Zadik, the lateral nail folds are excised and corresponding coaptation with sutures is performed if the lateral nail furrows are deep. As with certain other total nail ablation procedures, nail bed resection is directed proximally and the nail bed distal to the lunula is undisturbed (Fig. 33-10).

Varying reports of success reveal numbers as low as 16 percent symptomatic recurrence rate for onychocryptosis,[27] to a recurrence rate as high as 28 percent[26] or a 29 percent symptomatic recurrence rate when

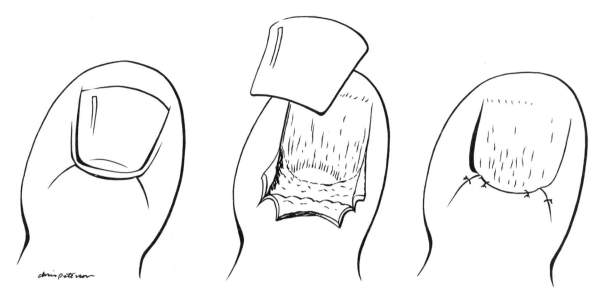

**Fig. 33-11.** Fowler procedure. (From Fowler,[2] with permission.)

performed on children with nail dystrophy of the hallux.[60]

### Fowler Procedure

Fowler described a procedure of onychogryphosis and "bilateral embedded nails" where three flaps are created to expose the germinal matrix[2] (Fig. 33-11). Three recurrences of nail growth were reported in 50 operations for onychogryphosis.

### Kaplan Procedure

In 1960, Kaplan published a procedure for total permanent nail avulsion in which no failures occurred in 369 cases.[61] The Kaplan procedure is performed as follows. After proper surgical preparation, the great toe is anesthetized and the nail avulsed. The foot is prepped and a tourniquet applied. Two 1.5-cm incisions are made in the medial and lateral aspects of the posterior eponychium and extended proximally. Sharp dissection "at the nail level depth" is performed to expose the nail matrix. Another incision connects the nail folds at the distal end of the toe. The entire nail bed including the matrix is removed from the phalanx using sharp dissection. Exposed exostoses are resected, and the eponychial flap is replaced and sutured.

Other modifications regarding the procedure have been reported.[62] Advantages of the Kaplan procedure are easy accessibility to the subungual exostosis if present, but disadvantages include wound healing by second intention or granulation tissue.

### Whitney Acisional Matrixectomy

A Whitney "acisional" total matrixectomy procedure involves two "Frost incisions" for exposure and resection of the nail matrix.[59] After nail avulsion, the nail bed proper is not routinely resected (Fig. 33-12).

### Suppan Nail Technique No. 2

To understand the technique behind the procedure, it is important to review Weisfeld's conception of the sagittal location of the nail matrix.[7] The nail matrix has a "wrap-around characteristic" (Fig. 33-13). This "envelope" is to be excised. A brief summation of the procedure as described by Weisfeld, referred to as the "Suppan Nail Technique No. 2," is as follows.

After proper prepping, anesthesia, and hemostasis, the nail is avulsed. The remaining areas of hyponychium are debrided to prevent postsurgical recurrence. A #15 blade is placed parallel to the corium at the medial margin of the posterior nail fold and the blade is kept just deep to the nail fold. The blade is drawn

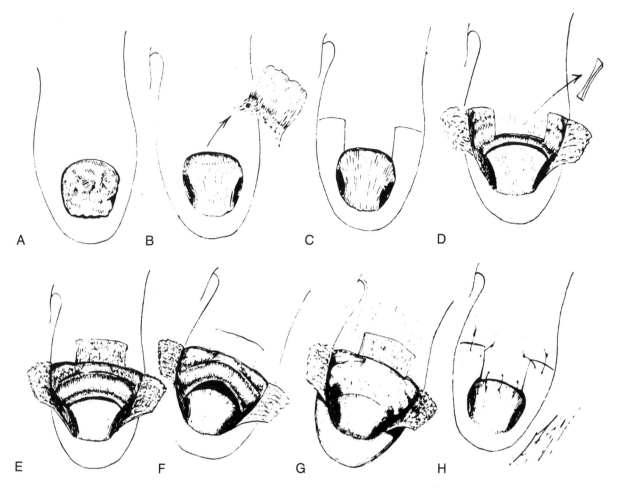

**Fig. 33-12.** (**A–H**) Whitney acisional matrixectomy. (From Whitney[59] with permission.)

laterally over the entire matrix (Fig. 33-14) and angled plantarly against the bone at the medial and lateral aspects of the incision. A transverse incision is made down to bone at the nail matrix and corium junction with the blade angled somewhat posteriorly. The matrix is resected in toto. The posterior nail fold may be sutured to the bed, after inspection and removal of any remaining matrix tissue. Obvious advantages of this procedure are that no skin incisions are made.

### Terminal Syme Procedure

Review of the literature reveals recurrences of ingrown nails to some extent, regardless of the procedure. One case report revealed the "ultimate solution"

as amputation for a ". . . physically distorted toe and hypertrophied toenail that has become inflamed, painful, and disabling."[63] In 1933, Lapidus described complete excision of the nail and its associated structures with removal of approximately one-half of the distal terminal phalanx[64] (Fig. 33-15).

Many modifications of the procedure have been described. Permanent removal of the nail with partial amputation of the distal phalanx has become known as the terminal Syme procedure. Indications for the procedure include onychocryptosis, subungual osteoma, onychauxis, glomus tumor, circulatory dystrophies, mallet toe deformities, and macrodactyly.[65]

With the advent of other techniques and specialized training, the terminal Syme procedure is usually re-

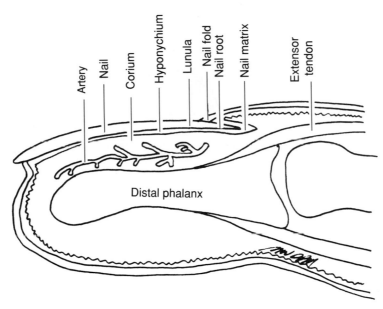

**Fig. 33-13.** Nail anatomy depicting "wrap-around characteristic" of the nail matrix. (From Weisfeld,[7] with permission.)

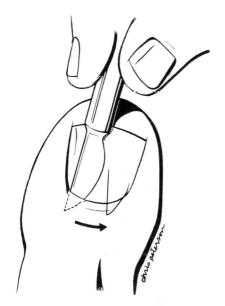

**Fig. 33-14.** Suppan nail technique no. 2.

served for special cases and not done routinely for recurrent ingrown nails.

## TOTAL NAIL AVULSION FOR TREATMENT OF ONYCHOMYCOSIS

Onychomycosis is a constant complaint in the podiatrist's office. Current treatments have led to limited success, if any. Application of topical antifungals for treatment of onychomycosis in general do not work. Oral antifungals have had some success, but the medication has to be taken for prolonged periods of time, and the patient must be monitored clinically and with laboratory tests to avoid possible serious side effects. However, in 1991 Hettinger and Valinsky reported very encouraging results for treatment of onychomycosis by nail avulsion and daily topical application of ketoconazole cream.[66]

Many clinicians have begun to avulse the nail, apply antifungal topicals to the nail bed and matrix, and begin an oral antifungal regime. This should resolve the onychomycosis in a shorter time period, increase the

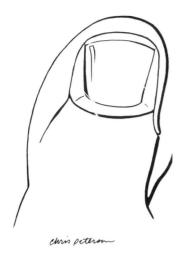 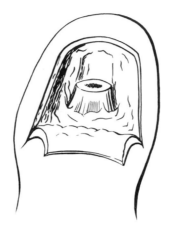 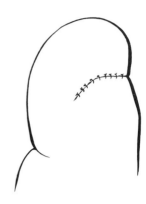

**Fig. 33-15.** The Lapidus procedure. (From Lapidus,[64] with permission.)

success rate of the treatment of fungal nails, and decrease the chance of side effects from prolonged use of medications. This method of treatment may therefore be an alternative that is much more attractive to the clinician and the patient.

A typical treatment regime for total nail avulsion with use of topical and oral antifungals involves nail avulsion and instructing the patient to begin foot soaks. Once the nail bed has stopped draining, Spectazole cream or Nizoral 2 percent cream is applied to the nail bed. The oral antifungal is started the same day as the nail avulsion, using Fulvicin P/G 330 or Nizoral. An intense history and physical examination should be performed, and the patient should not have a history of liver disease such as hepatitis or cirrhosis. Liver enzymes are monitored before nail avulsion and monitored every 3 months. Initial clinical results have been very promising (personal communication, Dr. Bruce Pichler). Other clinicians use the same basic protocol and stress the importance of a fungal culture and identification of the infecting fungus so the proper choice of topical and oral antifungal medications can be administered (personal communication, Dr. Robert Locastro).

Once again, it should be stressed that because of the risks, side effects, and long-term administration of oral antifungal medications, the patient who is considered to be a candidate for this therapy should be in good general health. Periodic monitoring of organ system function including renal, hepatic, and hematopoietic should be performed.[67] The patient should be instructed to report any signs and symptoms that may suggest liver dysfunction, which may include unusual fatigue, anorexia, nausea, vomiting, jaundice, dark urine, and pale stools. Some clinicians will prefer to consult the patient's internist to monitor the patient's health status. Further documentation and in-depth studies may shed more light in this treatment regimen.

## SUBUNGUAL EXOSTECTOMY

Many patients present to the clinic with nail pain without cryptosis of the nail borders. On reviewing radiographs, it may be discovered that the cause of the pain is a subungual exostosis that applies pressure to the nail bed from its inferior aspect (Fig. 33-16).

Debridement of the nail, if thickened and dystrophic, may being about adequate relief. However, if the nail is normal or debridement of the dystrophic nail is ineffective, then a subungual exostectomy should be performed. The procedure entails removing the nail after suitable prepping and anesthesia and rescrubbing the surgical area. The nail bed is incised in a linear fashion directly over the subungual exostosis and parallel to the longitudinal axis of the toe. Two incisions are effected at the distal end of the linear incision at approximately a 90° angle to the linear

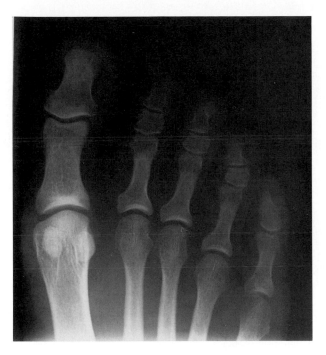

**Fig. 33-16.** Subungal exostosis.

incision to create two flaps and expose the exostosis (Fig. 33-17).

Careful tissue handling and dissection should be stressed to keep the nail bed, nail matrix, or both intact with minimal destruction. This will hopefully prevent postop nail pathology or prevent further nail pathology if already present. The exostosis is removed and sent for biopsy. This area should be saucerized to prevent recurrence of the exostosis from the periosteum. Nonabsorbable sutures are used to reapproximate the nail bed and are removed in 7 to 14 days to allow regrowth of the new nail. Advantages of this procedure are no visible skin incisions and easy accessibility of the exostosis. Disadvantages are possible extensive disruption of the nail matrix or nail bed, which may lead to the formation of a dystrophic nail if not already present, or regrowth of the nail in a "shoveled" or ingrown manner.

Another approach is a fish-mouth incision at the distal end of the toe without removal of the nail to remove the exostosis. This may lead to the formation of a subungual hematoma and therefore possible nail dystrophy. Also, because the exostosis is usually very close to the nail itself, exposure and adequate resection may be difficult. Once again, it should be stressed that removal of the exostosis is important to prevent exacerbation of the curvature of the nail and prevent onychocryptosis if not already present. This procedure is performed across the country, but unfortunately there are no studies available on results.

It should also be mentioned that proximal nail groove pain can be associated with an exostosis.[68] If the patient presents with this complaint by onychocryptosis is not evident, radiographs should be taken and appropriate surgical procedures performed.

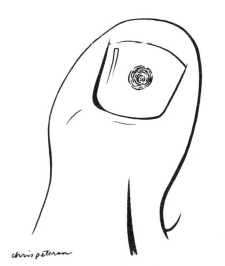
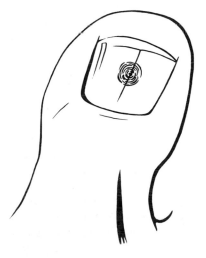

**Fig. 33-17.** Flaps created to remove subungal exostosis.

## SUMMARY

This chapter covered nail surgery with emphasis on procedures for permanent partial and total ablation of nails. The most routinely performed procedures were discussed in depth. New trends and techniques were also covered. Further research is expected to support new trends discussed here and advance nail surgery.

## REFERENCES

1. Burns SA, Ketai RS, Ketai NH: Onychocryptosis. J Am Podiatry Assoc 67:780, 1977

2. Fowler AW: Excision of the germinal matrix: a unified treatment for embedded toenail and onychocryptosis. Br J Surg 45:382, 1958

3. Zadik FR: Obliteration of the nail bed of the great toe without shortening of the terminal phalanx. J Bone Joint Surg Br 32:66, 1950

4. Travers GR, Ammon RG: The sodium hydroxide chemical matricectomy procedure. J Am Podiatry Assoc 70:476, 1980.

5. Bouche RT: Matricectomoy utilizing negative galvanic current. Clin Podiatr Med Surg 3:449, 1986

6. Whitney AK: An illustrated labiomatricectomy procedure. J Am Podiatry Assoc 57:169, 1967

7. Weisfeld M: Illustrated technique for the complete removal of nail matrix and hyponychium without skin incisions (Suppan nail technique n. 2). J Am Podiatry Assoc 65:481, 1975

8. Wee GC, Shieber W: Painless evacuation of subungual hematoma. Surg Gynecol Obstet 133:531, 1970

9. Palamarchuk HJ, Kerzner M: An improved approach to evacuation of subungual hematoma. J Am Podiatry Assoc 79:566, 1989

10. Albom MJ: Surgical gems: avulsion of a nail plate. J Dermatol Surg Oncol 3:34, 1977

11. Scher RK: Surgical avulsion of nail plates by a proximal to distal technique. J Dermatol Surg Oncol 7:296, 1981

12. Heifetz CJ: Ingrown toenail: a clinical study. Am J Surg 38:298, 1937

13. Dixon GL: Treatment of ingrown toenail. Foot Ankle 3:254, 1983

14. Herold HZ, Danial D: Radical wedge resection in the treatment of ingrowing toenail. Int Surg 49:558, 1968

15. Murray WR: Onychocryptosis. Principles of non-operative and operative care. Clin Orthop 142:96, 1979

16. Bartlett RW: Conservative operation for the cure of so called ingrown toenail. J Am Med Assoc 108:1257, 1937

17. Frost LA: Root resection for incurvated nail. J Am Podiatry Assoc 40:19, 1950

18. Perlman P: Don't take two aspirin. Johnson Publishing Company, Boulder, CO, 1982

19. Vandenbos KQ, Bowers WF: Ingrowing toenail: results of weight bearing on soft tissue. US Armed Forces Med J 10:1168, 1959

20. DuVries HL: Ingrown nail. Chiropody Rec 27:155, 1944

21. DuVries HL: Hypertrophy of unguilabia. Chiropody Rec 16:13, 1933

22. Newman RW: A simplified treatment of ingrown toenail. Surg Gynecol Obstet 89:638, 1949

23. Polokoff M: Ingrown toenail and hypertrophied nail lip surgery by electrolysis. J Am Podiatry Assoc 51:805, 1961

24. Frost L: A definite surgical treatment for some lateral nail problems. J Nat Assoc Chiropodists 47:493, 1957

25. Yale JF: Podiatric Medicine. 3rd Ed. Williams & Wilkins, Baltimore, 1987

26. Palmer BV, Jones A: Ingrowing toenails: the results of treatment. Br J Surg 66:575, 1979

27. Murray WR, Bedi BS: The surgical management of ingrowing toenail. Br J Surg 62:409, 1975

28. Steinberg MD: A simplified technique for the surgery of ingrowing nails. Surgery 36:1132, 1954

29. Perrone MA: Nail matricectomy by onychotripsy with airmotor. J Am Podiatry Assoc 60:92, 1970

30. Silverman SH: Cryosurgery for ingrowing toenail. J R Coll Surg Edinb 29:289, 1984

31. Vernon S: Ingrown toenail: operation by electrosurgery. Am J Surg 42:396, 1938

32. Dinesh D: Ingrowing toenail (letter to the editor). NZ Med J 89:494, 1979

33. Gardner P: Negative galvanic current in the surgical correction of onychocryptotic nails. J Am Podiatry Assoc 48:555, 1958

34. Linch AO: Treatment of ingrowing toenail. South Surg 8:173, 1939

35. Farnsworth FC: A treatment for convoluted nails. J Am Podiatry Assoc 62:110, 1972

36. Ilfeld FW, August W: Treatment of ingrown toenail with plastic insert. Orthop Clin North Am 5:95, 1974

37. Wallace WA, Milne DD, Andrew T: Gutter treatment for ingrowing toenails. Br Med J 2:168, 1979

38. Mercado OA: An Atlas of Foot Surgery. Vol. 1. Forefoot Surgery. Carolando Press, Oak Park, 1979

39. Winograd AM: A modification in the technique of operation for ingrown toenail. J Am Med Assoc 91:229, 1929

40. Winograd AM: Results in operation for ingrown toenail. Ill Med J 70:197, 1936

41. Gallocher J: The phenol alcohol method of nail matrix sterilisation. NZ Med J 86:140, 1977

42. Suppan RJ, Ritchlin JD: A non-disabilitating surgical pro-

cedure for ingrown toenail. J Am Podiatry Assoc 52:900, 1962
43. Robb JE, Murray WR: Phenol cauterisation in the management of ingrowing toenails. Scott Med J 27:236, 1982
44. Ross WR: Treatment of the ingrown toenail. Surg Clin North Am 49:1499, 1969
45. Shepherdson A: Nail matrix phenolization: a preferred alternative to surgical excision. Practitioner 219:725, 1977
46. Drago JJ, Jacobs AM, Oloff L: A comparative study of postoperative care with phenol nail procedures. J Foot Surg 22:332, 1983
47. McGlamry ED: Management of painful toes from distorted toenails. J Dermatol Surg Oncol 5:554, 1979
48. Yale JF: Phenol-alcohol technique for correction of infected ingrown toenail. J Am Podiatry Assoc 64:46, 1974
49. Greenwald L, Robbins HM: The chemical matricectomy. J Am Podiatry Assoc 71:388, 1981
50. Cooper C: Phenol-alcohol nail procedure: post-operative care. J Am Podiatry Assoc 55:661, 1965
51. Fulp M, McGlamry ED: New enzyme aids phenol technique in nail surgery. J Am Podiatry Assoc 62:395, 1972
52. Acker I: Preventing the postoperative sequelae to phenolization of nail bed and matrix. J Am Podiatry Assoc 58:351, 1968
53. Anton-Athens V, Ketai DL: Use of cortisporin otic solution in phenol nail surgery. J Am Podiatric Med Assoc 75:31, 1985
54. Rinaldi R, Sabia M, Gross J: The treatment and prevention of infection in phenol alcohol matricectomies. J Am Podiatry Assoc 72:435, 1982
55. Brown FC: Chemocautery for ingrown toenails. J Dermatol Surg Oncol 7:331, 1981
56. Apfelberg DB, Rothermel E, Widtfeldt A, et al: Progress report on use of carbon dioxide laser for nail disorders. Curr Podiatry 32:29, 1983
57. Borovoy M, Fuller TA, Holtz P, Kaczander BI: Laser surgery in podiatric medicine present and future. J Foot Surg 22:353, 1983
58. Farber EM, South DA: Urea ointment in the nonsurgical avulsion of nail dystrophies. Cutis 22:689, 1978
59. Whitney AK: Total matricectomy procedure. J Am Podiatry Assoc 58:157, 1968
60. Robb JE: The results of surgery for nail dystrophy of the hallux in children. Surg Infancy Child 39:131 1984.
61. Kaplan EG: Elimination of onychauxis by surgery. J Am Podiatry Assoc 50:111, 1960
62. Mercado OA, Dalianis G, Chulengarian J, et al: Kaplan nail revisited. Curr Podiatry 21:21, 1972
63. Field LM: An ultimate solution for a painful toe. J Dermatol Surg Oncol 5:402, 1979
64. Lapidus PW: Complete and permanent removal of toenail in onychogryphosis and subungual osteoma. Am J Surg 19:92, 1933
65. Gastwirth BW, Anton V, Martin RA: The terminal Syme procedure. J Foot Surg 20.95, 1981
66. Hettinger DF, Valinsky MS: Treatment of onychomychosis with nail avulsion and topical ketoconazole. J Am Podiatr Med Assoc 81:28, 1991
67. 1991 Physicians' Desk Reference. 45th Ed. p. 1119. Medical Economics Data, Montrale, NJ, 1991.
68. Chinn S, Jenkin W: Proximal nail groove pain associated with an exostosis. J Am Podiatr Med Assoc 76:506, 1986

# 34

# Rheumatoid Arthritis

*MICHAEL KORBOL*

Much of what has been presented in the previous chapters of this volume is also applicable to the patient with rheumatoid arthritis. Since Hoffman's[1] classic paper in 1911 on forefoot arthroplasty, however, little has changed in the practical management of crippling forefoot deformities. This chapter is concerned mainly with the surgical management of adult patients with rheumatoid arthritis in need of forefoot arthroplasty.

Vainio[2] reported 90 percent of adult patients with rheumatoid arthritis had variable degrees of symptoms in their feet. Additionally, the foot is the initial site of involvement in 16 percent of rheumatoid arthritis cases. Pedal involvement is nearly always bilateral. Those patients with arthritis of more than 10 years duration have significant involvement of their feet.

Typical symptoms and signs of the forefoot requiring surgery may include painful intractable plantar callouses or ulcers underlying metatarsal heads, painful ambulation, flatfeet, deformed and contracted toes with corns or ulcers, hallux abducto valgus, hallux varus, medial or lateral displaced lesser toes, painful limited joint motion, digital subluxations and dislocations, anterior displaced plantar fat pad, and inability to wear regular shoe gear (Figs. 34-1 and 34-2). Spreading of the toes secondary to rheumatoid nodules has now been shown to be a presenting symptom of rheumatoid arthritis[3] (Fig. 34-3).

Radiographic studies of late-stage arthritis may show severe destructive processes at the metatarsophalangeal joint (MTPJ), dorsally luxated or dislocated toes, hammer and claw toes, osteoporosis, metatarsal fatigue fractures, and sesamoid involvement (Fig. 34-4).

Of course, forefoot manifestations are just one part of a larger disease process with multilevel and multisystem involvement. It must be remembered this is often a progressive and unpredictable disease. An active, communicative team approach is essential in the management of such patients. Complications from inadequate preoperative planning can be devastating. The foot surgeon needs to be aware of the pathogenesis of the disease, its medical management, and other joint involvement to establish an appropriate temporal pattern for surgical intervention. Concomitant diseases may influence the surgical decisions.

## BIOMECHANICAL CONSIDERATIONS

The weight-bearing nature of the foot as well as the disease process subjects the foot to abnormal biomechanical influences that contribute to foot pain, deformity, and disability. Abnormal digital posturing arises mainly from synovitis, joint distention, ligament and skeletal muscle weakness, and cartilage erosion that results in intrinsic muscle destabilization.[4] Other factors, especially pronation forces, that contribute to foot deformity may include posterior tibial dysfunction, equinus, extremity structural valgus attitudes, and compensation for arthritic joints.[5]

Although a cavus-type foot with rheumatoid arthritis can exist, most arthritic feet demonstrate a flatfoot appearance.[5,6] Caution is advised when selecting patients with anterior cavus foot for forefoot arthroplasty because postoperative pain may continue from weight-bearing on the remaining metatarsal shaft.[7] Postoperatively, soft inner soles or soft custom foot orthoses are quite helpful in this patient.

The valgus foot, especially when resulting from hindfoot pathology, may contribute to knee valgus

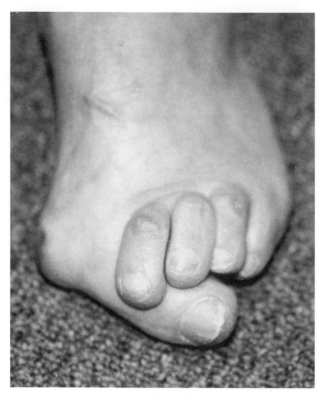

**Fig. 34-1.** Dorsal view of a typical rheumatoid forefoot.

alignment. It has been suggested that delaying or preventing hindfoot valgus may delay deformity in an otherwise normally aligned ipsilateral knee.[5] Also, it might be advisable to correct hindfoot malignment before knee arthroplasty to minimize abnormal stresses on an implant.[5] This author agrees with Schuberth[8] in that forefoot arthroplasty should be carried out before hindfoot arthrodeses if needed. In this manner, compensation for forefoot malignment can be accounted for by selective rearfoot wedging, whereas the converse is unlikely.

Clinical evaluation of both the static and dynamic foot with rheumatoid arthritis suggests abnormal plantar forces at work. The gait in late disease is often antalgic bilateral and of a flat, shuffling type.[5,9] Forefoot disability often arises from dorsally located toes with anterior fat pad displacement and resultant depressed metatarsal leading to great forces at the ball of the foot with resultant metatarsalgia, plantar callouses, and ulcerations. Forefoot arthroplasty will reduce abnormal pressure under the forefoot and may increase mobility.[9] A shuffling gait indicates an attempt to minimize joint motion and to increase the period of flat foot and area of weight-bearing to attain decreased peak plantar pressures in any one area.[10]

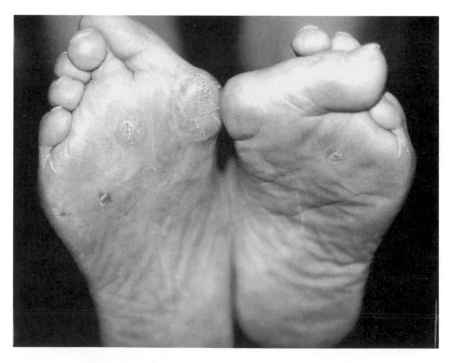

**Fig. 34-2.** Plantar view of typical rheumatoid forefeet.

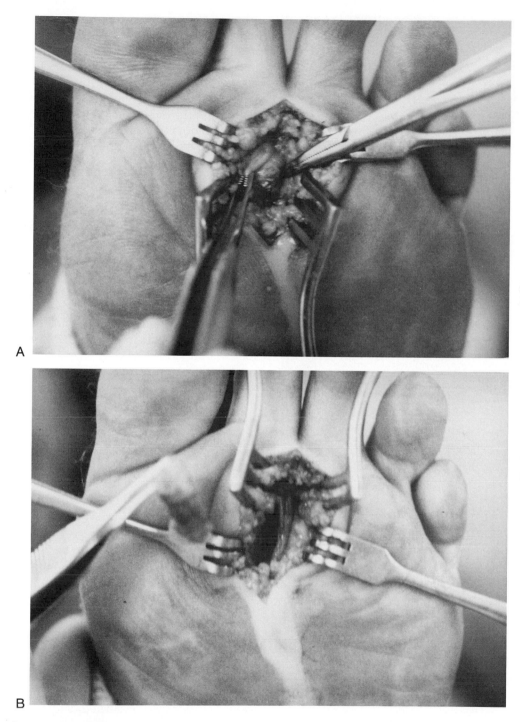

**Fig. 34-3.** Rheumatoid nodule. A 33-year-old white woman presented with complaints of spreading toes on both feet and neuroma-type pain. She also had bilateral carpal tunnel syndrome. Subsequent histologic analysis revealed a rheumatoid nodule and she eventually became seropositive. (**A**) The plantar common digital nerve is being retracted by forceps; the hemostat points to the underlying nodules. (**B**) The nodule is excised and the nerve is back in place. (*Figure continues.*)

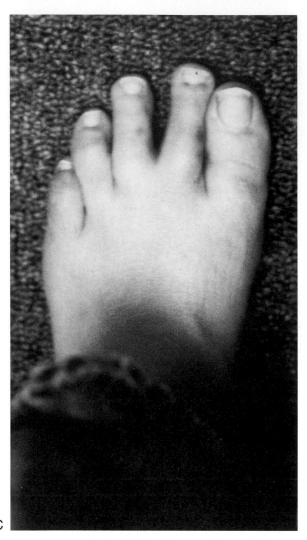

C

**Fig. 34-3** *(Continued)*. (**C**) Three weeks postoperative, with residual spreading of the toes.

## PROCEDURE OBJECTIVES

Pain relief is the primary goal in surgical management. This objective is achieved through deformity reduction and excision of diseased tissue. Secondary gains that can be expected include ease of wearing shoe gear, increased gait stability, improved function, avoidance of ulcerative lesions, and cosmetic appearance. Occasionally, surgery may be needed not for pain relief but more for recurrent ulcerative infections, espe-

cially in those patients requiring chronic or intermittent therapeutic use of immunosuppressive and antineoplastic drugs.

Functional improvement is not necessarily a prime objective and may not be achievable. Patients should be forewarned of this and, in fact, functional deterioration may ensue depending on the surgical procedures used and the disease process itself.[7,11–13]

## PATIENT SELECTION AND PREOPERATIVE CONSIDERATIONS

The candidate for forefoot arthroplasty usually already has an advanced disease process. Nonsurgical care has typically been exhausted or ineffective, and therefore deciding if surgery is actually required is straightforward. However, numerous considerations must be taken into account before proceeding. A thorough history and physical should be performed by an appropriate physician. Concurrent management of other systems pathology should be pursued. Concurrent orthopedic care may be necessary.

A preoperative evaluation of the patient is essential to identify and minimize risk factors. Although beyond the scope of this chapter, an excellent review has been given by White.[14] Salient points are presented here, especially in regard to reconstructive foot surgery.

Drug therapy at the time of surgical planning needs to be evaluated. Steroid use should be supplemented perioperatively to prevent adrenocortical crisis. Methotrexate therapy should be discontinued at least 1 week before surgery and not resumed until adequate skin healing has taken place. Surgery may need to be postponed until the active process is controlled by pharmacologic and physical means.

Surgery should be postponed in the patient with active rheumatoid vasculitis to avoid severe vascular and dermatologic consequences. Vasculitis may also indicate the rheumatoid disease is not under control. Organic occlusive arterial disease may exist and should be detected, evaluated, and treated if necessary, including the associated risk factors. Thromboembolism prophylaxis is not necessary unless the patient is immobilized and at risk. Otherwise, simple surveillance is mandatory.

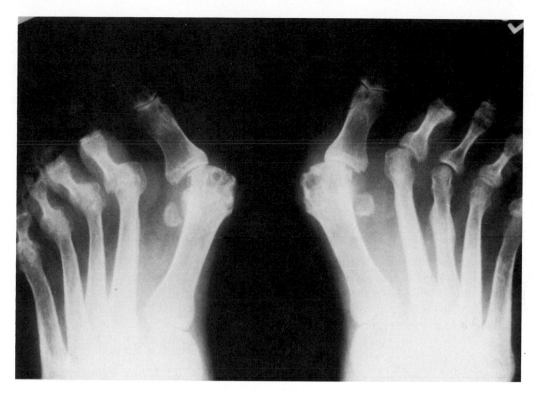

**Fig. 34-4.** Typical radiographic appearance of the forefoot requiring surgery. Note the dislocated toes, erosive joint changes, osteoporosis, and healing metatarsal fatigue fractures.

Wound healing can be a problem in the rheumatoid arthritis patient. For instance, corticosteroid and methotrexate can delay wound healing by diminishing the tensile strength. The skin is usually thinner in the older patient and may be exacerbated in the rheumatoid arthritis patient secondary to changes in collagen metabolism.[15] The presence of Felty syndrome (rheumatoid arthritis, splenomegaly, leukopenia) can increase the infection rate.[15] Other preoperative considerations include age of the patient, potential for rehabilitation, extent of deformity, location and extent of pain, activity level, motivation level, presence and location of rheumatoid nodules, and, of course, disease activity progression.

Prophylactic antibiotic use is almost routine in rheumatoid foot surgery. The reasons for antibiotics may include implant use, extensive exposure, multiple incisions, prolonged surgery, and a debilitated and immunocompromised host. The antibiotic benefits clearly outweigh the risks. Specific preoperative criteria for successful surgery typically include a patient older than 50 years, severe forefoot arthritis, severe metatarsalgia, toe deformity, and a painful apropulsive gait.

In my experience, local standby anesthesia is sufficient for forefoot arthroplasty in either ankle, midfoot, or ray infiltrative blocks. Bilateral forefoot surgery may require a lower percentage of a local anesthetic because of the greater volume necessary. There seems to be a poor "take" of local at lower percentages in the rheumatoid patient. In this case, epidural may be better suited, especially if prolonged surgery is anticipated. General anesthesia is rarely, if ever, recommended. If so, cervical flexion/extension radiographs should be obtained to evaluate cervical disease, and the anesthesiologist must be alerted.[14]

Extreme upper extremity involvement may limit surgery to one foot at a time to avoid unsafe use of ambulation aids. Home health care, family support, and home modifications (e.g., commode, wheelchair access, stairs) are necessary preoperative considerations for the patient's ease and safety.

# PROCEDURE SELECTION

The original Hoffman procedure from 1911 is still the gold standard in forefoot arthroplasty.[1] There have been several modifications of this procedure that merit review.

Hoffman[1] used a single, curved, transverse incision on the plantar foot distal to the metatarsal heads, and he excised the heads. This approach relieved the severe metatarsalgia, provided access to the plantar-flexed metatarsals, yet placed the incision distal to weight-bearing areas. This approach usually protects the vessels at this level that are deep in the intermetatarsal spaces.

Larmon[16] in 1951 used a three-incision, longitudinal, dorsal approach: the first incision was over the first metatarsophalangeal joint, the second between the second and third metatarsal heads, and a third between the fourth and fifth heads. A Keller procedure and removal of the plantar portion of the lesser metatarsal heads is performed.

Fowler[17] in 1959 made a dorsal transverse incision over the five metatarsals proximal to the toe webs. The proximal one-half of the proximal phalanges are removed, and the metatarsal heads are shortened and contoured. Anterior displacement of the fat pad is addressed by removing an ellipse of skin plantar and proximal to the metatarsal heads.

Clayton[18] in 1963 through a dorsal transverse approach excised all the metatarsal heads and bases of the proximal phalanges. Extensor tendons are transected without repair.

Kates et al.[19] in 1967 modified the original Hoffman approach. A single transverse plantar approach with the convexity proximal is made, and the metatarsal heads are excised. The phalangeal bases are left intact. A second proximal incision is then made forming an ellipse of skin that is excised to realign the fat pad. Sesamoids are excised if necessary.

Dwyer[20] in 1970 suggested a procedure to resect all the metatarsal heads and arthrodese the hallux meta-

tarsophalangeal joint and proximal interphalangeal joints of the lesser toes.

Swanson[21] in 1979 advocated using flexible stem silicone implants of the great toe. Cracchiolo[22] later also suggested using silicone implants in all metatarsophalangeal joints.

Hoder and Dobbs[23] in 1983 used a five-incision, dorsal longitudinal approach. Each incision is centered over a metatarsophalangeal joint. This approach presumably lessens the chance of vascular compromise and lymphatic obstruction.

Finally, in 1988 McGarvey and Johnson[12] modified Larmon's approach by modifying the lateral two incisions into Y-shaped incisions extending up the adjacent sides of the second and third as well as the fourth and fifth toes to the proximal interphalangeal joint (PIPJ) level. This technique is chosen to provide postoperative digital stabilization by syndactilization at closure.

## Procedure Selection: Key Points

A review of the already referenced sources demonstrates satisfactory reports, at least in the short term. The few long-term studies and literature reviews generally show a gradual deterioration of results over many years.[11–13,23–27] Recommendations based on all these papers are presented.

The incisional approach to the forefoot arthroplasty is essentially irrelevant as to the final outcome, but certain points regarding incisions should be made. Plantar incisions allow easy access to metatarsal heads with dorsally subluxed toes and should be made at or distal to the metatarsal heads to avoid vascular embarrassment and painful plantar scars. A plantar ellipse of skin to realign the fat pad is not necessary if digital reduction is obtained. Plantar incisions may require immediate, protected, postoperative weight-bearing to prevent dehiscence.

Dorsal incisions should be longitudinal because transverse incisions prolong the swelling; ambulation can be nearly immediate. The three-incision approach is most commonly recommended and provides good exposure. The five-incision approach is good for the novice surgeon for ease in dissection but should be used in caution in narrow or small feet because of potential vascular compromise in closely placed incisions. Dorsal incisions generally have more swelling

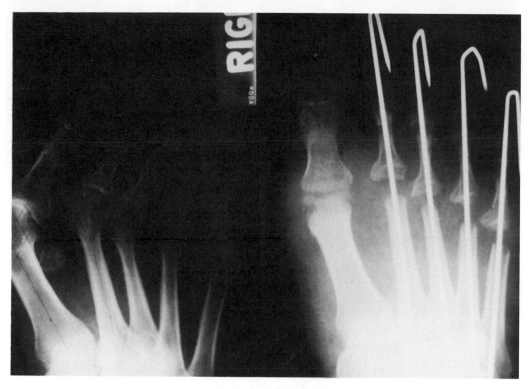

**Fig. 34-5.** Pre- and postoperative panmetatarsal head resection with implant and K-wire stabilization. Note the decrease in the intermetatarsal angle and the cascading metatarsal parabola.

than plantar incisions (personal observation). A combined dorsomedial approach for the first MTPJ and plantar approach under the lesser metatarsals is this author's favorite approach in patients without vascular disease.

Once the incision placement is determined, osseous procedures should be selected. Procedures for the first MTPJ should be some type of stabilizing option to prevent recurrence. Specifically, resection total hinged implant or resection arthrodesis should be considered (Figs. 34-5 and 34-6). Indications, techniques, and precautions outlined in other chapters of this book should be followed in choosing the technique to be used.

Resection arthroplasty has the greatest rate of failure and dissatisfaction and should be reserved for short-term relief (Fig. 34-7). Modular implants should not be used until long-term studies are completed.[28] Implants should not be used in the presence of abnormal biomechanical stresses or unreduced high intermetatarsal angles. Sesamoids should be excised if they pre-

vent reduction of deformities, contribute to plantar pain, or are severely diseased and displaced.

Reduction of the increased metatarsus primus adductus angle by osteotomy is suggested by some authors. This is not needed, as this increased intermetatarsal angle is positional and reduced by adequate decompression of the retrograde forces of the great toe. This is especially true with great toe arthrodesis.[29]

The lesser toe deformity and metatarsalgia should initially be addressed at the MTPJ level. Specifically, generous resection of the metatarsal heads should be carried out. The resulting metatarsal parabola length should generally be with the second the longest followed by the first, third, fourth, and fifth. I have observed no problem in leaving the first metatarsal as long or slightly longer than the second. In addition, the osteotomies should be angled from dorsal distal to proximal plantar. The first and fifth metatarsal shaft should be also angled proximal medial and proximal lateral, respectively. Resect either metatarsal heads or

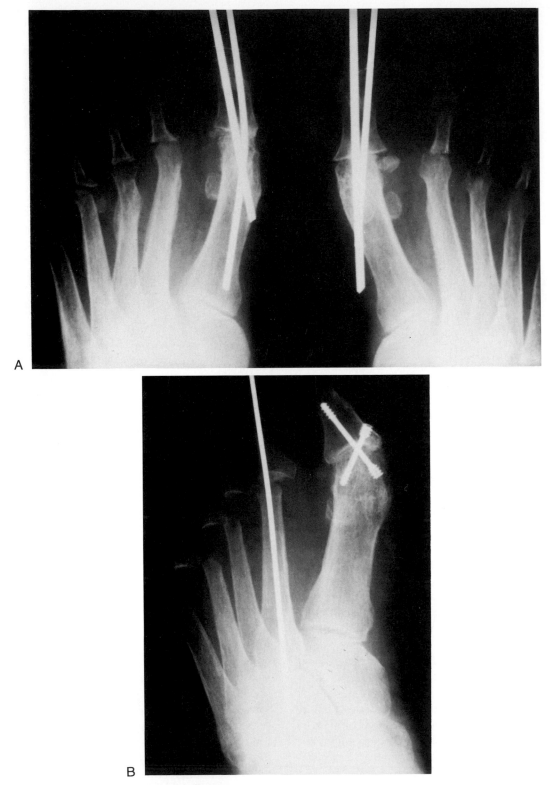

A

B

**Fig. 34-6.** Panmetatarsal head resection with arthrodesis. (**A**) Steinman pins are used with osteoporotic bone. (**B**) Internal screw fixation is used in relatively good bone stock.

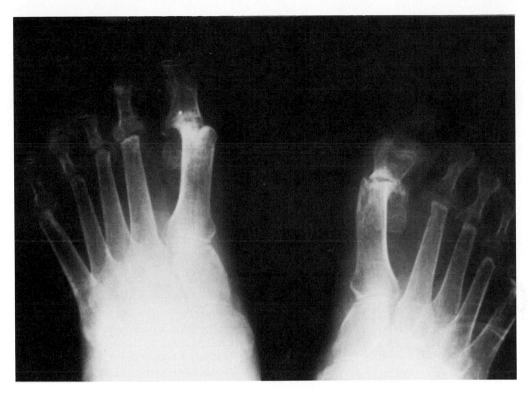

**Fig. 34-7.** Panmetatarsal head resection with resection arthroplasty of the first metatarsophalangeal joint in extremely osteoporotic bone.

none; the exception may be excising only the lesser metatarsal heads if the first is disease free. Single head resection is a poor choice. Total implants of the lesser MTPJ are generally not feasible because of the amount of bone resection needed.

Phalangeal bones, unless greatly enlarged or long, should be left in place. Digital reduction may require either manipulative reduction, resection arthrodesis, resection implant, or even resection arthroplasty at the PIPJ level. Each digit should be evaluated singly after MTPJ arthroplasty. The fifth should not be arthrodesed.

Kirschner wire (K-wire stabilization should be used for lesser toe arthrodesis. There is little evidence to show that K-wire stabilization of the MTPJ actually increases long-term stabilization. When used, however, wires should cross all interphalangeal and metatarsophalangeal joints and be left in place for 4 to 6 weeks. Digital syndactyly up to the PIPJ shows early promise for long-term stability. Naturally, syndactyly of both sides of a toe simultaneously is not recommended to avoid potential vascular embarrassment. Digital incisions should be longitudinal and may be elliptical to reduce excess skin.

Adjunct procedures, including tendon balancing and rheumatoic nodule excision, need to be addressed individually. Intraoperative radiographs should be taken to ascertain correct metatarsal parabola. Bone fragments remaining in the plantar region need to be removed. Silicone polyester metatarsal caps have yet to be demonstrated useful on a long-term basis.

## POSTOPERATIVE CARE

Postoperative care should include monitoring for vascular compromise, controlling edema by bed rest and elevation for 24 to 48 hours, and using drains as indicated. Sutures should be left in place for 3 weeks and augmented with adhesive wound bandages as needed to avoid discharge. K-wires are removed at about 4 weeks.

Ambulation can be resumed on a very limited basis at 24 to 48 hours after surgery using surgical shoes. These shoes should have a premolded soft arch support with a metatarsal pad to keep the fragile foot padded and toes plantar-flexed. Prolonged immbolization is to be avoided. Physical therapy is essential to aid in ambulation. Home care may be needed.

Long-term problems may include recurrence of abnormal digital posturing, recurrent hallux valgus or varus, plantar ulcers or lesions, implant or arthrodesis failure, recurrent pain, and difficulty with shoe gear. Long-term care includes use of custom-molded soft foot orthoses and extra-depth, stable shoes with rocker bottom soles. The patient should be followed for more than 5 years. Again, a team approach is essential in the postoperative management.

# REFERENCES

1. Hoffman P: An operation for severe grades of contracted or clawed toes. Am J Orthop Surg 9:441, 1911
2. Vainio K: Orthopaedic surgery in the treatment of rheumatoid arthritis. Ann Clin Res 7:216, 1975
3. Dedrick D, McCune W, Smith W: Rheumatoid arthritis presenting as spreading of the toes. J Bone Joint Surg AM 72:463, 1990
4. Manzi J, Pruzansky J: Digital foot deformities in the arthritic patient. Rheumatol Clin Podiatr Med Surg 5:1, 1988
5. Keenan M , Peabody T, Gronley J et al: Valgus deformities of the feet and characteristics of gait in patients who have rheumatoid arthritis. J Bone Joint Surg AM 73:237, 1991
6. Brown P: Rheumatoid flatfoot. J Am Podiatr Med Assoc 77:39, 1987
7. Oloff J, Sterns J: Forefoot arthroplasty in the arthritic patient. Rheumatol Clin Podiatr Med Surg 5:1, 1988
8. Schuberth J: Pedal fusions in the rheumatoid patient. Rheumatol Clin Prodiatr Med Surg 5:1, 1988
9. Betts R, Stockley I, Getty C et al: Foot pressure studies in the assessment of forefoot arthroplasty in the rheumatoid foot. Foot Ankle 8:315, 1988
10. Zhu H: Foot pressure distribution during waking and shuffling. Arch Phys Med Rehab 72:390, 1991
11. Saltrick K, Alter S, Catanzariti A: Pan metatarsal head resection: retrospective analysis and literature review. J Foot Surg 28:340, 1989
12. McGarvey S, Johnson K: Keller arthroplasty in combination with resection arthroplasty of the lesser metatarsophalangeal joints in rheumatoid arthritis. Foot Ankle 9:75, 1988
13. Hasselol L, Willkens R, Toomey H et al: Forefoot surgery in rheumatoid arthritis: subjective assessment of outcome. Foot Ankle 8:148, 1987
14. White R: Preoperative evaluation with rheumatoid arthritis. Semin Arthritis Rheum 14:287, 1985
15. O'Duffy J, Linscheid R, Peterson L: Surgery in rheumatoid arthritis: indications and complications. Arch Phys Med Rehab 70:2, 1972
16. Larmon W: Surgical treatment of deformities of rheumatoid arthritis of the forefoot and toes. Bull Northwestern Univ Med Sch 25:39, 1951
17. Fowler A: A method of forefoot reconstruction. J Bone Joint Surg 41B:507, 1959
18. Clayton M: Surgery of the lower extremity in rheumatoid arthritis. J Bone Joint Surg 45A:1517, 1963
19. Kates A, Kessel L, Kay A: Arthroplasty of the Forefoot. J Bone Joint Surg 49B:552, 1967
20. Dwyer A: Correction of severe toe deformities. J Bone Joint Surg 52:192, 1970
21. Swanson A, Lumsden R, Swanson G: Silicone implant arthroplasty of the great toe: a review of single stem and flexible hinge implants. Clin Orthop 142:30, 1979
22. Cracchiolo A: Management of the arthritic forefoot. Foot Ankle 3:17, 1982
23. Hoder L, Dobbs B: Pan metatarsal head resection: a review and new approach. J Am Podiatry Assoc 73:322, 1983
24. Watson M: A long term follow up of forefoot arthroplasty. J Bone Joint Surg 56:527, 1974
25. Gould N: Surgery of the forepart of the foot in rheumatoid arthritis. Foot Ankle 3:173, 1982
26. Gregory J, Childers R, Higgins K et al: Arthrodesis of the first metatarsophalangeal joint: a review of the literature and long term retrospective analysis. J Foot Surg 29:369, 1990
27. McLaughlin E, Fish C: Keller arthroplasty: is distraction a useful technique? A retrospective study. J Foot Surg 29:223, 1990
28. Koenig R: Koenig total great toe implant. J Am Podiatr Med Assoc 80:462, 1990
29. Mann R, Katcherian D: Relationship of metatarsophalangeal joint fusion on the intermetatarsal angle. Foot Ankle 10:8, 1989

# 35

# Methods for Assessing Stress under the Pathologic Forefoot

*RICHARD J. BOGDAN*

Pressure analysis of the foot while standing and walking has significantly progressed in the past decade. This is especially true for assessing the pattern and absolute dimensions of force and stress on the sole of the foot. Of considerable practical interest to podiatry, or any field that cares for the foot, is the evaluation of forefoot pain. In this chapter, various pressure analysis modalities are detailed. The author has found that no single current modality provides the ultimate pressure analysis. To assist readers in identifying which modality may be most appropriate for their needs, the benefits and limitations of those available is discussed. To illustrate the role of these devices, several case histories detailing use of the pedobarograph in forefoot pain are presented.

Early investigations provided pressure analysis of the general and nondiscrete patterns of stress affecting the foot. Recent advances have allowed identification of more discrete areas and different types of forces. Thus the first step in identifying foot pressures is to decide what type of stress and force are likely to be found. The force components are classified as vertical, anterior/posterior, shear, and mediolateral shear.

Force transducers have been used for several years to assess foot stress. These transducers are made of deforming materials such as polymers, crystals, and metallic rods. The best known is the force platform, which provides a general impression of the ground reaction forces on the entire foot. Earlier devices had inadequate resolution because of the small number of components assessing the stress under the selected area of the foot. Stresses recorded were low, implying that the results of these instruments could not be relied on or compared. The newer instruments have more components per area under the foot so that the stress pattern information is more accurate and reliable. There are however still difficulties with comparing results and in defining what is normal.

When evaluating these devices one has to be very critical of the engineering concepts by which they were developed[1]:

1. What is the dynamic range of the evaluating instrument? That is, does the device evaluate the range of high and low stresses you expect?
2. Does it evaluate the stress site well?
3. What is the sampling rate?
4. Does it have a high number of sampling cells to resolve the force into its components?
5. Does it respond to the frequency of the applied force?
6. Does it respond directly to the amount of force applied?
7. Is it temperature sensitive?
8. Is it reliable and user friendly?

As clinicians we are interested in evaluating the weight-bearing foot for several reasons. The following historical review will help in understanding the types of devices used in the past and those currently available in both clinical practice and research.

## MECHANICAL DEVICES

Devices to record the force or stress beneath the foot have existed since 1882 when Beely had subjects step on plaster-filled sacks, theorizing that the magnitude of pressure was proportional to the depth of the impression. This method and others like it tended to record the shape of the foot and not necessarily the pedal forces.[2–4] Another early method of recording stress was based on the deformation of pliable projections protruding from the underside of a mat upon which the subject walks or stands. This stress makes the projections collapse; the area of the mat in contact with the surface beneath increases, and produces a darkened area. The intensity of the inked area is proportional to the applied pressure. A pressure image is produced by an inked mat that leaves a single peak pressure picture on the paper below the sole imprint. The disadvantages of this method are twofold; one is the inability to provide any pressure versus time data, and the other is that the image reaches a maximum intensity after which no further increase in pressure can be detected.[2,4]

The first mechanical device was Morton's kinetograph. The projections on this device consisted of longitudinal ridges that pressed an inked ribbon onto a piece of paper and left a series of parallel lines that widened with increasing force.[5]

Elftman[2] used the principle of collapsing projections, but provided pressure-time data. His device consisted of a black rubber mat with pyramidal projections on the bottom that laid upon a glass plate. A white fluid filled the spaces between the pyramids and provided contrast when the pyramids spread. The image was recorded from below with a 16mm movie camera at 72 frames per second. This deformable projection principle is widely used today in the commercially available Harris mat. It has the advantages of being portable and providing better resolution than the previous devices, and is relatively inexpensive.[1] Brand in 1982[6] tried to utilize this device as an insole for patients with insensitive feet caused by Hansen's disease, but this simple method failed to provide quantitative data.

The Sheffield optical pedobarograph developed by Betts and Duckworth[7] after a proposal by Chodera[8] is the most advanced modification of the foregoing optical systems. The device consists of a glass plate illuminated at the edges by strip lights and covered at the top by a sheet of opaque white plastic with microscopic projections on the bottom. When unloaded, the light from the sides is reflected internally. When a subject steps onto the plastic, pressing it to the glass, the internal reflections are dispersed and a light is emitted with an intensity proportional to the pressure. Because the continuous gray scale emitted by the device makes it difficult to recognize subtle variations in pressure, the image is converted to a color contour map by a monochrome television camera, an electronic interface, and a color monitor.[9]

Brand and Ebner[6] used another simple concept and developed a pressure-sensitive device to provide artificial feedback to patients with insensitive hands and feet (Hansen's disease). The device consisted of socks and gloves made of 2 layers of thin polyurethane foam with microcapsules sandwiched between them. When previously established pressures were exceeded, the microcapsules ruptured, staining the socks. The microcapsules were manufactured to rupture at different pressures. The socks and gloves were used to retrain denervated individuals to apply appropriate pressures on their limbs during daily activities. The microcapsules were not reliable and would rupture depending on the hardness of the underlying tissue rather than applied pressure. Rupture also occurred with repeated use at low pressures. The devices failed to give any a warning if the stresses were in the dangerous level. The investigators suggested the use of some type of warning sensor in conjunction with the microcapsule devices.

## ELECTRONIC PRESSURE TRANSDUCERS

The failure to quantify stresses using mechanical techniques has resulted in the development and use of electronic transducers. Although the relative complexity and greater expense of electronic systems has previously confined them mainly to experimental use, increasing reliability and simplicity of operation are increasing their attractiveness as a clinical tool.[10]

Each type of electronic device has its own strengths and weaknesses. The suitability for a given application should be evaluated on the basis of performance in several important areas. Cavanagh and Ulbrecht[1] suggested the following guidelines when evaluating a transducer:

1. The presence of the device must not change the gait of the subject nor the quantity of pressure measured.

2. The system should be capable of measuring all magnitudes of pressure encountered in the observed activity.

3. The linearity or relation of input to output must be accounted for. A device that is linear produces a consistent increment of output per unit input over the measured range of values. If the device is nonlinear, this must be accounted for when analyzing the data.

4. The apparatus must be capable of recording data at the rate at which the measured phenomenon occurs. If a device with poor frequency response is loaded rapidly the output may be in error.

5. The sampling rate must be adequate.

6. The system should exhibit little hysteresis. The input/output curve should have the same shape loading, as unloading.

7. The spatial resolution of the device should be adequate. If you want the difference in pressure between two 1-cm$^2$ areas, you cannot find it with a single sensor of 10 cm$^{-2}$;

8. The system must distinguish between pressures that are close in amplitude.

9. Changes in temperature should not affect measured values.

10. There must be an adequate calibration procedure and the system divides it by the known area of that sensor. Therefore pressure values are very sensitive to transducer size. The larger the transducer the smaller the pressure for a given force. This is obvious for discrete sensors, but it must be remembered that matrix devices are also made up of functionally discrete transducers.

Because of the lack of studies comparing the different transducers and the values that result from them, as suggested by Lord[3] and Cavanagh and Ulbrecht,[1] "It is unwise to compare pressures read from different types of transducers."

## CAPACITANCE TRANSDUCERS

A capacitance transducer consists of two conductive plates or elements separated by a flexible dielectric. As the pressure is applied to the device, the distance between plates decreases; the capacitance then increases, and its resistance to alternating current decreases.[10] Capacitance transducers may consist of a single layer of compressible material sandwiched between two conductive layers, or they may contain several capacitors in parallel by stacking several alternating layers of plates and dielectrics. This type of device is inexpensive, stable, and produces fairly linear response, but tends to be thick, which makes it less adaptable for use in shoe transducers.[1,10]

Schwartz and Heath[11] created discrete "piczometric discs" of layers of paper and bronze that were taped to areas of interest on the soles of the feet. Bauman and Brand[12] reported that they were later discarded due to technical difficulties.

Holden and Muncey[13] used a single shield-shaped capacitance device about $\frac{1}{8}$ inch thick and 2 × 2 in. in area made of three layers of metal foil and two layers of pimpled rubber. The pressure-sensitive area was approximately 0.5 m.[2] This cumbersome device would fit into any shoe, but it was not demonstrated how it fit into the inside of the shoe. It developed a record by taking a photograph of a cathode ray spot.

Bauman and Brand[12] designed a capacitive system to evaluate areas of high pressure on the footsoles of Hansen's disease patients. They used the transducers designed by the Franklin Institute Laboratory[14] and taped them to regions of interest. The pressure transducer consisted of a 1-mm-thick capacitor with a 1-cm$^2$ pressure-sensitive area. The device was not accurate at pressures greater than 3.5 kg/cm$^2$, so the transducer was connected to a preamplifier. It was unstable with changes in temperature and necessitated zero pressure calibrations using a hydraulic device monitored by a precision strain gauge.

In 1978 Nicol and Hennig developed a flexible matrix of capacitance transducers using a 48 × 24 cm foam-rubber mat with 16 conductive strips on either side. The strips were oriented orthogonally to form 256 transducers, 1 at each intersection of strips. The entire array could be scanned in about 5 ms. The advantage of this system was its adaptability to curved surfaces and the ease with which it could be manufactured in different shapes. The disadvantages to this system, however, were cross-talk between transducers, the compression of the foam rubber, which resulted in nonlinear output with some hysteresis, and the fact that the mat could change the pressure under the foot because of its softness.[15] The nonlinearity problem has since been resolved. The refined device is sold today as the Novel's EMED system (Novel gmbh 1991).

Coleman[16] (1985) used four Hercules F4-4F capacitance transducers measuring 2 mm in thickness and 9 mm in diameter to quantify the reduction in pressures resulting from footwear modifications. The signals were fed to a thermal chart recorder where the peak pressures were measured with a micrometer.

A larger Hercules F4-4R capacitance sensor was tested by Kothari et al.[17] to determine its applicability for use in shoes. This sensor design could be subjected to high loads without harm because the metal did not yield when the corrugations were flattened out. The device was nearly linear up to 500 kPa.

## STRAIN GAUGES

A strain gauge transducer is created by bonding a conductive material to a mechanical member or beam. When the beam is deflected, the conductor is lengthened or compressed changing its cross section and its resistance.[3] The load-measuring devices of this type are many and varied, inexpensive, reliable, and have linear output. The devices may be fragile when smaller and be susceptible to temperature changes. When larger, they are bulky and require firm soft tissue to bend the beam.[1,10]

Hutton and Drabble[18] designed the first strain gauge device to observe the distribution of loads beneath the foot. Used by Stokes et al. in 1975,[19] the system measured stress medial to lateral aspects of the foot and could be rotated 90 degrees to observe anteroposterior loading.

Ctercteko et al.[20] appreciated the uses of the walkway system. Noting the poor resolution provided by the Hutton and Drabble system, they constructed one with better resolution. The Ctercteko device consisted of 128 load cells, capable of providing information on the medial to lateral and anteroposterior axes at the same time.

The first strain gauge used in the shoe was devised by Lereim and Serck-Hanssen[21] when producing a simple in-shoe device with linear output. The transducer was disc shaped, 2.5 mm thick, and covered by a membrane. As the foot contacted the beam it deformed the strain gauges connected to a Wheatstone bridge. The 2.5-mm thickness of the transducer was a significant disadvantage.

Soames et al.[22] used beam-type transducers similar to those of Leriem and Serck-Hanssen with the exceptions that they were square in shape and only 0.9 mm thick. The sensors were not set into the insole of the shoe, but were placed on the foot. These devices created an indentation in the foot that is inappropriate for the insensitive foot. However, these transducers could be calibrated by the manufacturer.

## PIEZOELECTRIC TRANSDUCER

A piezoelectric transducer functions on the principle that certain crystalline structures are piezoelectrically active and function as a bundle of dipoles, with positive charges grouped at one side and negative charges at the other. This surface charge disappears in a short period of time from to environmental factors; the advantage is this rapid discharge of the surface charge. When mechanical stress is applied to the material, separation of charge occurs proportional to the magnitude and orientation of the stress.[3,15] The advantages of this transducer are that smaller loads are produced under the foot and that output is linear and exhibits no hysteresis. Its disadvantages are that it is extremely sensitive to temperature changes. Also, the voltage decays with time so the device is not suitable for static data collection.

Hennacy and Gunther[23] used commercially available crystals (Vernitron PTZ-54) to build a piezoelectric pressure sensor that was easily calibrated, inexpensive, and capable of recording static and dynamic pressures. Hennig et al.[15] manufactured an insole-shaped piezoelectric transducer of separate 4 mm × 4 mm tiles in matrix form to resolve the problems inherent to the capacitance mat that they developed in 1978. This insole form was not used again. Cavanagh et al.[24] used this in a tiled form. Hennig and associates used it in a discrete sensor form for several studies involving running and other athletic events.[25,26] Bhat et al.[27] used commercially available piezo film to build a transducer that was thin, inexpensive, and durable. It would not register steady pressures at all, but the linearity of the device was good.

There are many problems inherent in piezoelectric

devices, problems which have discouraged clinical use of piezoelectric transducers.[1,10]

## FORCE-SENSING RESISTORS

Force-sensing resistors (FSR) are made by impregnating an elastic material such as foam rubber with a conductor such as metal or carbon powder. Two conducive sheets sandwich the conductive elastomer. When the sandwich is compressed, the elastic material gives and allows more surface contact of the powdered conductor, which results in decreased resistance proportional to the amount of compression.[28]

The main advantages of FSRs are their simplicity and very thin cross section. Most investigators who use these devices do so because they are thin and lightweight. The most widely used FSR is sold commercially as a complete pressure recording system called the Electrodynogram (EDG) (Langer Biomechanics Group, Deer Park, NY)[29] that was developed in 1979. Early users of the systems encountered difficulties. Misevich[30] chose the EDG for its small size and unobtrusiveness but found the early sensors were too thick and too variable to use in any reproducible experiments. In 1984 he used the newer Mylar sensors but cautioned others against using them without first performing rigorous calibration procedures. Brodsky et al.[31] using the EDG in 1987, reported it was inaccurate and that its results could not be reproduced. He cautioned investigators to be sceptical until its reliability was improved. Other investigators[32–34] used the system with no negative comments but did not discuss if they calibrated the device. It appears to be a good foot timing device.

## MAGNETO RESISTOR SENSORS

The magneto resistor uses a semiconductor the resistance of which varies with the strength of the magnetic field in which it is placed. The device was developed by Tappin et al.[35] to measure shear forces on the sole of the foot and was used by Pollard et al.[36] to examine shear forces in combination with normal stress. A similar smaller version of the sensor was recently developed by Laing et al.[37]

The Tappin transducer is constructed using two stainless steel disks 16 mm in diameter. The upper disk was grooved and attached to the subject's foot. The lower disk had a corresponding ridge which fit into the groove of the upper disk and allowed sliding translation between the two disks along one axis only. A magneto resistor was mounted flush with the floor of the groove, and a magnet was attached to the ridge. When assembled, the magnet and resistor would slide relative to each other. The disks were held together with silicone rubber, which allowed translation of the disks relative to each other and provided a recentering force. The electrical signal produced was proportional to the movement of the magnet, which was in turn proportional to the applied shear force.[35] The transducer is 2.7 mm thick and may be noticeable under the subject's foot; the device developed by Laing and associates is only 1 mm thick.

## CLINICAL APPLICATIONS

Clinical devices for the pressure measurement are of two categories, a discrete transducer and the matrix type. If you are interested in evaluating a discrete area of the foot, devices like the electrodynograph, magneto resistors, or piezoelectric devices should be considered. They are small, considerably less expensive, often portable, and easy to use for evaluation of the shoe–foot interface. Placement of the sensors is extremely important. Cavanagh and Ulbrecht[1] stated that the drawback of discrete sensors is that the investigator makes an assumption where the pattern of plantar pressure is before attaching the sensors to the foot. Lord[3] warned that discrete sensors might not give accurate measurements because of difficulty in accurately positioning the transducers. Care is required to position the sensors precisely at the intended location, which may be accomplished by radiography,[21] or by palpation of bony prominences or after location with inked pads.[38]

One must try to stop any movement of the sensor on the foot surface by applying tape or adhering the sensor. Misevich[30] reported that migration of the sensors on the sole of the foot ultimately required them to be in laid into the insole. The discrete transducer can act as a foreign body in the shoe, distorting pressures and affecting the subject's gait.[39,40] Lake et al.[41]

compared plantar pressures between transducers placed on top of the insole and those recessed into it, finding that transducers on top of the insole surface had increased recorded pressures.

When one requires an evaluation of the plantar aspect of the foot, the matrix devices are used. They evaluate the entire plantar aspect giving a relationship of discrete pressures to the entire distribution of plantar pressure. They can be used to determine the cause of a lesion (for example, diabetic) or to compare a pre- and postsurgical state. However, the matrices are likely to underestimate the peak pressure as the load may be borne on several sensors at once.[25]

The matrix devices are usually placed in a walkway (e.g., the EMED-SF, Musgrave FSR, Pedobarograph BTE) or in the shoe (the F-Scan or Micro EMED). The difficulty when the modality is in a walkway or set in the ground is that this only allows for bare foot or outer shoe conditions to be evaluated. Another difficulty is the collection of successive trials, the mid gait collection technique versus the first-step collection technique (which may avoid the targeting problem of midgait collection).[1,42] The circuitry and subsequent expense of these devices is considerable when compared to the discrete sensor.[9,15,25]

## THE PRACTICAL EVALUATION OF SUBJECTS WITH FOREFOOT DEFORMITY AND PAIN

Four examples utilizing the pedobarograph plantar pressure assessment are presented to show the use of this device in the decision-making process for treatment of the painful forefoot. Significant numbers of surgical forefoot corrections are attempted every year, and many of them are resurgeries because past procedures have failed. As detailed in the first case study, use of the pedobarograph may help to reduce the number of surgical failures from poor subject selection.

## CASE STUDIES
### Case Study 1

An 18-year-old caucasian woman presented with complaints of pain in the great toe joints during the past

**Table 35-1.** Results of Arthrometric Examination

| Anatomic Site | Left | Right |
|---|---|---|
| Hip | 11° external | frontal plane |
| Hamstrings | Zero | Zero |
| Malleolar torsion | 18° external | 18° external |
| Ankle dorsiflexion | 10° | 10° |
| Subtalar joint | 13° inv/8° ev | 19° inv/9° ev |
| Forefoot to rearfoot | 6° varus | 4° varus |
| RCSP | 4° ev | 1° ev |
| NCSP | 10° inv | 10° inv |
| Limb length | Equal | Equal |
| Tibial influence | 9° mv | 9° mv |

*Abbreviations:* inv, inversion; ev, eversion; RCSP, resting calcaneal stance position; NCSP, neutral calcaneal stance position.

year. Wearing high-heeled shoes causes aching in the great toe joint. Table 35-1 shows the results of her arthrometric examination.

Visual gait analysis noted a pronated stance phase, with heel contact phase demonstrating rapid heel eversion past the vertical. This heel eversion appeared to continue into late midstance, resulting in an everted heel lift and propelling with a medial rolloff. The hallux valgus functional deficit became very evident in the pedobarograph results for both the left and right foot.

The lack of proper forefoot loading is first noticed from the medial to the lateral column. The first ray demonstrates that the load is inappropriate on the right side until the middle of midstance phase of gait (0.35 s). This type of function is seen in the pronated foot. The hallux valgus deformity creates a lack of forefoot stability at the end of forefoot loading phase. The unstable medial column is related to the forefoot varus, demanding the rear foot continue pronating to enable the forefoot to reach the ground. The compensation of the rearfoot varus also continues the instability of the lateral and the medial columns. The pronation continues about the midtarsal joint until the second through fourth metatarsals are stable in the sagittal plane.

The preparation of the forefoot stability takes three-quarters of the stance period. The demand for stability creates a plantar flexion of the hallux to resist the lateral to medial weight transfer. This occurs in conjunction with the sagittal plane stress that results from body movement. The hallux stress is larger than the load under the first metatarsal head. The pattern of increased hallux and second metatarsal stress is associated with a decreased first metatarsal stress, defined as a functional hallux limitus (FHL). A functional or structural metatarsus primus elevatus will exhibit pressure findings similar to that described as FHL.

Radiography and clinical evaluation will distinguish between the two conditions. As seen in this case, on x-ray the first metatarsal was elevated; however, it was not short and a tongue-and-groove configuration was noted in the first metatarsal head. The majority of the hallux valgus angle was formed by the distal abductus angulation.

Orthotic functional control of this case should focus on the heel lift period of stance. Control at this time would enable the foot to adequately prepare for the next stance phase. This would be achieved by using an aggressive rearfoot and forefoot varus post, 18-mm heel cup height, and a Morton's forefoot extension. The control and balance of the forefoot loading would be required up to 85 percent of the stance phase (early propulsive phase) of gait.

In this case, what surgical procedure would you contemplate to correct the functional assymetries in the medial and the lateral columns of the foot? Would a procedure to lower the first ray be sufficient? Would a procedure to elevate the second and third metatarsals also be appropriate to avoid future problems? Could a more aggressive surgical plan such as derotation of the navicular be best? In conjunction with the surgery, would the orthotic therapy be sufficient to support the foot after the procedure?

The answers to these questions become very important when considering the surgical intervention on the functional hallux limitus or metatarsus primus elevatus (MPE) foot type via the first metatarsophalangeal joint arthroplasty with or without implant. One can realize the stress that would develop under the central rays of the foot in the MPE foot type after such a procedure.

## Case Study 2

This example is a 61-year-old black man who complained of a painful hallux valgus deformity of his left foot. This subject demonstrates a severe limited ankle dorsiflexion of 90° of both feet with the knees extended. He also presents with a moderate rearfoot

varus and inverted forefoot to rearfoot. Observation of his gait notes an inverted heel at heel strike while at midstance his midtarsal joint is compensated by a fixed pronated position.

Biomechanical function was further assessed while the subject walked over the pedobarograph matrix platform. The forefoot loading is caused by the deviation of the first metatarsophalangeal joint; first metatarsophalangeal joint loading notes practically no stress in the left foot and minimal stress in the right. Severe stress is present under the second metatarsal with a supportive stress by the hallux. The loading characteristic of the hallux and the second ray is seen during the late stages of midstance and the propulsive phase of gait. This represents a hallux limitus and non-supportive function of the first ray. Is this the sign of instability of the first ray or the sign of hypermobility or an adapted elevatus of the first ray? Correlated to the biomechanical findings, a large range of first-ray dorsiflexion and lesser first-ray plantar flexion was noted. The first metatarsophalangeal joint was also restricted in its dorsiflexion (25°).

How much would the orthosis manipulate the patients propulsive function? Would it reduce the need for surgery? Would a plantar-flexory surgery of the first metatarsal assist the balance of the stresses at the forefoot?

## Case Study 3

A 32-year-old Caucasian male warehouse worker complained of a painful left foot in the area of the ball of the foot near the third metatarsal head. The tyloma was noted to be concentrated under the site of pain with a fibrous base. The patient described his pain being localized and having a burning/shooting character. He ambulated with a slight antalgic gait; overactivity of the anterior tibial muscle and lesser extensors musculature was also noted. In biomechanical examination, a compensated moderate rearfoot varus and forefoot varus in association with a low axis of the subtalar joint were noted. Ambulation throughout stance was with an everted relaxed calcaneal stance position.

The pedobarograph notes loading of the forefoot that is out of the normal sequence of the fifth to the first metatarsal loading sequence. The loading of the forefoot begins at the time of maximum load (0.20 s) for the heel, which is about 50 percent of the maximum load to the forefoot. The concentration of the vertical force is under the second through the fourth metatarsal heads. The load under the second and the third metatarsal heads and halluces is at their maximum (at 0.65 s) of the foot during late propulsive phase. The center of pressure line of this patient suggests a moderately pronated function in this foot as well. Similar function is noted in the right foot.

Questions arise as to what therapy would be best to relieve the neuritic symptoms as well as the tyloma in the area of maximum stress. Would a forefoot to rearfoot balance be sufficient in the positive cast or would it be better to use an extrinsic post? Will soft tissue supplementation with accommodation of a 4-mm depth be required? Or would it be best to elevate or shorten the metatarsals along with excision of the entrapped nerve?

## Case Study 4

The final example is a patient who had previous metatarsal surgery of the area of interest, the third metatarsal of both feet. The lesions were present for several years before surgical intervention. There was no preoperative pedobarographs. The lesions were not altered by the surgical intervention. No orthotic therapy was utilized after surgery.

Now the patient presented for a second opinion with deep callused lesions under the fourth metatarsal heads of both feet. In addition she presented biomechanically with compensated forefoot varus of 5 degrees, a rearfoot varus of 4 degrees, and contracted third and fourth metatarsophalangeal joints.

A pedobarograph examination was conducted before and after debridement of these lesions. Debridement of the lesions reduced the abrupt contact of the area of interest. The vertical stress in this area was reduced approximately 70 percent, and the patient's antalgic ambulation improved dramatically.

Therapeutic concerns for these lesions would be further surgical intervention to reduce the contracted metatarsophalangeal joints, an elliptical plantar skin revision with appropriate midtarsal and forefoot orthotic control, or elevation of another metatarsal.

## SUMMARY

The aim of this brief review of pressure-evaluating tools is to develop an awareness of the types of mechanical devices available for better evaluation of painful complaints of the forefoot and better patient care. Deformity is generally very obvious, but more depth of thought and insight into function are needed to provide correction. The tools are available now to investigate and to establish the biomechanical parameters of surgical therapy.

## REFERENCES

1. Cavanagh PR, Ulbrecht JS: Biomechanics of the diabetic foot: a quantitative approach to the assessment of neuropathy, deformity and plantar pressure. p. 1864. In Jahss MH (ed): Disorders of the Foot and Ankle, 2nd Ed. WB Saunders, Philadelphia, 1991
2. Elftman HO: A cinematic study of the distribution of pressure in the human foot. The Anatomical Record 59:481, 1934
3. Lord M: Foot pressure measurement: a review of methodology. J Biomed Eng 3:91, 1981
4. Masson EA, Boulton AJM: Pressure assessment methods in the foot. In Frykberg RG (ed): The High Risk Foot in Diabetes Mellitus. Churchill Livingstone, New York, 1991
5. Morton DJ: Structural factors in static disorders of the foot. Am J Surg 93:15, 1930
6. Brand PW, Ebner JD: Pressure sensitive devices for denervated hands and feet. J Bone Joint Surg Am 51:109, 1969
7. Betts RP, Duckworth T: A device for measuring the plantar pressures under the sole of the foot. Eng Med 7:223, 1978
8. Chodera JD, Hard M: Examination methods of standing in man. FU CSAV Praha, 1, 1957
9. Betts RP, Franks CI, Duckworth T, Burke J Static and dynamic foot-pressure measurement in clinical orthopedics. Med Biol Eng Comput 18:674, 1980
10. Alexander IJ, Chao EYS, Johnson KA: The assessment of dynamic foot-to-ground contract forces and plantar pressure distribution: a review of the evolution of current techniques and clinical applications. Foot Ankle, 11:152, 1990
11. Schwartz RP, Heath AL: The definition of human locomotion on the basis of measurement: with description of oscillographic method. J Bone Joint Surg 29:203, 1947
12. Bauman JH, Brand PW: Measurement of pressure between foot and shoe. Lancet 2:629, 1963

13. Holden TS, Muncey RW: Pressures on the human foot during walking. Aust J Appl Sci 4:405, 1953

14. Frank WE, Gibson RJ: A new pressure-sensing instrument. Franklin Institute Report F-2385 T1.F8:21. Philadelphia, 1954

15. Henning EM, Cavanagh PR, Albert HT, Macmillan, NH: A piezoelectric method of measuring the vertical contact stress beneath the human foot. J Biomed Eng 4:213, 1982

16. Coleman WC: The relief of forefoot pressures using outer shoe sole modifications. p. 29. In Mothirami Patil K, Srinivasa H (eds): Proceedings of the International Conference on Biomechanics and Clinical Kinesiology of Hand and Foot, Madras, India. Indian Institute of Technology, Madras, 1985

17. Kothari M, Webster JG, Tompkins WJ, et al: Capacitive sensors for measuring the pressure between the foot and shoe. In 10th Annual International Conference. IEEE Engineering in Medicine and Biology Society, New York, 1988

18. Hutton WC, Drabble GE: An apparatus to give the distribution of vertical load under the foot. Rheumatol Phys Med 11:313, 1972

19. Stokes IAF Faris IB, Hutton WC: The neuropathic ulcer and loads on the foot in diabetic patients. Acta Orthop Scand 46:839, 1975

20. Ctercteko GC, Dhanendran MK, Hutton WC, Le Quesne LP: Vertical forces acting on the feet of diabetic patients with neuropathic ulceration. Br J Surg 68:608, 1981

21. Lereim P, Serck-Hanssen F: A method of recording pressure distribution under the sole of the foot. Bull Prosthet Res 10:118, 1973

22. Soames RW, Stott JRR, Goodbody A, et al: Measurement of pressure under the foot during function. Med Biol Eng Comput 20:489, 1982

23. Hennacy RA, Gunther A: A piezoelectric crystal method for measuring static and dynamic pressure distributions in the feet. J Am Podiatry Assoc 65:444, 1975

24. Cavanagh PR, Valiant GA, Misevich KW: Biological aspect of modeling shoe interaction during running. p. 24. In Frederick EC (ed): Sport Shoes and Playing Surfaces. Human Kinetics Publishers, Champaign, 1984

25. Henning EM, Milani TL: Pressure distribution measurement techniques for the prevention of athletic injuries. p. 183. In Proceedings of the First I.O.C. World Congress. United States Olympic Committee, 1989

26. Milani TL, Hennig EM: Pressure distribution patterns inside a running shoe during up-and downhill running (abstract). J Biomech 22:1050, 1989

27. Bhat S, Webster JB, Tompkins WJ, Wertch JJ: Piezoelectric sensor for foot pressure measurement. p. 1435. In 11th Annual International Conference, IEEE Engineering in Medicine & Biology Society, New York, 1989

28. Maalej N, Bhat S, Zhu H, et al: A conductive polymer pressure sensor. In 10th Annual International Conference, p. 770. IEEE Engineering in Medicine & Biology Society, 1988

29. Langer S, Polchaninoff M, Hoerner EF: Principles and Fundamentals of Clinical Electrodynography. Langer Corp., Deer Park, NY, 1984

30. Misevich KW: The evaluation of force/time distributions in athletic equipment with pressure sensors. In ASME Engineering Foundation Conference, Sports Biomechanics, 1985

31. Brodsky JW, Kourosh S, Mooney V: Objective evaluation and review of commercial gait analysis systems. In Proceedings, The American Orthopaedic Foot and Ankle Society 19th Annual Meeting, Las Vegas, NV, 1989

32. D'Amico JC, Dinowitz HD, Polchaninoff M: Limb length discrepancy. An electrodynographic analysis. J Am Podiatric Med Assoc 75:639, 1985

33. Smith L, Plehwe W, McGill M et al: Foot bearing pressure in patients with unilateral diabetic foot ulcers. Diabetic Med 6:573, 1989

34. Gastwirth BW, O'Brien TD, Nelson RM, et al: An electrodynographic analysis of foot function in shoes of varying heel heights. J Am Podiatric Med Assoc 81:463, 1991

35. Tappin JW, Pollard J, Beckett EA: Method of measuring "shearing" forces on the sole of the foot. Clin Phys Physiol Measur 1:83, 1980

36. Pollard JP, Le Quesne LP, Tappin, JW: Forces under the foot. J Bio-med Eng 5:37, 1983

37. Laing P, Cogley D, Crerand S, Klenerman L: The liverpool shear transducer (abstract). In The Diabetic Foot, First International Symposium and Workshop, The Netherlands, 1991

38. Bauman JH, Girling E, Brand PW: Plantar pressures and trophic ulceration—an evaluation of footwear. J Bone Joint Surg 45B:652, 1963

39. Collis WJMF, Jayson MIV: Measurement of pedal pressures. An illustration of a method. Ann Rheum Dis 31:215, 1972

40. Brodsky JW, Kourosh S, Stills M, Mooney V: Objective evaluation of insert material for diabetic and athletic footwear. Foot Ankle 9:111, 1988

41. Lake MJ, Lafortune MA, Perry SD: Heel plantar pressure distortion caused by discrete sensors. (abstract). J Biomech 25:768, 1992

42. Rodgers MM: Plantar pressure distribution during barefoot walking: normal and predictive equations. Doctoral dissertation, The Pennsylvania State University, University Park, PA, 1985

# 36

# Rationale for Prophylactic Surgery in the Diabetic Foot

*RICHARD M. STESS*
*MARILYN J. WALLER*

The Diabetes Control Activity has established diabetes control programs in 20 states. Each program has investigated the extent and nature of diabetes morbidity within its state by means of a descriptive analysis of selected health status indicators. In a 1983 study by Most and Sinnock, data from six states were pooled to provide a profile of lower extremity amputations (LEA) in diabetic individuals.[1] Results indicated that 45 percent of all LEAs were performed in patients with diabetes. An age-adjusted LEA rate of 59.7 per 10,000 diabetic individuals was computed. Diabetes-related amputation rates increase with age and are higher in males. The overwhelming majority of LEAs were either toe or above the knee (AKA), with few performed on the foot. The relative risk of LEAs for diabetic patients compared with the nondiabetic population was highest in the under-45 age group, although the attributable risk was highest in the older population, 191.5 per 10,000 diabetic individuals.

Overall diabetic persons have a 15-fold higher risk of LEA than nondiabetic individuals.[2] According to Bild et al., the direct cost of an amputation including hospitalization, surgery, and anesthesia is $8,000 to $12,000 per case.[3,4] It is estimated that the annual yearly outpatient costs for diabetes sufferers is $1.7 billion, of which $372 million is expended on 13.4 million visits to physicians.[5] This information, provided by the National Center for Health Statistics, does not show the costs or percentage of the total figure for foot-related conditions. Some have estimated this figure to be as high as 20 percent of hospitalizations for diabetic foot-

related conditions.[6] Approximately half the amputations performed in Veterans Affairs hospitals occurred in individuals with diabetes.[1] The 3-year survival for people with diabetes who have undergone an LEA is only 50 percent.[7] It is further estimated that more than 50 percent of the amputations within the diabetic population could be prevented by reducing risk factors for amputation and improving foot care. Integral to many programs for preventative foot care, prophylactic surgery in the diabetic foot has been advocated for the treatment of forefoot and midfoot deformities that are predisposed to concentrated pressures on localized areas.[8–10] There appear to be no studies to date correlating reduction in the number of LEAs performed on diabetic individuals who have previously undergone prophylactic surgery of the foot specifically to change deforming forces once identified as a risk factor for LEA.

In reviewing literature and statistics related to surgery in the diabetic foot, prophylactic surgery appears to be a small percentage of all diabetic foot surgery.[11–13] In a 5-year review at the University of Chicago Hospital and clinics, prophylactic surgery was only 12.3 percent of all diabetic foot surgery. It was found that most surgery in diabetic patients was ablative in nature and was usually performed to debride infected soft tissue or bone.[14] Their study indicated the rate of complications from prophylactic diabetic foot surgery approached 31.2 percent even with a thorough preoperative workup. Most of these complications occurred when ulcerations had been previously present for more than 1 year and had been localized to a weight-bearing metatarsal head surface. Deformities that place a diabetic individual at significant risk for ulceration include ingrown toenails, digital contractures, bunion and tailor's bunion, and midfoot protrusion secondary to muscle imbalance or Charcot joint.[6] With nearly all LEAs in diabetic patients being directly or indirectly related to ulceration, it would be prudent from concerns about both health care costs and patient morbidity to identify those diabetic individuals who are at risk for tissue breakdown and consider prophylactic surgical reduction of deformities among the treatment plans. The success rate of prophylactic foot surgery should be able to achieve the success level of surgeries performed on the non-diabetic foot, provided the high-risk patient can be identified and treated appropriately by means of preoperative criteria and analysis before complications occur.[14]

Surgery of the foot in patients with diabetes mellitus should not be considered taboo but it does require specific criteria that must be strictly followed. Careful and comprehensive preoperative assessment and strictly scheduled preoperative management are the hallmarks of successful care of the diabetic foot. A close working relationship with the diabetologist or internist responsible for medical management of the patient is of utmost importance for a successful outcome of any foot pathology correction. This becomes a cardinal rule when discussing the surgical management of the diabetic foot, and one that the competent practioner will never break.

The podiatric physician and internist must be well versed in perioperative protocols for diabetic patients because of the surgical stresses placed on either insulin-dependent diabetics (IDDM, type I) or non-insulin-dependent diabetic patients (NIDDM, type II). Impaired renal function and macrovascular disease significantly increase the morbidity and mortality among diabetic patients,[6,9] and become an issue when the podiatric physician becomes involved in extensive reconstructive foot surgery, in neuropathic osteoarthropathy (Charcot foot deformity) or when amputation is considered. Urinary tract infections, pneumonia, and wound infections are common in the postoperative period particularly in cases of persistent hyperglycemia. Blood glucose greater than 240 mg/dl can result in impaired fibroblast function, which may then cause incisional dehiscence.

Patients who are undiagnosed for diabetes may be prone to excessive hyperglycemic osmotic diuresis and dehydration following a prolonged foot procedure.[15,16] It therefore becomes essential that all patients be adequately evaluated preoperatively and that all diabetic patients are carefully controlled via an approved perioperative diabetic surgical protocol. The true meaning of the multidisciplinary team approach to patient management is realized in effective management in the care of the diabetic foot.

One of the conditions most often seen and just as commonly mismanaged is diabetic foot ulceration.[18] Two of the more widely published authorities on diabetic foot care have diverging opinions in the issue of foot soaks. One believes that the foot should be well hydrated to maintain the normal skin integrity, stating that the best way to accomplish this is to get water to the keratin layer via soaking in water for 15 to 20 min/day.[18] The other author believes that excessive soaks lead to excessive dryness, fissuring, and cracking of the skin. He states that "foot soaks lead to more complications in diabetes than any other home remedy."[19] This controversy points out the larger differences and often empirical methods employed in managing the diabetic foot. Limited objective research exists that firmly establishes a causal effect of a particular treatment modality. As a result, management of diabetic foot ulcerations is placed in the hands of practitioners who often employ techniques passed down from generations of clinicians whose treatment protocols lack scientific scrutiny. The time has come to investigate the simplest of methods and to firmly establish proven and successful techniques in the management of the diabetic foot ulcer. Recent introduction of wound healing factors has added another dimension to the treatment of the diabetic foot wounds. Careful scrutiny of these newer modalities must be made by the podiatrist as the claims of the manufacturer may be somewhat optimistic. It appears unclear to many who have taken the responsibility of treating the diabetic foot whether the wound healing factors are responsible for the enhanced rates of healing or if the more intensive comprehensive care being used is the determining factor. At this junction it would appear that research into the efficacy of wound healing factors must be carefully viewed and the results of double-blind, placebo-controlled protocols be scrutinized before final judgment passed on use of such factors in the management of foot ulcerations.

Guidelines for minor foot surgery were reviewed by Gavin.[22] Table 36-1 indicates an approved protocol for both type I (IDDM) and type II (NIDDM). Minor foot surgery is considered that form of surgery requiring only local anesthetic agents. Major cases, those

**Table 36-1.**  Guidelines for Diabetes Control: Minor Surgery and Invasive Diagnostic Procedures

| Insulin-Treated Patient | Oral Hypoglycemic Agent (OHA)-Treated Patient |
|---|---|
| NPO Day of Surgery | |
| • IDDM:  Cover with insulin-glucose infusion  Check fasting blood glucose (FBG) q2h–q4h with bedside meter.  • NIDDM: Hold *morning* NPH/ Lente.  Check FBG and administer regular insulin q4h–q6h as shown below. | • Hold morning OHA  • Check FBG pre- and post-surgery.  • Give evening OHA.  • Insulin *rarely* needed. If necessary, use regular human insulin as shown below. |

| Blood Glucose (BG) (mg/dl) | Subcutaneous Regular Insulin (U) |
|---|---|
| <180 | 0 |
| 181–220 | 5 |
| 221–260 | 6 |
| 261–300 | 8 |
| 300 | 10 |

| | |
|---|---|
| • After the procedure, give usual evening dose of insulin if dinner allowed. If patient remains NPO, continue the selected regimen. | |
| Breakfast on Day of Surgery | |
| • Give normal morning insulin dose: Check BG q2h–q4h.  • Supplement with regular insulin: BG >220, 5 U, etc.  • Avoid hypoglycemia. | • Give normal morning OHA.  • Check BG pre-and post-surgery.  • Given evening OHA. |

performed under general anesthetic agents, may require continuous insulin infusion that should be planned to begin the night before surgery. Good metabolic control can be maintained via this method in a procedure that may be somewhat prolonged. Most forefoot cases including amputations can be performed under local anesthesia whether or not there is evidence of peripheral neuropathy, and consequently it would be doubtful that insulin infusion would be utilized. More extensive rearfoot cases would be classified as major surgery as these are often performed under general anesthesia.

An understanding of the disease process in diabetes is mandatory to being able to analyze treatment choices and identify preoperative criteria when prophylactic surgery is being considered for the diabetic patient. Vascular disease combined with neuropathy leads to a significant portion of the morbidity we see in the lower extremities of diabetic individuals.[6,23–25] Progressive symmetrical distal polyneuropathy of motor and sensory nerves causes sensory deficits, which can lead to significant anesthesia so that the skin cannot handle repetitive stress.[15] Consequently skin and underlying tissues may break down and become an attractive environment for infection.

It is believed that during repetitive stress the normal sensate individual is aware of subsequent repeated trauma to the skin and underlying tissues.[26] As a result, gait and stride may be altered as a means of protection. The patient who has lost this protective sensation threshold and continues to traumatize local regions of the foot is predisposed to callus formation, foot ulceration, and possibly amputation.[27] Polyneuropathy begins distally and spreads proximally with initial sensory deficits in a stocking distribution. These patients show varying degrees of diminished touch, pain, vibration, and joint position sense, with depressed reflexes. It is interesting to note that the achilles reflex is often absent in the early stages of diabetes and neuropathy. Motor nerve changes also lead to rapid increases in the formation of digital, forefoot, and midfoot deformities, and in certain circumstances neuropathic osteoarthropathy.[28] Mononeuropathy is believed to be the result of vascular occlusion of an arterial supply to a peripheral nerve.[10] Peroneal palsy is the most common disorder. Clinically the patient may present with a motor, sensory, and reflex impair-

**Table 36-2.** Signs and Symptoms Associated With the Insensitive Foot

Paresthesias
Hypesthesia
Anesthesia
Nocturnal cramping
Diminished or absent deep tendon reflexes
Diminished or absent vibratory sensation
Diminished or absent temperature or pain sensation
Anhidrosis
Callus formation
Ulceration
Intrinsic muscle atrophy
Digital deformity
Cavus foot deformity or pes valgus deformity
Increased skin temperature
Edema
Change in function (foot-drop)

**Table 36-3.** Perioperative Risks of Diabetic Patients

Autonomic neuropathy
  Difficulty in maintaining stable blood pressure
  Postural hypotension
  Painless myocardial infarction
Increased sensitivity to drugs
Coronary artery disease (three to four times as frequent in age-matched population)
Nephropathy
  Difficulty metabolizing and excreting drugs
  Fluid and electrolyte imbalance
Nutritional imbalance

ment in the distribution of a specific peripheral nerve (Table 36-2).

Vascular changes in the diabetic extremity can be the result of three mechanisms: occlusive peripheral vascular disease, autonomic neuropathy, and microvascular insufficiency, most likely caused by basement membrane hypertrophy.[15,29] The development of arterial occlusive diseases is approximately five times more common in diabetics than nondiabetics. Pathologic changes occur within the walls of the small, medium, and large blood vessels of diabetic persons, causing lesions in lower extremity vessels.[30] The diabetic patient often develops arterial occlusion in both large and small vessels, as evidenced by calcification of larger arteries in the tunica media as well as hemorrhagic plaques and calcification in the intima. The process occurs more frequently, at an earlier age, and with more complications for the diabetic patient.[15] Arteriosclerosis in the diabetic person appears to occur more distally and progresses in distal to proximal fashion, resulting in the development of a less effective collateral circulation[14] (Table 36-3).

Local manifestations of autonomic neuropathy in the diabetic foot can be manifest as medial vascular calcification and neuropathic edema.[6,14,15,31] It has been associated with an increased incidence of ulceration and the development of a painful neuropathy. Long-term sympathetic denervation has been shown to cause structural damage to the peripheral arteries.[28] The effects of long-term sympathectomy include smooth muscle atrophy in the vessels, leading to ulti-

mate structural changes in the arterial tree. This increase in blood flow has been implicated as an important factor in the development of Charcot joint and pedal ulceration. Ward et al.[16] postulated that, flow in the small distal vessels is inadequate as a result of faster flow from ateriovenous shunting. Abnormally high blood flow, vasodilation, and arteriovenous shunting that results from sympathetic denervation lead to abnormal venous pooling.[16] The neuropathic edema that develops interferes with the normal mechanism of skin function and predisposes the patient to the development of pedal ulcerations.

Biomechanical processes are significantly altered with diabetes.[15] It has been shown by sonographic examination that diabetic patients who suffer from neuropathy have atrophic plantar fat pads.[17] Brand conducted an experiment that suggested that tissue will most likely break down at those areas of high pressure with repetitive stress.[18] Stokes and coworkers found, in diabetic patients, that peak loads were shifted laterally on the foot and that increasing abnormalities in loading occurred with a corresponding evidence of peripheral neuropathy. Their most striking factor was a reduction of load of the toes. Stokes theorized that lateral shifting and weight-bearing could be caused by weakness of the muscles or loss of coordination from loss of physiologic impulses from the tendon receptors and denervation of the intrinsic muscles. This would result in overpowering of the extrinsic extremity muscles, contributing to significant digital contracture and leading to hammer toes and submetatarsal head lesions.[20,21]

Several authors have demonstrated the importance in the accumulation of dynamic plantar pressure data in the diabetic foot.[32,33] Recent technologic advances by instruments such as the EMED (Novel), Pedobarograph (Biokenitics), and Tekscan (Physical Support Systems, Inc.) now can provide reproducible vertical force and pressure data invaluable in the comprehensive care of the diabetic patient. Although no "normal" values or normal feet have been firmly established in the literature, several studies have demonstrated the force and pressure data of diabetic feet and how these differ from nondiabetic subjects.[32,33] A recent chapter by Cavanagh and Ulbrecht[32] concluded, "Circumstantial evidence has shown that elevated plantar pressure is a risk factor for ulceration in the diabetic foot. Elevated plantar pressure, however, even in the presence of sensory neuropathy, has not been proved to cause a plantar ulcer." Despite this we can unequivically state that peak plantar pressure is one factor in plantar ulcer development and that this pressure must be determined if we hope to be in the position of prospective determination of the likelihood of a neuropathic diabetic patient to develop a foot ulcer. At this point prophylactic intervention via custom orthotic devices, custom footwear, and routine lesion debridement will be irrefutable as to their importance in ulcer prevention.

It requires more than technologic sophistication to achieve a well-coordinated plan for perioperative care. Careful integrated planning as well as collaboration by all care-givers will achieve optimal results. Without this effort by the podiatric surgeon, internist, endocrinologist, anesthesiologist, and nursing and other staff members, the result would be only an increase in morbidity and unsatisfactory surgical outcomes.

# REFERENCES

1. Most RS, Sinnock: The epidemiology of lower extremity amputations in diabetic individuals. Diabetes Care 6:87, 1983
2. Kozac GP, Hoar C, Rowbotham JL, et al: Management of Diabetic Foot Problems. WB Saunders, Philadelphia, 1984
3. Jacobs J: The economic impact of diabetes. In Conference preceding ADA 48th Meeting, August 1988
4. Bild DE, Selby JV, Sinnock P, et al: Lower extremity amputations in people with diabetes. Epidemiology and prevention. Diabetes Care 12:24, 1989
5. Penn I: Diabetes mellitus and the surgeon. Curr Probl Surg 24:546, 1987
6. Levin ME, O'Neal LW: The Diabetic Foot. CV Mosby, St. Louis, 1983
7. National Diabetes Advisory Board: The Prevention and Treatment of Five Complications of Diabetes. A Guide for Primary Care Practitioners. HHS Publ. No. 82-14680, Centers for Disease Control, Atlanta, 1983
8. Martin WJ, Wail LS, Smith SD: Surgical management of neuropathic ulcers in the diabetic foot. J Am Podiatry Assoc 65:365, 1975
9. Towne JE: Management of foot lesions in the diabetic patient. Vasc Surg, November, 1985
10. Wagner FW Jr: The dysvascular foot: a system for diagnosis and treatment. Foot Ankle 2:64, 1981
11. Baker WH, Barnes RW: Minor forefoot amputations in patients with low ankle pressures. Am J Surg 133:331, 197
12. Gianfortune P, Pulla RJ, Sage R: Ray resections in the intensive or dysvascular foot: a critical review. J Foot Surg 24:103, 1985
13. Pinzur MS, Sage R, Schwaegle P: Ray resection in the dysvascular foot: a retrospective review. Clin Orthop 191:323, 1984
14. Gudas, CJ: Prophylactic surgery in the diabetic foot. Clin Podiatr Med Surg 4:445, 1987
15. Stess RM, Hetherington VJ: The diabetic and insensitive foot, p. 523. In Principles and Practice of Podiatric Medicine. Churchill Livingstone, New York, 1990
16. Ward JD, Simms JM, Knight, et al: Venous distention in the diabetic neuropathic foot (physical sign of arteriovenous shunting). JR Soc Med 76:1011, 1983
17. Gooding GAW Stress RM, Graf PM, et al: Sonography of the sole of the foot: evidence of loss of foot pad thickness in diabetics and its relationship to ulceration of the foot. Invest Radiol 21:45, 1986
18. Brand PW: The diabetic foot. p. 829. In Ellenberg M, Rifken H (eds): Diabetes Mellitus, Theory and Practice, 3rd Ed. Medical Examination Publishing, 1983
19. Rowbotham JL, Gibbons GW, Kozak GP: The diabetic Foot. p. 221. In Kozak GP (ed): Clinical Diabetes. WB Saunders, Philadelphia, 1982
20. Stokes IAF, Hutton WC: The effect of the diabetic ulcer on the load-bearing function of the foot. p. 245. In Kenedi RM, Cowden JM (eds): Bedsore Biomechanics. University Park Press, Baltimore, 1976
21. Stokes IAF, Faris IB, Hutton WC: The neuropathic ulcer and loads on the foot in diabetic patients. Acta Orthop Scand 46:839, 1975
22. Gavin L: The Diabetic Surgical Patient. Practical Aspects of Diabetes Management. HP Publishing, New York, 1989
23. Fagerberg SE: Diabetic neuropathy, a clinical and histo-

logical study on the significance of vascular affectations. Acta Med Scand 164(Suppl 345), 1959

24. Ferrier TM: Comparative study of arterial disease in amputated lower limbs from diabetics and nondiabetics. Med J Aust 1:5, 1967

25. Gibbon GW, Freeman D: Vascular evaluation and treatment of the diabetic. Clin Podiatr Med Surg 4, 1987

26. Bauman, J, Girling J, Brand P: Plantar pressures and trophic ulcerations. J Bone Joint Surg 45B:652, 1963

27. Gazivoda P, Sollitto RJ, Slomowitz H; Diabetic foot amputations. J Foot Surg 29:72, 1990

28. Pedersen J, Olsen S: Small vessel diseases of the lower extremity in diabetes mallitus: on the pathogenesis of foot lesion in diabetics. Acta Med Scand 171:551, 1962

29. LoGerfo FW, Coffman JD. Vascular and microvascular disease of the foot in diabetics. Med Intell 311:1615, 1984

30. Ferguson BD, Kozak GP: Clinical Diabetes Mellitus. WB Saunders, Philadelphia, 1982

31. Schustek S, Jacobs AM: Diabetic autonomic neuropathy in the surgical management of the diabetic foot. J Foot Surg 21:16, 1982

32. Cavanagh PR, Ulbrecht JS: Plantar pressure in the diabetic foot. Chap. 5. In Sanmarco GJ (ed): The Foot in Diabetes. Lea & Febiger, Philadelphia, 1991

33. Wolfe L, Stess RM, Graf PM: Dynamic pressure analysis of the diabetic Charcot foot. J Am Podiatr Med Assoc 81, 1991

# Appendix 36-1.
# University of California, San Francisco, Diabetes Service

## PERIOPERATIVE MANAGEMENT OF DIABETES GENERAL GUIDELINES

☐ Admit patient the evening before surgery and schedule early surgery.
☐ Physician, anesthesiologist and surgeon liaison to plan regimen.
☐ Aim to keep blood glucose (BG) in a safe range (120–240 mg/dl).
☐ Bedside monitoring of BG with METER must be available.

**DEFINITIONS:**
IDDM: Insulin-dependent diabetes mellitus. These patients (pts.) need frequent (q4–6h) insulin to prevent DKA.

NIDDM: Non-insulin-dependent diabetes mellitus. Generally treated with diet ± oral hypoglycemic agent (OHA). However, many (30%) take insulin to achieve optimum control.

MAJOR SURGERY: General anesthesia–Invasion of body cavity—Duration > 2 h – NPO > 24 h.

MINOR SURGERY: Mild Sedation—Short duration (<2 h)—Food OK post-op.

**NEED FOR INSULIN DURING MAJOR SURGERY:**
All insulin-treated diabetic pts. (IDDM and NIDDMs)
NIDDMs (not on insulin) with average FBG > 180 during elective major and emergency surgery.
Variable: NIDDMs with average FBG < 180 on diet ± OHA. These may not need insulin for short-duration major surgery not invading a body cavity and when allowed food post-op.

**INSULIN REGIMENS:** INSULIN **DRIP** (Regular [R] Human[Novolin] 25 u in 250 ml N-Saline): This provides excellent flexibility for elective major and emergency surgery in all insulin-treated diabetic pts. Required for CABG, organ transplant (Tx).

---

INSULIN-GLUCOSE **INFUSION** (Regular [R] Human [Novolin] 7–15 u in 1000 ml of 5% D.W.): Suitable for NIDDM pts. during elective major surgery, except CABG and Organ Tx.

Pre-Op **INTERMEDIATE** INSULIN (NPH 30–50% AM dose): Reasonable for NIDDM but *not* IDDM during elective major surgery. These pts. should be taken to OR early and receive 5% D.W. (100 ml/h) in order to avoid potential hypoglycemia during a protracted NPO period.

**INSULIN DOSE:** Individualize re type of DM, FBG control, renal status and stress of surgery. Average normal dose: NPO, 0.3 u/Kg/day (dose needs may increase 2–3 fold during severe stress). Food OK—0.6 u/kg/day.

REGIMEN DURING MINOR SURGERY AND INVASIVE DIAGNOSTIC PROCEDURES (**Bedside Meter for BG Test**):
NPO: IDDM: Cover with "Insulin-Glucose Infusion." Check BG q4–6h.
    NIDDM: Hold (AM) DM med, Rx Regular (sc) q4–6h for BG > 180.
FOOD OK: Give usual (AM) DM med: OHA or insulin.
Post-surgery, if food OK give (PM) DM med., if NPO continue regimen.

**DKA—EMERGENCY SURGERY:**
1. Diagnosis: BG > 300 mg/dl, pH < 7.3, $HCO_3$ < 15, and plasma (urine) positive for ketones.
2. Stabilize patient prior to surgery with rehydration (fluid and electrolytes) and BG correction (BG < 240). This generally requires 3–4 h.
3. Insulin is best delivered by DRIP. Insulin needs are high during the initial phase (0.1 u/kg/h). Once stabilized, the insulin drip can be used for perioperative control as per detailed guidelines.
4. Glucose should be added to maintenance fluids once BG < 240 mg/dl.
5. Check serum potassium q2–4h to determine ongoing needs.

**TPN** should be considered in pts. **NPO** > 72h:
1. Most diabetic pts. will need insulin cover during TPN.
2. Nondiabetic pts. develop hyperglycemia (10–15%) and need insulin.
3. The safest insulin regimen is to add Regular Human (Novolin) directly to the standard TPN solution (Dextrose 25%, Amino Acids 4.25%).
4. Guidelines for initial insulin dose for diabetes based on pre-TPN BG:

| Blood Glucose (mg/dl): | < 120 | 121–180 | 181–240 | > 240 |
|---|---|---|---|---|
| Regular/Liter TPN: | 10 u | 15 u | 25 u | 35 u |

5. Supplement with Regular (sc) q4h for BG > 240 mg/dl. Make adjustments to Regular dose in subsequent bottles.
6. If insulin needs exceed 50 u/TPN liter, control BG with an Insulin Drip.

**DETAILED GUIDELINES**
**WRITE INSULIN ORDERS** the evening before surgery, and send to IV Additives.
1. The evening before surgery administer usual diabetes medication.

2. Hold morning diabetes medication.
3. Obtain 6 AM STAT FBG. (Lab and Bedside) (split sample).
4. Check BG hourly (bedside meter) perioperatively until patient is stable.
5. Assess potassium needs daily.

**INSULIN DRIP:** Regular (R) 25 u in 250 ml N-saline (1 u per 10 ml).

**A.** Begin INSULIN DRIP as per sliding scale (*see* B) for BG > 80.

Use a Microdrip (60 drops/ml), infusion pump. Flush 50 ml through line before connecting "piggyback" to the maintenance IV fluids.

Maintenance fluids must contain glucose (5%) infused at a constant rate.

**B.** SLIDING SCALE FOR DRIP RATE ADJUSTMENT

| Blood Glucose (mg/dl) | Insulin Drip (*IV*) U/H |
|---|---|
| <80 | 0.0 _____ |
| 81–100 | 0.5 _____ |
| 101–140 | 1.0 _____ |
| 141–180 | 1.5 _____ |
| 181–220 | 2.0 _____ |
| 221–260 | 2.5 _____ |
| 261–300 | 3.0 _____ |
| 301–340 | 4.0 _____ |
| >340 | 5.0 _____ |

BG + 100 gives a reasonable estimate of insulin dose (U/H).
Individualized dose re type of DM, renal status and stress.

**C. HYPOGLYCEMIA:** BG < 80 but > 60 mg/dl, STOP Insulin Drip. Once BG > 80, restart Insulin Drip. If BG < 60 mg/dl but pt. conscious, bolus with 25 cc of 50% D.W. If comatose, give 50 cc of 50% D.W., call M.D. and recheck BG in 15 minutes.
**D. HYPERGLYCEMIA:** Persistent BG > 340 mg/dl, despite 5 u/h insulin, call M.D. for reevaluation.
**E. If HIGH-DOSE INSULIN:** (>5 u/h) is anticipated (e.g., CABG, Organ Tx), use a more concentrated Insulin Drip. A special **DRIP** may also be needed to avoid excess fluids and for pediatrics.

**INSULIN-GLUCOSE INFUSION:** Base Regular (R) insulin (Novolin) dose on average FBG during the previous week. Begin infusion at 100 ml/h.
**A.** FBG 120–180 mg/dl: Add 7 u R to 1000 ml of 5% D.W. (0.7 u/h).
   FBG 181–240 mg/dl: Add 10 u R to 1000 ml (1.0 u/h)
   FBG > 240 mg/dl:   Add 15 u R to 1000 ml (1.5 u/h).
   FBG < 120 mg/dl:   Do not add insulin to infusion for NIDDM.
   However, for IDDM add 5 u R to 1000 ml (0.5 u/h).
   To avoid hypokalemia add KCl (20 mEq/L) except in renal failure.
**B.** During post-op period check BG q4h once patient stable. BG < 80, STOP infusion and treat as above in "Insulin Drip," C. Should BG > 240 mg/dl supplement with R (Novolin) sc.
   Adjust insulin dose in subsequent infusions as per supplements.

**POST-OP TRANSITION FROM NPO TO FOOD INTAKE** (Need Lab FBG and 4 PM BG qd):

**A.** Pre-op **INTERMEDIATE** INSULIN (NPH) Regimen: If post-op food OK—Rx usual pm Meds. If NPO-Rx R (sc) q6h for BG > 180 as per BG sliding scale (bedside meter).

**B.** Peri-op DRIP/INFUSION Regimen: Continue infusion (IV) until normal feeding established, then plan new regimen. Do not routinely give insulin by IV push. Its biological action is too short-lived (15 min.).

1. NIDDM previously treated with diet ± OHA: Rx pre-op medication if BG < 180. Higher BG may required transient R (sc) q6h.

2. Insulin-treated Diabetic patients: Use pt's usual insulin regimen or develop a new **BASIC DOSE** regimen:

The dose selected should be 60–80% of the previous day's total insulin dose. Needs may be higher during persistent stress (infection, pain, steroids, etc.) or high food intake (TPN, etc.).

The selected BASIC DOSE may be given as pre-meal [Breakfast (25%), Lunch (25%), Dinner (25%)] Regular (sc) and NPH at Bedtime (25%).

Use BG sliding scale to ADJUST the **PREMEAL BASIC DOSE.**

| **BG PREMEAL** | **BASIC DOSE** |
|---|---|
| (*Bedside Meter*) | *Regular Insulin* |
| <80 mg/dl | 4 units less |
| 81–120 mg/dl | 3 units less |
| 121–180 mg/dl............GIVE............BASIC DOSE | |
| 181–240 mg/dl | 2 units more |
| 241–300 mg/dl | 3 units more |
| >300 | 4 units more |

Aim to keep BG in safe range (120–240).

The **BASIC DOSE** should be regularly modified (1–2 days) according to the sliding scale needs.

Additional doses of R may be needed at other times, e.g., 10 PM, 2 AM.

**C.** Prior to discharge establish the most suitable insulin regimen.

# SUGGESTED READINGS

Gavin LA: Management of the diabetic patient during surgery. West J Med 151:525, 1989

Rosenstock J et al: Practical guidelines for diabetes management. Clinical Diabetes 5:49, 1987

Schuman CR: Controlling diabetes during surgery. Diabetes Spectrum 2:263, 1989

# 37

# International Perspectives

# Hallux Valgus in Japan

*TADAO ISHIZUKA*

## DEFINITION

Hallux valgus is a forefoot deformity in which the great toe, at the metatarsophalangeal joint takes a valgus position toward the fifth toe (Fig. 37-1A).

There is no clear agreement as to how many degrees the great toe must deviate from the normal position in order to be called hallux valgus. However, treatment of the condition must be considered even with only slight deviation if the patient is suffering severe pain or if the patient's daily life and activities are affected.

As the degree of valgus position increases, the metatarsophalangeal joint of the great toe becomes dislocated, the first metatarsal bone shifts to the medial side, and the great toe becomes deformed in the shape of the Japanese "kana" character *ku* (<), hooking toward the lateral side (Fig. 37-1B). In many cases, this process results in a bunion, with symptoms such as redness, swelling, and pain.

Hallux valgus deformity of the foot occurs both with and without pain; today many people consult their doctors simply for cosmetic reasons.

## FREQUENCY OF HALLUX VALGUS CASES IN JAPAN

In comparison with Western countries, the frequency of hallux valgus cases in Japan is quite low. The reason is that the traditional Japanese *geta* or *zori* footwear is unconfining, being much like modern sandals. Even today, the custom in Japan is to remove the shoes inside the home. However, with the rapid westernization of the nation's life style following World War II, many women joined the commercial work force, and the traditional Japanese geta and zori have been almost completely abandoned and replaced by fashionable Western shoes. This has caused a rapid increase of hallux valgus cases in Japan in recent years.

Table 37-1 shows the number of hallux valgus patients and operations performed at Jonan Hospital, Tokyo. During the 6-year period from January 1, 1985 to December 31, 1990, the total number of such patients visiting our hospital was 1,077, of which 70 were men and 1,007 women. Of that number, 166 patients were treated surgically with procedures being performed on 309 feet. In 1985, only 12 feet were operated on, while in 1989 the number had reached 118. Over the 6-year period, patients suffering from hallux valgus visiting Jonan Hospital increased tenfold, just as the number of surgical cases also increased (see Table 37-1).

## SURGICAL PROCEDURES

All the operations I performed were on patients complaining mainly of pain, but whose daily lives were also adversely affected by difficulty in walking.

The surgical procedures can be roughly divided into two types: treatment primarily of the soft tissues, and treatment of the bones.

529

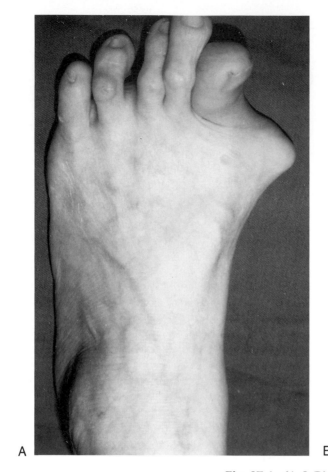
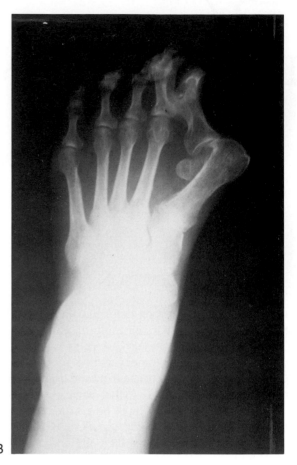

A    B

**Fig. 37-1. (A & B)** Hallux valgus.

In Japan, bone treatment is generally practiced. There are four methods of correcting hallux valgus through bone procedures:

1. Treatment of the distal phalanx of the great toe, the middle phalanx and the proximal phalanx
2. Treatment of the metatarsal bones
3. Treatment at the same time of both the tendon soft tissues and bones
4. Implantation of artificial joints

## Treatment Primarily of Soft Tissues

### McBride Procedure

The salient feature of the McBride procedure is the relocation of the adductor hallucis muscle (Fig. 37-2). First, the bunion is removed and the joint capsule is sutured, thereby shortening the capsule. Then the adductor hallucis muscle, which is attached to the bottom part of the proximal phalanx of the hallux, is resected and reattached, together with the flexor hallucis brevis muscle, to the lateral side of the metatarsal head by means of implantation in a drilled hole. At the same time, the sesamoid bone on the lateral side is removed. For patients with only slight to moderate hallux valgus and for those with relatively flexible metatarsal joints, considerable benefit from this approach can be obtained.

### Relocation of the Abductor Hallucis and Chiseling of the Medial Side of the First Metatarsal Head

It is often the case with hallux valgus patients that the abductor hallucis muscle is located more toward the

**Table 37-1.** Hallux Valgus Patients Surgeries Performed at Jonan Hospital, Tokyo, 1985–1990

| | 1985 | | 1986 | | 1987 | | 1988 | | 1989 | | 1990 | | | | |
|---|---|---|---|---|---|---|---|---|---|---|---|---|---|---|---|
| | M | F | M | F | M | F | M | F | M | F | M | F | M | F | Total |
| <10 years of age | 0 | 0 | 0 | 0 | 0 | 1 | 0 | 1 | 0 | 0 | 0 | 0 | 0 | 5 | 5 |
| 10–20 years of age | 1 | 3 | 0 | 4 | 0 | 15 | 0 | 19 | 1 | 26 | 0 | 19 | 2 | 86 | 88 |
| 21–30 years of age | 0 | 16 | 1 | 18 | 4 | 35 | 1 | 28 | 1 | 40 | 1 | 37 | 8 | 174 | 182 |
| 31–40 years of age | 1 | 9 | 0 | 13 | 4 | 29 | 1 | 20 | 1 | 39 | 2 | 25 | 9 | 135 | 144 |
| 41–50 years of age | 0 | 17 | 1 | 12 | 0 | 30 | 5 | 33 | 1 | 60 | 1 | 32 | 8 | 184 | 192 |
| 51–60 years of age | 3 | 31 | 2 | 22 | 4 | 54 | 2 | 51 | 5 | 75 | 4 | 50 | 20 | 283 | 303 |
| 61–70 years of age | 1 | 5 | 2 | 14 | 4 | 16 | 5 | 21 | 5 | 37 | 1 | 17 | 18 | 110 | 128 |
| >71 year of age | 1 | 4 | 1 | 3 | 2 | 5 | 0 | 8 | 1 | 9 | 0 | 1 | 5 | 30 | 35 |
| Total | 7 | 85 | 7 | 86 | 18 | 185 | 14 | 181 | 15 | 286 | 9 | 184 | 70 | 1,007 | 1,077 |
| No. of surgeries performed one side | 0 | 0 | 0 | 0 | 0 | 2 | 0 | 5 | 0 | 8 | 3 | 5 | 3 | 20 | 23 |
| No. of surgeries performed both sides | 1 | 5 | 2 | 9 | 5 | 10 | 3 | 29 | 2 | 53 | 2 | 22 | 15 | 128 | 143 |
| Total no. of surgeries performed | 1 | 5 | 2 | 9 | 5 | 12 | 3 | 34 | 2 | 61 | 5 | 27 | 18 | 148 | 166 |
| Total no. of feet on which surgeries performed | 2 | 10 | 4 | 18 | 10 | 22 | 6 | 63 | 4 | 114 | 7 | 49 | 33 | 276 | 309 |

*Abbreviations:* M, male; F, female.

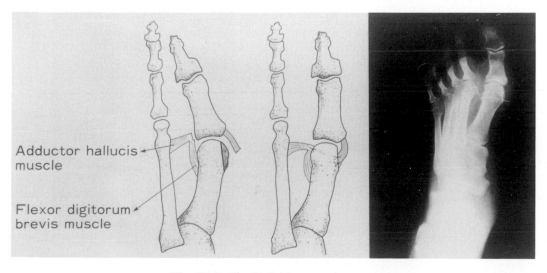

**Fig. 37-2.** The McBride procedure.

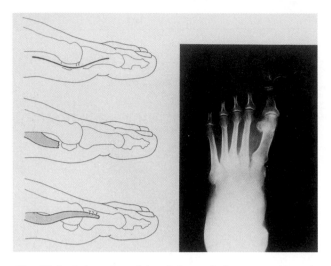

**Fig. 37-3.** Relocation of the abductor hallucis muscle, with chiseling of the medial side of the first metatarsal head.

plantar side of the foot than is normal. In this procedure, the abductor hallucis muscle tendon is detached and then implanted into the proximal phalanx (Fig. 37-3). This method is effective for relatively moderate valgus cases with flexible and mobile metatarsophalangeal joints. Implantation of the abductor muscle

tendon shows better results when it is used in conjunction with osteotomy of the lower section of the metatarsal head, as described below.

## Treatment of the Bones

### Keller Procedure

In the Keller procedure (Fig. 37-4) the first metatarsal joint capsule is opened and one-third to one-half of the proximal edge of the proximal phalanx of the hallux is removed, including the end facing the joint. If the medial side of the metatarsal head is protruding, a part of it is removed and suturing is done in such a way that the great toe is fixed in its normal position. This method has proven highly effective in severe cases of hallux valgus. However, patients have subsequently had difficulty in the toe-pressure and roll-over phases of walking. Another observed shortcoming is that stability of the joint at the point of resection is reduced.

### Hohmann Osteotomy

The Hohmann osteotomy (Fig. 37-5) is performed in the first metatarsal head and parallel to the longitudinal axis of the metatarsal bone. The metatarsal head is

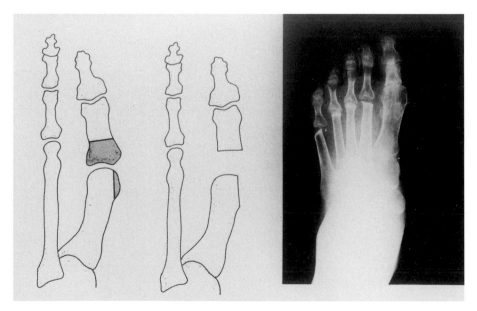

**Fig. 37-4.** The Keller procedure.

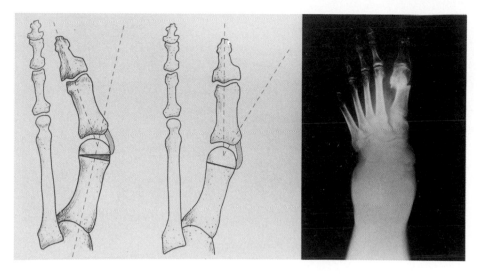

**Fig. 37-5.** The Hohmann osteotomy.

shifted slightly to the lateral side and secured in that position. At present, this procedure is widely practiced internationally and has the advantage of correcting abnormal rotation (rotatory position) of the great toe. Kato et al. have reported good results using this procedure together with relocation-implantation of the abductor hallucis muscle.

## Gibson Oblique Osteotomy

As with Hohmann, the Gibson osteotomy is performed below the first metatarsal head. The difference is that the osteotomy is done obliquely, higher on the medial side and lower on the lateral side (Fig. 37-6). In this procedure the metatarsal head is slightly shifted to the

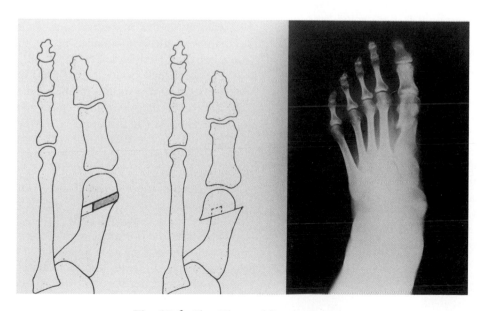

**Fig. 37-6.** The Gibson oblique osteotomy.

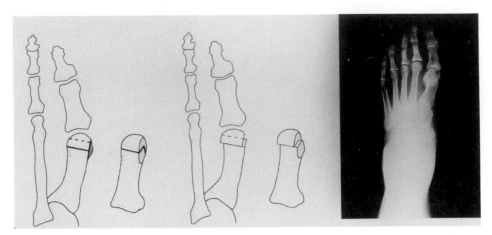

**Fig. 37-7.** The Chevron osteotomy.

lateral side precisely in line with the oblique cut in the bone and secured accordingly. In the original version of this procedure, a portion of the medial side of the metatarsal bone is removed and the remaining spike or post is then inserted into the head of the metatarsal bone (see Fig. 37-6).

### Chevron Osteotomy

In the Chevron osteotomy (Fig. 37-7) the metatarsal joint capsule is opened from the medial side, the protruding medial portion of the metatarsal bone is excised, and the osteotomy is performed with an inverted **V**-cut on the lateral side of the metatarsal bone. With strong lateral pressure, the head of the metatarsal bone is shifted to the lateral side and secured in the new position.

The disadvantages of this procedure are the difficulty in determining the angle and size of the inverted **V**-cut and the complexity of the manual techniques required. Unless the operation is performed with great attention and care, it is not possible to achieve the correct hallux angle. If performed satisfactorily, the metatarsophalangeal joint face is retained and a thoroughly acceptable degree of correction is achieved with respect to the metatarsal bones. This procedure is excellent from the cosmetic point of view.

### Mitchell Osteotomy

In the Mitchell osteotomy (Fig. 37-8), which is widely used internationally, the metatarsophalangeal joint

capsule is opened up with a **Y**-shaped incision. The protruding medial part of the metatarsal head is removed, and holes are drilled at two different points. Below the metatarsal head, a wedge-type osteotomy is performed, after which the metatarsal head is shifted internally. The previously removed pieces of bone are then implanted in the new position and are firmly secured with silk thread through the drilled holes.

### Z-Shaped Osteotomy (Ishizuka Osteotomy)

The **Z**-shaped osteotomy (Figs. 37-9 and 37-10) is an osteotomy of the metatarsal bone and represents a variation of the combination procedure of Hawkins, Mitchell, and Hendrick. The head and trunk portions of the metatarsal bone are exposed, after which the deformed and protruding medial section of the metatarsal head is removed with a chisel and the bone face is filed smooth. The **Z**-shaped osteotomy is carried out in the head of the metatarsal with a small bone saw. The length of the cut is usually slightly less than one centimeter.

The head of the metatarsal bone is then shifted laterally to the proper position, almost directly in line with the longitudinal axis of the leg (see Fig. 37-10). In other words, the proximal edge of the metatarsal bone is positioned as if it were embedded in the medial side of the metatarsal head. It is then secured in that position with Kirschner wire (K-wire) (see Fig. 37-10).

Examination of the abductor hallucis muscle is essential. If it has slipped down to the plantar side, it must be detached and transferred to a more dorsal

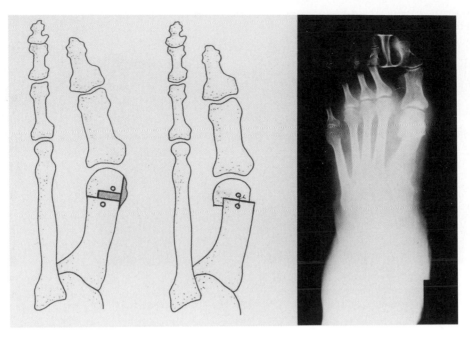

**Fig. 37-8.** The Mitchell osteotomy.

position and sutured under the periosteum of the proximal phalanx of the great toe. This procedure must be carried out simultaneously with the osteotomy.

When using the osteotomy procedure, it is absolutely essential that the bones be successfully grafted.

With the bone cut in a **Z** shape, the contact surface area of the graft is greater than with other methods and the bone graft occurs more readily. Another advantage is that it results in a shortening of the great toe and can therefore be used to adjust great toe length for patients with Egyptian toe (in which the great toe is

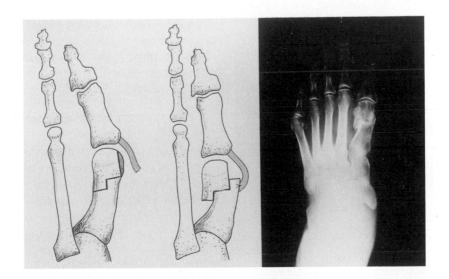

**Fig. 37-9.** Z-shaped osteotomy.

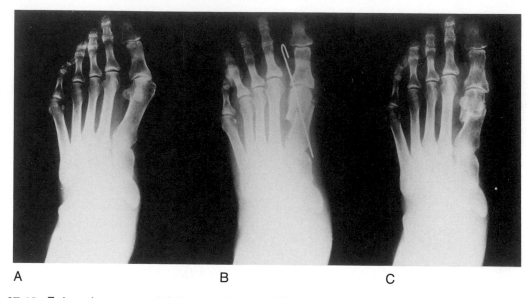

**Fig. 37-10.** Z-shaped osteotomy. (**A**) Preoperative view. (**B**) Postoperative view. (**C**) View 1 year postoperatively.

longer than the second toe). Conversely, for patients with Greek toe (in which the second toe is longer than the great toe), it has the cosmetic disadvantage of further shortening the great toe. It is therefore necessary to properly counsel the patient on this point before performing the operation.

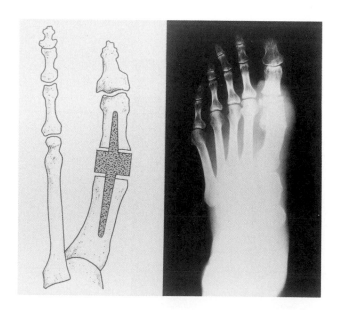

**Fig. 37-11.** The Swanson double-stem artificial joint.

Recovery from this surgery is very satisfactory, and the degree of valgus angle correction is also quite acceptable.

### Swanson Artificial Joint

In the application of artificial joints for hallux valgus surgery, two Swanson joints are available: the Swanson single stem joint, and the double stem joint (Fig. 37-11). In addition, there are the artificial joints developed by Wenger and Whalley. At the present time, osteotomy of the metatarsal head has become a generally satisfactory procedure for correcting valgus. Those cases in which use of an artificial joint is an absolute necessity are rare.

## CASE STUDIES

To think of hallux valgus as a disorder limited to the great toe is to understand it in only a very narrow sense. Other toes can also acquire a valgus position, as typified by the following cases.

### Phalangeal Valgus

The patient was a 51-year-old housewife in good health with no history of disease that might cause de-

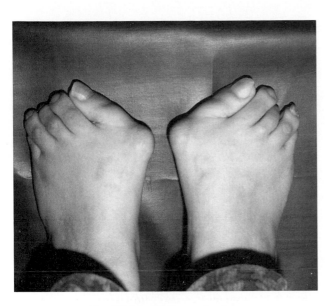

**Fig. 37-12.** Phalangeal valgus.

In both feet, all toes manifest the valgus position. In my opinion, such cases should be called phalangeal valgus instead of hallux valgus. Radiographs show deformity, especially of the metatarsal bone head, as well as atrophy of the bones themselves.

All ten toes were treated surgically. For both great toes, a Keller proximal phalanx procedure was performed; for the second to fifth toes of both feet, Lipscomb metatarsal bone head arthrectomy (metatarsal head resection) was used. In this particular case, I operated in such a way as to avoid resection of the proximal phalanx, leaving the face of the joints and excising only the metatarsal bone heads. Postoperative progress was satisfactory. The large tylosis with pain in the plantar that existed before the operation also showed improvement. The tylosis itself resolved almost completely after 6 months.

formity of the feet, such as rheumatism or diabetes. However, she had been forcing herself to wear shoes about two sizes smaller than her actual size in order to make her feet appear more dainty. Furthermore, for the previous 5 to 7 years she wore fashionable, high-heeled shoes with pointed toes. The results are shown in Figure 37-12.

## Serious Deformity of the Forefoot Caused by Rheumatism

The following very unusual case of extreme severity involved a 52-year-old woman (Fig. 37-13). The patient was suffering from hallux valgus, hammer toe, and a large tylosis accompanied by pain in the plantars of both feet, caused by rheumatism. In this case as well, the great toe was treated by a Keller procedure, while

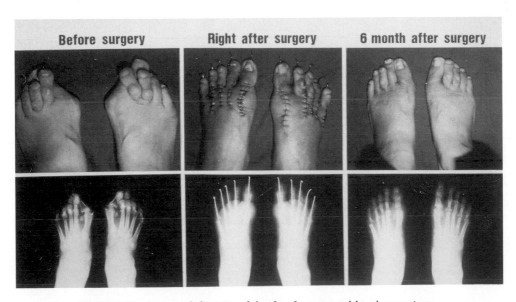

**Fig. 37-13.** Severe deformity of the forefoot caused by rheumatism.

in the other toes, the metatarsal head was removed by a Lipscomb procedure (metatarsal head resection). The operation was concluded with insertion of K-wire in all ten toes. Four weeks after the operation, the K-wire was removed and physical therapy was begun. Therapy involved both self-movement and assisted movement of the affected members. The results were quite satisfactory.

After the operation, the patient was equipped with a modified Thomas heel, known in Japan as the *Ishizuka heel*. In addition, by placing a bar beneath the metatarsal head, some protection was provided at the site of the excision. At the same time, attention was given to maintaining flexibility of the metatarsal joints. Furthermore, cushioning material was put inside the patient's shoes.

Once so equipped, the patient was allowed to stand and walk. The results were quite satisfactory, with the patient experiencing greater relief from the operation than had been anticipated.

## EVALUATION OF RESULTS

The following are considered to be the essential criteria for evaluating the results of the surgery:

1. The degree of patient satisfaction
2. Whether abnormal sensory response or feeling are observed in areas near the point of surgery
3. The degree of functionality of the great toe (muscle strength for up and down movement, as well as the ability to stand on one's tiptoes)
4. The results of treatment of additional complications (i.e., whether or not tylosis, clavus, plantar myostis, or metatarsal head pain have been eliminated)
5. How well shoes can be made to fit after the operation

Figure 37-14 shows the results of the operations performed on the patients described above from 6 months to 5 years after surgery. Results are classified as excellent, good, fair, and poor. "Excellent" means that the patient is very pleased with the results and that there have been almost no complaints. "Good" means that the patient is satisfied with the results of the operation; however, muscle strength is slightly reduced from its preoperative state. Also, slight sensory abnormality is experienced in walking and tylosis with pain still persists in the plantar. "Fair" means that there may be complaints of medium-level pain while walking in shoes and when attempting to stand on tiptoe, and inadequate strength in the great toe. "Poor" means that the patient obtained no satisfaction.

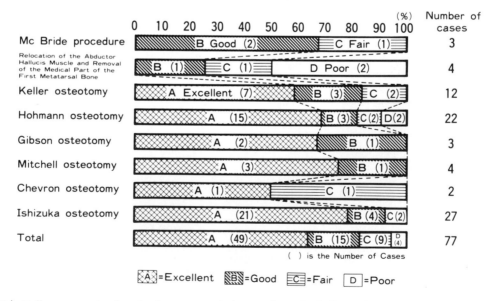

**Fig. 37-14.** Follow-up study of each of seven surgical procedures for hallux valgus. The observation period was from 6 months to 2 years postsurgery.

## CONCLUSIONS

There is quite a variety of surgical procedures currently under development in addition to those described above. Regardless of the procedure of choice, it is not possible with a single approach to address all possible problems. It is therefore recommended that the surgeon select from among the already developed procedures the one that is most suitable to that particular patient. At the same time, the surgeon should consider applying two or three different procedures concurrently.

Based on my experience, I consider the most critical element to be the postoperative fitting of shoes. Even if the operation has been successful, its evaluation should not be based only on appearance. Patients may complain that they cannot find shoes that fit their feet after the operation. The physician who performs the surgery must always provide shoes that satisfy the patient and that enable the patient to function well in daily life. Assessment of surgical success should also include the degree to which postoperative shoes can be fitted comfortably to the feet.

Japan's post-World War II economic development has been remarkably successful and the country is becoming an affluent society. Compared with the past, peoples' material wishes are more easily satisfied and they tend to have a great deal of freedom. In recent years, there has been a tendency for them to damage their bodies through incorrect health care as they abuse such freedom.

At the same time, physicians are inclined to concentrate on treatment of the condition, and it is doubtful that they are giving proper guidance and advice to patients with problems that could easily have been prevented. Physicians must not only concern themselves with treating illnesses after they have appeared. They must also recognize their responsibility to provide their patients with guidance on how to maintain healthy feet and to improve their patients' innate human capacity for standing and walking.

## SUGGESTED READINGS

Cleveland W, Winant M: An end result study of the Keller operation. J Bone Joint Surg Am 32:163, 1950

Crenshaw AH: Campbell's Operative Orthopaedics. Vol. 2. CV Mosby, St. Louis, 1987

Gibson J, Piggott H: Osteotomy of the neck of the first metatarsal in the treatment of hallux valgus: a follow-up study of 82 feet. J Bone Joint Surg Br 44:349, 1962

Hammond G: Mitchell osteotomy-bunionectomy for hallux valgus and metatarsus primus varus. In: American Academy of Orthopaedic Surgeons Instructional Course Lectures. Vol. 21. CV Mosby, St. Louis, 1972

Hattrup SJ, Johnson KA: Chevron osteotomy: analysis of factors in patients' dissatisfaction. Foot Ankle 5:327, 1985

Hohmann G: Symptomatische oder physiologische Behandlung des Hallux valgus. Munch Med Wochen 33:1042, 1921

Kato T, Watanabe S: The etiology of hallux valgus in Japan. Clin Orthop 157:78, 1981

Mann R: Surgery of the foot. 5th Ed. CV Mosby, St. Louis, 1986

McBride E: Hallux valgus bunion deformity. In: American Academy of Orthopaedic Surgeons Instructional Course Lectures. Vol. 9. CV Mosby, St. Louis, 1952

Mitchell CL, Fleming J, Allen R et al: Osteotomy-bunionectomy for hallux valgus. J Bone Joint Surg Am 40:41, 1958

Regnauld B: The Foot. Springer-Verlag, New York, 1986

Wilson DW: The Foot. Vol. 1. Churchill Livingstone, New York, 1988

Wenger RJ, Whalley RC: Total replacement of the first metatarsophalangeal joint. J Bone Joint Surg Br 60:88, 1978

# The Treatment of Hallux Abducto Valgus in China

*BAO-XING CHEN*

Podiatry as a health care specialty does not exist in China today, where most foot problems are cared for by orthopaedic surgeons. In this country with its vast population dependent upon their feet for walking or for pedaling bicycles, foot problems are naturally more prevalent than in the West. Following a modernization drive by the state, women in China began wearing high-heeled and pointed shoes; as a result, hallux abducto valgus has become one of the most common foot disorders in China today. Since these cases are treated by orthopaedists, hallux abducto valgus is to a certain extent underestimated or even neglected; the Chinese literature dealing with its treatment is very limited. To meet the current demand of foot care and to take advantage of visits of the American delegations of podiatrists in recent years, Sino-American conferences on foot disorders were held in 1987 and 1990 respectively in Beijing. From the Chinese participants, a total of ten papers on the treatment of hallux abducto valgus and two on clinical research from ten major hospitals were presented.[1–12]. A collective review of these articles described 676 cases (979 feet) of hallux abducto valgus treated with surgery by orthopaedic surgeons in Beijing, Shanghai, and Nanjing. Although far from a nationwide survey of the problem, these studies shed some light on the current status of management of hallux abducto valgus in China today.

## CLINICAL DATA

Of the 676 cases (979 feet) 122 were men and 554 women, giving a male-to-female ratio of approximately 1 : 4.5. Sixty-nine cases (10 percent) had a family history of hallux abducto valgus and 120 cases (18 percent) were associated with hammer toe deformity. The ages ranged from 16 to 85 with an average of 42. Of all cases, 525 (77.7 percent) were between the age range of 20 to 35; among the 412 women in this age group (77.7 percent), 339 cases (82.3 percent) had a history of wearing high-heeled and pointed shoes. Classification of hallux abducto valgus was done by five authors.[1,2,5,6,10] Measurements were made of the hallux abductus and intermetatarsal (IM) angles and the congruity of metatarsophalangeal joint (MPJ). The lesions were grouped into mild (HA, 20° to 30°, IM, 8° to 10°, congruous MPJ); moderate (HA, 30° to 40°, IM, 10° to 15°, deviated MPJ); and severe (HA, 40°+; IM, 15°+, subluxated MPJ). Accordingly, among the 333 feet treated by these five authors, there were 257 feet of the mild, 49 of the moderate, and 27 of the severe types. Osteoarthritis changes of the first MPJ were seen in 31 cases, all above the age of 60. In 615 cases (90.9 percent) patients were treated surgically for pain relief; in 25 cases (3.7 percent) in the age of 20 to 30 years, the patients had the deformity corrected for cosmetic purposes.

## ETIOLOGY AND PATHENGENSIS OF HALLUS ABDUCTO VALGUS

Over the years, efforts have been made to establish the etiologic factors in the development of hallux abducto valgus. Currently those factors can be grouped into two categories: predisposing structural factors and mechanical factors.

## Predisposing Structural Factors

Predisposing structural factors include splay foot, metatarsus primus adductus, general ligamentous laxity, and muscular imbalance of the forefoot. These are all hereditary factors. Three authors[1,2,5] have clinical data showing family histories of hallux abducto valgus in 20 to 30 percent of their cases. However, none of these authors made in-depth observations as to the genetic abnormalities. Zhao[11] studied radiographs of 140 adults in two age groups with equal numbers of men and women. Observations were made on the shape of the cuneometatarsal joint, the base and distal shaft of the first metatarsal, the base and shaft of the hallucal phalanx, the MPJ, the sesamoid positions, the distal and the proximal articular set angles (PASAs), and the shape of the head of the first metatarsal. Bony structural abnormality of the first ray were always present in cases of hallux abducto valgus deformity.

## Mechanical Factors

Mechanical factors mainly involve the wearing of shoes that force the hallux into a deviated position. The first metatarsal head acts as one of the three points of balance for the entire foot. It has a greater diameter and is able to bear twice the weight of any of the other metatarsals. High-heeled shoes adversely affect the first ray. Dorsiflexion and inversion of the first MPJ, deviation of the sesamoids, and rotation of the first MPJ are the compensatory processes of the first metatarsal to the wearing of the high-heeled shoes. This is the primary etiology of many cases of hallux abducto valgus. Five authors[1,2,5,6,8] recorded a history of inappropriate footwear among more than 60 percent of women aged 25 to 35. According to He et al.,[8] one-third of the patients aged 25 to 35 years (75 cases, 105 feet) had a history of wearing high-heeled and pointed shoes. In the out-patient department of the foot section of the Institute of Orthopaedics, 60 percent of the cases were sufferers of hallux abducto valgus. Among them more than 70 percent had a history of wearing the high-heeled shoes. Chen and Tian[12] studied the modified dynamics of the feet with hallux abducto valgus. The ratio of the amplitude of the electromyographic action potential of the abductor hallucis and the adductor hallucis were reversed from 2:1 in normal persons wearing flat shoes to 1:3 in patients with hallux abducto valgus wearing the same kind of shoes. When both groups wore high-heeled shoes, the ratios were 2:1 and 1:6. The abductor hallucis undergoes a reduction of function in feet with hallux abducto valgus and the action potential of the adductors is intensified, making the deformity worse. The results indicate that muscular imbalance of the forefoot chiefly involving both the abductor hallicis and adductor hallucis may present a predisposing factor, and the wearing of high-heeled shoes makes the condition worse (Table 37-2).[6]

## METHODS AND RESULTS OF TREATMENT OF HALLUX VALGUS

The surgical procedures used in the ten hospitals consisted of simple bunionectomy (Silver procedure; 39 feet), Keller procedure (344 feet) McBride procedure (239 feet) and a variety of osteotomies of the first metatarsal (in 295 feet). The Joplin and Lapidus procedures were used by only one author, in 5 and 2 cases respectively.[1] The results of the treatment were evaluated on the basis of the relief of bunion pain, the

**Table 37-2.** Action Potential of Abductor and Adductor Hallucis in Forefoot Weight-Bearing Position

| | Normal Persons | | | | Patients With Hallux Valgus | | | |
| | Flat Shoes[a] | | High-Heeled Shoes[a] | | Flat Shoes[a] | | High-Heeled Shoes[a] | |
| | Amp. | Fr. | Amp. | Fr. | Amp. | Fr. | Amp. | Fr. |
|---|---|---|---|---|---|---|---|---|
| Abd. h. | 624 | 12 | 640 | 14 | 30 | 5 | 20 | 10 |
| Add. h. | 316 | 10 | 395 | 12 | 90 | 11 | 120 | 30 |
| Ratio of abd. h to add. of h. | 2/1 | 6/5 | 2/1 | 7/6 | 1/3 | 1/2 | 1/6 | 1/3 |

*Abbreviations:* Amp., amplitude; Fr., frequency; Abd. h., abductor hallucis; Add. h., adductor hallucis.
[a] $n = 11$.

**Table 37-3.** Methods and Results of Treatment of Hallux Valgus

| Reference | 1 | 2 | 3 | 4 | 5 | 6 | 7 | 8 | 9 | 10 |
|---|---|---|---|---|---|---|---|---|---|---|
| No. of patients | 100 | 100 | 60 | 28 | 59 | 60 | 89 | 104 | 62 | 14 |
| No. of feet | 143 | 132 | 70 | 34 | 86 | 76 | 148 | 180 | 85 | 25 |
| Bunionectomy | | | | | | | 32 | 7 | | |
| Keller procedure | 43 | 95 | 70 | | | 16 | 9 | 11 | | |
| McBride procedure | 36 | 37 | | | | 30 | 74 | 62 | | |
| Osteotomy of 1st metatarsal | 57 | | | | | | | | | |
| Wilson procedure | | | | | 86 | | | | | |
| Simond procedure | | | | | | | 16 | | | |
| Mitchell procedure | | | | | | | 17 | | | |
| Ball-and-Socket | | | | 34 | | | | | | |
| Impacted | | | | | | | | | 85 | |
| Lapidus procedure | 2 | | | | | | | | | |
| Joplin procedure | 5 | | | | | | | | | |
| Minimal incision surgery | | | | | | | | | 30 | 25 |
| Follow-up (yr) | 14 | 11 | 4.2 | 4.2 | 6 | 4.2 | 4.6 | 4 | 11 | 3 |
| Excellent to good results (%) | 95 | 86 | 80 | 90 | 90 | 90 | 90 | 90 | 85 | 85 |

appearance of the feet postoperatively, the free choice of the types of shoes worn by the patient, the improvement of walking ability, and the occurrence of the postoperative complications. Overall excellent to good results were obtained in 609 cases (90 percent) by the 10 authors during a follow-up period extended from 1 to 14 years (Table 37-3).

## PROCEDURES

Well over 100 different surgical procedures have been described for the treatment of hallux abducto valgus. This procedural diversity leads one to believe that no procedure has been entirely satisfactory by itself, and the surgeon must study each individual case and apply a method or a combination of procedures to suit that particular case. In this review of 676 cases (979 feet) treated with surgery by ten different Chinese orthopaedic surgeons, the most commonly used procedures are the Keller procedure, osteotomies of the first metatarsal with different modifications, and the McBride procedure. The Keller procedure was used on 344 feet; osteotomy of the first metatarsal was used on 295 feet; and the McBride operation was used on 239 feet. A simple bunionectomy is indicated only in elderly patients; often it was used in combination with the other procedures.

The Keller procedure[13] involves the amputation of the proximal half of the first phalanx and is indicated in severe cases of hallux abducto valgus with arthritic changes in the MPJ. The base of the proximal hallucal phalanx is resected. It basically decompresses the MPJ, corrects the deformity, and overcomes the bowstring effect of the tendons after excision of the base of the proximal phalanx. The toe remains comfortable for the rest of the patient's life. If however the big toe is shortened too much, the patient is left with a floppy toe and persistent weakness. Simultaneously, the second toe may be left too long and hammer toe may develop, which may need correction. Dorsal displacement or rotational deformity of the great toe may also occur and requires intrinsic tenotomy. The advantage of the Keller procedure is its simplicity and the ease with which it is carried out. Both Lu[1] of Beijing and Zhu[2] of Nanjing obtained satisfactory results in 95 percent and 86 percent of their cases, respectively, by carrying out the procedure in the elderly with osteoarthritic changes in the MPJ. Zhao[3] of Beijing reported 60 cases treated with Keller's operation with an average follow-up period of 4.2 years. This procedure gave excellent to good results in 80.0 percent. Surgical correction of hallux valgus involving the distal aspect of the first metatarsal shaft had been devised by Wilson, Austin, Reverdin, Mitchell, and others. Osteotomy of the first metatarsal is done with the purpose of realigning the great toe and reducing the medial bony hump without disturbing the MPJ. It is useful for adolescent cases. In a review of the surgery for hallux valgus, Helal[14] found that metatarsal shaft osteotomy is the most successful operation, since it narrows the forefoot, relaxes the soft tissue, and maintains excellent mobility of the first MPJ. The osteotomy can be performed at the head and neck, the shaft, and the base of the first metatarsal. Jiang and Gu[5] of Shanghai performed 86 osteotomies of the first metatarsal similar to Wilson's technique and obtained satisfactory results in 90 percent of the cases during a follow-up period of 6 years. Similarly, Zhao[4] of Shanghai performed 34 ball and socket osteotomies over the neck of the first metatarsal, and Shi et al.[9] of Beijing performed 85 cases of impacted osteotomies over the shaft. They obtained satisfactory results in 90 percent and 85 percent, respectively. In 89 cases (148 feet) Fang and Ma[7] of Beijing, obtained the best results in those cases treated with the Simmond and Michell osteotomies. These results indicated that in the treatment of hallux valgus, especially in the adolescent cases, attention must be paid to the correction of pathologic changes of the first metatarsal.

McBride's (1928)[15] and Joplin's (1950)[16] procedures are the so-called conservative procedures for the correction of hallux abducto valgus. In McBride's operation, the adductor hallucis tendon is transferred onto the first metatarsal after simple bunionectomy. In order to make the anchoring of the adductor tendon secure over the metatarsal head, Zhao[4] of Shanghai modified McBride's procedure by making a drill hole transversely through the metatarsal head and a through-and-through suture was used for the fixation. Zhu[2] of Nanjing and Lu[1] and He et al.[8] of Beijing had successful results using McBride's procedure in young individuals without arthritic changes in the MPJ.

Joplin's operation[16] is a plantar sling technique valuable for hallux valgus associated with splay foot. The long extensor tendon of the fifth toe is divided and passed under the metatarsal heads. Together with the tendon of the adductor hallucis, it is then threaded through a drill hole in the first metatarsal head and sutured to the capsule on the tibial side. This is used only occasionally in China. Lu[1] of Beijing had reported 5 cases with good results.

The Lapidus procedure (1934)[17] is an arthrodesing operation. It was originally designed for the correc-

tion of varus deformity of the first metatarsal. The Lapidus technique for correction of hallux abducto valgus involves a closing abductory wedge osteotomy and arthrodesis at the first cuneometatarsal joint. This procedure is most useful when the first metatarsal is in extreme varus in adult cases of hallux abducto valgus. Lu[1] of Beijing reported two successful cases.

The minimal incision surgery for the treatment of hallux abducto valgus has been described only rarely in the orthopaedic literature, and controversies still exist as to its use. Since the introduction of minimal incision surgery for the treatment of foot disorders by podiatrists to China in 1983, the Chinese orthopaedic surgeons began using this technique in decompression osteotomies of the os calcis and for treatment of heel pains. Some also used the method for the treatment of hallux valgus. The minimal incision technique used in China is not completely the same as that practiced by the American surgeons. Li and Nu[10] of Beijing reported 14 cases (24 feet) of hallux valgus in patients ranging in age from 20 to 35 years. The patients were treated with an incision of 1 cm for bunionectomy and osteotomy of the distal end of the first metatarsal. Ten cases were followed for more than 1 year; excellent to good results were seen in all. Tian and Chen had reported 30 cases treated with the minimal incision technique for the treatment of hallux abducto valgus. They concluded that the minimal incision method must be done with utmost care and the patients must be observed carefully after surgery. For the severe cases of hallux abducto valgus with the HA angle of 40+°, IM angle 15+°, and a subluxated MPJ, the conventional method using the regular incisions is still preferable.

# REFERENCES

1. Lu HS, Zhao ZY, Feng CH, et al: Surgical treatment of hallux valgus; podiatrics. p. 23. In Chen BH (ed): Current Concepts and Recent Advance. Institute of Orthopaedics and Traumatology, China Academy of TCM. Beijing, Sept, 1987

2. Zhu LH, Li ZQ, Han ZB, et al: Surgical treatment of hallux valgus in adults. p. 28. In Chen BH (ed): Current Concepts and Recent Advance. Institute of Orthopaedics and Traumatology, China Academy of TCM. Beijing, Sept, 1987

3. Zhao DT, Liu RB, Sun JH, et al: Keller's operation for the treatment of hallux valgus. p. 31. In Chen BH (ed): Cur-

rent Concepts and Recent Advance. Institute of Orthopaedics and Traumatology, China Academy of TCM. Beijing, Sept, 1987

4. Zhao DL: A new operative procedure for the treatment of hallux valgus. p. 17. In Chen BH (ed): Current Concepts and Recent Advance. Institute of Orthopaedics and Traumatology, China Academy of TCM. Beijing, Sept, 1987

5. Jiang ZJ, Gu XJ: Oblique lateral displacement osteotomy of the first metatarsus for the treatment of hallux valgus. p. 34. In Chen BH (ed): Current Concepts and Recent Advance. Institute of Orthopaedics and Traumatology, China Academy of TCM. Beijing, Oct, 1987

6. Chen BX, Tian DH: Evaluation of different methods for the treatment of hallux valgus. p. 15. In Chen BH (ed): Current Concepts and Recent Advance. Institute of Orthopaedics and Traumatology, China Academy of TCM. Beijing, Oct, 1987

7. Fang ZW, Ma ZT: A comparative analysis of five operative methods for the treatment of hallux valgus. p. 11. Proceedings of the Second Sino-American Conference on Foot Disorders. Institute of Orthopaedics and Traumatology, China Academy of TCM. Beijing, 1990

8. He RC, Chen KD, Wang RD, et al: A review of the operative results for 104 cases of hallux valgus, with a description of a modified procedure of McBride's operation. p. 8. Proceedings of the Second Sino-American Conference on Foot Disorders. Institute of Orthopaedics and Traumatology, China Academy of TCM. Beijing, 1990

9. Shi SS, Deng HD, Wei TD, et al: A new method for surgical of the treatment of hallux valgus: oblique impacted osteotomy of the neck of metatarsus. p. 20. Proceedings of the Second Sino-American Conference on Foot Disorders. Institute of Orthopaedics and Traumatology, China Academy of TCM. Beijing, 1990

10. Li DZ, Nu LS: Investigation on the method of operative procedures for hallux valgus. p. 5. Proceedings of the Second Sino-American Conference on Foot Disorders. Institute of Orthopaedics and Traumatology, China Academy of TCM. Beijing, 1990

11. Zhao DT, Wang J: Hallux valgus of the adults: role of the skeletal structure. p. 30. Proceedings of the Second Sino-American Conference on Foot Disorders. Institute of Orthopaedics and Traumatology, China Academy of TCM. Beijing, 1990

12. Tian DH, Chen BX: Electromyographic study of the feet in high heel and narrow tipped shoes and its relationship with the development of hallux abducto valgus. p. 40. Proceedings of the Second Sino-American Conference on Foot Disorders. Institute of Orthopaedics and Traumatology, China Academy of TCM. Beijing, 1990

13. Keller WL: Surgical treatment of bunions and hallux valgus. NY State J Med 80:741, 1904

14. Helal B: Surgery for adolescent hallux valgus. Clin Orth Rel Res 157:50, 1981

15. McBride ED: A conservative operation for bunions. J Bone Joint Surg 10:735, 1928

16. Joplin RJ: Sling procedure for correction of splay-foot, metatarsus primus varus, and hallux valgus. J Bone Joint Surg Am 32:779, 1950

17. Lapidus PW: The operative correction of the metatarsus varus primus in hallux valgus. Surg Gyn Obst 58:183, 1934

# Cerclage Techniques for the Treatment of Hallux Valgus

*DAVID STANLEY*
*T.W.D. SMITH*

Although more than 100 different operations have been devised to correct hallux valgus, the majority are varieties of osteotomy, arthrodesis, or arthroplasty. Soft tissue techniques are less frequently performed and with the exception of McBride's procedure are also probably less well known.

In this chapter part we describe another type of soft tissue procedure designed to approximate the first and second metatarsals. Thus the metatarsus varus is reduced and the valgus deformity of the great toe corrected. However, before describing the salient features of the operation and postoperative management we give a brief historical review of other similar types of procedure that have been described.

## HISTORICAL REVIEW

Cerclage procedures appear to have originated in Europe and have one of two main conformations. The hallux valgus deformity is either corrected by approximating the first to the second metatarsal, or by fashioning a sling between the first and fifth metatarsals. Lexer (1919)[1] (Fig. 37-15A) employed the first technique, while Lenggenhager (1935)[2] described a similar procedure except that fixation was achieved by passing the suture through rather than around the first metatarsal (Fig. 37-15B). Goeball (1927)[3] used fascia to secure the first to the fifth metatarsals (Fig. 37-16A), and Joplin (1950)[4] (the first non-European, who worked in Boston, MA), achieved his correction by rerouting the detached proximal end of the fifth toe extensor tendon. This was taken across the sole of the foot and

through a drill hole made in the first metatarsal neck. In addition, adductor hallucis was detached from its insertion and also passed through the drill hole. Both tendons were sutured to the capsule over the medial aspect of the first metatarsophalangeal joint (MPJ) (Fig. 37-16B). More recently, Botteri and Castellana (1961)[5] and Pagella and Pierleoni (1971)[6] described a distal osteodesis of the first two metatarsal bones. In this operation, the adductor hallucis was detached from its insertion and the lateral sesamoid excised. The opposing surfaces of the first and second metatarsal necks were scarified and two double threads of chromic cat gut passed through holes in the neck of the first metatarsal and around the second metatarsal. The threads were firmly tied, producing approximation of the metatarsal heads with correction of the deformity (Fig. 37-17). Although the authors obtained excellent results by this technique, osteodesis between the first and second metatarsals might theoretically be expected to interfere with normal forefoot function.

The technique we describe approximates the first and second metatarsals and incorporates some of the features from these earlier operations.

## CRITERIA FOR SURGERY

Since 1980 this technique has been our preferred operation for all teenage patients presenting with bunion pain and deformity of the hallux. In addition, it has also been performed on older patients providing that on examination there is no restriction of MPJ movement and no evidence of degenerative changes radio-

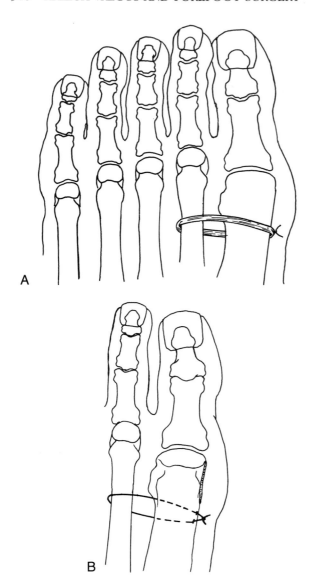

A

B

**Fig. 37-15.** (**A**) Lexer's[1] single suture approximations of the first and second metatarsals. (**B**) Lenggenhager[2] passed his suture through the shaft of the first metatarsal.

logically. The severity of intermetatarsal and hallux valgus angulation has not been regarded as a contraindication to surgery, although it should be noted that in our experience this is usually not excessive in teenagers, and in adults with marked angulation there is often associated arthritic changes at the MPJ, which does preclude the procedure.

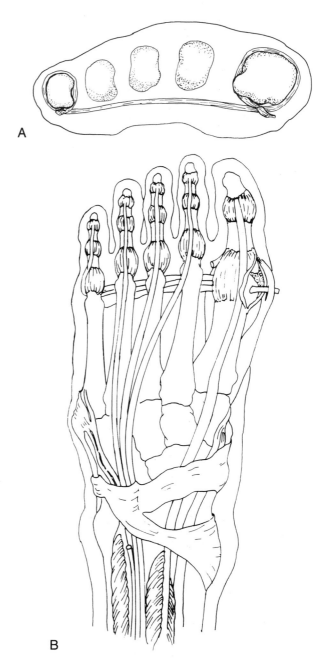

A

B

**Fig. 37-16.** (**A**) Goeball[3] used fascia to approximate the first and fifth metatarsals. (**B**) The detached proximal end of the fifth extensor tendon is passed across the sole of the foot and with adductor hallucis through the first metatarsal neck (Joplin [1950][4]).

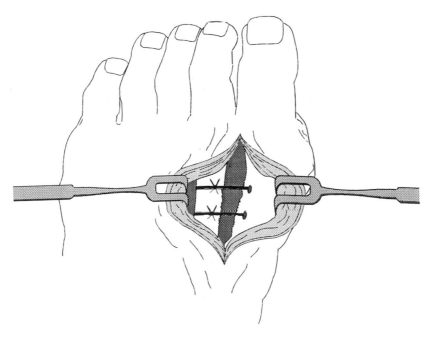

**Fig. 37-17.** Distal osteodesis of the first two metatarsal bones.

## SURGICAL TECHNIQUE

Under tourniquet control a 4- to 5-cm straight incision is made on the dorsal surface of the foot between the first and second metatarsals (Fig. 37-18). The skin edges are retracted, superficial veins ligated, and the small cutaneous nerve branches protected. This reduces the risk of subsequent sensory disturbance or painful neuromata formation. The space between the first and second metatarsals is then opened and the first dorsal interosseous muscle freed along its attachment to the first metatarsal and displaced laterally. A self-retaining retractor should then be inserted and opened out between the adjacent metatarsal bones. This improves visualization of the adductor hallucis, which can then be released from its insertion (Fig. 37-19). Unlike the McBride procedure[7] no attempt is made to reattach the muscle more proximally. Care must be taken during the release of adductor hallucis since the medial plantar nerve will be seen in the wound and must not be divided. It is now possible to approximate the first and second metatarsals and when this is done the valgus deviation of the great toe is automatically corrected. To hold the metatarsals in

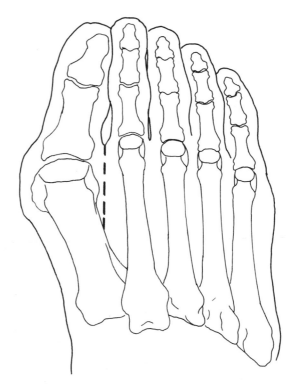

**Fig. 37-18.** Skin incision for the cerclage technique that we have used.

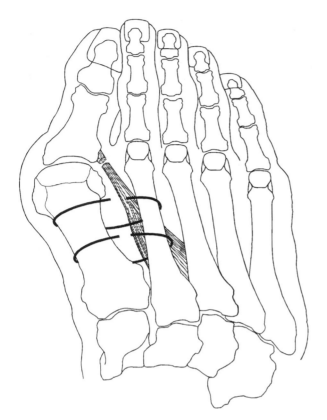

**Fig. 37-19.** Adductor hallucis has been detached from its insertion and double nylon sutures carefully passed around the first and second metatarsals.

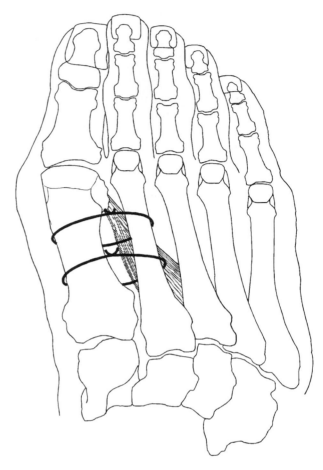

**Fig. 37-20.** The nylon sutures have been firmly tied, correcting the metatarsus deformity and realigning the hallux.

the new position a double thickness #2 nylon suture is passed carefully around the shaft of both bones and firmly tied (Fig. 37-20). The suture must pass between both the extensor tendon and bone and the flexor tendons and bone. If either tendons are trapped by the suture the patient will be unable to flex or extend the affected toe. Although we have found the steela suture passer to be the most useful instrument in aiding passage of the suture around the bones, an alternative that can also be used is an appropriately sized aneurysm needle.

Absorbable suture is used to repair the subcutaneous tissues and cover the approximation suture, while nylon is used to close the skin. A below-the-knee walking plaster is applied; it provides external splintage, holding the foot in the corrected position. The wound is inspected and sutures removed at 2 weeks, but the walking plaster must be maintained for a total of 6 weeks.

## SURGICAL RESULTS

All the patients who have undergone this procedure have had their hallux valgus deformity improved. Review of our early cases showed the mean preoperative hallux valgus angle of 38° (range, 25° to 48°) to be reduced to 14° postoperatively (range, 2° to 30°), with a commensurate decrease in the intermetatarsal angle from a mean of 15° preoperatively (range, 13° to 18°) to 9° postoperatively (range, 7° to 12°). This gave a 93 percent excellent or good result as judged by Bonney and MacNab's classification. Symptomatic pain relief based on the same classification was also impressive with 86 percent of patients having either an excellent result (no pain) or good result (occasional pain). Figure 37-21 shows the pre- and postoperative radio-

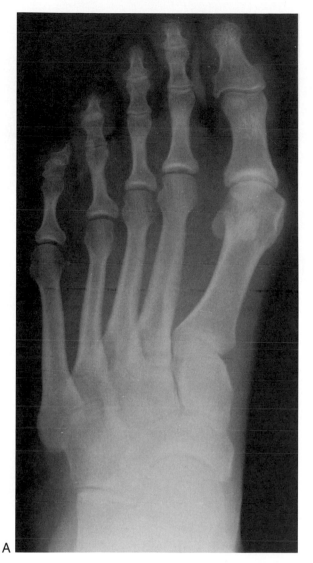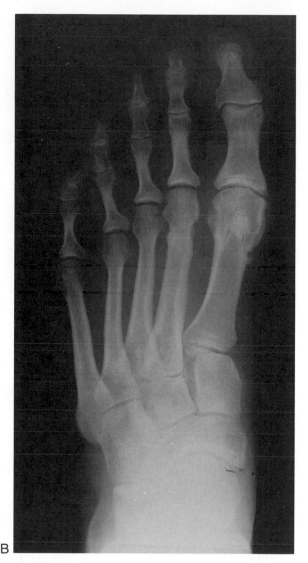

**Fig. 37-21.** (**A**) Preoperative and (**B**) postoperative radiographs of a typical patient. The follow-up period in this case is 6 years. The indentation that the suture makes on the bone can be clearly seen in the post operative radiograph.

graphs of a typical patient, while Figure 37-22 shows one of our best results.

## COMPLICATIONS

The only complications we have experienced have been tenderness over the knot of the approximation suture and the occasional stitch abscess at the same site. Where this has occurred removal of the approxi-

mation suture has been performed. Subsequent follow-up has failed to show clinical or radiographic evidence of a loss of correction.

## CONCLUSIONS

The merits of this operation, apart from patient satisfaction, are that the procedure is limited, requiring

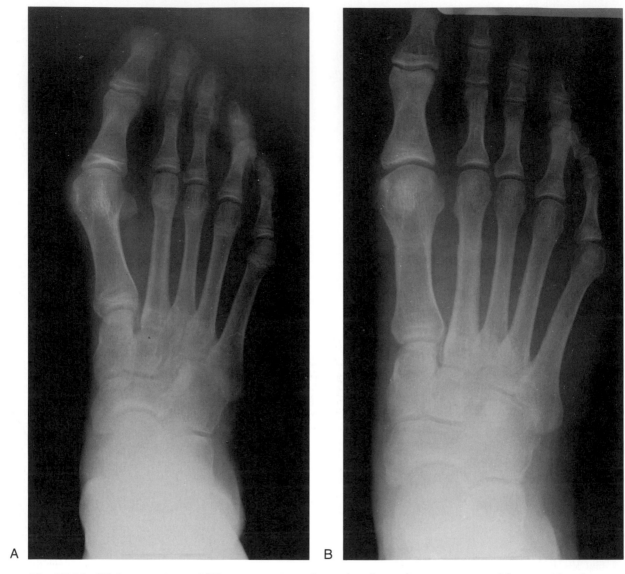

A   B

**Fig. 37-22.** (**A**) Preoperative and (**B**) postoperative radiographs of one of our most successful cases with a three year follow-up.

minimal soft tissue release and no bony correction or destruction. This is of particular importance in skeletally immature patients since it avoids the risk of bone growth disturbance. In addition, since the MPJ is not violated the patients are able to wear shoes of variable heel height. Further, if at any stage failure occurs, all other surgical options remain open.

## REFERENCES

1. Lexer E: Die Freien Transplantationen. Neue Deutsche Chirurgie, Stuttgart, 1919
2. Lenggenhager K: Eine Neue Operations Methode Zur Behandlung Des Hallux Valgus. Chr Z 7:689, 1935
3. Goebell R: Uber Arthroplastische Freie Fascien und Apo-

neurostransplantation Nach Martin Kirschner. Arch Klin Chir 146:462, 1927

4. Joplin RJ: Sling procedure for correction of splay foot, metatarsus primus varus and hallux valgus. J Bone Joint Surg Am 32:779, 1950

5. Botteri G, Castellana A: L'Osteodesi distale dei due primi metatarsi nella cula dell'alluce valgo. La Clinica Orthopedica 13:139, 1961

6. Pagella P, Pierleoni GP: Hallus valgus and its correction. LO Scalpello 1:55, 1971

7. McBride ED: A conservative operation for bunions. J Bone Joint Surg 10:735, 1928

# Surgical Treatment of Hallux Valgus

## BERNARD REGNAULD

Hallux valgus is a predominantly transverse plane deformity occurring at the first metatarsophalangeal joint (MPJ). Important in the evaluation and treatment of this malalignment is that consideration be given to the forefoot as a whole in order to properly correct the hallux valgus and associated forefoot syndromes. Without precise reconstruction of these disorders the deformity of hallux valgus is doomed to recurrence.

Hallux valgus is a disorder that is both structural and functional in nature. The varus deformity of the first metatarsal is reflected by the increase in intermetatarsal (IM) angle which may be increased as high as 20°. Hallux valgus increases gradually from 10° and may advance to a rather large angle approaching 90° with dislocation of the MPJ. The deformity is accompanied with displacement of the sesamoids into the first metatarsal space.

Functionally, the deformity is precipitated by a dynamic imbalance of the musculotendinous structures of the first MPJ. This imbalance results in contracture of the long toe flexor and extensor. There is shortening of the abductor and short flexor of the great toe accompanied by apparent elongation of adductor tendon and medial capsule, causing essentially a contraction of the joint dorsally and laterally with elongation of the medial anatomic structures.

At the joint level the disorder is brought about by simultaneous flexion and abduction of the great toe, which may be accompanied with axial rotation. It may also be associated with contracture and malalignment of the lesser toes. Symptomatology, especially, with weight-bearing is characteristic of this disorder. Plantar callosities beneath the second metatarsal associated with the pathologic varus of the first metatarsal is

also associated. A medial bursitis may be present with inflammation, and plantar callouses of the hallux may be present as a result of the axial rotation of the great toe.

Morphologically there is an absence of the aesthetic appearance of the foot because of the appearance of the hallux valgus, digital deformities and contractions, and other malalignments of the forefoot.

Deformity of hallux valgus is characterized and classified in three degrees. The first degree is characterized by a metatarsus primus varus with an IM angle ranging from 5° to 20° and a hallux valgus (HV) angle of 10° to 20°, usually with isolated inflammatory symptoms (e.g., pain) limited to the first ray. Inflammation may also be associated with metatarsalgia due to friction.

The second degree of deformity is characterized by a varus of the first metatarsal from 20° to 30° associated with an HV angle of 20° to 40°. This is complicated by joint aches and painful malalignment of one or several of the lesser rays. It is often associated with clawing of the second toe and the appearance of dorsal digital corns. Contraction and prominence of the extensor tendons may be visualized and there is an increase of pressure in weight-bearing borne by the central three metatarsals.

Third-degree deformity is characterized by varus of the first metatarsal. It is reflected by an increase of the IM angle of more than 30° and an HV angle greater than 40° associated with a global deformity of the forefoot. This is associated with uniform or disorganized digital malalignments in either varus or valgus, with contraction of the tendons dorsally and laterally, and subluxation of the MPJs. There is a syndrome of hy-

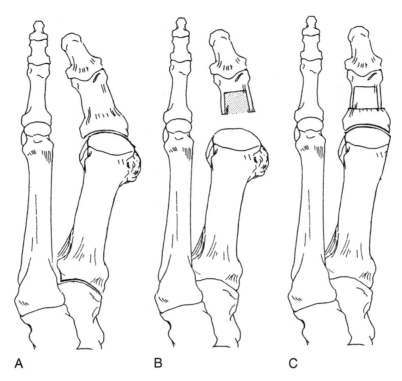

**Fig. 37-23.** (**A–C**) Graphic representation of the osteocartilagenous graft procedure for the management of hallux valgus.

perpressure on one or two of the metatarsals—either the second or the third, second and third, or else the third or fourth. There may also be association with forefoot syndromes such as the anterior round or flat triangular forefoot.

The deformity of hallux valgus can appear and be associated with any of the classic forefoot morphologies; however, the frequency of occurrence is highest with the Egyptian, then Greek, and lastly the squared forefoot configurations. As mentioned previously, treatment must not be directed only to the first ray as an isolated pathology, but the deformity of the whole forefoot must be taken into consideration. It is important to perform a complete examination of the foot to identify factors that would contribute to the foot deformity, such as inflammatory or arthritic conditions.

Surgical treatment must do the following: (1) address and correct the varus of the first metatarsal and the valgus of the great toe but respect physiologic diversion of the first metatarsal; (2) reconstitute the articular anatomy by implantation of an osteocartilage-

nous graft; (3) reestablish function; and (4) correct associated deformities of the other rays to avoid occurrence.

The specific operative criteria are chronic pain and discomfort, the inability to ambulate in conventional shoe gear, and recurrent inflammation regardless of the degree of the hallux valgus deformity. Surgical intervention is not necessary if there is no pain or functional disability. The operation must correct the deformity, reestablish the regularity of the weight-bearing of the forefoot, and recreate our aesthetic forefoot.

The operative technique is one of the metatarsophalangeal arthroplasty with implantation of osteocartilagenous graft to the proximal phalanx, represented graphically in Figure 37-23. The technique is the same in all cases of hallux valgus except those that are accompanied by arthritis within the joint, thereby necessitating an interpositional prosthesis for one year period. The operative technique is performed in the following manner.

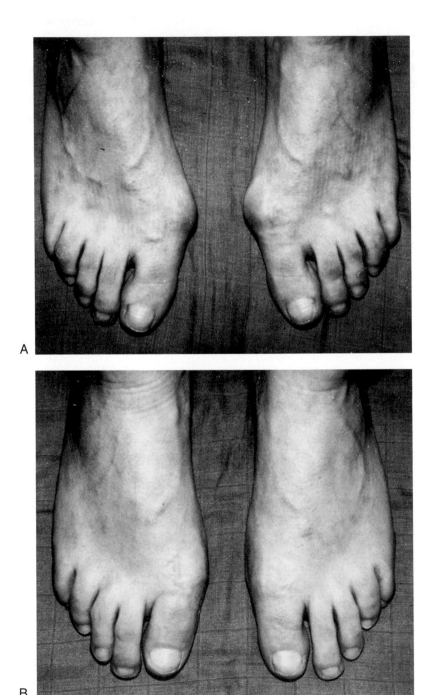

**Fig. 37-24.** First degree hallus valgus. (**A**) Preoperative view. (**B**) Postoperative result.

# TECHNIQUE

A medial skin incision is performed with deepening of the dissection through the subcutaneous tissues. A capsular incision is also produced medially. The capsular tissue are dissected around the base of the proximal phalanx. Care is taken to preserve the dorsal attachments of the metatarsal capsular plane in order to permit a good point for reattachment to reduce the sesamoid subluxation. Care must be taken to respect the posterior medial attachments of the metatarsal capsule in order to avoid sesamoid retraction. The base of proximal phalanx is resected at an appropriate level so that when inserting the osteocartilagenous graft the length of toe will be restored, giving the Greek forefoot configuration. The canal is then reamed carefully into the base of the proximal phalanx. The medial exostosis of the metatarsal head is resected without damaging the medial cortical bone or extending too far onto the medial cortical bone. Next, by means of an osteotome or elevator at the lateral and plantar surface of the metatarsal head, the sesamoids are freed to help reduce their external subluxation. This allows reduction of the varus of the first metatarsal and repositioning of the sesamoids and first metatarsal head.

The osteocartilagenous graft from the resected proximal phalanx is most frequently fashioned in a hat shape because this confers excellent stability (see Fig. 37-24). The hat-shaped graft is implanted into the premade canal of the phalanx. During the impaction of the graft great care must be taken to avoid damage to cartilagenous surface. One must avoid tapping the graft and manipulating to check the impaction of the graft.

The capsule of the joint is then repaired initially by three relaxed sutures. One plantar sesamoid-phalangeal suture passes backwards in the substance of the capsule between the two sesamoid and the remaining capsule-periosteal tissue of the phalanx. This point approximates the plantar capsular plane of the sesamoid apparatus to resist retraction.

A second metatarsophalangeal suture reduces the hallux valgus, and lastly a simple capsular suture is attached into the dorsal plane of the metatarsal head and into the medial capsule including the medial sesamoid. This suture replaces the sesamoid under the metatarsal head and also corrects the varus of the first metatarsal. While correcting the varus it is important to preserve the vertical and lateral amplitude of movement of the first metatarsal by allowing sufficient freedom between the first and second metatarsal heads. Additional sutures close the joint and the skin is closed.

The key points of the procedure of this operation is the size of the osteocartilagenous graft and graft stability when implanted into the phalanx.

# RESULTS

The desired results are incorporation of the osteocartilagenous graft, physiologic mobility, and suppleness of the first MPJ, normal amplitude of dorsiflexion and plantar flexion of the great toe, absence of pain, and the aesthetic appearance of the forefoot.

# COMPLICATIONS

Although they are rare, complications due occur. They include rigidity of the joint, which follows an osteophytic reaction around the graft. Pseudoarthrosis, lysis, fracture, necrosis, luxation, and dislocation of the graft may occur when the osteocartilagenous graft is poorly implanted into the phalanx or when the grafted bone was of poor quality.

Osteomyelitis is unusual but usually results in complete failure of the procedure. Recurrence of the deformity is unusual, but is felt to occur due to high-heel shoes or wearing of shoes with a triangular sole postoperatively. Recurrence is associated with the correction of the first ray problem without total evaluation of the forefoot as a whole. This procedure provides a reconstruction to a functional foot, repair with uniformity of metatarsal weight-bearing, mobility, and suppleness with painless motion of the first MPJ.

Postoperatively management is accomplished with a dressing change 48 hours after the operation on the eighth and twelfth day postoperatively for the removal of sutures. Protection from loading for 30 days is followed by walking with special shoes. Active rehabilitation by the patient obviates the need for passive mobilization through physical therapy. Restitution of nor-

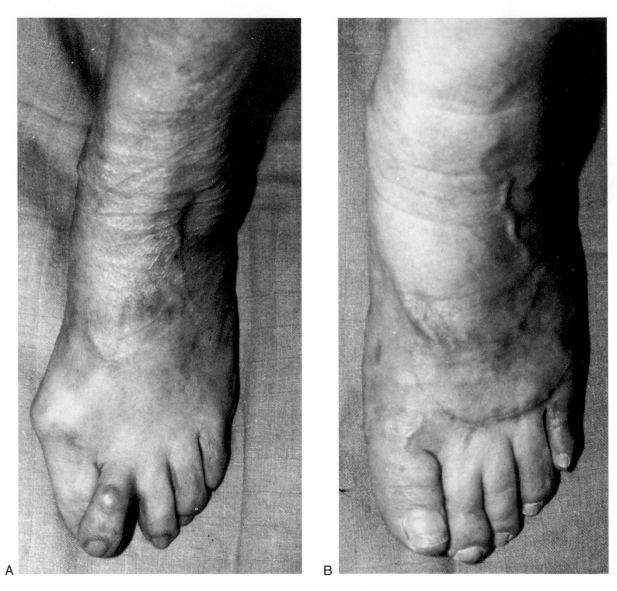

**Fig. 37-25.** Second degree hallux valgus. (**A**) Preoperative view. (**B**) Postoperative result after osteocartilagenous graft and forefoot reconstruction.

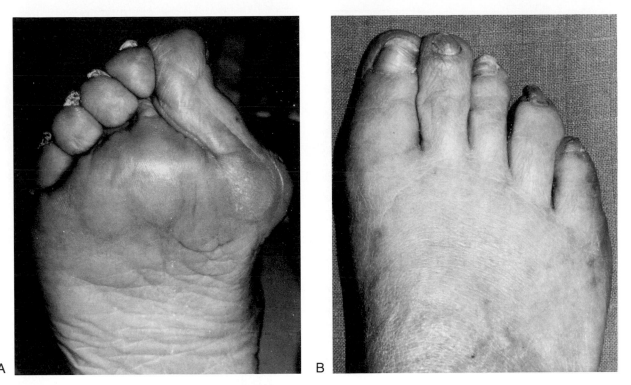

**Figure 37-26.** Third degree hallux valgus with flat triangular forefoot. (**A**) Preoperative view. (**B**) Postoperative result after hallux valgus correction and forefoot reconstruction.

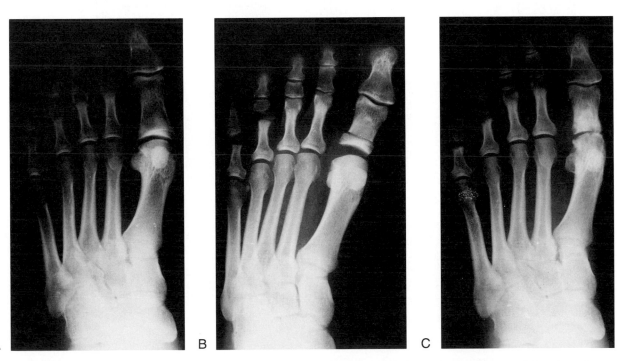

**Fig. 37-27.** First degree hallux valgus of the left foot treated by metatarsophalangeal arthroplasty with hat-shaped graft. (**A**) Preoperative view. (**B**) Four days postoperative. (**C**) Eleven months postoperative.

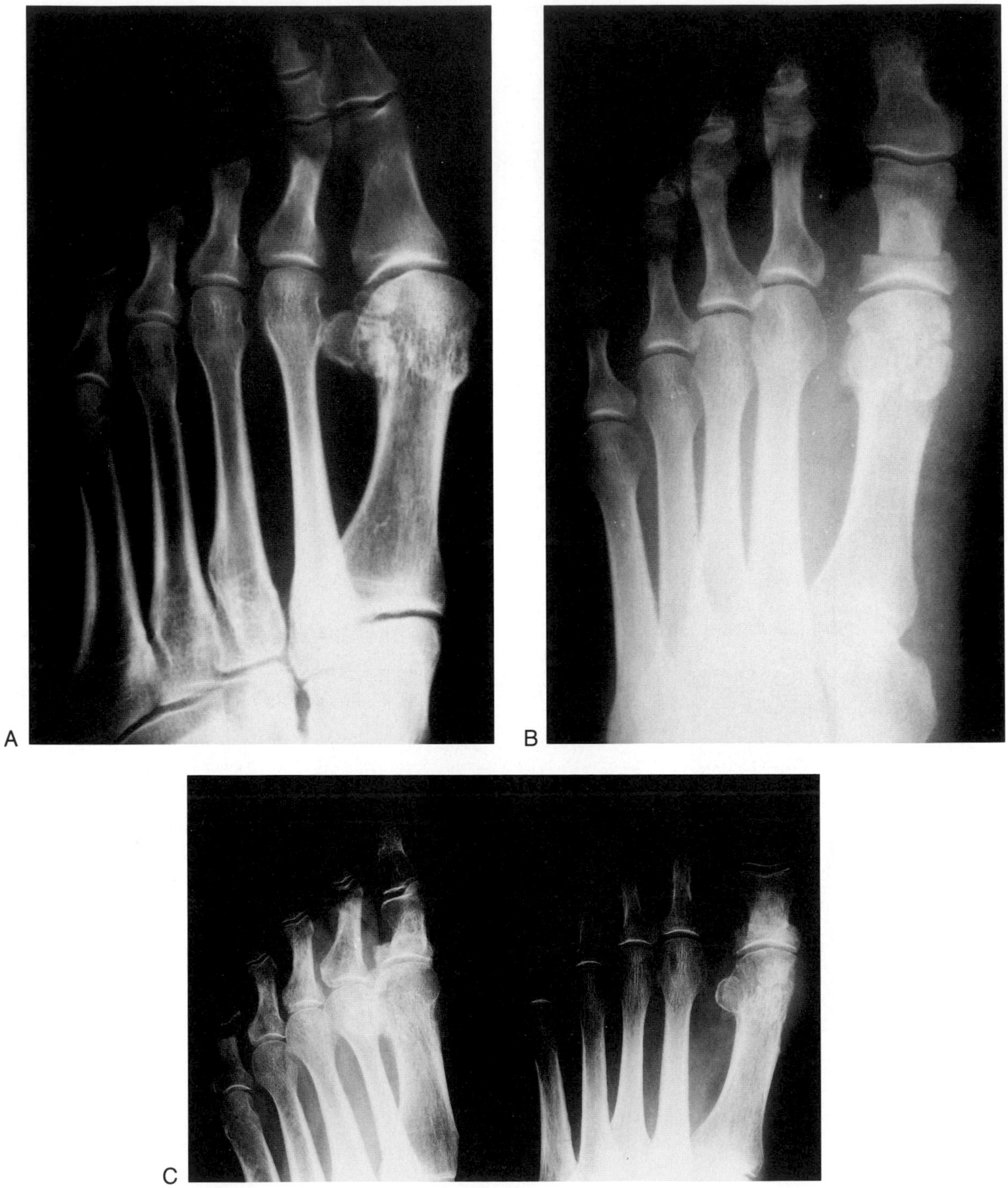

**Fig. 37-28.** Second degree hallux valgus of the left foot treated by metatarsophalangeal arthroplasty with hat-shaped graft. (**A**) Preoperative view. (**B**) Four days postoperative. (**C**) One year postoperative.

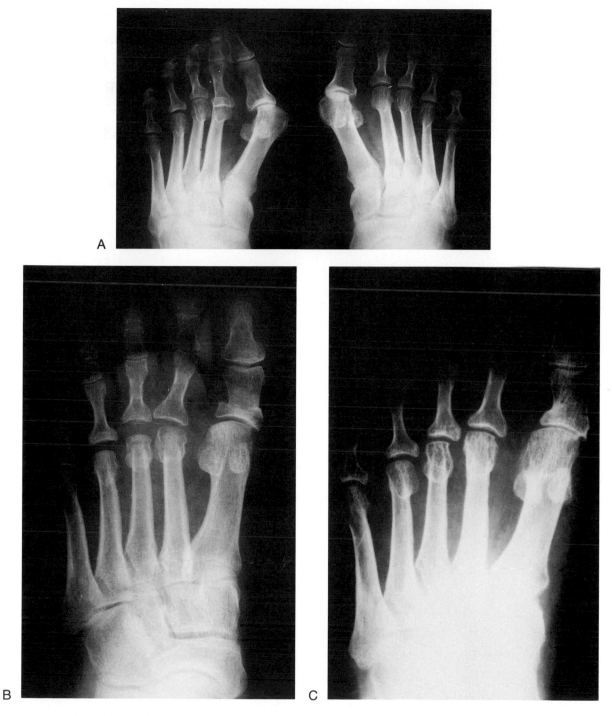

**Fig. 37-29.** Third degree hallux valgus associated with a convex triangular forefoot, frontal protrusion, equinus of the central metatarsal and dorsal subluxation of the second toe. Treatment included metatarsophalangeal joint arthroplasty with hat-shaped graft, metatarsal head-shaft enclavement of central metatarsals, arthroplasty of the fifth digits, and extensor tendon lengthening. (**A**) Preoperative view. (**B**) Four days postoperative. (**C**) Eleven months postoperative.

mal walking is encouraged as soon as possible postoperatively for the resolution of the postoperative edema. Radiographs are usually taken to allow postoperative assessment at 8 days, 3 months, and 6 months postoperatively with personal follow-ups at the first, second, and fifth year postoperatively.

This procedure of metatarsophalangeal arthroplasty with osteocartilagenous grafts has proven to be successful in the management of the hallux valgus deformity. Clinical and radiographic examples are demonstrated in Figures 37-24 to 37-29.

## SUGGESTED READING

Regnauld B: The Foot. Springer-Verlag, New York, 1986

# Surgery of Hallux Valgus and Metatarsalgia

## GUNTHER STEINBÖCK

## PROCEDURES

In searching for optimal methods for the treatment of hallux valgus, we aimed for sound, joint-preserving procedures, and tried to improve techniques for resection arthroplasties.[1]

The Hohmann procedure[2] was abandoned because of postoperative complications involving plaster casts as well as the necessity of internal fixation.

With Regnauld's replantation of the base of the phalanx[3] we experienced technical difficulty, dislocation and fracture of the replant, and stiffening of the joint.

The Mitchell procedure[4] was technically difficult. There was marked shortening of the first metatarsal and occasional tilting upward of the metatarsal head, creating transfer metatarsalgia.

The Kramer osteotomy,[5] a Hohmann-type distal osteotomy that is stabilized by a Kirschner wire (K-wire) that is inserted transcutaneously into the medullary space, was associated with pin-track infections and was therefore abandoned. As joint-saving procedures there remained a modification of Silver's operation, which we named after Petersen,[6] who was the first to recommend a lateral release; the chevron osteotomy of Austin,[7] which was introduced to us by Dr. Hetherington in 1983; and a minimal incisional technique of the Akin[8] type that was tought to us by Dr O.T. New in 1983.

If proximal osteotomies of the metatarsal appeared to be necessary, an opening-wedge type procedure after Trethowan[1] was used.

To the Keller procedure a fibrous cerclage of the capsule was added, in the manner of Lelievre.[9] With larger intermetatarsal angles we combined the Keller procedure with a proximal opening wedge osteotomy according to Trethowan, which was popularized by Gore.[10]

## MATERIAL AND METHODS

While following patients whose halluces had been treated with different methods, we developed guidelines for establishing appropriate indications in respect of the size of the valgus and metatarsal angles by evaluating the best results that were possible with the largest angles in the respective group.

## OPERATIVE PROCEDURES

### Petersen Procedure

At the medial side of the joint a distally pedunculated capsular flap is developed, the width of which being directly proportional to the malalignment of the metatarsal head and the sesamoid apparatus (Fig. 37-30A). After removal of the exostosis, the lateral capsule is dissected and a transverse capsular incision is carried down to sever the insertion of the adductor hallucis tendon at the base of the phalanx (Fig. 37-30B). Medial capsulorraphy is performed by suturing the capsule from proximal to distal while the metatarsal head is held laterally (Fig. 37-30C). The remaining flap is sewn over the suture (Fig. 37-30D).

### New's Procedure

New's procedure[11] represents a minimal incision technique based on the principles of Akin.[8] It consists of the removal of the pseudoexostosis with a burr and a

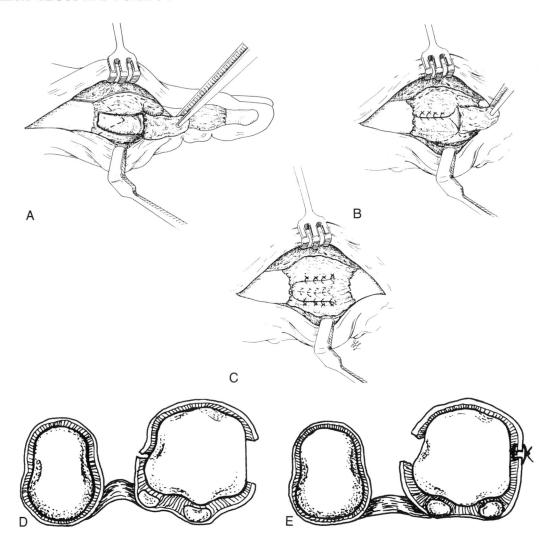

**Fig. 37-30.** (**A–C**) Treatment of capsuloligamentous apparatus in reconstructive surgery of hallux valgus. A distally pedunculated capsuloligamentous flap is formed. After dissection of the insertion of the adductor tendon at the phalanx the lateral capsule and ligaments are dissected longitudinally. Capsuloligamentous defect is sewn medially, the metatarsal head is replaced upon the sesamoids. With the suture completed, the flap can be sewn over the suture. (**D & E**) Transverse sections.

corrective osteotomy near the base of the first phalanx, using a side cutter.

## Austin Procedure

Austin's operation[7,12] is a **V**-shaped transpositional osteotomy of the metatarsal head. The exostosis is removed. After completion of the osteotomy and a lat-

eral capsular release, the metatarsal head is shifted laterally and the capsule is reefed medially.

## Trethowan Procedure

Trethowan's opening wedge osteotomy[13] near the base of the first metatarsal with insertion of a wedge-shaped part of the removed base of the phalanx was used in combination with a lateral release and a medial reconstruction of the ligaments at the metatarsophalangeal joint (MPJ).

## Keller's Procedure[14]

Keller's procedure was always combined with a fibrous cerclage after Lelièvre[9]. This consists of a lateral capsuloligamentous release, mobilization of the sesamoid apparatus, and a medial reefing after resecting a longitudinally oriented strip out of the medial capsule.

## Gore Procedure

The Gore procedure,[10] used to control large intermetatarsal angles, was performed in the same way as the Keller, adding a proximal Trethowan osteotomy.

The follow-up period ranged from 1 to 8 years. Pain at the first MPJ, metatarsalgia, shoe conflict, mobility of the joint, and size of hallux valgus and intermetatarsal angles served as criteria for the evaluation of the results. A joint without pain and shoe problems and the reduction of the valgus angle below 20° and an intermetatarsal angle below 10° was considered an excellent result. A dorsiflexion of 50° after the Petersen, New, and Trethowan procedures, 40° after the Austin procedure, and 30° after resection arthroplasties were considered sufficient for an excellent outcome of the operation. Concessions were necessary after New's operation because this method does not aim at reducing the intermetatarsal angle.

## RESULTS

Of 55 Petersen procedures, 13 were graded as excellent. In these the average valgus angle was reduced from 26° (20° to 40°) to 11° (0° to 20°), the intermetatarsal angles from 10° (5° to 16°) to 8° (5° to 10°).

Although in this group excellent results were achievable, with preoperative valgus angles up to 40°, we do not recommend the method with valgus angles larger than 30° preoperatively because the results were very inconsistant.

With New's operation 11 excellent results were found among 72 operated feet.[11] The mean reduction of the valgus angle in these cases was from 27° preoperatively to 14° postoperative. The intermetatarsal angle remained unchanged. Therefore, a reduction of

the valgus angle of approximately 13° is possible. According to our experience it is not recommended to use this technique on a valgus angle exceeding 30° because in these cases subluxation of the phalanx is usually already induced and is prone to proceed after the operation.

Assuming the intermetatarsal angle is not addressed, 12° is the maximum intermetatarsal angle tolerable for this procedure.

The V-shaped transpositional osteotomy of the metatarsal head after Austin gave 21 excellent results out of 31 feet.[12] In these the mean valgus angle of 31° (15° to 37°) was diminished to 14° (0° to 20°), the intermetatarsal angle averaging 14.5° (11° to 19°) to 6.6° (4° to 10°).

When the extreme 37° valgus angle is not considered, it seems realistic to limit the indications to a valgus angle up to 35° and an intermetatarsal angle of 15°.

Two Trethowan's osteotomies combined with removal of the exostosis and a capsular reconstruction at the joint gave 1 good and 1 excellent result. In the latter an intermetatarsal angle of 25° was reduced to 8° and the valgus angle of 40° to 12°. Extension exceeded 50°. Although few data are available, this method might be the solution in cases of an intermetatarsal angle significantly greater than 15° provided there is good mobility and healthy cartilage of the joint.

With the Keller resection arthroplasty plus the fibrous cerclage of Lelièvre, 20 of 74 operated feet were graded as excellent. A preoperative valgus angle averaging 37° (25° to 50°) was opposed by a postoperative angle of 14° (0° to 20°). By reduction of the mean intermetatarsal angle from 16° (12° to 20°) to 8° (7° to 10°) it was normalized. Perhaps until now the efficiency of the fibrous cerclage was underestimated since in some cases we indicated the proximal opening wedge osteotomy with an intermetatarsal angle of 14°. It seems justifiable to aim for a good result with intermetatarsal angles up to 18° if there is no concomitant metatarsalgia found preoperatively.

With larger intermetatarsal angles the Keller procedure was combined with an opening wedge adduction osteotomy near the base of the first metatarsal according to recommendations of Gore. Even here the cerclage fibreux was added, although surprisingly enough the first metatarsal head was reposed on the sesamoids without it in individual cases.

In 12 excellent results out of a series of 30 Gore operations the mean preoperative valgus was reduced from 41° (32° to 55°) to 8.7° (0° to 16°), the intermetatarsal angle from 17.3° (14° to 22°) to 6.2° (0° to 10°).

# CONCLUSIONS

Thirteen excellent results out of 55 feet (24 percent) in the Petersen group were contrusted with 21 excellent outcomings out of 31 feet (64 percent) in the Austin group. There was no excellent result in the Petersen group when the preoperative valgus angle exceeded 30°. Results of surgical treatment of the capsuloligamentous apparatus were the same. The reason for the discrepancy of the results seems to be the beneficial effect of shortening of the first metatarsal by 3 to 4 mm on the tension of the tendons. The shortening is compensated by directing the V-osteotomy obliquely plantar-ward at an angle of approximately 20°.

We therefore abandoned the Petersen technique and indicated the Austin procedure at valgus angles up to 35° and intermetatarsal angles up to 15°. With a skilful technique and internal fixation with a K-wire we were able to be successful with this technique in valgus angles up to 40° and intermetatarsal angles up to 20°. If the latter is exceeded the proximal metatarsal osteotomy combined with a distal reconstruction of the capsuloligamentous apparatus is appropriate.

New's procedure was recently used rather infrequently and cannot be considered as a routine method. With New's procedure, a valgus angle over 30° and an intermetatarsal angle over 12° are limiting factors.

In joints damaged by osteoarthritis the Keller operation can be tried with intermetatarsal angles up to 18° when the cerclage fibreux is added. Above 18° the procedure should be combined with a proximal metatarsal osteotomy as recommended by Gore, especially if metatarsalgia of the lesser metatarsals is present.

According to the overall results the most successful type of operation in the joint-preserving group was the chevron osteotomy designed by Austin.[12] With larger intermetatarsal angles we used a proximal horizontal V-osteotomy after Kotzenberg, as described by Schotte,[15] combined with a lateral release and a medial capsular reconstruction. This method avoids lengthening of the first metatarsal as in opening wedge procedures, which can lead to undesired tension of tendons.

If the MPJ cannot be preserved the Keller operation is combined with a fibrous cerclage[9,16,17] This provides for correction of intermetatarsal angles up to 18° and improves the results compared with a simple Keller procedure.[16,17]

When there is a rigid first ray or an intermetatarsal angle larger than 18° an opening wedge osteotomy is recommended. Especially in index minus cases of hallux valgus the lengthening of the first metatarsal will be of biomechanical benefit. A summary of indications and procedure choice is demonstrated graphically in Figure 37-31.

# METATARSALGIA

Metatarsalgia is a consequence of disturbed function of the foot. Insufficiency of the first ray is followed by overload of the lesser rays. The connections of the second to fourth metatarsals with the tarsus are more stable than those of the first and fifth rays. This along with muscular imbalance leads to overload of the lesser metatarsals accompanied by transmittal of shear forces to the tissues between the ground and the metatarsal heads, resulting in painful callosities.

In the pronated foot an orthotic device aiming at controlling movement of the subtaler joint about its neutral position and preventing excessive pronation during the stance phase of gait is an efficient treatment. Sometimes this requires much patience of the patient, the technician, and the physician.

Gross deformity of the foot such as cavus deformity may have to be addressed surgically. The function of an insufficient first ray in severe hallux valgus or sequelae of inadequate hallux valgus surgery must be improved before osteotomies at the metatarsals are planned.

Lesser metatarsals that are too long and that cause "dynamic" callosities distal to the metatarsal heads must be shortened. It must be kept in mind that all shortening along the longitudinal axis of the metatarsal always leads to elevation of the metatarsal heads.

Static callosities situated directly under the metatarsal heads are treated by elevation of the metatarsal heads. This can be accomplished by distal or proximal

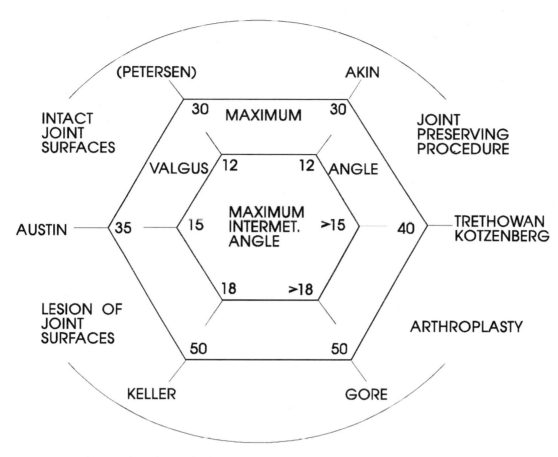

**Fig. 37-31.** Selection chart for method of operation depending on intermetatarsal and hallux valgus angles.

dorsiflexion osteotomies. Metatarsalgia in the elderly caused by atrophy of the adipose cushion over the metatarsal heads must be treated by soft orthotics. We indicate an operation if conservative measurements fail or are rejected by the patient and if dislocated hammertoes are present. Many methods have been developed to treat metatarsalgia surgically; for none of them are the results are clearly predictable.

## METHODS

### Helal's Telescoping Osteotomy

Helal's telescoping osteotomy has been used at the Orthopedic Hospital of Vienna since 1978. Of 87 patients operated on between 1979 and 1983, 62 were seen at follow-up presenting 75 operated feet. Using

Helal's[18] score, of the 75 feet 56 (75 percent) were graded as good, 11 (14 percent) as fair, and 8 (11 percent) as poor. Patients were very satisfied with 44 feet (59 percent), satisfied with minor complaints with 20 (27 percent), and unhappy with 11 (14 percent).

The technique of the operation was as described by Helal (Fig. 37-32). In all but 2 feet all three central metatarsals were osteotomized. At radiologic and clinical evaluation the following reasons for the unfavorable results were identified.

In 9 feet there was insufficient elevation of the metatarsal heads, which resulted in persistent keratomas and pain. In 4 feet painful keratomas developed under the first and fifth metatarsal heads.

In 6 osteotomized metatarsals pseudarthrosis developed, but were painful in only one. The nonunions were caused without exception by an osteotomy

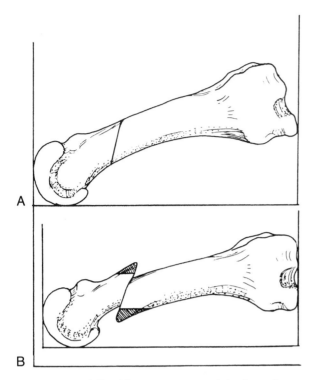

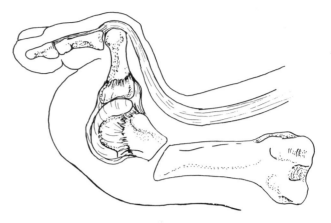

**Fig. 37-33.** If metatarsal head is not mobilized sufficiently the metatarsal tilts upward rather than slides. If there are contractures at the metatarsophalangeal and interphalangeal joints the whole complex moves up, inducing the toes to float.

**Fig. 37-32.** Helal's oblique osteotomy. (**A**) The inclination is 45° to the longitudinal axis of the metatarsal. (**B**) The metatarsal head moves dorally and proximally.

placed too far proximally. Only one of them caused pain.

Floating toes occurred in 57 feet. If at the time of the operation a dorsiflexion contracture of the MPJ, subluxation, or dislocation is not corrected, the whole

complex of the clawing toe and metatarsal head will be elevated and no contact of the toe with the ground will be possible (Fig. 37-33).

With 89 percent good and fair results in the Helal score and 86 percent of the patients satisfied, this method may be recommended as a comparatively simple and sound way to treat metatarsalgia if conservative measurements are not successful. Factors for success include a metaphyseal position of the osteotomy, an angle of the osteotomy of 45°, plantar mobilization of the metatarsal heads to allow their gliding up and proximally, and correction of contractures and dislo-

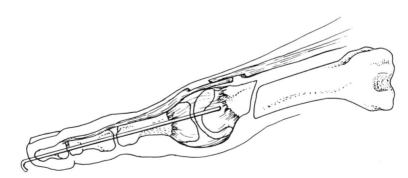

**Fig. 37-34.** Correction of contractures, subluxations, and dislocations, including resection of the head of the first phalanx; dissection of the extensor hood; lengthening of the extensor tendons; dorsal, medial, and lateral capsulotomy; oblique osteotomy; and transfixation by K-wire.

cations of the MPJ (Fig. 37-34). Early weight-bearing seems to be of good influence on results.

## Shortening Osteotomy by Reverse Helal

The direction of the "reverse Helal" osteotomy is from distal dorsal to proximal plantar (Fig. 37-35). The procedure is indicated if metatarsalgia is caused by overly long lesser metatarsals. The advantage is that upward movement of the metatarsal heads is controlled, especially if internal fixation with a K-wire is provided. Sometimes a tilting upward of the metatarsal heads can be detected radiographically, but this tilting aligns the metatarsal heads in a frontal plane. Although follow-up of the thirty operated feet has not yet been initiated, early results appear favorable.

## Regnauld's Reenclavement of the Metatarsal Heads

In Regnauld's reenclavement,[19] the metatarsal heads are removed, shelled out, and replaced onto the remaining shaft of the metatarsals (Fig. 37-36). The oper-

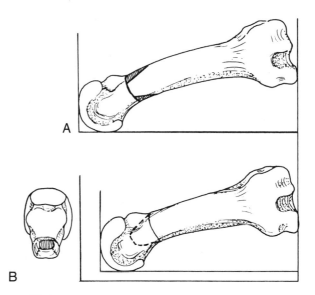

**Fig. 37-36.** Regnauld's reenclavement. (**A**) The metatarsal head is removed and shelled out and the metatarsal shaft is trimmed. (**B**) The metatarsal head is replanted on the shaft. It is elevated, the metatarsal head shortened.

ation requires much skill, but if properly performed the results are good. Occasionally partial osteonecrosis of the metatarsal heads is evident radiographically, but this does not influence the results. We rarely use the technique because it is difficult. Because of the transverse incision and mobilization of soft tissues, swelling of the forefoot persists for several months.

## Forefoot Correction

Forefoot correction refers to metatarsal head resections, usually performed in rheumatoid arthritis. The U-shaped, distally convex incision is at the plantar aspect of the foot for the metatarsals and medial for the hallux. An ellipse of skin 1.5 cm wide containing the plantar keratomas is resected. Thus a plantar dermodesis can be performed, pulling the distally dislocated adipose cushion over the metatarsal stumps after mobilization. We aim at an alignment of the metatarsals in a manner such that the length of the first equals the second, the third is shorter than the second, and so on (Lelievre).[21] Hammer toes and claw toes are manipulated straight and a special foot orthosis is worn dur-

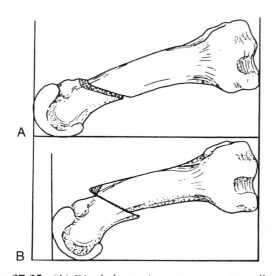

**Fig. 37-35.** (**A**) Distal shortening osteotomy. A small segment of bone is removed, the metatarsal head is gliding proximally without elevation of the metatarsal head. (**B**) The dorsal spur is removed from the proximal fragment. The osteotomy can be stabilized by a K-wire.

ing the first 2 weeks and after this for 3 months at night.

The results are good and long lasting in feet with a low arch. In cavus feet the cavus would have to be addressed first. Recently the first MPJ was arthrodesed after equalizing the length of the first metatarsal to the stump of the second to provide for more stability of the first ray.

# REFERENCES

1. Steinböck G: Differential indication for the treatment of hallux valgus. p. 203. In Mann G (ed): Sports Injuries: Proceedings of the Fourth Jerusalem Symposium 1988. Freund Publishing, London, 1991
2. Hohmann G: Über Hallux valgus und Spreizfuβ, ihre Entstehung und physiologische Behandlung. Arch Orthop Unfallchir 21;524, 1923 524–550.
3. Regnauld B: Le Pied. p. 307. Springer Verlag, Berlin, 1986
4. Mitchell CL, Fleming JL, Allen R, et al: Osteotomy-bunionectomy for hallux valgus. J Bone Joint Surg Am 40:41, 1958
5. Kramer J: Die Kramer-Osteotomie zur Behandlung des Hallux valgus und des Digitus quintus varus. Operat Orthop Traumatol 2;29, 1990
6. Roy-Camille R, Lelievre JF: Cure de l'hallux valgus par la technique de Petersen. La Nouvelle Presse Medicale 3;294, 1974
7. Austin DW, Leventen EO: A new osteotomy for hallux valgus. Clin Orthop 157;25, 1981
8. Akin OF: The treatment of hallux valgus: a new operative procedure and its results. Med Sentinel 33:678, 1925
9. Levievre J, Lelievre JF: Pathologie du Pied. 5th Ed. p. 477. Masson, Paris, 1981
10. Gore DR, Knavez J, Schaefer WW, et al: Keller bunion-ectomy with opening wedge osteotomy of the first meta-tarsal. p. 148. In Bateman JE, Trott AW (eds): The Foot and Ankle. Decker, Thieme-Stratton, New York, 1980
11. Steinböck G, Leder K: Operation des hallux valgus nach Akin-New. Z Orthop. 126;420, 1988
12. Steinböck G, Hetherington V.: Austin bunionectomy. J Foot Surg. 27;211, 1988
13. Trethowan J: Hallux valgus. p. 1046. In Choyce CC (ed): A System of Surgery. PB Hoeber, New York, 1923
14. Keller WL: The surgical treatment of bunions and hallux valgus. Medical Record 80;741, 1904
15. Schotte M: Zur operativen Korrektur des Hallux valgus im Sinne Ludloffs. Klin Wschr. 8; 2333, 1919
16. Steinböck G: Die Cerclage fibreux als zusätzliche Maβnahme bei der Operation des Hallux valgus. Orthop Praxis 10;840, 1981
17. Vitek M, Steinböck G: Value of cerclage fibreux for the Keller-Brandes procedure. Arch Orthop Trauma Surg 108;104, 1989
18. Helal B, Greiss M: Telescoping osteotomy for pressure metatarsalgia. J Bone Joint Surg. 66;213, 1984
19. Regnauld B: Techniques chirurgicales du pied. Masson, Paris, 1974
20. Hoffmann P: An operation for severe grades of contracted or clawed toes. Am J Orthop Surg 9:441, 1912
21. Lelièvre J, Lelièvre JF: Pathologie du pied. 5th Ed. Masson, Paris, 1981

# Index

*Page numbers followed by* f *indicate figures; those followed by* t *indicate tables.*

Reverdin procedure *(Continued)*
   base wedge osteotomy with, 253
   disadvantages of, 204, 207
   operative technique in, 203–204, 205f
   postoperative care in, 204
   proximal articular set angle in, 204
   radiographic criteria for, 203, 204f
Reverdin-Todd procedure, 210f–211f,
   211–212
Reverse osteotomies
   Austin, 465, 465f
   in hallux varus, 311
   Helal, 567, 567f
   Juvara, 243
Rheumatism, severe deformity from, 537f,
   537–538
Rheumatoid arthritis, 499–508, 500f–502f
   arthroplasty in, 504–508, 505f–507f
      patient selection in, 502
      preoperative considerations in,
         502–504
   biomechanical aspects of, 499–500
   gait in, 500
   implant arthroplasty in, 333, 335
   juvenile, hallux valgus in, 119
   postoperative care in, 507–508
   procedure selection in, 504–507
   radiographic features of, 71–72, 72f,
      499, 503f
Richards implant, 351, 351f
Riedel arthroplasty, 295, 296t
Rocyn Jones osteotomy, 258–259, 259f
Rose arthroplasty, 295, 296t
Roux osteotomy, 163, 164f, 295, 296t

## S

Sagittal plane V sliding osteotomy in tai-
   lor's bunion, 465, 465f
Salvage procedures in hallux
   limitus/rigidus, 333, 334t
Saphenous nerve, 26, 27f, 404f
Saphenous vein, lesser, 36
Scarf-Meyer Z osteotomy, 221–224,
   222f–224f
Schede soft-tissue procedure, 126t
Schink metatarsal spreader, 419, 421f
Schwann cells, 402
Sciatic nerve, 405f
Sclerotic disorders, radiographic features
   of, 84–86, 85f–86f
Second metatarsal bone, 12
   infraction of. *See* Freiberg's disease
Second toe overlap, acquired, 375f,
   375–376
   relocation of digit in, 375–376, 376f
Seeburger implant, 347–349, 348f
Septa
   intermuscular, medial and lateral, 23
   sagittal, 19

Sesamoid bones, 14, 42, 153–161
   anatomy of, 154, 155f
   arterial supply of, 35, 154
   disorders of, 155–156
   embryology of, 153–154
   fibular, 14
      release of, 129, 129f
      removal of, hallux varus from, 129,
         134, 308, 308f
   fracture of, 159, 160f, 161f
   functional role of, 156
   hypertrophy of, 158, 159f
   infection of, 156, 157f
   lateral movement of, 50–52, 51f
   normal function of, 155
   ossification of, 153, 158
   osteochondritis of, 157f, 158
   partitions of, 158f, 158–159
      compared to fractures, 159
      etiology of, 158–159
      incidence of, 158
   pathomechanics of, 155–156
   tibial, 14
      articulation preservation with angled
         cut, 127, 129f
      peaking after medial eminence resec-
         tion, 129, 130f, 134
      position measurements, 115, 115f
      subluxation after adductor hallucis
         tendon transfer, 309–310, 310f
   trauma of, 156
Sesamoidectomy, Austin osteotomy with,
   176
Sesamoideophalangeal ligaments, 16f, 17
   biomechanical alterations in, 108
Sesamoiditis, 156–157
Shoes
   adjustments after hallux amputation,
      475f
   affecting shape of foot, 40f
   and hallux valgus formation, 1, 2,
      39–41, 60–61, 61f, 541, 541t
   and Morton's neuroma development,
      414
   postoperative fitting of, 539
   selection of, 388–389, 393f
   test of padding material in, 386, 388,
      390f–392f
Shortening metatarsal osteotomy in
   Freiberg's disease, 455f–456f, 456
"Shoveling" of nail, postoperative, 482,
   482f
Silicone implants, 327, 330
   host reactions to, 344
Silver bunionectomy, 125, 131, 132f–133
Simmond osteotomy, 542t, 543
Skeletal structure of foot, 9f, 9–14
Skin examination, 103
Sodium hydroxide chemical matrixectomy
   in onychocryptosis, 489

Soft-tissue procedures, 125–134
   adductor hallucis tendon transfer in,
      130–131, 133
   capsulorraphy in, 130
   capsulotomy in, 127
   cerclage techniques in, 545–550
   complications of, 134
   criteria for, 131–133
   in digital deformities, 359
   extensor hallucis brevis tenotomy in,
      130
   extensor hallucis longus lengthening in,
      130
   fibular sesamoid release in, 129, 129f
   fibular sesamoid removal in, 129, 133
      hallux varus from, 129, 134, 308, 308f
   historical aspects of, 125–126
   in Japan, 530–532
   in juvenile hallux valgus, 121
   lateral release in, 127–131
   medial eminence resection in, 127, 128f
   objectives of, 126–127
   osseous procedures with, 131, 132f
   postoperative analyses in, 133–134
   postoperative course in, 134
   preservation of tibial sesamoid articula-
      tion in, 127, 129f
   recurrence of deformity after, 134
   release of adductor tendons in, 128–129
   techniques in, 127–131
   tibial sesamoid peaking in, 129, 130f,
      134
      prevention of, 127, 129f
Spiculectomy, nail, 488
Splayfoot with tailor's bunion, 459
Splints, digital, 389, 397f
   hallux night splint, 393, 398f
Spondyloarthropathies, radiographic features of, 72–75, 73f–75f
Stein soft-tissue procedure, 126t
Steindler stripping of os calcis, 147, 148
Strain gauges, 512
Stress assessment under pathologic forefoot, 509–516. *See also* Pressure
   analysis of foot stress
Subtalar joint pronation, and tailor's
   bunion, 459–460
Suppan nail technique No.2, 491–492, 493f
Sural nerve, 28, 403f, 405f
   entrapment of, 409
Swanson implants
   in hallux limitus/rigidus, 324–325
   hemi-implants, 330, 331t, 345, 347, 349,
      349f
      titanium, 354, 354f
   hinged, 350f, 350–351
      titanium grommets for, 345, 350, 351f
   in Japan, 536, 536f
   placement of, 339f
   in rheumatoid arthritis, 504
   total, 331, 331t, 345